IMMUNOLOGY AND SEROLOGY IN LABORATORY MEDICINE

IMMUNOLOGY
AND
SEROLOGY
IN
LABORATORY
MEDICINE

MARY LOUISE TURGEON
Ed.D., M.T. (ASCP)

Assistant Director of Medical Education
Guthrie Medical Center
Sayre, Pennsylvania

Research Assistant Professor
College of Medicine
State University of New York
Health Science Center at Syracuse
Syracuse, New York

Assistant Clinical Professor
University of North Dakota
School of Medicine
Grand Forks, North Dakota

With 107 illustrations

THE C. V. MOSBY COMPANY

St. Louis • Baltimore • Philadelphia • Toronto   1990

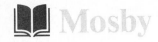

Editor: Stephanie Bircher
Assistant Editor: Anne Gunter
Production Editor: Radhika Rao Gupta
Designer: Susan E. Lane

Cover Photo: Macrophages, red blood cells and T-lymphocytes (2500×)
© Manfred Kage/Peter Arnold, Inc.

Printed in the United States of America

The C. V. Mosby Company
11830 Westline Industrial Drive, St. Louis, Missouri 63146

Library of Congress Cataloging-in-Publication Data

Turgeon, Mary Louise.
  Immunology and serology in laboratory medicine.

  Includes bibliography references.
    1. Serum diagnosis. 2. Serology. 3. Immunology.
I. Title. [DNLM: 1. Allergy and Immunology—
laboratory manuals. 2. Immunologic Technics.
3. Immunologic tests. 4. Serology—laboratory
manuals. QW 525 T936i]
RB46.6.T87 1990   616.07′9   89-13448
ISBN 0-8016-5131-X

C/VH/VH   9 8 7 6 5 4 3 2

Preface

Immunology and Serology in Laboratory Medicine has been written primarily for undergraduate students in a clinical laboratory science program. This book is intended to fulfill the needs of medical laboratory technology (clinical laboratory technician—CLT) and medical technology (clinical laboratory science—CLS) students, and their instructors for an entry-level text that encompasses theory, practice, and clinical applications in the fields of immunology and serology. Practicing medical technologists, medical students and medical residents, nursing students and practitioners, students and practitioners in other allied health disciplines such as medical assisting, physician assistants, and practicing physicians such as general internists and family medicine specialists can use this text as a reference.

The purpose of this book is to describe the basic theoretic concepts in immunology, to explain the underlying theory of procedures performed in immunology and serology laboratories, to summarize clinical features of relevant selected disorders, and to detail procedures applicable to specific disorders. The major topical areas are organized into four primary sections. The initial two sections progress from basic immunologic mechanisms and serologic concepts to the theory of laboratory procedures including automated techniques. The latter two sections emphasize medical applications. The latter sections contain representative disorders of infectious and immunologic origin as well as topics such as transplantation and tumor immunology.

The sequence of the sections is designed to accommodate the core needs of clinical laboratory technology and clinical laboratory science students in basic concepts, the underlying theory of procedures, and immunologic manifestations of infectious diseases. Because the needs of medical technology students are more advanced in the area of immunopathology, these topics are presented in the latter part of the book in order to allow students to analyze and evaluate abnormalities based upon their knowledge of the preceding sections. Students may study specific components of the book depending upon the length and objectives of the course.

In order to achieve clarity, a topical outline is presented at the beginning of each chapter. These outlines should be of value to students in the organization of the material and may be of convenience to instructors in preparing lectures. Illustrations, photographs, and summary tables are used to visually clarify various conceptual themes and arrange detailed information. Chapter highlights and multiple-choice licensure-type review questions are provided at the conclusion of each chapter.

Procedures are organized according to the format suggested by the National Commission for Clinical Laboratory Standards (NCCLS). This format introduces students to the typical procedural write-up encountered in a working clinical laboratory. This format includes a brief statement of procedural theory and purpose; specimen requirements, handling and storage; reagents, supplies and equipment; quality control requirements; procedural steps; calculations; normal values; procedural notes, including sources of error, clinical applications, and limitations of the procedure; and procedural references.

The field of immunology has exploded with new information over the past decade. For example, two diseases (AIDS and Lyme disease) have been discovered or more fully described during the research and writing phases of this book. The subspecialty areas within the field have proliferated to the extent that a substantial body of knowledge unique to each particular subspecialty exists. Most current texts attempt to comprehensively include this enormous body of theoretic knowledge into a single book. Consequently, most books begin at an advanced level and fail to recognize the needs of the novice for basic information as well as medical applications that are of particular importance to students in the health professions. A few textbooks are more simplistic in presentation but are actually serology texts with limited immunology content.

Immunology and Serology in Laboratory Medicine has been written for beginning students in immunology, who need an emphasis on the medical aspects of the discipline. No attempt has been made to replace books written at more sophisticated reference levels. This text should provide students with a basic foundation in the theory and practice of clinical immunology during a one-term course.

Mary L. Turgeon

Acknowledgments

My objective in writing *Immunology and Serology in Laboratory Medicine* was to integrate basic science concepts and procedural theory in immunology and serology with relevant medical applications. Because of the rapidly expanding body of knowledge in immunology, writing a book that addresses the holistic needs of those in the clinical sciences has been a challenge. In addition, this book has provided me with the opportunity to share my experience and insight as a medical educator with others.

I would like to express gratitude to Rodney F. Hochman, M.D., Associate in Rheumatology, Guthrie Clinic/Guthrie Medical Center, Sayre, Pennsylvania; Steven Villaneuwava, M.D., Internal Medicine Resident, Robert Packer Hospital/Guthrie Medical Center, Sayre, Pennsylvania; and James A. Terzian, M.D., Chief Pathologist, St. Joseph's Hospital, Elmira, New York, who generously gave of their time to review portions of the manuscript. In addition, I appreciate the efforts of the members of the editorial and production staff at the C.V. Mosby Company.

Finally, special thanks to Don Turgeon for his forbearance during the period of manuscript preparation, and for once again contributing to the artistic elements of this, my third book.

To
Don
for his unwavering support of my pursuits

Contents

PART I

Basic Immunologic Mechanisms

An Overview of Immunology

*I*mmunology is defined as the study of the molecules, cells, organs, and systems responsible for the recognition and disposal of foreign (nonself) material, of how body components respond and interact, of the desirable and undesirable consequences of immune interactions, and of the ways in which the immune system can be advantageously manipulated to protect against or treat diseases. Immunologists in the Western Hemisphere generally exclude from the study of immunology the relationship between cells during embryonic development.

The function of the immune system is to recognize self from nonself and to defend the body against nonself. Such a system is necessary for survival in all living organisms. Nonself substances can be as diverse as life-threatening infectious microorganisms or a lifesaving organ transplant. The desirable consequences of immunity include natural resistance, recovery, and acquired resistance to infectious diseases. A deficiency or dysfunction of the immune system can cause many disorders. Undesirable consequences of immunity include allergy, rejection of a transplanted organ, or an *autoimmune* disorder (a condition in which the body's own tissues are attacked as if they were foreign).

BODY DEFENSES: RESISTANCE TO MICROBIAL DISEASE

Before a pathogen can invade the human body, it must overcome the resistance provided by the body's immune system, which consists of nonspecific and specific defense mechanisms (Fig. 1-1).

First Line of Defense

The *first line of defense* or first barrier to infection is unbroken skin and mucosal membrane surfaces. These surfaces are of utmost importance in forming a physical barrier to many microorganisms because this is where foreign materials usually first contact the host. Keratinization of the upper layer of the skin, and the constant renewal of the skin's epithelial cells which repairs breaks in the skin, assist in the protective function of skin and mucosal membranes. In addition, the *normal flora* (microorganisms normally inhabiting the skin and membranes) deter penetration or facilitate elimination of foreign microorganisms from the body.

Secretions are also an important component in the first line of defense against microbial invasion. Mucus adhering to the membranes of the nose and nasopharynx traps microorganisms, which can be expelled by coughing or sneezing. Sebum (oil) produced by the sebaceous glands of the skin and lactic acid contained in sweat possess antimicrobial properties. The production of ear wax is another example of a process that guards the auditory canals of the ear from infectious disease. Secretions produced in the process of eliminating liquid and solid wastes (e.g., the urinary and gastrointestinal processes) are important in physically removing potential pathogens from the body. The acidity and alkalinity of the fluids of the stomach and intestinal tract as well as the acidity of the vagina can destroy many potentially infectious microorganisms. Additional protection is provided to the respiratory tract by the constant motion of the cilia of the tubules.

In addition to the physical ability to wash away

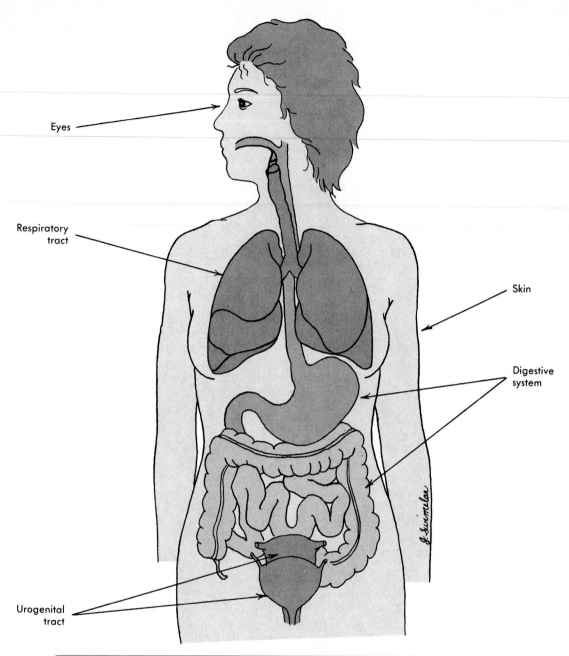

FIGURE 1-1

Natural body defenses. Body fluids, specialized cells, fluids, and resident bacteria (normal flora) allow systems such as the respiratory, digestive, urogenital, and integumentary systems to naturally defend the body against microbial infection.

potential pathogens, tears and saliva also have chemical properties that are of value in defending the body. The enzyme, *lysozyme*, is found in tears and saliva. Lysozyme attacks and destroys the cell wall of susceptible bacteria, particularly certain gram-positive bacteria. *IgA antibody* is another protective substance of importance in tears and saliva.

Thus the body has a wide variety of barrier-assisting defenses that protect against disease as the first line of defense. Although these barriers vary between individuals, they do assist in the general resistance to infectious organisms.

Natural Immunity

Natural (innate or inborn) *resistance* is one of the two ways that the body resists infection after microorganisms have penetrated the first line of resistance. The second form, *acquired resistance*, which specifically recognizes and selectively eliminates exogenous (or endogenous) agents, is discussed later in this chapter.

Natural immunity is characterized as a nonspecific mechanism. If a microorganism penetrates the skin or mucosal membranes, a second line of cellular and humoral defense mechanisms (see box below, left) becomes operational. The elements of natural resistance include *phagocytic cells, complement,* and *acute inflammatory reaction.* Despite their relative lack of specificity, these components are essential because they are largely responsible for natural immunity to many environmental microorganisms. Phagocytic cells (see Chapter 3), which engulf invading foreign material, constitute the major cellular component. Complement proteins (see Chapter 5) are the major humoral (fluid) component of natural immunity. Other substances of the humoral component are lysozymes and *interferon,* which are sometimes described as "natural antibiotics." Interferon is a family of proteins produced rapidly by many cells in response to viral infection. It functions to block the replication of virus in other cells.

Tissue damage produced by infectious or other agents results in inflammation, a series of biochemical and cellular changes that facilitate the *phagocytosis* (the engulfing and destruction) of microorganisms or damaged cells. If the degree of inflammation is sufficiently extensive, it is accompanied by an increase in the plasma concentration of *acute-phase proteins or reactants,* a group of glycoproteins. Acute-phase proteins (see Chapter 3) are sensitive indicators of the presence of inflammatory disease and are especially useful in monitoring such conditions.

Adaptive Immunity

If a microorganism overwhelms the body's natural resistance, a third line of defensive resistance exists. *Acquired* or *adaptive immunity* is a more recently evolved mechanism. It allows the body to recognize, remember, and respond to a specific stimulus, an *antigen.* Adaptive immunity can result in the elimination of microorganisms and recovery from disease and frequently leaves the host with specific immunologic memory. This condition of memory or recall, acquired resistance, allows the host to respond more effectively if reinfection with the same microorganism occurs.

Adaptive immunity, like natural immunity, is composed of cellular and humoral components (see box below, right). The major cellular component of this mechanism is the *lymphocyte* (see Chapter 4);

the major humoral component is the *antibody* (see Chapter 2). Lymphocytes selectively respond to nonself materials, antigens, which leads to immune memory and a permanently altered pattern of response or adaptation to the environment. The majority of the actions of the two categories of the adaptive response, humoral-mediated and cell-mediated immunity (Table 1-1), are exerted by the interaction of antibody with complement and the phagocytic cells of natural immunity, and of *T cells* with *macrophages.*

Humoral-Mediated Immunity

If specific antibodies have been formed to antigenic stimulation, they are available to protect the body against foreign substances. The recognition of foreign substances and subsequent production of antibodies to these substances are the specific meaning of immunity. *Antibody-mediated immunity* to infection is acquired if the antibodies are formed by the host or received from another source. These two types of acquired immunity (Table 1-2) are called *active* and *passive* immunity, respectively.

Active immunity can be acquired by natural exposure in response to an infection or natural series

TABLE 1-1

Characteristics of Humoral- and Cell-Mediated Immunity

	Humoral-mediated immunity	Cell-mediated immunity
Mechanism	Antibody-mediated	Cell-mediated
Cell type	B lymphocytes	T lymphocytes
Mode of action	Antibodies in serum	Direct cell-to-cell contact or soluble products secreted by cells
Purpose	Primary defense against bacterial infection	Defense against viral and fungal infections, intracellular organisms, tumor antigens, and graft rejection

Components of the Natural Immune System

Cellular	Mast cells
	Neutrophils
	Macrophages
Humoral	Complement
	Lysozyme
	Interferon

Components of the Adaptive Immune System

Cellular	T lymphocytes
	B lymphocytes
	Plasma cells
Humoral	Antibodies
	Lymphokines

TABLE 1-2

Comparison of the Types of Acquired Immunity

Type		Mode of acquisition	Antibody produced by host	Duration of immune response
Active	Natural	Infection	Yes	Long
	Artificial	Vaccination	Yes	Long*
Passive	Natural	Transfer in vivo or colostrum	No	Short
	Artificial	Infusion of serum/plasma	No	Short

*Immunocompetent host.

of infections, or it may be acquired by an intentional injection of an antigen. This intentional injection of antigen, *vaccination,* is an effective method of stimulating antibody production and memory (acquired resistance) without suffering from the disease. Suspensions of antigenic materials used for immunization are varied and may be of animal or plant origin. These products may be composed of living suspensions of weak or attenuated cells or viruses, killed cells or viruses, or extracted bacterial products such as the altered and no longer poisonous toxoids used to immunize against diphtheria and tetanus. The selected agents should stimulate the production of antibodies without clinical signs and symptoms of disease in an *immunocompetent* (a host that is able to recognize a foreign antigen and build specific antigen-directed antibodies) and cause permanent antigenic memory. Booster vaccinations may be needed in some cases to expand the pool of memory cells. The mechanism of antigen recognition and antibody production is discussed in Chapter 2.

Artificial passive immunity is achieved by infusion of serum or plasma containing high concentrations of antibody. This form of passive immunity provides immediate antibody protection against microorganisms, such as hepatitis A, by administering preformed antibodies. These antibodies have been produced by another person or animal that has been actively immunized, but the ultimate recipient has not produced them. The recipient will only temporarily benefit from passive immunity for as long as the antibodies persist in their circulation.

In addition, passive immunity can be acquired naturally by the fetus because of the transfer of antibodies by the maternal circulation in utero. Maternal antibodies are also transferred to the newborn after parturition in the prelactation fluid, *colostrum.* In order for the newborn to have lasting protection, active immunity must occur.

Immediate hypersensitivity comprises a subset of the body's antibody-mediated mechanisms. This subset consists of the reactions primarily mediated by *immunoglobulin E (IgE),* a class of immunoglobulins with unique biologic properties. Expression of immediate hypersensitivity results from the following:

1. Exposure to antigen (allergens)
2. Development of an IgE antibody response to the antigen

3. Binding of the IgE to mast cells
4. Reexposure to the antigen
5. Antigen-interaction with antigen-specific IgE bound to the surface membrane of mast cells
6. Release of potent chemical mediators from sensitized mast cells
7. Action of these mediators on various organs

Atopic diseases are processes mediated by or related to IgE-immediate hypersensitivity. The most dramatic and devasting systemic manifestation of immediate hypersensitivity is *anaphylaxis.* Anaphylaxis is an immediate (type I) hypersensitivity reaction characterized by local reactions, such as *urticaria* (hives) and *angioedema* (redness and swelling), or systemic reactions in the respiratory tract, cardiovascular system, gastrointestinal tract, or skin. This type of reaction can be fatal. Other types of atopic diseases include allergic rhinoconjunctivitis, urticaria, angioedema, asthma, gastrointestinal allergy, and atopic dermatitis, an eczematous skin eruption.

In addition to IgE-dependent hypersensitivity, two other immunoglobulin-dependent (antibody-dependent) mechanisms and a fourth, cell-mediated, delayed hypersensitivity mechanism exist. These clinical reactions are discussed in detail in Chapter 23. An alternate system of classification for hypersensitivity was developed by Gell and Coombs over two decades ago. Characteristics of this classification of hypersensitivity are presented in Table 1-3.

Cell-Mediated Immunity

Cell-mediated immunity consists of immune activities that differ from antibody-mediated immunity (Table 1-1). Cell-mediated immunity is moderated by the link between T lymphocytes and phagocytic cells, i.e., *monocytes-macrophages.* Lymphocytes (T cells) do not recognize the antigens of microorganisms or other living cells such as *allografts* (a graft of tissue from a genetically different member of the same species, e.g., a human kidney) directly, but rather when the antigen is present on the surface of an antigen-presenting cell, the macrophage. Lymphocytes are immunologically active through various types of direct cell-to-cell contact and by the production of soluble factors, *lymphokines,* for specific immunologic functions such as the recruitment of phagocytic cells to the site of inflammation. The roles of various types and subset

TABLE 1-3

Classification of Hypersensitivity Reactions

	Type I	Type II	Type III	Type IV
Antibody	Anaphylactic IgE	Cytotoxic IgG Possibly other	Immune complex IgG IgM	T-cell dependent None
Complement Involved	No	Yes	Yes	No
Cells Involved	Mast cells Basophils	Red cells White cells Platelets	Host tissue cells	T cells Macrophages
Examples	Anaphylaxis Hay fever Food allergy	Transfusion reactions Hemolytic disease of newborn Thrombocytopenia	Arthus reaction Serum sickness Pneumonitis	Allergy of infection Contact dermatitis

Modified from Barrett JT: Textbook of immunology, St Louis, 1988, The CV Mosby Co.

types of lymphocytes are discussed in Chapter 4.

The term *delayed hypersensitivity* is often used synonymously with the term *cell-mediated immunity. Delayed hypersensitivity,* however, refers to the slow appearance of a secondary response in the skin and dates back to the time when antibody responses were detected by immediate hypersensitivity and reflected the subtle difference in the length of time that it took for a delayed response to occur (e.g., tuberculin skin test). Cell-mediated immunity is responsible for the following immunologic events:

1. Contact sensitivity (e.g., poison-ivy dermatitis caused by binding of substance to the skin)
2. Delayed hypersensitivity (e.g., contact dermatitis)
3. Immunity to viral and fungal antigens
4. Immunity to intracellular organisms
5. Rejection of foreign-tissue grafts
6. Elimination of tumor cells bearing neoantigens
7. Formation of chronic granulomas (undegradable material such as tubercle bacilli, streptococcal cell walls, asbestos, or talc, sequestered in a focus of concentric macrophages that also contains some lymphocytes and eosinophils)

Under some conditions, the activities of cell-mediated immunity may not be beneficial. Suppression of the normal adaptive immune response *(immunosuppression)* by drugs or other means is necessary in conditions such as organ transplantation, hypersensitivity, and autoimmune disorders.

FACTORS ASSOCIATED WITH IMMUNOLOGIC DISEASE

Many of the same factors, such as general health and the age of an individual, are important in the development of immunologic as well as infectious disease. In the case of noninfectious diseases or disorders, however, additional factors may be of importance. These factors can include genetic predisposition to many disorders, nutritional status, and the individual's method of coping with stress.

Effect of Age on Immunity

Although nonspecific and specific body defenses are present in the unborn and newborn infant, many of these defenses are not completely developed in this group. Therefore young children are at greater risk for diseases, particularly infectious diseases.

A loss of immune defenses, not disease itself, may be the cause of death in at least 30% of people over 85 years of age. In the elderly, certain natural barriers to infection break down. Changes in the skin due to the normal aging process allow it to be breached more readily. In the lung, many of the specialized defenses against foreign invasion are weakened, including the cough reflex and bronchotracheal ciliary action. Other age-related changes include incomplete emptying of the bladder that can lead to infection and alteration in the normal flora of the intestine, caused by immobilization or as a result of drug therapy. In addition, some age-associated diseases exert detrimental effects on the immune system. Diabetes, which is increasing in incidence in older persons, results in greater susceptibility to diseases such as septicemia and gangrene.

The ability to respond immunologically to disease is age related. It has been suggested that faulty immunologic reactions are involved in the aging process; however, the effect of aging on the immune response is highly variable. In studies of the cells of the immune system, a general decline in the quantity of some types of lymphocytes in the blood has been observed in some elderly persons. A decrease in lymphocyte subset types and aberrant functioning of immunoregulatory cells have been implicated as potential causes of many age-related immunologic dysfunctions that contribute to poor immunity in the aged. It is not known if enhancement of the immune response with methods such as tissue removal, dietary manipulation, cell grafting, and chemical intervention in the elderly will be associated with clinical benefits; but immunomodulation may be a formidable tool to combat aging of the immune system in the future.

Role of Nutrition and Immunity

The importance of good nutrition to good health has always been emphasized. Good nutrition is known to be important to growth and development, and it is now suggested that a healthy diet is important in the aging process and in the triad of nutrition, immunity, and infection. The consequences of diet, however, in many aspects of the immune response have been documented in multiple disorders. Every constituent of body defenses, including phagocytosis and humoral and cellular immunity, appears to be influenced by nutritional intake. Deficient or excessive intake of some dietary components, such as vitamins and minerals (Table 1-4), can exert negative effects on the immune response. Therefore a healthy diet is important to maximum functioning of the immune system.

Effects of a Proper Diet

The study of the relationship of nutrition to immunity is complex because of factors such as the diversity of the food we eat and the influence of environment on specific nutritional needs. Some nutritional associations hold true for the risk of malignancy and immune function but others do not. The role of nutrition in the risk and treatment of malignancy has been studied. For example, low intake of vitamin A and high intake of fats have been associated with an increased risk of malignancy in humans. Both constituents also have a marked effect on the immune response. It has been suggested that the balance and absolute intake of multiple nutrients have an influence on susceptibility to in-

TABLE 1-4

Examples of the Effects of Increased or Decreased Levels of Vitamins and Minerals

Constituent	Effect	Constituent	Effect
Water-soluble vitamins		**Water-soluble vitamins—cont'd**	
Folic acid	Deficiency has a profound effect on cell-mediated immunity.	Vitamin B$_{12}$ (Cobalamin)	Congenital deficiency of transcobalamin II,* associated with decreased white cells; the absence of immunoglobulins; impaired phagocytosis.
Pantothenic acid	A deficiency in conjunction with pyridoxine deficiency is associated with the absence of antibodies.	Vitamin C (Ascorbic acid)	Increased or decreased amounts may negatively affect phagocytosis.
Vitamin B$_1$ (Thiamin)	Deficiency can produce abnormal phagocytosis, e.g., Schwachman-Diamond syndrome.	**Fat-soluble vitamins and congeners**	
Vitamin B$_2$ (Riboflavin)	No disease associated with deficiency. Specific role in human malignancy is unclear but believed to play a role in tumorigenesis.	Vitamin A	Decreased intake of vitamin A and a high intake of fats is associated with an increased risk of malignancy.
Vitamin B$_6$ (Pyridoxal, pyridoxine)	Deficiency during prenatal and postnatal development affects organs of the immune system, spleen, and thymus respectively. Deficiency in children and adults can cause mild impairment, e.g., decreased lymphocytes; decreased hormones produced by immune organs (e.g., thymus); inability to produce antibodies to various antigens; and depression of delayed hypersensitivity. If simultaneous deficiency in pantothenic acid, complete absence of antibody production will occur.	**Minerals**	
		Cadmium Lead	Excess but subtoxic amounts have a negative effect on normal immune function.
		Copper	Deficiency associated with increase in severity of inflammatory lesion and antibody-forming cell response.
		Iodine	In excess has a dose-dependent immunosuppressive effect.
		Iron	Deficiency probably increases susceptibility to infection because iron is an integral part of microbicidal process.
		Selenium	Deficiency impairs T cell–dependent antibody responses, particularly in association with vitamin E deficiency.

*Proteins that deliver vitamin B$_{12}$ to the tissues.

fection, to host immune response, and possibly on susceptibility to and treatment of autoimmune disorders.

Food is a complex mixture of organic and inorganic substances and metals in varying proportions. Within each group of nutrients, each chemical can have a different effect on various physiologic functions. Specific components of food may impair or cause an abnormality in immune function by the following mechanisms:
1. Deficiency of nutrient
2. Excess of nutrient
3. An error of metabolism
4. Direct toxic effect and/or an allergic reaction

Deficiency of a Nutrient

Malnutrition caused by extremely reduced caloric intake or a deficiency, complete or partial, of a specific nutrient can produce abnormal immune function. Malnutrition has also been implicated in cancer risk and in abnormalities of immune function.

Protein deficiency is an example of a disorder that compromises the immune system. Patients with such deficiency have altered immune defenses, such as decreased levels of IgA in secretions and decreased total levels and abnormal ratios of lymphocytic white cells. Abnormalities of immune function and increased susceptibility to infection are seen in alcoholics due to an improper diet, but it is unclear as to what degree dietary imbalance influences these abnormalities. These patients do have increased zinc and B-complex vitamin requirements.

Imbalanced intake of minerals can also cause immunologic abnormalities. For example, the amount of molybdenum in the diet has an influence on the effect of copper intake. If molybdenum is deficient, the quantity of copper ingested can result in death if copper is deficient, or death from toxicity if copper is excessive, or maintenance of good health if normal levels of copper are ingested.

Excess of a Nutrient

An excess of total calories or the increase of a specific nutrient can have immunologic consequence. Obesity, for example, has been implicated in cancer risk and in abnormalities of immune function. Obesity has been associated with a high incidence of infections, and infection-related mortality is higher in obese patients than in normal persons. Obese children have alterations in cell-mediated immune functions and white cell (neutrophil) function.

An example of the dire effects of an excess quantity of a specific nutrient is seen in cases of rapid repletion of iron in malnourished children. If iron is replaced rapidly before resolution of their malnourished state, death or other serious complications from overwhelming sepsis can result. Although iron appears to be important for immune competence, the effect of iron on any specific individual depends on a balance between the host's iron-dependent immunocompetence and microbial need for iron.

Errors of Metabolism

Innate or acquired errors of metabolism that result in the inability to degrade or synthesize intermediate metabolites of a nutrient can lead to immune dysfunction or deficiency. The best examples are patients with the syndrome associated with the abnormal metabolism of purines.

In some cases, a deficiency of adenosine deaminase has been associated with severe combined (cellular and humoral) deficiency caused by abnormal lymphocyte function. Children with a deficiency of adenosine deaminase have markedly depressed cellular and humoral immunity and are considered to have a defect at the level of the stem cell from which T and B cells are derived. At the present time, treatment to replace this enzyme involves red blood cell transfusion, which restores immunocompetence in most patients.

Another example of metabolic insufficiency that affects the immune system is the absence of the enzyme *purine nucleoside phosphorylase*, in the purine salvage pathway. This absence is associated with the loss of cellular immunity only. Patients with this disorder have normal humoral immunity, however.

Direct Toxic Effect or Allergic Reaction

Besides contaminants that can be present in food, naturally occurring toxins of plant or animal origin such as food additives (nitrates, nitrites, and dyes) and chemicals produced during food processing or cooking (nitrosamines, etc.) can produce adverse effects. Although many natural toxins have medicinal properties, some types (Table 1-5) are associated with immunologic abnormalities or precipitate the manifestation of signs and symptoms of immune disorders, or both. Food allergies are common and are believed to represent (type I) hypersensitivity reactions. Man-made chemical food

TABLE 1-5

Examples of Naturally Occurring Toxins

Type of toxin	Effect on humans
Allergens	Target organs may be skin, lungs, gastrointestinal tract, nervous system or musculoskeletal system.
Carcinogens and mutagens	Aflatoxins are suspected in the pathogenesis of some malignancies.
Nonphysiologic amino acids	L-canavanine can induce or exacerbate the lupus syndrome.
Protease inhibitors	IgE antibodies to the Kunitz soybean inhibitor produce anaphylaxis and angioedema.

additives are particularly hazardous to asthmatics. When exposed to agents such as sulfites, asthmatics and others may manifest such signs as itching and hives or anaphylactic shock, or death may result. Denatured rapeseed oil causes toxic oil syndrome. As the result of ingesting this toxin, an autoimmune disorder can develop.

Role of Proteins, Carbohydrates, and Lipids in Immunity

Proteins

Protein deficiency can have serious effects on the immune response and the ability of tumors and infections to prosper in a host. Malnutrition caused by lack of protein in children before 7 months of age produces decreased levels of antibody production. Children suffering from malnutrition secrete low levels of IgA and produce low levels of IgA in response to viral vaccines. The production of substances such as lysozyme and interferon is also decreased. These children fail to demonstrate an inflammatory reaction in response to infection; and the degree of suppression of cell-mediated immunity correlates with the severity of the protein deficiency. Changes in phagocytosis are also noticed.

In patients with *anorexia nervosa*, an eating disorder that is prevalent in adolescent females, the consequences of protein depletion express themselves in immunologic terms. Anorexia nervosa causes depressed levels of proteins synthesized by the body such as IgM and IgG antibodies, *transferrin*, and various complement components. Defects in phagocytosis are also observable. In adults, chronic malnourishment is the cause of higher incidences of postoperative wound infection, bacteremia, and/or pneumonia. Fasting, however, can be beneficial in certain conditions associated with autoimmune disorders.

Amino acids, the building blocks of proteins, are important to body defenses. Excess or decreased concentrations of specific amino acids in the diet appear to have an effect on immunity. For example, tryptophan and phenylalanine appear to be necessary for optimal production of antibodies. Depressed serum levels of the amino acid histidine in patients with disorders such as rheumatoid arthritis have been found to correlate with disease activity.

Lectins are additionally important to immunity. These proteins, many of which are glycoproteins, are immunologically important because of their ability to bind specific sugars on cell membranes. This binding thereby triggers cellular events, such as mitosis.

Carbohydrates

Studies of carbohydrates support the concept that sugars such as glucose play a role in immunity. In humans, the increased susceptibility of diabetics to infection has long been known. In persons with diabetes, impaired phagocytosis has been demonstrated. Children with galactosemia are also

at an increased risk of bacterial infection. Increased levels of sugar, however, may not be the exclusive reason for these manifestations. Ketoacidosis, rather than hyperglycemia may be important in susceptibility to infection.

Lipids

Both the total intake of specific fats and the relative balance of various dietary fats appear to play a major role in immunologic functions. In the skin, for example, long-chain saturated lipids and waxes provide a barrier to the outside environment. Essential fatty acid deficiency symptoms cause changes in the skin and impaired wound healing.

Fish oils have been suggested as having a possible antiinflammatory role. High-fat diets have been correlated with promoting the action of carcinogens, however.

Role of Vitamins and Minerals in Immunity

Multiple vitamin deficiencies occurring alone or in combination are particularly prevalent among the elderly and the sick. Vitamin deficiencies can compromise body defenses in various ways. Vitamin A, for example, is of major importance in maintaining the integrity of anatomic barriers, i.e., skin and mucosal membranes. Through their role in cell differentiation, vitamin A congeners and natually occurring provitamins may play a significant role in susceptibility to cancer.

In the early 1970s, the relationship between vitamin deficiencies and antibody formation was noted. A deficiency of vitamins such as pyridoxine, pantothenic acid, and folate causes profound impairment of antibody response. Moderate impairment is noted in deficiencies of riboflavin, thiamin, biotin, niacin-tryptophan, and vitamin A. Antibody response has not been observed as being defective in the presence of deficiencies of either vitamin B_{12} or vitamin D. Cellular immunity is affected profoundly by decreased levels of pyridoxine, folic acid, and vitamin A. Phagocytosis, however, may be specifically affected by the availability of some vitamins such as vitamin C.

Excessive quantities of most of the heavy metals, even essential trace elements like zinc, depress immunity and increase susceptibility to infections. Mineral deficiencies, as well, produce markedly impaired cell-mediated immunity. Minerals such as calcium are important in the activation of complement. Calcium also has a regulatory effect on lymphocyte and phagocytic cell function. It is likely that calcium may indirectly affect critical sites of immune processes. Calcium intake and supplementation, however, do not appear to play a role in immune function. The role of fiber in immune function is not defined.

Relationship of the Brain and Immune System

Increasing scientific evidence supports age-old observations that psychosocial factors are closely associated with the development of certain physical and mental illnesses. The relationship between psychologic stress, such as bereavement, and the occurrence of illness is illustrated by the fact that rates of illness and death tend to be higher among those who have recently lost a spouse. Abnormalities of immune functions have been found in bereavement, major affective disorders, and schizophrenia. In contrast, a positive mental state may favorably influence health and longevity. Response to stress, however, is often variable. Studies support both negative and positive effects of stress.

Psychoneuroimmunology

During the past decade, research findings have begun to confirm that the mind and body interact in remarkable ways. Studies are demonstrating that stressful emotions can be translated into altered responses in the cells, glands, and organs of the immune system. The scientific discipline of *psychoneuroimmunology* combines research in basic science with psychologic and psychosocial investigations to study the complex relationship of mind and body. This relationship may explain the correlation between increased susceptibility to certain diseases and psychologic events; however, the interrelationship of the various components of the immune system and psychologic reactions is complex.

Stress and Disease

The ability of an individual to control stress both psychologically and neurochemically appears to be as critical a factor as the nature of stress itself. A patient's personality and coping style, the meaning of the stress, the presence of social supports, and other environmental factors determine how an individual will respond to any life event. Psychosocial factors are believed to influence susceptibility to infectious diseases as part of the response each organism has to a pathogenic microorganism.

Studies support the concept that stress, per se, is not oncogenic; however, the inability to cope with stress may allow for the development and proliferation of tumor cells. The immune system appears to play a primary mediating role. Acute stress may initiate a transient, immunologically protective response, but prolonged or poorly controlled pychosocial stresses may result in depression of different components of the immune system.

Hormonal Regulators of Stress and Immunity

Stress has a direct effect on hormone production. For example, deprivation of sleep causes elevations of stress-related hormones. In addition, several scientific observations support a hormonally mediated link between psychosocial stressors and impaired immune function. Hormones and catecholamines are also known to be a mediating mechanism regulated by the central nervous system and having an influence on immune suppression as well as on the pathogenesis of disease. Stimulation of the cortical-hypothalamic-pituitary axis leads to alteration in immune function, either indirectly by changes in secretion of hormones or neurotransmitters or directly, by the less well-documented *bidirectional neuronal* stimulation of lymphoid tissue.

Indirect endocrine system responses to stress include stimulation of the hypothalamus, which then initiates a response in the adrenal medulla with the subsequent release of *catecholamines*. The catecholamines, in turn, stimulate the release of a variety of other stress-related hormones. Alterations in concentrations of hormones, e.g., aldosterone, calcitonin, growth hormone, adrenocorticotropin, melanocyte-stimulating hormone, prolactin, thyrotropin, vasopressin, parathyroid hormone, thyroxine, glucagon, renin, erythropoietin, and gastrin, have also been documented in association with stress.

The autonomic nervous system, which is highly responsive to stress, in conjunction with corticosteroids, generally has an inhibitory effect on cell-mediated immunity. The impact on the immune system of other hormones released in response to stress is less clear. These responses, however, may be related to, or independent of, changes in the neuroendocrine system.

Immune Consequences of Stress

Lymphocyte metabolism and proliferation are inhibited by increased production of the hormone *corticosteroid*, but lymphocytes have been observed to be elevated transiently with alterations of lymphocyte functions during periods of stress. Lymphoid organs are known to atrophy as a result of chronic stress, resulting in a decreased number of lymphocytes. In addition, certain kinds of lymphocytes, natural killer cells, are affected by corticosteroids and catecholamines. Other blood cells are also affected by hormonal changes. Phagocytosis, for example, is decreased by stress reactions.

In experimental observations, secretions of IgA were observed to be lower in high-stress times and higher in low-stress periods. A higher incidence of respiratory disease was also noted following a period of stress.

An increased risk of infection, autoimmune disease, and cancer has been noted in depressed patients. In these patients, inhibition of phagocytosis can be demonstrated. Because patients with major depressive disorders have decreased lymphocytic mitotic activity, an altered immune response is suspected. Elevated levels of corticosteroids may play a mediating role.

Chapter Review

HIGHLIGHTS

Immunology is defined as the study of the molecules, cells, organs, and systems responsible for the recognition and disposal of nonself material; of how body components respond and interact; of the desirable or undesirable consequences of immune interactions; and of the ways in which the immune system can be advantageously manipulated to protect against or treat diseases.

The function of the immune system is to recognize self from nonself and to defend the body against nonself. The first line of defense against infection is unbroken skin and mucosal membrane surfaces. Secretions are also an important component in this first line of defense. Natural resistance is one of the two ways that the body resists infection if microorganisms penetrate the first line of resistance. Acquired resistance specifically recognizes and selectively eliminates exogenous or endogenous agents. Tissue damage produced by infectious or other agents results in inflammation, a series of biochemical and cellular changes that facilitates the phagocytosis of microorganisms or damaged cells. If the degree of inflammation is sufficiently extensive, it is accompanied by an increase in the plasma concentration of acute-phase proteins, a group of glycoproteins.

If a microorganism overwhelms the body's natural resistance, a third line of defensive resistance exists. Acquired or adaptive immunity is a more recently evolved mechanism; it allows the body to recognize, remember, and respond to a specific stimulus, an antigen. Adaptive immunity can result in the elimination of microorganisms and recovery from disease, and it frequently leaves the host with specific immunologic memory. This condition of memory or recall, acquired resistance, allows the host to respond more effectively if reinfection with the same microorganism occurs. Antibody-mediated immunity to infection is acquired if the antibodies are formed by the host or received from another source. These two types of acquired immunity are called active and passive immunity respectively.

Immediate hypersensitivity comprises a subset of the body's antibody-mediated effector mechanisms. This subset consists of the reactions primarily mediated by immunoglobulin E (IgE). Cell-mediated immunity consists of immune activities that differ from antibody-mediated immunity. Cell-mediated immunity is moderated by the link between T lymphocytes and phagocytic cells. T lymphocytes do not recognize the antigens of microorganisms or other living cells, such as allografts, but do so when the antigen is present on the surface of an antigen-presenting cell, the macrophage. Lymphocytes are immunologically active through various types of direct cell-to-cell contact and by the production of lymphokines for specific immunologic functions, such as the recruitment of phagocytic cells to the site of inflammation. The term delayed hypersensitivity is often used synonymously with the term cell-mediated immunity. Delayed hypersensitivity, however, refers to the slow appearance of a secondary response in the skin.

Many of the same factors, such as general health and the age of an individual, are important considerations in the development of immunologic as well as infectious disease. These factors can include genetic predisposition to many disorders, nutritional status, and the individual's method of coping with stress. Studies in the scientific discipline of psychoneuroimmunology additionally demonstrate that stressful emotions can be translated into altered responses in the cells, glands, and organs of the immune system. This relationship may explain the correlation between increased susceptibility to certain diseases and psychologic events; however, the interrelationship of the various components of the immune system and psychologic reactions is complex.

REVIEW QUESTIONS

1. The desirable consequences of immunity include:
   A. natural resistance
   B. acquired resistance
   C. allergies
   D. rejection of transplanted organs
   E. both A and B
2. Components of the first line of defense against infection include:
   A. intact skin
   B. phagocytosis
   C. complement activation
   D. production of antibodies
   E. recognition of foreign antigens
3. The major cellular component of adaptive immunity is the:
   A. mast cell
   B. neutrophil
   C. macrophage
   D. basophil
   E. lymphocyte
4. The major humoral component of adaptive immunity is:
   A. complement
   B. antibody
   C. lysozyme
   D. interferon
   E. lymphokine
5. The majority of the actions of the two categories of the adaptive response are exerted by the interaction of:
   A. antibody with complement and phagocytic cells
   B. T cells with macrophages
   C. B cells with lymphokines
   D. plasma cells and T cells
   E. both A and B
6. Which of the following statements is (are) true about active immunity?
   A. antibodies are formed by the host
   B. antibodies are received from infusion of antibody-containing serum or plasma
   C. results from vaccination
   D. results from infection with a specific organism
   E. all of the above except B
7. Immediate hypersensitivity primarily consists of reactions mediated by:
   A. complement
   B. IgM antibody
   C. IgG
   D. IgE
   E. IgD

8. The term *delayed hypersensitivity* is often used synonymously with:
   A. antibody-mediated immunity
   B. cell-mediated immunity
   C. anaphylactic shock
   D. both A and B
   E. both B and C
9. Some naturally occurring toxins can:
   A. produce anaphylaxis
   B. produce angioedema
   C. induce lupus syndrome
   D. be the cause of pathogenesis in some malignancies
   E. all of the above

Questions 10-14
Match a deficiency of each of the following vitamins with the associated condition. Use an answer only once.
10. Folic acid
11. Vitamin C
12. Vitamin B_1-Thiamin
13. Vitamin B_6
14. Vitamin B_{12}
   A. can produce abnormal phagocytosis, e.g., Schwachman-Diamond syndrome
   B. if a simultaneous deficiency occurs with pantothenic acid, a complete absence of antibody production results
   C. a deficiency of transcobalamin II is associated with the absence of immunoglobulins
   D. has a profound effect on cell-mediated immunity
   E. increased or decreased amounts may negatively affect phagocytosis

15. Lymphocyte metabolism and proliferation are inhibited by increased production of the hormone:
   A. catecholamine
   B. corticosteroid
   C. aldosterone
   D. calcitonin
   E. glucagon

Answers

1. E 2. A 3. E 4. B 5. E 6. E 7. D 8. B 9. E 10. D 11. E 12. A 13. B 14. C 15. B

BIBLIOGRAPHY

Barrett JT: Textbook of immunology, ed 5, St Louis, 1988, The CV Mosby Co.
Bellanti JA: Immunology: basic processes, Philadelphia, 1979, WB Saunders Co.
Corman LC: Effects of specific nutrients on the immune response, Med Clin North Am 69(4):759, 1985.
Delafuente JC: Immunoenescence, Med Clin North Am 69(3):475, 1985.
Edwards NL: Immunodeficiencies associated with errors in purine metabolism, Med Clin North Am 69(3):505, 1985.
Gelman D and Hager M: Body and soul, Newsweek, p 88, Nov 7, 1988.
Playfair JHL: Immunology at a glance, Oxford, England, 1979, Blackwell Scientific Publications, Inc.
Roitt, IM: Essential immunology, ed 5, Oxford, England, 1984, Blackwell Scientific Publications, Inc.
Roitt, IM: Immunology, London, 1985, Gower Medical Publishing.
Rudbach JA ed: How aging affects immunity, Infectious Disease and Immunology Forum, Chicago, Dec 1984, Abbott Laboratories.
Schindler BA: Stress, affective disorders, and immune function, Med Clin North Am 69(3):585, 1985.

CHAPTER 2

Antigens and Antibodies

ANTIGEN CHARACTERISTICS
General Characteristics of Antigens

Foreign substances can be immunogenic or *antigenic* (capable of provoking an immune response) if their membrane or molecular components contain structures that are recognized as foreign by the immune system. These structures are called *antigenic determinants*, or *epitopes*. Not all surfaces, however, act as antigenic determinants. Only prominent determinants on the surface of a protein are normally recognized by the immune system, and some of these are much more immunogenic than others. An immune response is directed against specific determinants, and resultant antibodies will bind to them with much of the remainder of the molecule being nonimmunogenic.

The cellular membrane of mammalian cells chemically consists of proteins, phospholipids, cholesterol, and traces of polysaccharide. Polysaccharides (carbohydrates) in the form of either glycoproteins or glycolipids can be found attached to the lipid and protein molecules of the membrane. Most of these proteins are immunogenic when a different individual of the same species is exposed to cells or tissues containing them, such as erythrocytes and body tissues. Outer surfaces of bacteria such as a

capsule or the cell wall, as well as the surface structures of other microorganisms, are immunogenic.

Cellular antigens of importance to immunologists include *histocompatibility* (HLA) *antigens*, *autoantigens*, and *blood group antigens*. The normal immune system responds to foreignness by producing antibodies. For this reason, microbial antigens are also of importance to immunologists in the study of the immunologic manifestation of infectious diseases.

Histocompatibility Antigens

Nucleated cells, such as leukocytes and tissues, possess many *cell-surface-protein* antigens that readily provoke an immune response if transferred into a genetically different (allogenic) individual of the same species. Some of these antigens, which constitute the major *histocompatibility complex*, are much more potent than others in provoking an immune response. This major histocompatibility complex (MHC) is referred to as *HLA system* because its gene products were originally identified on white blood cells *(human leukocyte antigens)*. These antigens are second only to the ABO antigens in influencing the survival or graft rejection of transplanted organs. HLA antigens are the subject of numerous scientific investigations because of the strong association between individual HLA antigens and immunologic disorders. The HLA system is discussed in further detail in Chapter 28.

Autoantigens

The evolution of a recognition system that can recognize and destroy nonself material must also have safeguards to prevent damage to self-antigens. The body's immune system usually exercises tolerance to self-antigens, but in some situations antibodies may be produced in response to normal self-antigens. This failure to recognize self-antigens can result in autoantibodies directed at hormones, such as thyroglobulin. Cell-membrane antigens are discussed in detail in Chapter 25.

Blood Group Antigens

Blood group substances are widely distributed throughout the tissues, blood cells, and body fluids. When foreign red cell antigens are introduced to a host, a transfusion reaction or hemolytic disease of the newborn can result. The subject of blood group antigens and antibodies is described in detail in *Fundamentals of Immunohematology*. A brief description of these disorders is presented in this book in Chapter 23. In addition, certain antigens, especially those of the Rh system, are integral structural components of the erythrocyte membrane. If these antigens are missing, the erythrocyte membrane is defective and results in hemolytic anemia. When antigens do not form part of the essential membrane structure, e.g., A, B, and H antigens, the absence of antigen has no effect on membrane integrity.

CHEMICAL NATURE OF ANTIGENS

Antigens, or *immunogens*, are usually large organic molecules that are either proteins or large polysaccharides and rarely, if ever, lipids. Antigens, especially cell surface or *membrane-bound* antigens, can be composed of combinations of the biochemical classes, e.g., glycoproteins or glycolipids. For example, histocompatibility (HLA) antigens are glycoprotein in nature and are found on the surface membranes of nucleated body cells comprising both solid tissue and most circulating blood cells, e.g., granulocytes, monocytes, lymphocytes, and thrombocytes.

Proteins are excellent antigens because of their high molecular weight and structural complexity; *lipids* are considered to be inferior antigens because of their relative simplicity and lack of structural stability. However, when lipids are linked to proteins or polysaccharides, they may function as antigens. Nucleic acids are poor antigens because of relative simplicity, molecular flexibility, and rapid degradation. Antinucleic acid antibodies can be produced by artificially stabilizing them and linking them to an immunogenic carrier. Carbohydrates (polysaccharides) by themselves are considered too small to function as antigens. However, in

the case of erythrocyte blood group antigens, protein or lipid carriers may contribute to the necessary size and the polysaccharides present in the form of side chains confer *immunologic specificity*.

PHYSICAL NATURE OF ANTIGENS

In order to function as effective antigens, several factors are important: foreignness, degradability, molecular weight, structural stability, and complexity.

Foreignness

Foreignness is the degree to which antigenic determinants are recognized as nonself by an individual's immune system. The immunogenicity of a molecule depends to a great extent on its degree of foreignness. Normally, an individual's immune system does not respond to self-antigens.

Degradability

In order for an antigen to be recognized as foreign by an individual's immune system, sufficient antigens to stimulate an immune response must be present. Foreign molecules, which are rapidly destroyed, will not be present long enough to provide adequate antigenic exposure.

Molecular Weight

The higher the molecular weight, the better the molecule will function as an antigen. The number of antigenic determinants on a molecule is directly related to its size. Although large foreign molecules (molecular weight greater than 10,000) are better antigens, *haptens*, which are very small molecules, can bind to a larger carrier molecule and behave as an antigen. If a hapten is chemically linked to a large molecule, a new surface structure is formed on the large molecule, which may function as an antigenic determinant.

Structural Stability

If a molecule is an effective antigen, structural stability is mandatory. If a structure is unstable, e.g., gelatin, the molecule will be a very poor antigen. Similarly, totally inert molecules are poor antigens.

Complexity

The more complex an antigen is, the more effective it will be. Complex proteins are better antigens than large repeating polymers such as lipids, carbohydrates, and nucleic acids, which are relatively poor antigens.

GENERAL CHARACTERISTICS OF ANTIBODIES

Antibodies are specific glycoproteins referred to as *immunoglobulins*. Many antibodies can be isolated in the gamma globulin fraction of protein by *electrophoresis separation* (Fig. 2-1). The term *immunoglobulin* (Ig), however, has replaced *gamma globulin* because not all antibodies have gamma electrophoretic mobility. Antibodies can be found in

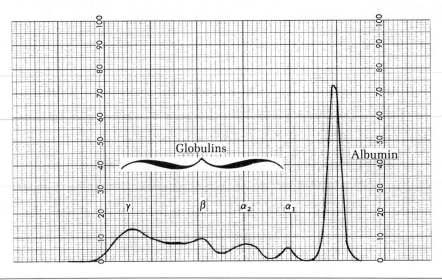

FIGURE 2-1

A tracing of the electrophoretic pattern of normal serum.
(From Barrett JT: Textbook of immunology, ed 5, St. Louis, 1988, The CV Mosby Co.)

TABLE 2-1

Characteristics of immunoglobulin classes

	IgM	IgG	IgA	IgE	IgD
Molecular weight	900,000	160,000	360,000	200,000	160,000
Sedimentation coefficient	19S	7S	11S	8S	7S
Percent carbohydrate	12	3	7	12	12
Subclasses	None	IgG1-4	Alpha 1,2	None	None
Serum concentration*(mg/dL; adults)	50-200	800-1600	150-400	0.002-0.05	1.5-40
Half-life (days)	5	21	6	2	3

*Conversion factors
IgG 1 mg= 11.5 IU   IgM 1 mg= 117.0 IU
IgA 1 mg= 57.7 IU   IgD 1 mg= 709.0 IU

blood plasma and many body fluids such as tears, saliva, and colostrum.

The primary function of an antibody in body defenses is to combine with antigen, which may be enough to neutralize bacterial toxins or some viruses. A secondary interaction of an antibody molecule with another effector agent, such as complement, is usually required to dispose of larger antigens, such as bacteria.

Determination of the concentration of immunoglobulin can be of diagnostic significance in infectious and autoimmune diseases. Test methods to detect the presence and concentration of immunoglobulins (discussed in Chapters 7 to 11 and in chapters relating to specific diseases) include agglutination reactions, radial immunodiffusion, and nephelometry.

IMMUNOGLOBULIN CLASSES

Five distinct classes of immunoglobulin molecules are recognized in most higher mammals: IgG, IgM,

IgA, IgD, and IgE. These immunoglobulin classes differ from each other in characteristics such as molecular weight, sedimentation coefficient, and carbohydrate content (Table 2-1). In addition to the differences between classes, the immunoglobulins vary within each class.

IgG

The major immunoglobulin in normal serum is IgG. This immunoglobulin diffuses more readily than other immunoglobulins into the extravascular spaces and neutralizes toxins or binds to microorganisms in extravascular spaces. It is capable of crossing the placenta. In addition, when IgG complexes are formed, complement can be activated. IgG accounts for 70% to 75% of the total immunoglobulin pool. It is a 7S molecule with a molecular weight of approximately 150,000. One of the subclasses, IgG_3, is slightly larger (MW 170,000) than the other subclasses.

Normal human adult serum values of IgG are

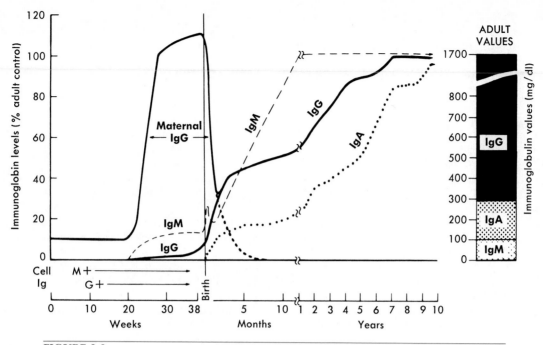

<u>FIGURE 2-2</u>

Immunoglobulin concentration in newborns, infants, and children.
(From Bauer JD: Clinical laboratory methods, ed 9, St. Louis, 1982, The CV Mosby Co.)

800 to 1800 mg/dL (90 to 210 IU/mL). At 3 to 4 months of age, the level of IgG is approximately 350 to 400 mg/dL (40 to 45 IU/mL), and it gradually increases to 700 to 800 mg/dL (80 to 90 IU/mL) by the end of the first year of life (Fig. 2-2). The average adult level is achieved before the age of 16 (Fig. 2-3). Other body fluids containing IgG include cord blood and cerebrospinal fluid (CSF). Cord blood contains 800 to 1800 mg/dL and CSF contains from 2 to 4 mg/dL of IgG.

Decreased levels of IgG can be manifested in primary (genetically determined) or secondary (acquired disorders associated with certain diseases) immunoglobulin deficiencies. Significant increases of IgG can be demonstrated in a variety of diseases and disorders. These include the following:
1. Infectious diseases, e.g., hepatitis, rubella, infectious mononucleosis
2. Collagen disorders, e.g., rheumatoid arthritis, systemic lupus erythematosus
3. Hematologic disorders, e.g., polyclonal gammopathies, monoclonal gammopathies, monocytic leukemia, Hodgkin's disease

Subclasses of IgG

Within the major immunoglobulin classes, there exist variants known as *subclasses* and *subtypes.* These subclasses differ in their heavy-chain composition and in some of their characteristics such as biologic activities (see Table 2-2). Four IgG subclasses (IgG$_1$, IgG$_2$, IgG$_3$, IgG$_4$) exist. The subclasses

TABLE 2-2

Characteristics of IgG subclasses

	IgG$_1$	IgG$_2$	IgG$_3$	IgG$_4$
Percentage of serum	65	24	7	4
Complement fixation	4+	2+	4+	(+)
Half-life (days)	23	23	8	23
Placental passage	+	?	+	+

occur in the approximate proportions of 66%, 23%, 7%, and 4%, respectively, in humans.

IgM

IgM accounts for about 10% of the immunoglobulin pool, and it is largely confined to the intravascular pool because of its large size. This antibody is produced early in an immune response and is largely confined to the blood. IgM is effective in agglutination and cytolytic reactions. In humans, it is found in smaller concentrations than IgG or IgA. The molecule has five individual heavy chains with an MW of 65,000; the whole molecule has an MW of 900,000 and has a sedimentation coefficient of 19S.

Normal values of IgM are 60 to 250 mg/dL (70 to 290 IU/mL) for males and 70 to 280 mg/dL (80 to 320 IU/mL) for females. Fifty percent of the adult levels are present at 4 months of age, and adult levels are obtained between 8 to 15 years of age. Cord blood contains <20 mg/dL. IgM is usually undetectable in cerebrospinal fluid (CSF).

IgM is decreased in primary (genetically determined) or secondary (acquired) immunoglobulin disorders. It can be increased in a wide variety of diseases and disorders. These conditions include:
1. Infectious diseases, e.g., subacute bacterial endocarditis, infectious mononucleosis, leprosy, trypanosomiasis, malaria, actinomycosis
2. Collagen disorders, e.g., scleroderma
3. Hematologic disorders, e.g., polyclonal gammopathies, monocytic leukemia, and monoclonal gammopathies such as Waldenstrom's macroglobulinemia

IgA

IgA represents 15% to 20% of the total circulatory immunoglobulin pool. It is the predominant immunoglobulin in secretions such as tears, saliva, colostrum, milk, and intestinal secretions. IgA is synthesized largely by plasma cells located on body surfaces. If the IgA is produced by cells in the intestinal wall, it may pass directly into the intestinal lumen or diffuse into the blood circulation. As IgA is transported through intestinal epithelial cells or hepatocytes, it binds to a glycoprotein called the *secretory piece*. The secretory piece protects IgA from digestion by gastrointestinal proteolytic enzymes and forms a complex molecule named *secretory IgA* (SIgA).

Secretory IgA is of critical importance in protecting body surfaces against invading microorganisms. It provides external surfaces of the body with protection from microorganisms because of its presence in seromucous secretions such as tears, saliva, nasal fluids, and colostrum.

IgA monomer is present in relatively high concentrations in human serum. It is present in a concentration of 90 to 450 mg/dL (55 to 270 IU/mL) in normal adult humans. Twenty-five percent of the adult IgA level is reached at the end of the first year of life and 50% at 3½ years of age. The average adult level is attained by age 16. IgA concentration in cord blood is <1 mg/dL, and CSF contains 0.1 to 0.6 mg/dL.

This immunoglobulin is decreased in primary (genetically determined) or secondary (acquired) immunoglobulin deficiencies. Significant increases in the concentration of serum IgA increases are associated with:
1. Infectious diseases, e.g., tuberculosis and actinomycosis
2. Collagen disorders, e.g., rheumatoid arthritis
3. Hematologic disorders, e.g., polyclonal gammopathies, monocytic leukemia, and the monoclonal gammopathy (IgA myeloma)
4. Liver disease, e.g., Laënnec's cirrhosis and chronic active hepatitis

IgD

IgD is found in very low concentrations in plasma, accounting for less than 1% of the total immunoglobulin pool. It is very susceptible to proteolysis and is primarily a cell membrane immunoglobulin found on the surface of B lymphocytes in association with IgM.

IgE

IgE is a trace plasma protein found in the blood plasma of unparasitized individuals. It has an MW of 188,000. IgE is of major importance because it mediates some types of hypersensitivity (allergic) reactions, allergies, and anaphylaxis and is generally responsible for an individual's immunity to invading parasites. The IgE molecule is unique in that it binds strongly to a receptor on mast cells and basophils and, together with antigen, mediates the release of histamines and heparin from these cells.

ANTIBODY STRUCTURE

Antibodies exhibit diversity among the different classes, which suggests that they perform different functions in addition to their primary function of antigen binding. Essentially each immunoglobulin molecule is bi-functional; one region of the molecule is concerned with binding to antigen while a

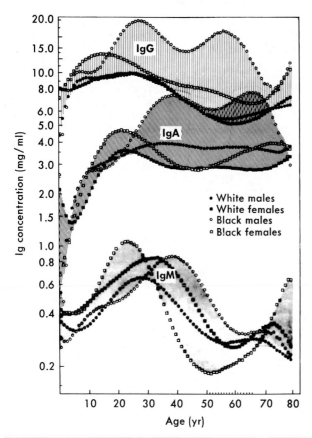

FIGURE 2-3

Serum immunoglobulins in 800 apparently healthy patients.
(From Bauer JD: Clinical laboratory methods, ed 9, St. Louis, 1982, The CV Mosby Co.)

different region mediates binding of the immunoglobulin to host tissues, including cells of the immune system and the first component (C1q) of the classic complement system.

The primary structure of a protein is based on the sequence of amino acid residues linked by the peptide bond. All antibodies have a common basic polypeptide structure that has a three-dimensional configuration. The polypeptide chains are linked by

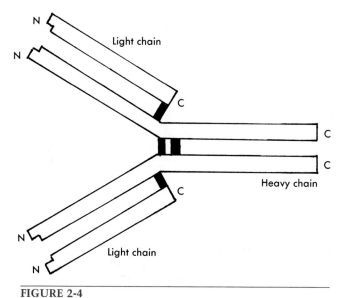

FIGURE 2-4

Basic immunoglobulin configuration.
(From Fundamentals of immunohematology, Philadelphia, 1989, Lea & Febiger.

covalent and noncovalent bonds, which produce a unit composed of a four-chain structure based on pairs of identical heavy and light chains. The immunoglobulins IgG, IgD, and IgE occur only as monomers of the four-chain unit; IgA occurs in both monomeric and polymeric forms; IgM occurs as a pentamer with five four-chain subunits linked together.

Typical Immunoglobulin Molecule

The basic unit of an antibody structure is the homology unit or *domain*, of which a typical molecule has 12, arranged in two heavy and two light (H and L) chains, linked through cysteine residues by disulfide bonds so that the domains lie in pairs (Fig. 2-4). Variations between the domains of different antibody molecules are responsible for differences in antigen binding and in biologic function. The antigen-binding portion of the molecule (N-terminal end) shows such heterogeneity that it is known as the *variable* region; the remainder is relatively *constant*, but some heterogeneity in form is observed in classes and subclasses. This diversity results in a variety of molecules being able to bring any antigen into contact with any one of several body defenses. Species differences do exist, especially in the heavy chain subclasses.

A classic model of antibody structure is displayed by the IgG molecule. Using electron microscopy, it can be seen to be Y-shaped (Fig. 2-5). If the molecule is chemically treated to break interchain disulfide bonds, the molecule separates into four separate polypeptide chains. The basic molecule consists of two identical light polypeptide chains

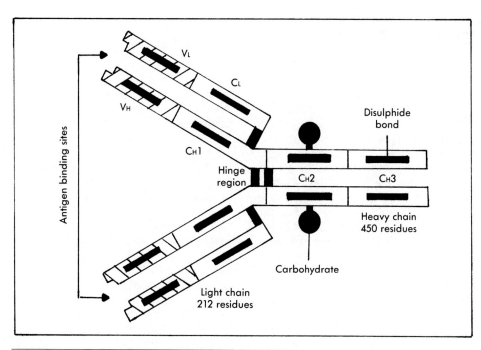

FIGURE 2-5

The basic structure of IgG.
(From Fundamentals of immunohematology, Philadelphia, 1989, Lea & Febiger.)

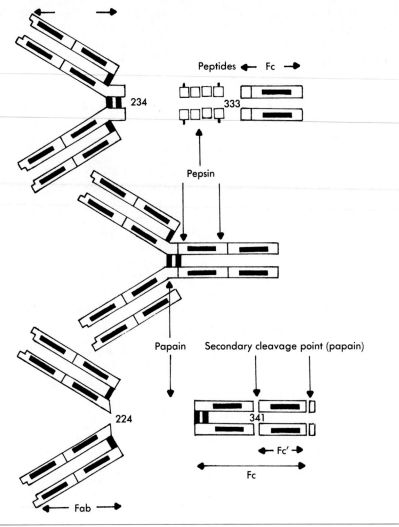

FIGURE 2-6

Enzymatic cleavage of human IgG 1.
(From Fundamentals of immunohematology, Philadelphia, 1989, Lea & Febiger.)

and two identical heavy polypeptide chains linked by disulfide bonds. The light chains are found in the N-terminal half of the molecule. Light chains are small chains (MW 25,000) and are common to all classes of immunoglobulins. The light chains are of two subtypes, termed *kappa* (κ) and *lambda* (λ), which have very different amino acid sequences and are antigenically different. In humans, about 65% of immunoglobulin molecules have kappa chains, while 35% have lambda chains. The larger heavy chains (MW 50,000 to 77,000) extend the full length of the molecule.

A general feature of the immunoglobulin chains is their amino acid sequence. The first 110 to 120 amino acids of both the light and heavy chains have a variable sequence and form the variable (V) region; the remainder of the light chains represents a constant (C) region with an amino acid sequence that is similar for each type and subtype. The remaining portion of the heavy chain is also constant

for each type and has a hinge region. The class and subclass of an immunoglobulin molecule are determined by its heavy chain type.

Fab, Fc, and Hinge Molecular Components

A typical monomeric IgG molecule consists of three globular regions (two Fab regions and an Fc portion) linked by a flexible hinge region. If the molecule is digested with a proteolytic enzyme (Fig. 2-6) such as papain, it splits into three approximately equal-size fragments. Two of these fragments retain the ability to bind antigen and are called the *antigen-binding fragments* (Fab fragments). The third fragment, which is relatively homogeneous and is sometimes crystallizable, is called the *Fc portion*. If IgG is treated with another proteolytic enzyme, *pepsin*, the molecule separates in a somewhat different manner. The Fc fragment is split into very small peptides and thus completely destroyed. The two Fab fragments remain

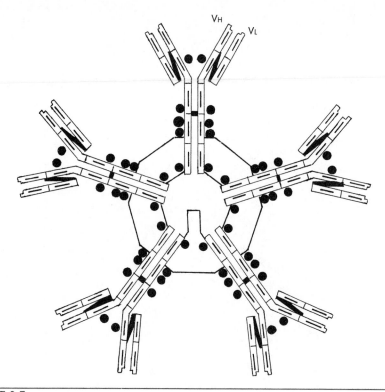

V_H V_L

FIGURE 2-7

Pentameric polypeptide chain structure of human IgM.
(From Fundamentals of immunohematology, Philadelphia, 1989, Lea & Febiger.)

joined to produce a fragment called *F(ab)'2*. This fragment possess two antigen binding sites. If F(ab)'2 is treated to reduce its disulfide bonds, it breaks into two Fab fragments, each of which has only one antigen binding site. Further disruption of the interchain disulfide bonds in the Fab fragments demonstrates that each contains a light chain and half of a heavy chain, which is called the *Fd fragment*.

Electron microscopy studies of IgG reveal that the Fab regions of the molecule are mobile and can swing freely around the center of the molecule as if it were hinged. This hinge consists of a group of about 15 amino acids located between the C_{H1} and C_{H2} regions. The exact sequence of amino acids in the hinge is variable and unique for each immunoglobulin class and subclass. Because amino acids can rotate freely around peptide bonds, the effect of closely spaced proline amino acid residues is production of a universal joint around which the immunoglobulin chains can freely swing. A remarkable feature of the hinge region is the presence of a large number of hydrophilic and proline residues. The hydrophilic residues tend to open up this region and thus make it accessible to proteolytic cleavage with enzymes such as pepsin and papain. This region also contains all of the interchain disulfide bonds except for IgD, which has no interchain links.

Structure of Other Immunoglobulins
IgM

The IgM molecule is structurally composed of five basic subunits. Each basic subunit consists of two kappa or two lambda light chains and two μ heavy chains. The individual monomers of IgM are linked together by disulfide bonds in a circular fashion (Fig. 2-7). A small cysteine-rich polypeptide, the *J chain*, must be considered an integral part of the molecule. IgM has carbohydrate residues attached to the C_{H3} and C_{H4} domains. The site for complement activation by IgM is located on this C_{H4} region. IgM is more efficient than IgG in activities such as the activation of complement cascade and agglutination.

IgA

In humans, more than 80% of IgA occurs as a typical four-chain structure consisting of paired kappa or lambda chains and two heavy chains (Fig. 2-8). The basic four-chain monomer has an MW of 160,000; however, in most mammals plasma IgA occurs mostly as a *dimer*. In dimeric IgA, the molecules are joined by a J chain linked to the Fc regions. Secretory IgA exists mainly in the 11S dimeric form and has an MW of 385,000 (Fig. 2-9). This form of IgA is present in fluids and is stabilized against proteolysis when combined with another protein called the *secretory component*. In

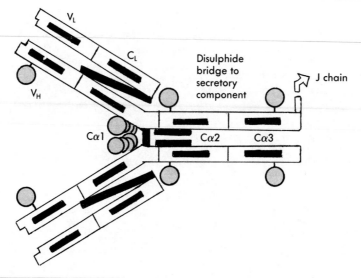

FIGURE 2-8
A molecule of IgA.

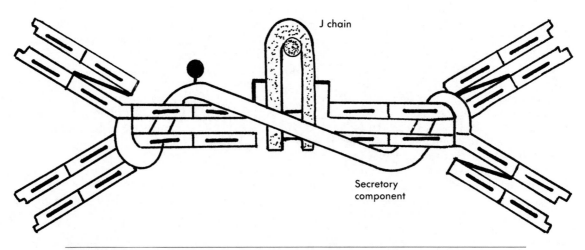

FIGURE 2-9
A molecule of secretory IgA.

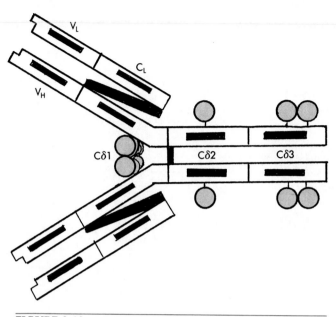

FIGURE 2-10
A molecule of IgD.

humans, variations in the heavy chains account for the subclasses IgA_1 and IgA_2.

IgD

The *IgD* molecule has an MW of 184,000 and consists of two kappa or lambda light chains and two delta (δ) heavy chains (Fig. 2-10). It has no interchain disulfide bonds between its heavy chains and an exposed hinge region.

IgE

The IgE molecule is composed of paired kappa or lambda light chains and two *epsilon* (ε) heavy chains (Fig. 2-11). It is unique in that its Fc region binds strongly to a receptor on mast cells and basophils and, together with antigen, mediates the release of histamines and heparin from these cells.

IMMUNOGLOBULIN VARIANTS

An antigenic determinant is the specific chemical determinant group or molecular configuration against which the immune response is directed. Immunoglobulins themselves can function as very effective antigens when used to immunize mammals of a different species because they are proteins. When the resulting anti-immunoglobulins or antiglobulins are analyzed, three principal categories (Table 2-3) of antigenic determinants can be recognized: *isotype, allotype,* and *idiotype* (Fig. 2-12).

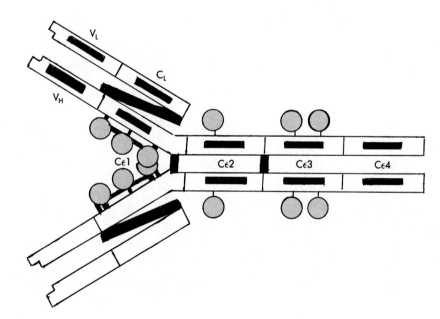

FIGURE 2-11
A molecule of IgE.

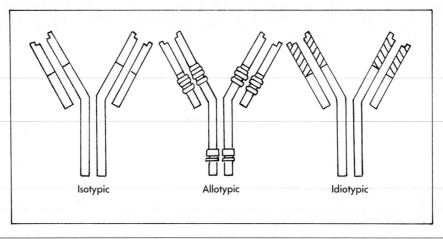

FIGURE 2-12
Variants of antibodies.
(From Fundamentals of immunohematology, Philadelphia, 1989, Lea & Febiger.)

TABLE 2-3

Immunoglobulin Variants

Variant	Distribution	Variant	Location	Examples
Isotypic	All variants in normal persons	Classes	C_H	IgM, IgE
		Subclasses	C_H	IgA_1, IgA_2
		Types	C_L	Kappa
				Lambda
Allotypic	Genetically-controlled alternate forms—not present in all persons	Allotypes	Mainly C_H/C_L Sometimes V_H/V_L	Gm groups in humans
Idiotypic	Individually specific to each immunoglobulin molecule	Idiotypes	Variable regions	Probably one or more hypervariable regions forming the antigen-combining site

Modified from Roitt IM: Essential immunology, ed 5, Oxford, England, 1984, Blackwell Scientific Publications, Inc.

Isotype Determinants

This class of antigenic determinants is the dominant type found on the immunoglobulins of all animals of a species. The heavy-chain, constant-region structures associated with the different classes and subclasses are termed *isotypic variants.* Genes for isotypic variants are present in all healthy members of a species. Determinants in this category include those specific for each immunoglobulin class, such as gamma for IgG, mu for IgM, and alpha for IgA, as well as the subclass-specific determinants kappa and lambda.

Allotype Determinants

The second principal group of determinants is found on the immunoglobulins of some, but not all, animals of a species. Antibodies to these allotypes (alloantibodies) may be produced by injecting the immunoglobulins of one animal into another member of the same species. The allotypic determinants are genetically determined variations representing the presence of allelic genes at a single lo-

cus within a species. Typical allotypes in humans are the *Gm specificities* on IgG (Gm is a marker on IgG). In humans, five sets of allotypic markers have been found: Gm, Km, Mm, Am, and Hv.

Idiotype Determinants

Idiotypes exist as a result of the unique structures on light and heavy chains. These individual determinants characteristic of each antibody are termed the *idiotypes.* The idiotypic determinants are located in the variable part of the antibody associated with the hypervariable regions that form the antigen-combining site.

ANTIBODY SYNTHESIS

Production of antibodies is induced when the host's immune system comes into contact with a foreign antigenic substance and reacts to this antigenic stimulation. When an antigen is initially encountered, the cells of the immune system (see Chapters 3 and 4) recognize the antigen as nonself and either elicit an immune response or become tolerant to it,

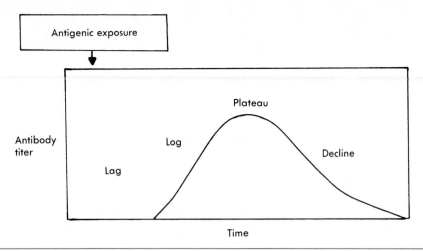

FIGURE 2-13

The four phases of an antibody response.
(From Fundamentals of immunohematology, Philadelphia, 1989, Lea & Febiger.)

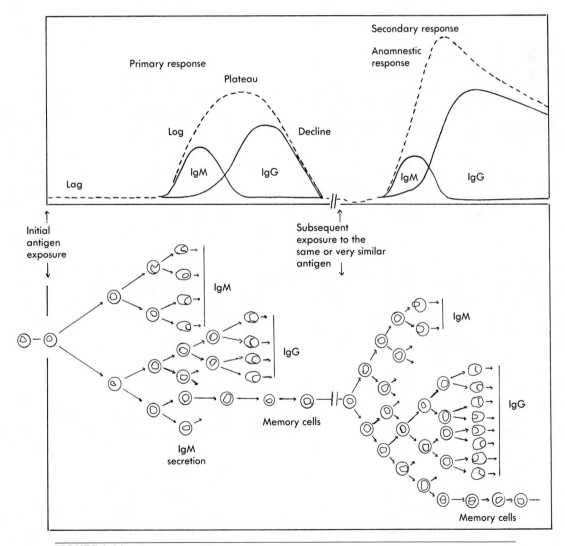

FIGURE 2-14

Primary and secondary antibody response.
(From Fundamentals of immunohematology, Philadelphia, 1989, Lea & Febiger.)

depending on the circumstances. An immune reaction can take the form of *cell-mediated immunity* (immunity dependent on T cells and macrophages) or involve the production of antibodies directed against the antigen. Whether a cell-mediated response or an antibody response takes place depends on the way in which the antigen is presented to the lymphocytes; many immune reactions display both kinds of responses. The antigenicity of a foreign substance is also related to the route of entry. Intravenous and intraperitoneal routes are stronger stimuli than subcutaneous and intramuscular routes. Subsequent exposure to the same antigen produces a memory response, or *anamnestic response*, and reflects the outcome of the initial challenge. In the case of antibody production, both the quantity and class of immunoglobulins produced vary.

Primary Antibody Response

Following a foreign antigen challenge, an IgM antibody response proceeds in four phases (Fig. 2-13), but the actual time period and levels of antibody (titer) depend on the characteristics of the antigen and the individual. The four phases are:
1. A *lag* phase when no antibody is detectable
2. A *log* phase in which the antibody titer rises logarithmically
3. A *plateau* phase during which the antibody titer stabilizes
4. A *decline* phase in which the antibody is catabolized

Secondary (Anamnestic) Response

Subsequent exposure to the same antigenic stimulus produces an antibody response that exhibits the same four phases as the primary responses (Fig. 2-14). Repeated exposure to an antigen can take place many years after the initial exposure, but clones of the T memory cells will be stimulated to proliferate with subsequent production of antibody by the individual. However, an anamnestic response differs from a primary response in several important aspects. These differences are:
1. *Time.* A secondary response has a shorter lag phase, a longer plateau, and a more gradual decline.
2. *Type of antibody.* IgM-type antibodies are the principal class formed in the primary response. Although some IgM antibody is formed in a secondary response, the IgG class is the predominant type formed.

3. *Antibody titer.* In a secondary response, antibody levels attain a higher titer. The plateau levels in a secondary response are typically ten-fold, or more, than the plateau levels in the primary response.

FUNCTIONS OF ANTIBODIES

The principal function of an antibody is to bind antigen. However, antibodies may exhibit secondary effector functions as well as behaving like antigens. The significant secondary effector functions of antibodies (Table 2-4) are complement fixation and placental transfer. The activation of complement (discussed in Chapter 5) is one of most important effector mechanisms of IgG$_1$ and IgG$_3$ molecules. IgG$_2$ seems to be less effective in activating complement; IgG$_4$, IgA, IgD, and IgE are ineffective in terms of complement activation. In humans, most of the IgG subclass molecules are capable of crossing the placental barrier. It is not universally agreed whether or not IgG$_2$ crosses the placenta. Passage of antibodies across the placental barrier is important in the etiology of hemolytic disease of the newborn (see Chapter 23) and in conferring passive immunity to the newborn during the first few months of life.

ANTIGEN-ANTIBODY INTERACTION AND IMMUNE COMPLEXES

The ability of a particular antibody to combine with one antigen instead of another is referred to as its *specificity*. This property resides in the portion of the Fab molecule called the *combining site*, a cleft formed largely by the hypervariable regions of heavy and light chains. There is evidence, however, that an antigen may bind to larger, or even separate, parts of the variable region. The closer the fit between this site and the *antigen determinant*, the stronger will be the noncovalent forces such as hydrophobic or electrostatic bonds between them, and the higher the affinity between the antigen and antibody. Binding depends on a close three-dimensional fit, allowing weak intermolecular forces to overcome the normal repulsion between molecules. When more than one combining site interacts with the same antigen, the bond has greatly increased strength.

ANTIBODY SPECIFICITY AND CROSS-REACTIVITY

Antigen-antibody reactions can show a high level of specificity. Specificity refers to the fact that the

TABLE 2-4

A Comparison of Properties of Immunoglobulins

	IgG$_1$	IgG$_2$	IgG$_3$	IgG$_4$	IgM	IgA	IgD	IgE
Complement fixation	2+	1+	3+	0	3+	0	0	0
Placental transfer	1+	+/−	+	1+	0	0	0	0

binding sites of antibodies directed against determinants of one antigen are not complementary to determinants of another, dissimilar antigen. When some of the determinants of an antigen are shared by similar antigenic determinants on the surface of apparently unrelated molecules, a proportion of the antibodies directed against one kind of antigen will also react with the other kind of antigen. This is called *cross-reactivity.* Antibodies directed against a protein in one species may also react in a detectable manner with the homologous protein in another species, which is another example of cross-reactivity.

Examples of cross-reactivity occur between bacteria that possess cell-wall polysaccharides in common with mammalian erythrocytes. Intestinal bacteria as well as other substances found in the environment possess A- or B-like antigens similar to the A and B erythrocyte antigens. If A or B antigens are foreign to an individual, production of anti-A or anti-B occurs, despite lack of previous exposure to these erythrocytic antigens. Cross-reacting antibodies of this type are *heterophile* antibodies.

Antibody Avidity

Each four polypeptide chain antibody unit has two antigen-binding sites, which allows them to be potentially multivalent in their reaction with an antigen. The strength with which a multivalent antibody binds a multivalent antigen is termed *avidity,* in contrast to *affinity* (the bond between a single antigenic determinant and an individual combining site). When a multivalent antigen combines with more than one of an antibody's combining sites, the strength of the bonding is significantly increased. In order for the antigen and antibody to dissociate, all of the antigen-antibody bonds must be broken simultaneously.

Decreased avidity can result from the fact that an antigen has only one antigenic determinant (monovalent). Additionally, a hapten is monovalent; therefore, it can only react with one antigen-combining site.

Immune Complexes

The noncovalent combination of antigen with its respective, specific antibody is called an *immune complex.* An immune complex may be of the small (soluble) or large (precipitating) type, depending on the nature and proportion of antigen and antibody. Under conditions of antigen or antibody excess, small soluble complexes tend to predominate. If equivalent amounts of antigen and antibody are present, a precipitate may form. All antigen-antibody complexes, however, will not precipitate, even at equivalence.

Antibody can react with antigen that is fixed or localized in tissues or with antigen that is released or present in the circulation. Once formed in the circulation, the usual fate of an immune complex is its removal by phagocytic cells of the body, through the interaction of the Fc portion of the antibody

Factors Determining Immune Complex Level

Nature of the antigen
  Quantity of available antigen
  Number of determinants (epitopes) per molecule
  Size
Nature of the antibody
  Quantity
  Affinity
  Class
    Valence
    Complement-fixing properties
    Reactivity with cellular receptors
Degree of lattice formation*
  Size of the complex
  Solubility properties
  Complement-fixing properties
  Clearance and distribution properties
Rate of formation
  Antigen availability
  Antibody synthesis rate
Rate of clearance
  Degree of lattice formation*
  Nature of the antigen
  Ability of the complex to react with complement or cellular receptors
  Condition of the mononuclear phagocytic system

*Lattice formation is the cross-linking between sensitized particles and antibodies resulting in aggregation (clumping). Adapted from McDougal JS and McDuffie FC: Detection and significance of immune complexes. In Spiegel HE ed: Advances in clinical chemistry, New York, 1985, Academic Press, Inc.

with complement and with cell-surface receptors. Under normal circumstances, this process does not lead to pathologic consequence, and may be viewed as a major host defense against the invasion of foreign antigens. It is only in unusual circumstances that the immune complex persists as a soluble complex in the circulation, escapes phagocytosis and is deposited in endothelial or vascular structures where it causes inflammatory damage, the principal characteristic of immune complex disease; or is deposited in organs such as the kidney; or inhibits useful immunity, such as to tumors or parasites. The level of circulating immune complex is determined by factors such as the rate of formation, the rate of clearance, and, most importantly, the nature of the complex formed (see accompanying box). Detection of immune complexes and the identification of the associated antigens are important to the clinical diagnosis of immune complex disorders (see Chapters 25 to 27).

MOLECULAR BASIS OF ANTIGEN-ANTIBODY REACTIONS

The basic Y-shaped immunoglobulin molecule is a bifunctional structure. The V regions are primarily concerned with antigen binding. When an antigenic determinant and its specific antibody combine, they interact through the chemical groups found on the surface of the antigenic determinant and on the surface of the *hypervariable* regions of the immunoglobulin molecule. Although the C regions do not form the antigen binding sites, the arrangement of the C regions and hinge region give the molecule segmental flexibility, which allows it to combine with separated antigenic determinants.

Types of Bonding

Bonding of an antigen to an antibody takes place because of the formation of multiple, reversible, intermolecular attractions between an antigen and amino acids of the binding site. These forces require proximity of the interacting groups. The optimum distance separating the interacting groups varies for different types of bond; however, all of these bonds act only across a very short distance and weaken very rapidly as that distance increases.

The bonding of antigen to antibody is exclusively noncovalent. The attractive force of noncovalent bonds is weak when compared to covalent bonds, but the formation of multiple noncovalent bonds produces considerable total binding energy. The strength of a single antigen-antibody bond is termed *antibody affinity,* and it is produced by the summation of the attractive and repulsive forces. The types of noncovalent bonds involved in antigen-antibody reactions are:
1. Hydrophobic bonds
2. Hydrogen bonding
3. Van der Waals forces
4. Electrostatic forces

Hydrophobic Bonds

The major bonds formed between antigens and antibodies are hydrophobic. Many of the nonpolar side chains of proteins are hydrophobic. When antigen and antibody molecules come together, these side chains interact and exclude water molecules from the area of the interaction. The exclusion of water frees some of the constraints imposed by the proteins, which results in a gain in energy and forms an energetically stable complex.

Hydrogen Bonds

Hydrogen bonding results from the formation of hydrogen bridges between appropriate atoms. Major hydrogen bonds in antigen-antibody interactions are O-H-O, N-H-N, and O-H-N.

Van der Waals Forces

Van der Waals forces are nonspecific attractive forces generated by the interaction between electron clouds and hydrophobic bonds. These bonds occur as a result of a minor asymmetry in the charge of an atom as a result of the position of its electrons. They rely on the association of nonpolar, hydrophobic groups so that contact with water molecules is minimized. Although Van der Waals forces are very weak, they may become collectively important in an antigen-antibody reaction.

Electrostatic Forces

Electrostatic forces result from the attraction of oppositely charged amino acids located on two proteins' side chains. The relative importance of electrostatic bonds is unclear.

Goodness of Fit

The strongest bonding develops when antigens and antibodies are close to each other and when the shapes of both the antigenic determinants and the antigen-binding site conform to each other. This complementary matching of determinants and binding sites is referred to as *goodness of fit* (Fig. 2-15).

A good fit will create ample opportunities for the simultaneous formation of several noncovalent bonds and few opportunities for disruption of the bond. If a poor fit exists, repulsive forces can overpower any small forces of attraction. Variations from the ideal complementary shape will produce a decrease in the total binding energy due to increased repulsive forces and decreased attractive forces. Therefore goodness of fit is important in determining the binding of an antibody molecule for a particular antigen.

Detection of Antigen-Antibody Reactions

In vitro tests detect the combination of antigens and antibodies. Tests such as agglutination tests are widely used in immunology to detect and measure the consequences of antigen-antibody interaction. Other test types include precipitation reac-

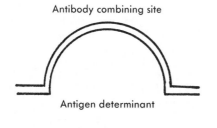

Antibody combining site

Antigen determinant

Good fit

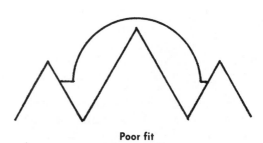

Poor fit

FIGURE 2-15
Goodness of fit.

TABLE 2-5

Role of Specific Immunoglobulins
in Diagnostic Tests

	IgG	IgM	IgA
Agglutination	1+	3+	1+
Complement fixation	1+	3+	Neg
Time of appearance after exposure to antigen (days)	3-7	2-5	3-7
Time to reach peak titer (days)	7-21	5-14	7-21

tions, hemolysis testing, and inhibition of agglutination. Tests such as the radioimmunoassay (RIA) and enzyme-linked immunoabsorbent assay (ELISA) measure immune complexes formed in an in vitro system. The principles of immunologic methods are discussed in Section II.

Detection and quantitation of immunoglobulins are important in the manifestation diagnosis of infectious disease as well as in immunologic disorders (Table 2-5).

Influence of Antibody Types on Agglutination

Immunoglobulins are relatively positively charged, and following sensitization or coating particles, they reduce the *zeta potential* (the difference in electrostatic potential between the net charge at the cell membrane and the charge at the surface of shear). Antibodies can bridge charged particles by extending out beyond the effective range of the zeta potential, which results in the erythrocytes closely approaching each other, binding together, and agglutinating.

Antibodies differ in their ability to agglutinate. IgM type antibodies, sometimes referred to as *complete antibodies*, are considerably more efficient than IgG or IgA antibodies in exhibiting in vitro agglutination when the antigen-bearing erythrocytes are suspended in physiologic (0.85%) sodium chloride (saline). Antibodies that do not exhibit visible agglutination of saline-suspended erythrocytes, even when bound to the cell's surface membrane, are considered to be nonagglutinating antibodies and may be called *incomplete antibodies*. Incomplete antibodies may fail to exhibit agglutination because the antigenic determinants are located deep within the surface membrane or may demonstrate restricted movement in their hinge region, causing them to be functionally *monovalent*.

MONOCLONAL ANTIBODIES

Monoclonal antibodies are purified antibodies cloned from a single cell. These antibodies are engineered to bind to a single specific antigen. Monoclonal antibodies bound to cell surface antigens now provide a method for classifying and identifying specific cellular membrane characteristics, such as in the typing of erythrocyte and leukocyte antigens, and as a reagent in the detection of coating of

erythrocyte antigens in the anti–human globulin test (AHG) test.

Discovery of the Technique

In 1975, George Kohler, a postdoctoral student at Cambridge University, was examining cell hybrids made between different lines of cultured myeloma cells (plasma cells derived from malignant tumor strains) by using Sendai virus to induce the cells to fuse. Sendai virus is an influenza virus that characteristically causes cell fusion.

Initially Kohler immunized donors with sheep erythrocytes in order to provide a marker for the normal cells. After making the hybrids, he tested them to see if they still produced antibodies against the sheep erythrocytes. He discovered that some of the hybrids were manufacturing large quantities of specific antisheep erythrocyte antibodies.

This technique is referred to as *somatic cell hybridization.* The resulting hybrid cells secrete the antibody that is characteristic of the parent cell, e.g., antisheep erythrocyte antibodies. The multiplying hybrid cell culture is called a *hybridoma.* Hybridoma cells can be cloned (the process in which single cells are selected and grown). The immunoglobulins derived from a single clone of cells are termed *monoclonal antibodies.*

Monoclonal Antibody Production

Modern methods (Fig. 2-16) for producing monoclonal antibodies are refinements of the original technique developed by Kohler. Basically, hybridoma technique enables scientists to inoculate crude antigen mixtures into mice and then select clones producing specific antibodies against a single cell-surface antigen. The process of producing monoclonal antibodies takes from 3 to 6 months.

Mice are immunized with a specific antigen. Several doses of the antigen are given to ensure a vigorous immune response. After 2 to 4 days, spleen cells are mixed with cultured mouse myeloma cells. Myeloma parent cells that lack the enzyme *hypoxanthine phosphoribosyl transferase* are selected because these cells cannot use hypoxanthine derived from the culture medium to manufacture purines and pyrimidines and, if unfused, will not survive in the culture medium. Additionally, the mouse myeloma cell lines usually do not secrete immunoglobulins so this simplifies the purification process.

Polyethlene glycol, rather than Sendai virus, is added to the cell mixture to promote cell-membrane fusion. Only one in every 200,000 spleen cells actually forms a viable hybrid with a myeloma cell. Normal spleen cells do not survive in culture. The fused-cell mixture is placed in a medium containing hypoxanthine, aminopterin, and thymidine (HAT medium). Aminopterin is a drug that prevents myeloma cells from making their own purines and pyrimidines, and since they cannot use hypoxanthine from the medium, they will die.

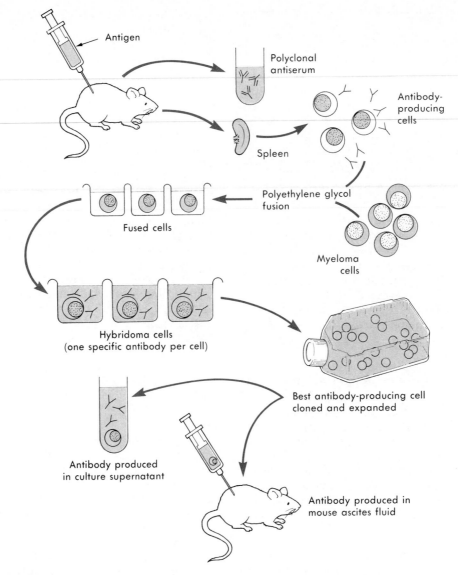

FIGURE 2-16

Production of monoclonal antibody.
(From Baron EJ and Finegold SM: Bailey and Scott's Diagnostic microbiology, ed 8, St. Louis, 1990, The CV Mosby Co.)

Hybrids resulting from the fusion of spleen cells and myeloma cells contain transferase provided by the normal spleen cells. Consequently, the hybridoma cells are able to use the hypoxanthine and thymidine in the culture medium and survive. They divide rapidly in HAT medium, doubling their numbers every 24 to 48 hours. About 300 to 500 different hybrids can be generated from the cells of a single mouse spleen, although not all will be making the desired antibodies. After the hybridomas have been growing for 2 to 4 weeks, the supernatant is tested for specific antibody, using methods such as ELISA or RIA. Clones that produce the desired antibody are grown in mass culture and recloned to eliminate nonantibody producing cells.

Antibody-producing clones lose their ability to synthesize or secrete antibody after being cultured for several months. It is usual to freeze and store hybridoma cells in small aliquots. They may then be grown in mass culture or injected intraperitoneally into mice. Because hybridomas are tumor cells, they grow rapidly and induce the effusion of large quantities of fluid into the peritoneal cavity. This ascites fluid is rich in monoclonal antibody and can be easily harvested.

The greatest impact of monoclonal antibodies in immunology has been on the analysis of cell-membrane antigens. Because monoclonal antibodies have a single specificity compared to the range of antibody molecules present in the serum, they are useful in erythrocyte typing, leukocyte typing (lymphocyte subsets), and tissue typing.

Chapter Review

HIGHLIGHTS

Foreign substances can be immunogenic if their membrane or molecular components contain structures that are recognized as foreign by the immune system. These structures are called antigenic determinants or epitopes. Cellular antigens of importance to immunologists include histocompatibility (HLA) antigens, autoantigens and blood-group antigens. The normal immune system responds to foreignness by producing antibodies. For this reason, microbial antigens are also of importance in the study of the immunologic manifestation of infectious diseases.

Nucleated cells possess many cell-surface-protein antigens, which readily provoke an immune response if transferred into an (allogenic) individual of the same species. Some of these antigens, e.g., the major histocompatibility complex, are much more potent than others in provoking an immune response. This major histocompatibility complex (MHC) is referred to as the HLA system. The body's immune system usually exercises tolerance to self-antigens, but in some situations antibodies may be produced in response to normal self-antigens. Antigens are usually large organic molecules that are either proteins or polysaccharides and rarely, if ever, lipids. In order to function as effective antigens, several factors are important: foreignness, degradability, molecular weight, structural stability, and complexity. Although large foreign molecules are better antigens, haptens, which are very small molecules, can bind to larger carrier molecules and behave as antigens.

Agglutination of particles to which soluble antigen has been absorbed produces a serum method of demonstrating precipitins. Examples of artificial carriers include latex particles and colloidal charcoal. Antibodies are specific glycoproteins referred to as immunoglobulins. Many antibodies can be isolated in the gamma globulin fraction of protein by electrophoresis separation. The term *immunoglobulin* (Ig), however, has replaced *gamma globulin* because not all antibodies have gamma electrophoretic mobility.

Antibodies can be found in blood plasma and many body fluids such as tears, saliva, and milk. The primary function of an antibody in body defenses is to combine with antigen, which may be enough to neutralize bacterial toxins or some viruses. A secondary interaction of an antibody molecule with another effector agent, such as complement, is usually required to dispose of larger antigens, such as bacteria.

Five distinct classes of immunoglobulin molecules are recognized in most higher mammals: IgM, IgG, IgA, IgD, and IgE. These immunoglobulin classes differ from each other in characteristics such as molecular weight, sedimentation, coefficient, and carbohydrate content. Antibodies exhibit diversity among the different classes, which sug-

gests that they perform different functions in addition to their primary function of antigen binding. Each immunoglobulin molecule is essentially bifunctional: one region of the molecule is concerned with binding to antigen while a different region mediates binding of the immunoglobulin to host tissues, including cells of the immune system and the first component (C1q) of the classic complement system.

The primary structure of a protein is based on the sequence of amino acid residues linked by the peptide bond. The basic unit of an antibody structure is the homology unit or domain, of which a typical molecule has 12, arranged in two heavy and two light (H and L) chains, linked through cysteine residues by disulfide bonds so that the domains lie in pairs.

Variations between the regions of different antibody molecules are responsible for differences in antigen binding and in biologic function. The antigen-binding portion of the molecule (N-terminal end) shows such heterogeneity that it is known as the variable region; the remainder is relatively constant, but some heterogeneity in form is observed in classes and subclasses.

A typical monomeric IgG molecule consists of three globular regions (two Fab regions and a Fc portion) linked by a flexible hinge region. If the molecule is digested with a proteolytic enzyme such as papain, it splits into three approximately equal-size fragments. Two of these fragments retain the ability to bind antigen and are called the *antigen-binding* (Fab) *fragments*. The third fragment, which is relatively homogeneous and sometimes crystallizable, is called the Fc portion.

An antigenic determinant is the specific chemical determinant group or molecular configuration against which the immune response is directed. Immunoglobulins themselves can function as very effective antigens when used to immunize mammals of a different species because they are proteins. When the resulting antiimmunoglobulins or antiglobulins are analyzed, three principal categories of antigenic determinants can be recognized: isotype, allotype, and idiotype determinants.

Production of antibodies is induced when the host's immune system comes into contact with a foreign antigenic substance and reacts to this antigenic stimulation. When an antigen is initially encountered, the cells of the immune system recognize the antigen as nonself and either elicit an immune response or become tolerant to it, depending on the circumstances. An immune reaction can take the form of cell-mediated immunity (immunity dependent on T cells and macrophages) or involve the production of antibodies directed against the antigen.

Following a foreign antigen challenge, an IgM antibody response proceeds in four phases, but the actual time period and titer depend on the characteristics of the antigen and the individual. The four phases are the lag, log, plateau, and decline. Subsequent exposure to the same antigenic stimulus produces an antibody response that exhibits the same four phases as the primary responses.

Repeated exposure to an antigen can take place many years after the initial exposure, but clones of the T memory cells will be stimulated to proliferate with subsequent production of antibody by the individual. An anamnestic response, however, differs from a primary response in several important aspects. These differences are time, type of antibody produced, and the titer of antibody.

The ability of a particular antibody to combine with one antigen instead of another is referred to as its specificity. This property resides in the portion of the Fab molecule called the combining site, a cleft formed largely by the hypervariable regions of heavy and light chains. There is evidence, however, that an antigen may bind to larger, or even separate, parts of the variable region. The closer the fit between this site and the antigen determinant, the stronger will be the noncovalent forces, such as hydrophobic or electrostatic bonds, between them, and the higher the affinity between the antigen and antibody.

Binding depends on a close three-dimensional fit, allowing weak intermolecular forces to overcome the normal repulsion between molecules. When more than one combining site interacts with the same antigen, the bond has greatly increased strength. When some of the determinants of an antigen are shared by similar antigenic determinants on the surface of apparently unrelated molecules, a proportion of the antibodies directed against one kind of antigen will also react with the other kind of antigen. This is called cross-reactivity.

The strength with which a multivalent antibody binds a multivalent antigen is termed *avidity*, in contrast to *affinity*. When a multivalent antigen combines with more than one of an antibody's combining sites, the strength of the bonding is significantly increased. In order for the antigen and antibody to dissociate, all of the antigen-antibody bonds must be broken simultaneously. Decreased avidity can result from an antigen having only one antigenic determinant (monovalent). Additionally, a hapten is monovalent; therefore, it can only react with one antigen combining site.

The noncovalent combination of antigen with its respective, specific antibody is called an immune complex. An immune complex may be of the small (soluble) or large (precipitating) type, depending on the nature and proportion of antigen and antibody. Bonding of antigen to antibody is exclusively noncovalent and may be of several types: hydrophobic bonds, hydrogen bonding, Van der Waals forces, or electrostatic forces.

In vitro tests detect the combination of antigens and antibodies. Tests such as agglutination tests are widely used in immunology to detect and mea-

sure the consequences of antigen-antibody interaction. Other test types include precipitation reactions, hemolysis testing, and inhibition of agglutination. Tests such as the radioimmunoassay (RIA) and enzyme-linked immunoabsorbent assay (ELISA) measure immune complexes formed in an in vitro system.

Antibodies differ in their ability to agglutinate. IgM-type antibodies, sometimes referred to as *complete antibodies*, are considerably more efficient than IgG or IgA antibodies in exhibiting in vitro agglutination when the antigen-bearing erythrocytes are suspended in physiologic (0.85%) sodium chloride. Antibodies that do not exhibit visible agglutination of saline-suspended erythrocytes, even when bound to the cell's surface membrane, are considered to be nonagglutinating antibodies and may be called incomplete antibodies.

Monoclonal antibodies are purified antibodies cloned from a single cell. These antibodies are engineered to bind to a single specific antigen. Monoclonal antibodies bound to cell surface antigens now provide a method for classifying and identifying specific cellular membrane characteristics, such as in the typing of erythrocyte and leukocyte antigens, and as a reagents in the detection of coating of erythrocyte antigens in the anti–human globulin test (AHG) test.

REVIEW QUESTIONS

1. A synonym for an antigenic determinant is:
   A. immunogen
   B. epitope
   C. binding site
   D. polysaccharide
   E. histocompatibility antigen
2. Genetically different individuals are referred to as:
   A. allogenic
   B. heterogenic
   C. autogenic
   D. isogenic
   E. immunogenic
3. Antigenic substances are usually composed of:
   A. carbohydrates
   B. proteins
   C. lipids
   D. glycoproteins
   E. all of the above, except C
4. Which of the following characteristics of an antigen is the least important?
   A. Foreignness
   B. Degradability
   C. Molecular weight
   D. Complexity
   E. The presence of large, repeating polymers
5. The chemical composition of an antibody is:
   A. protein
   B. lipid
   C. carbohydrate
   D. glycolipid
   E. glycoprotein

Questions 6-10. Match the following characteristics with the appropriate antibody subclass (use an answer only once).
6. IgM
7. IgG
8. IgA
9. IgE
10. IgD
    A. the highest in plasma/serum concentration in normal individuals
    B. has the shortest half-life
    C. 19S
    D. can exist as a dimer
    E. has no known subclasses

Questions 11-15. Match the following characteristics with the appropriate antibody.
11. IgG
12. IgM
13. IgA
14. IgD
15. IgE
    A. predominant immunoglobulin in secretions
    B. increased in infectious diseases, collagen disorders, and hematologic disorders
    C. mediates some types of hypersensitivity reactions
    D. primarily a cell-membrane immunoglobulin
    E. produced early in an immune response

Questions 16-18. Match each of the following antigenic determinant terms with its appropriate definition.
16. isotype
17. allotype
18. idiotype
    A. found on the immunoglobulins of some, but not all, animals of a species
    B. dominant type found on immunoglobulins of all animals of a species
    C. individual determinants characteristic of each antibody

Questions 19-24. Arrange the sequence of events of a typical antibody response
19. _ _ _
20. _ _
21. _ _ _
22. _ _ _
    A. plateau
    B. lag phase
    C. log phase
    D. decline
23. Which of the following characteristics is *not* true of an anamnestic response compared to a primary response?
    A. has a shorter lag phase
    B. has a longer plateau
    C. antibodies decline more gradually
    D. IgM antibodies predominate
    E. antibody levels attain a higher titer
24. Which type of antibody is capable of placental transfer?
    A. IgM
    B. IgG
    C. IgA
    D. IgD
    E. IgE

Questions 25-28. Match the following terms and their respective definitions.
25. specificity
26. affinity
27. avidity
28. immune complex
    A. the bond between a single antigenic determinant and an individual combining site
    B. the noncovalent combination of an antigen with its respective specific antibody
    C. the ability of an antibody to combine with one antigen instead of another
    D. the strength with which a multivalent antibody binds to a multivalent antigen
29. Which of the following type(s) of bonding is (are) involved in antigen-antibody reactions?
    A. hydrophobic
    B. hydrogen
    C. Van der Waals
    D. electrostatic
    E. all of the above
30. Monovalent antibodies may also be referred to as:
    A. complete antibodies
    B. incomplete antibodies
31. Which of the following is an accurate statement about monoclonal antibodies? Monoclonal antibodies are:
    A. antibodies engineered to bind to a single specific cell
    B. purified antibodies that are cloned from a single cell
    C. used to classify and identify specific cellular membrane characteristics
    D. derived from a single hybridoma clone of cells
    E. all of the above

Answers

1. B 2. A 3. E 4. E 5. E 6. C 7. A 8. D 9. B 10. E 11. B 12. E 13. A 14. D 15. C 16. B 17. A 18. C 19. B 20. C 21. A 22. D 23. D 24. B 25. C 26. A 27. D 28. B 29. E 30. B 31. E

BIBLIOGRAPHY

Barrett JT: Textbook of immunology, ed 5, St Louis, 1988, The CV Mosby Co.

Bellanti JA: Immunology: basic processes, Philadelphia, 1979, WB Saunders Co.

McDougal JS and McDuffie FC: Detection and significance of immune complexes, Adv Clin Chem 24:4, 1985.

Ritzmann SE and Daniels JC eds: Serum protein abnormalities, Boston, 1985, Little, Brown & Co.

Ritzmann SE ed: Physiology of immunoglobulins, New York, 1982, Alan R Liss, Inc.

Roitt IM: Essential immunology, ed 5, Oxford, England, 1984, Blackwell Scientific Publications, Inc.

Turgeon ML: Fundamentals of immunohematology, Philadelphia, 1989, Lea & Febiger.

The Cells and Cellular Activities of the Immune System

Granulocytes and Mononuclear Cells

The entire leukocytic cell system is designed to defend the body against disease. Each cell type, however, has a unique function and behaves both independently and, in many cases, in cooperation with other cell types. Leukocytes can be functionally divided into the general categories of granulocyte, monocyte-macrophage and lymphocyte-plasma cell. The primary phagocytic cells are the polymorphonuclear neutrophilic (PMN) leukocytes and the mononuclear monocytes-macrophages. The lymphocytes participate in body defenses primarily through the recognition of foreign antigen and/or production of antibody. Plasma cells are antibody synthesizing cells.

ORIGIN AND DEVELOPMENT OF BLOOD CELLS

Embryonic blood cells, excluding the lymphocyte type of white blood cell, originate from the mesenchymal tissue that arises from the embryonic germ layer, the mesoderm. The sites of blood cell development, *hematopoiesis,* follow a definite sequence in the embryo and fetus:

1. The first blood cells are primitive red blood cells (erythroblasts) formed in the islets of the *yolk sac* during the first 2 to 8 weeks of life.
2. Gradually, the *liver* and *spleen* replace the yolk sac as the sites of blood cell development. By the second month of gestation, the liver becomes the major site of hematopoiesis,

and granular types of leukocytes have made their initial appearance. The liver and spleen predominate from about 2 to 5 months of fetal life.

3. In the fourth month of gestation, the bone marrow begins to function in the production of blood cells. After the fifth fetal month, the bone marrow begins to assume its ultimate role as the primary site of hematopoiesis.

The cellular elements of the blood are produced from a common, multipotential, hematopoietic (blood-producing) cell, the stem cell. Following stem cell differentiation, blast cells arise for each of the major categories of cell types: erythrocytes, megakaryocytes, granulocytes, monocytes-macrophages, lymphocytes, and plasma cells. Subsequent maturation of these cells will produce the major cellular elements of the circulating blood, the erythrocytes, thrombocytes, and specific types of leukocytes. In normal peripheral or circulating blood, the following types of leukocytes can be found in order of frequency: neutrophils, lymphocytes, monocytes, eosinophils, and basophils.

GRANULOCYTIC CELLS

Granulocytic leukocytes can be further subdivided on the basis of morphology into neutrophils, eosinophils, basophils. The neutrophil, basophil, and eosinophil each begin as the multipotential stem cell in the bone marrow. The major role of each of these cells in body defenses is unusual.

Neutrophils

The neutrophilic leukocyte, particularly the neutrophilic polymorphonuclear (PMN) type, provides an effective host defense against bacterial and fungal infections. Although the monocytes-macrophages and other granulocytes are also phagocytic cells, the neutrophil is the principal leukocyte associated with *phagocytosis* (Fig. 3-1) and a localized inflammatory response. The formation of an inflammatory exudate (pus), which develops rapidly in an inflammatory response, is primarily composed of neutrophils and monocytes.

Mature neutrophils are found in two, evenly divided pools, the circulating and the marginating pool. The marginating granulocytes adhere to the vascular endothelium. In the peripheral blood, these cells are only in transit to their potential sites of action in the tissues. The movement of granulocytes from the circulating pool to the peripheral tissues occurs by a process called *diapedesis* (movement through the vessel wall). Once in the peripheral tissues, the neutrophils are able to carry out their function of phagocytosis.

The granules of segmented neutrophils contain various antibacterial substances including lysosomal hydrolases, lysozyme, and peroxidase. Some of these granules are typical lysosomes. During the phagocytic process, however, the powerful antimicrobial enzymes that are released also disrupt the integrity of the cell itself. Neutrophils are also steadily lost to the respiratory, gastrointestinal, and urinary systems, where they participate in generalized phagocytic activities. An alternate route for the removal of neutrophils from the circulation is phagocytosis by cells of the mononuclear-phagocytic system.

Signs and Symptoms of Abnormal Neutrophil Function

The importance of the neutrophil to body defenses is illustrated by the fact that patients with quantitative or qualitative defects of neutrophils have a high rate of infection. Individuals having a marked decrease of neutrophils (neutropenia) or severe defects in neutrophil function frequently suffer from recurrent systemic bacterial infections, such as pneumonia, disseminated cutaneous pyogenic lesions, and other types of life-threatening bacterial and fungal infections.

Leukocyte mobility may be impaired in diseases such as rheumatoid arthritis, cirrhosis of the liver and *chronic granulomatous disease.* Defective locomotion or leukocyte immobility can also be seen in patients receiving steroids and in those with *lazy leukocyte syndrome.* A marked defect in the cellular response to chemotaxis, an important step in phagocytosis, can be seen in patients suffering from *diabetes mellitus, Chediak-Higashi anomaly,* sepsis, and in those with high levels of antibody IgE, such as in *Job's syndrome.*

Congenital Abnormalities of Neutrophil Structure and Function

A small number of patients have congenital abnormalities (see box below) of neutrophil structure and function.

Chediak-Higashi Syndrome

The Chediak-Higashi syndrome represents a qualitative disorder of neutrophils. It is a rare familial disorder inherited as an autosomal recessive trait and expressed as an abnormal granulation of neutrophils. Neutrophils having giant granules display impaired chemotaxis and delayed killing of of ingested bacteria.

Chronic Granulomatous Disease (CGD)

The chronic granulomatous diseases are a genetically heterogeneous group of disorders of oxidative metabolism affecting the cascade of events required for hydrogen peroxide production by phagocytes. Multiple types of inheritance of the disorder have been described, including sex-linked (X-chromosome linked) in 66% of cases, an autosomal recessive in 34% of cases, and an autosomal dominant in <1% of cases. Patients with the autosomal recessive form may have a less severe clinical course than patients with the X-linked form.

The onset is during infancy with one third of patients dying before the age of 7 because of infections. In 1966, it was observed that in the presence of normal or elevated leukocyte counts the neutrophilic granulocytes "in vitro" ingested (Fig. 3-2) but only destroyed streptococci, not staphylococci. Subsequent testing revealed that the cells from CGD patients can phagocytize non–hydrogen-peroxide producing bacteria such as *Staphlococcus aureus* and gram-negative rods, the *Enterobacteriaceae,* but they cannot destroy them. In the X-linked form the defective leukocytes fail to exhibit increased anaerobic metabolism during phagocytosis because of a cytochrome b_{558} deficiency (which expresses itself as a defect in the 91,000-dalton glycoprotein membrane anchor of the cytochrome complex), or produce hydrogen peroxide as the result of a deficiency of the enzyme, myeloperoxidase.

Patients with this abnormality suffer from infections with catalase-positive bacteria and fungi affecting the skin, lungs, liver, and bones. They also develop granuloma resulting from a lack of resolution of inflammatory foci even after the infection has been eliminated. This leads to extensive granuloma formation and, in some circumstances, im-

---

Congenital Abnormalities of Neutrophil Structure and Function

> Chediak-Higashi syndrome
> Chronic granulomatous disease
> CR 3 (iC3b receptor) deficiency
> Myeloperoxidase deficiency
> Specific granule deficiency

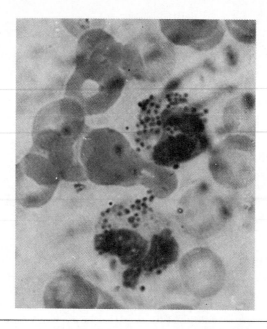

FIGURE 3-1

The two phagocytic cells have engulfed numerous *Staphylococcus aureus* cells.
(From Barrett JT: Textbook of immunology, ed 5, St. Louis, 1988, The CV Mosby Co.)

pairment of physiologic processes, such as obstruction of the esophagus or urinary tract.

The Nitroblue Tetrazolium (NBT) test (described at the end of the chapter) is useful in the diagnosis of this disorder. Defective neutrophils demonstrate no spontaneous reduction of the NBT dye. In normal individuals, NBT is precipitated as a dark blue salt in the neutrophils during the process of phagocytosis. The neutrophils from patients with CGD fail to produce a color change.

CR3 (iC3b Receptor) Deficiency

The CR3 disorder is a rare condition inherited as an autosomal recessive trait on chromosome 21. There is an absence of deficiency of the cell-surface glycoproteins CR3, LFA-1 and p150,95. This deficiency affects the adherence-related functions of neutrophils, monocytes, and lymphocytes.

A CR3 deficiency in neutrophils is associated with marked abnormalities of adherence-related functions, including decreased aggregation of neutrophils to each other after activation, decreased adherence of neutrophils to endothelial cells, poor adherence and phagocytosis of opsonized microorganisms, defective spreading, and decreased diapedesis and chemotaxis. Patients with this disorder may also lack an intravascular marginating pool of neutrophils. Defects in T-lymphocytes are characterized by faulty lymphocyte-mediated cytotoxicity with poor adherence to target cells. Abnormalities of B lymphocytes have also been observed.

Clinically, a deficiency can manifest itself by delayed separation of the umbilical cord. Other signs and symptoms include the early onset of bacterial infections, including skin infections, mucositis, otitis, gingivitis, and periodontitis. A depressed inflammatory response and neutrophilia can be observed.

Myeloperoxidase Deficiency

A deficiency of myeloperoxidase is inherited as an autosomal recessive trait on chromosome 17. Myeloperoxidase is an iron-containing heme protein responsible for the peroxidase activity characteristic of azurophilic granules and accounts for the greenish color of pus. Human neutrophils contain many granules of various sizes that are morphologically, biochemically, and functionally distinct. The azurophilic granules normally contain myeloperoxidase. In this disorder azurophilic granules are present but myeloperoxidase is decreased or absent. If phagocytes are deficient in myeloperoxidase, the patient's phagocytes manifest a mild-to-moderate defect in bacterial killing and a marked defect in fungal killing in vitro.

Persons with a myeloperoxidase deficiency are generally healthy and do not have an increased frequency of infection. The absence of increased susceptibility to infection is probably because other microbicidal mechanisms compensate for the deficiency. Patient with diabetes and myeloperoxidase deficiency, however, may have deep fungal infections caused by *Candida* species.

Specific Granule Deficiency

Specific granule deficiency is believed to be an autosomal recessive disease. It is caused by a fail-

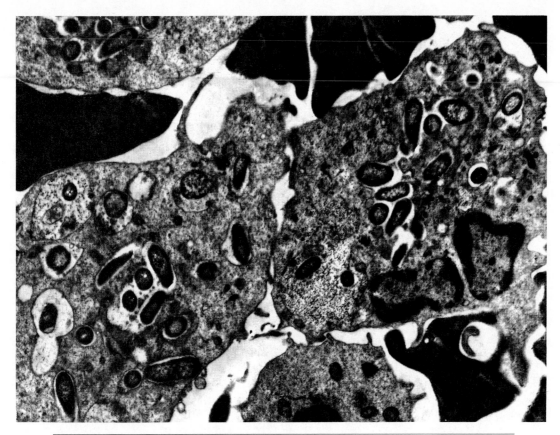

FIGURE 3-2
Undigested bacteria are numerous within the phagosomes of these phagocytes taken from a patient with chronic Granulomatomous disease.
(From Barrett JT: Textbook of immunology, ed 5, St. Louis, 1988, The CV Mosby Co.)

ure to synthesize specific granules and some contents of other granules during differentiation of neutrophils in the bone marrow. Persons with specific granule deficiency suffer from recurrent, severe bacterial infections of the skin and deep tissues. A depressed inflammatory response is also manifested.

Eosinophils and Basophils

Although eosinophils and basophils are capable of participating in phagocytosis, they possess less phagocytic activity. The ineffectiveness of these cells results from both the small number of cells in the circulating blood and the lack of powerful digestive enzymes. Both the eosinophils and basophils, however, are functionally important in body defense.

Eosinophils

The eosinophil is considered to be a homeostatic regulator of inflammation. Functionally, this means that the eosinophil attempts to suppress an inflammatory reaction to prevent the excessive spread of the inflammation. The eosinophil may also play a role in the host defense mechanism because of its ability to kill certain parasites.

A functional property related to the membrane receptors of the eosinophil is the ability of the cell to interact with the larval stages of some helminth parasites and to damage them by way of oxidative mechanisms. Certain proteins released from eosinophilic granules damage antibody-coated Schistosoma parasites and may account for damage to endothelial cells in hypereosinophilic syndromes.

Basophils

Basophils have high concentrations of heparin and histamine in their granules, which play an important role in acute, systemic, hypersensitivity reactions (see Chapter 23). Degranulation (Fig. 3-3) occurs when an antigen, such as pollen, binds to two adjacent IgE antibody molecules located on the surface of mast cells. The events resulting from the release of the contents of these basophilic granules include increased vascular permeability, smooth muscle spasm, and vasodilation. If this reaction is severe, it can result in anaphylactic shock.

A newly identified class of compounds, the leukotrienes, mediate the inflammatory functions of leukocytes. The observed systemic reactions related to this compound were previously attributed to the slow reacting substance of anaphylaxis (SRS-A).

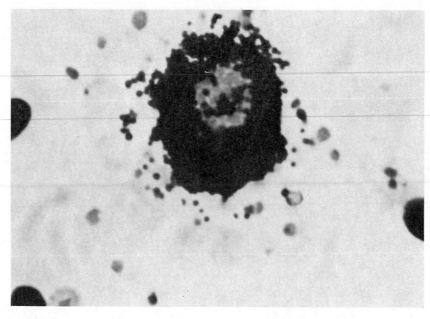

FIGURE 3-3

A mast cell that has begun to discharge its granules. The light area in the center of the cell, partially shielded by granules, is the nucleus.
(From Barrett JT: Textbook of immunology, ed 5, St. Louis, 1988, The CV Mosby Co.)

Monocytes and Macrophages

In the past the mononuclear monocyte-macrophage was known only as a scavenger cell. Only recently has its role as a complex cell of the immune system in the host defense against infection been recognized.

The Mononuclear-Phagocyte System

The macrophage and its precursors are widely distributed throughout the body (Fig. 3-4). These cells are considered to constitute a physiologic system, the *mononuclear-phagocyte system*, which includes promonocytes and their precursors in the bone marrow, monocytes in the circulating blood, and macrophages in tissues. This collection of cells is considered to be a system because of their common origin, similar morphology, and common functions, including rapid phagocytosis mediated by receptors for IgG and the major fragment of the third component of complement, C3.

Macrophages and their known precursor, the monocytes, migrate freely into the tissues from the blood to replenish and reinforce the macrophage population (Fig. 3-5). Macrophages exist as either *fixed* or *wandering* cells. Specialized macrophages, such as the pulmonary alveolar macrophages, are the dust phagocytes of the lung that function as the first line of defense against inhaled foreign particles and bacteria. Fixed macrophages line the endothelium of capillaries and the sinuses of organs such as the bone marrow, spleen and lymph nodes. These cells along with the network of reticular cells of the spleen, thymus, and other lymphoid tissues, comprise the mononuclear-phagocyte system (Fig. 3-6). The term *mononuclear-phagocyte system* should replace the older term, "reticuloendothelial system."

Development of Monocytes-Macrophages

Cells of the macrophage system originate in the bone marrow from the multipotential stem cell. This common, committed progenitor cell can differentiate into either the granulocyte or monocyte-macrophage pathway depending on the microenvironment and chemical regulators. Maturation and differentiation of these cells may be in various directions. Circulating monocytes may continue to have a multipotential and give rise to different types of macrophages.

Functionally, the most important step in the maturation of macrophages is the lymphokine-drive conversion of the normal *resting macrophage* to the *activated macrophage*. Macrophages can be activated during infection by the release of macrophage-activating lymphokines, such as interferon gamma and granulocyte-colony–stimulating factor, from T lymphoycytes specifically sensitized to antigens from the infecting microorganisms. This interaction constitutes the basis of *cell-mediated immunity*. In addition, macrophages exposed to an endotoxin release a hormone, tumor necrosis factor-alpha-cachectin, which can itself activate macrophages under certain in vitro conditions.

The terminal stage of development in the mono-

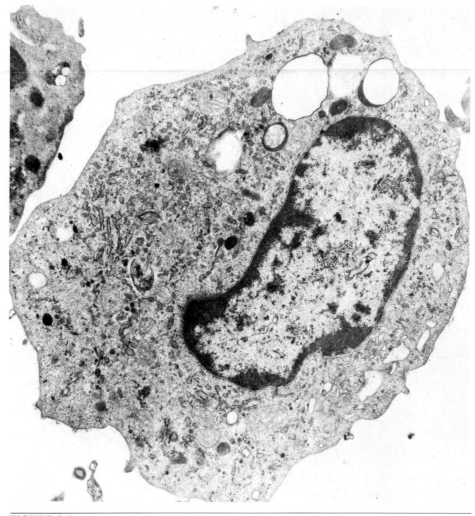

FIGURE 3-4

Electron micrograph of a macrophage.
(From Barrett JT: Textbook of immunology, ed 5, St. Louis, 1988, The CV Mosby Co.)

nuclear-phagocyte cell line is the multinucleated giant cell, which characterizes granulomatous inflammatory diseases such as tuberculosis. Both monocytes and macrophages can be demonstrated in the lesions in these disease before the formation of giant cells; they are thought to be the precursors to the multinucleated cells.

FUNCTIONS OF MONOCYTES-MACROPHAGES IN HOST DEFENSE

Functionally, monocytes-macrophages have phagocytosis as their major role. These cells, however, perform at least three distinct but interrelated functions in host defense. The categories of host defense functions of monocytes-macrophages include:

1. Phagocytosis
2. Antigen presentation and induction of the immune response
3. Secretion of biologically active molecules.

The principal functions of mononuclear phagocytes in body defenses result from the changes that take place in these functions when the macrophage is activated. These changes are presented in the box on p. 41.

Phagocytosis

Macrophages carry out the fundamental function of ingesting and killing invading microorganisms, such as intracellular parasites, *Mycobacterium tuberculosis*, and some fungi. In addition, macrophages also remove and eliminate such extracellular pathogens as pneumococci from the blood circulation. It is also known that the macrophage has the capacity to phagocytize particulate and aggregated soluble materials. This process has shown to be enhanced by the presence of receptors on the surface of the Fc portion of IgG and the C3 complement component. The ability to internalize soluble substances undoubtedly supports the increased microbicidal and tumoricidal ability of activated macrophages. Another important phagocytic function of macrophages is their ability to dispose of dam-

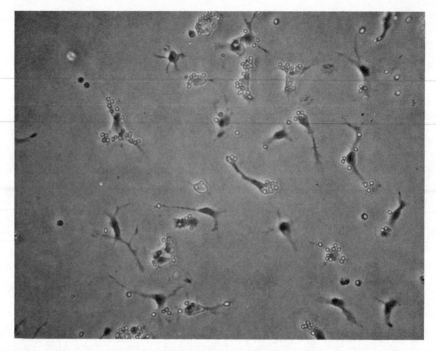

FIGURE 3-5

Macrophages in culture. Note their elongated form, indicative of their motility. The cellular refractile bodies are erythrocytes that the macrophages are phagocytosing.
(From Barrett JT: Textbook of immunology, ed 5, St. Louis, 1988, The CV Mosby Co.)

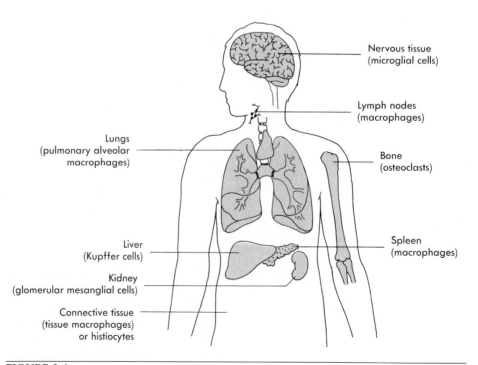

FIGURE 3-6

The mononuclear phagocytic system.
(From Turgeon ML: Clinical hematology: theory and procedures, Boston, 1988, Little, Brown and Co.)

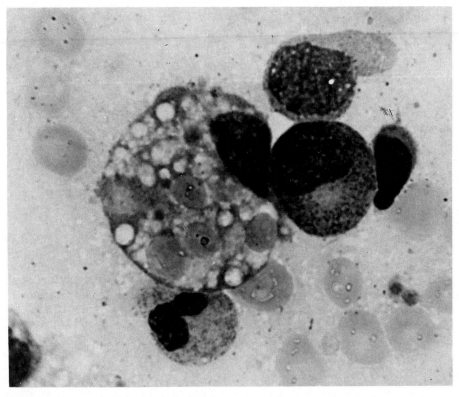

FIGURE 3-7

Bone marrow macrophage showing erythrophagocytosis.
(From Bauer JD: Clinical laboratory methods, ed 9, St. Louis, 1982, The CV Mosby Co.)

Functions of Mononuclear Phagocytes

Increased activity in activated macrophages

Antigen presentation
Chemotaxis
Glucose transport and metabolism
Microbicidal activity
Phagocytosis (variable activity depending on particle)
Phagocytosis-associated respiratory burst
Pinocytosis
Tumoricidal activity

Increased constituents in activated macrophages

Acid hydrolases
Angiogenesis factor
Arginase
Collagenase
Complement components[1]
Cytolytic proteinase

Increased constituents in activated macrophages—cont'd

Fibronectin
Interleukin-1
Interferon (alpha and beta)
Plasminogen activator
Tumor necrosis factor—cachectin[2]

Decreased constituents in activated macrophages

Apolipoprotein E and lipoprotein lipase
Elastase
Prostaglandins, leukotriennes

Constituent demonstrating no change in activated macrophages

Lysoenzyme

[1]Increased or no change
[2]When stimulated
Adapted from Johnston RB: Monocytes and macrophages, New Engl J Med 318(12):749, March 1988.

aged or dying cells (Fig. 3-7). Macrophages lining the sinusoids of the spleen are particularly important in ingesting aging erythryocytes. They are also involved in removing tissue debris and repairing wounds, and in removing debris as embryonic tissues replace one another.

Phagocytic activity increases when there is tissue damage and inflammation, which releases substances that attract macrophages. Activated macrophages migrate more vigorously in response to chemotactic factors and should enter sites of inflammation, e.g., locations of infection or cancer, more efficiently than resting macrophages. Migration of monocytes into different body tissues appears to be a random phenomenon in the absence of localized inflammation. An essential factor in the protective function of monocytes is the capacity of the cell to move through the endothelial wall of blood vessels (diapedesis) to the site of microbial invasion in tissues. The attracting forces, chemotactic factors, for monocytes include complement products and chemoattractants derived from neutrophils, lymphocytes, or cancer cells.

The activity of mononuclear phagocytes against cancer cells in humans is less well understood than the phagocytosing of microorganisms. Phagocytes are thought to suppress the growth of spontaneously arising tumors. The ability of these cells to control malignant cells may not involve phagocytosis, but it may be related to secreted cellular products, such as lysosomal enzymes, oxygen metabolites, e.g., hydrogen peroxide; proteinases, and tumor necrosis factor-cachectin. The proteolytic enzymes present on the surface membrane of monocytes could also have a role in tumor rejection.

Antigen Presentation and Induction of the Immune Response

The phagocytic property of the macrophage is particularly important in the processing of antigens as part of the immune response. Macrophages are believed to process antigens and physically present this biochemically modified and more reactive form of antigen to lymphocytes (particularly T-helper cells) as an initial step in the immune response. Recognition of antigen on the macrophage surface by T-lymphocytes, however, requires an additional match of the surface class II gene product of the major histocompatibility complex. This gene product is the Ia product in the mouse and D gene region product in humans. With proper recognition, the macrophage secretes a lymphocyte-activating factor (interleukin-1), lymphocyte proliferation ensues, and the immune response (T- and/or B-cell response) is facilitated.

Secretion of Biologically Active Molecules

It has recently been discovered that monocytes-macrophages release many factors associated with host defense and inflammation. In this role, these cells serve as supportive "accessory" cells to lymphocytes, at least partly by releasing soluble factors. In cellular immunity, monocytes assume a "killer role" in that they are activated by sensitized lymphocytes to phagocytize offending cells or antigen particles. This is important in fields such as tumor immunology.

In addition to their phagocytic properties, monocytes-macrophages are able to synthesize a number of biologically important compounds, including transferrin, complement, interferon, pyrogens, and certain growth factors. Approximately 100 distinct substances have been identified as being secreted by monocytes-macrophages.

Blood monocytes and tissue macrophages are primary sources of the polypeptide hormones termed *interleukin-1 (IL-1)*, which have a particularly potent effect on the inflammatory response. Interleukin-1 also supports B-lymphocyte proliferation and antibody production, as well as T-lymphocyte production of lymphokines. The increased synthesis of interleukin-1 by activated macrophages could contribute to enhancement of the immune response. Endotoxin also induces the synthesis of interleukin-1. This effect is achieved at least partly by stimulation of the macrophages to release tumor necrosis factor-cachectin, which then stimulates the production of interleukin-1 by endothelial cells and macrophages. Activated macrophages release much more tumor necrosis factor-cachectin than do resting macrophages that are exposed to endotoxin. Both tumor necrosis factor-cachectin and interleukin-1 can induce the fever and synthesis of acute-phase reactants (discussed later in this chapter) that characterize inflammation.

Monocyte-Macrophage Disorders

Monocyte-macrophage has been demonstrated to be abnormal in a variety of diseases (Table 3-1). The abnormality is partial, and no related association with increased susceptibility to infection has been established. In cases of severely depressed migration of monocytes, however, it is likely that this dysfunction predisposes a patient to infection because other defects of host defense coexist in these disorders.

The signs and symptoms of abnormalities of monocyte-macrophage function are extremely evident in some conditions. The profound defect of phagocytic killing exhibited by patients with CGD results in the formation of subcutaneous abscesses and abscesses in the liver, lungs, spleen, and lymph nodes. Cancer patients with a defective monocyte cytotoxicity may develop this defect because tumors have the ability to release factors that suppress the generation of toxic oxygen metabolites by macrophages. In newborn infants depressed chemotaxis and killing, and decreased synthesis of the phagocytosis-promoting factors fibronectin, C3, and complement factor B have been observed. In addition, the newborn infant's macrophages may not respond effectively to infection because his/her lymphocytes have impaired the production of the macrophage activator interferon gamma.

Qualitative disorders of monocytes-macrophages

TABLE 3-1

Primary and Secondary Abnormalities
of Monocyte-Macrophage Function

Abnormality	Condition
Defect in phagocytic killing	Chronic granulomatous disease (CGD); corticosteroid therapy; newborn infants; viral infections
Defective monocyte cytotoxicity	Cancer; Wiskott-Aldrich syndrome
Defective release of macrophage-activating factors	Acquired immunodeficiency syndrome (AIDS); intracellular infections, e.g., lepromatous leprosy, tuberculosis, visceral leishmaniasis
Depressed migration	Acquired immunodeficiency syndrome (AIDS); burns; diabetes; immunosuppressive therapy; Newborn infants
Impaired phagocytosis	Congenital deficiency of CD11-CD18; monocytic leukemia; systemic lupus erythematosus (SLE)

reflect themselves as lipid storage diseases including a number of rare autosomal recessive disorders. In these conditions the expression in macrophages of a systemic enzymatic defect permits the accumulation of cell debris normally cleared by macrophages. The macrophages are particularly prone to accumulate undegraded lipid products. Resistance to infection can be impaired, at least partially, because of an impairment in macrophage function. Disorders of this type include *Gaucher's disease* and *Niemann-Pick disease.*

Gaucher's disease. Gaucher's disease is an inherited disease caused by a disturbance in cellular lipid metabolism. It is most frequently discovered in children, and the prognosis varies from patient to patient. If the disease is mild, the patient may live a relatively normal life. If the disease is severe, the patient may die prematurely.

The disorder represents a deficiency of beta-glucocerebrosidase, the enzyme that normally splits glucose from its parent sphingolipid, glucosylceramide. As the result of this enzyme deficiency, cerebroside accumulates in histiocytes (macrophages). Gaucher's cells are rarely found in the circulating blood. The typical Gaucher cell is large with one to three eccentric nuclei and a characteristically wrinkled cytoplasm. These cells are found in the bone marrow, spleen, and other organs of the mononuclear-phagocyte system. Production of erythrocytes and leukocytes decreases as these abnormal cells infiltrate into the bone marrow.

Niemann-Pick disease. Niemann-Pick disease is similar to Gaucher's disease because it is also an inherited abnormality of lipid metabolism. Niemann-Pick disease afflicts infants and children

with the average patient's life expectancy being 5 years.

This disorder represents a rare autosomal recessive deficiency of the enzyme sphingomyelinase. It is characterized by massive accumulation of sphingomyelin in the mononuclear phagocytes. The characteristic cell in this disorder, Pick's cell, is similar in appearance to Gaucher's cell; however, the cytoplasm of the cell is foamy in appearance.

Phagocytosis and Acute Inflammation

Tissue damage results in inflammation, a series of biochemical and cellular changes that facilitate the phagocytosis of invading microorganisms or damaged cells. If inflammation is sufficiently extensive, it is accompanied by an increase in the plasma concentration of acute phase reactants. Because acute phase protein changes are sensitive indicators of the presence of inflammatory disease, they are especially useful in monitoring such conditions. They are less valuable, however, as a diagnostic tool.

The Process of Phagocytosis

Phagocytosis (methodology is described at the end of the chapter) can be divided into several stages (Fig. 3-8): the movement of cells, engulfment, and digestion. If bacteria are not effectively immobilized, subsequent phagocytic activity may take place.

Initiation. The physical occurrence of damage to tissues, either by trauma or because of microbial multiplication, releases substances, such as activated complement components and/or the products of infection. This leads to an increase in the chemoattractants, C5a, formyl-methionyl-leucyl-phenlyalanine, and LTB_4, which activate phagocytic cells as well as promote diapedesis and chemotaxis. The activated phagocyte has an increase in surface receptors (CR3, formyl-methionyl-leucyl-phenylalanine receptors, and laminim receptors), which promotes adherence.

Movement of cells. The various phagocytic cells continually circulate throughout the blood, lymph, gastrointestinal system, and respiratory tract. When trauma occurs, the neutrophils arrive at the site of injury and can be found in the beginning exudate in less than 1 hour. Monocytes are slower in moving to the inflammatory site.

Segmented neutrophils are able to gather at the site of injury quickly because they are actively motile. The marginating pool of neutrophils, adhering to the endothelial lining of nearby blood vessels, migrates through the vessel wall to the interstitial tissues. This ameboid movement is called *diapedesis.* Cells are guided to the site of injury by the chemoattractant substances. This event is termed *chemotaxis.*

Engulfment. After the phagocytic cells have arrived at the site of injury, the bacteria can be engulfed through active membrane invagination. Phagocytosis is mediated predominantly by Fc receptors and CR3. It is important to realize that

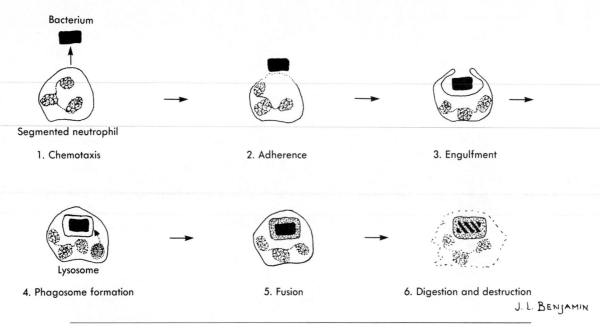

Bacterium

Segmented neutrophil

1. Chemotaxis

2. Adherence

3. Engulfment

Lysosome

4. Phagosome formation

5. Fusion

6. Digestion and destruction

J. L. BENJAMIN

FIGURE 3-8

The process of phagocytosis.
(From Turgeon ML: Clinical hematology: theory and procedures, Boston, 1988, Little, Brown and Co.)

phagocytosis is an active process requiring a large expenditure of cell energy. The required energy is primarily provided by anaerobic glycolysis.

However, the principal factor in determining whether or not phagocytosis can occur is the physical nature of the surface of both the bacteria and the phagocytic cell. The bacteria must be more hydrophobic than the phagocyte. Some bacteria, such as *Diplococcus pneumoniae*, possess a hydrophilic capsule and are not normally phagocytized. Most nonpathogenic bacteria are easily phagocytized because they are very hydrophobic. The presence of certain soluble factors such as complement, a plasma protein, coupled with antibodies, and chemicals, such as acetylcholine, enhance the phagocytic process. Enhancement of phagocytosis through the process of opsonization, the coating of a particle with certain plasma factors, can speed up the ingestion of particles. If the surface tensions are conducive to engulfment, the phagocytic cell membrane invaginates. This invagination leads to the formation of an isolated vacuole, a *phagosome*, within the cell.

Digestion. Digestion follows ingestion of particles with the required energy being primarily provided by anaerobic glycolysis. The vacuole formed during the engulfment process fuses with one or more lysosomal granules that contain various lytic enzymes. Degranulation of the neutrophil (Fig. 3-9) releases substances from the granules of neutrophils with antibacterial substances such as lactoferrin, lyso-zyme, defensins, and bactericidal-permeability–increasing protein. Elastase, which is one of several substances that can damage host tissues, is also released. The myeloperoxidase granules are responsible for the action of the oxygen-dependent, myeloperoxidase-mediated system. Hydrogen peroxide and an oxidizable cofactor serve as major factors in the actual killing of bacteria within the vacuole. Other oxygen-independent systems such as alterations in pH, lysozymes, lactoferrin, and the granular cationic proteins also participate in the bactericidal process. Monocytes are particularly effective as phagocytic cells because of the large amounts of lipase in their cytoplasm. Lipase is able to attack those bacteria, such as *Mycobacterium tuberculosis*, with a lipid capsule. Monocytes are further able to bind and destroy cells coated with onocomplement-fixing antibodies because of the presence of membrane receptors for specific components or types of immunoglobulin.

As the result of the release of lytic enzymes, the neutrophils die and are in turn phagocytized by macrophages. Macrophage digestion proceeds without risk to the cell unless the ingested material is toxic. However, if the ingested material damages the lysosomal membrane, the macrophage will also be destoyed because of the release of lysosomal enzymes.

Subsequent phagocytic activity. If invading bacteria are not phagocytized at entry into the body, they may establish themselves in secondary sites, such as the lymph nodes or various body organs. These undigested bacteria produce a secondary inflammation where neutrophils and macrophages again congregate. If bacteria escape from secondary tissue sites, a bacteremia will develop. In patients who are unresponsive to antibiotic intervention, this situation can prove fatal.

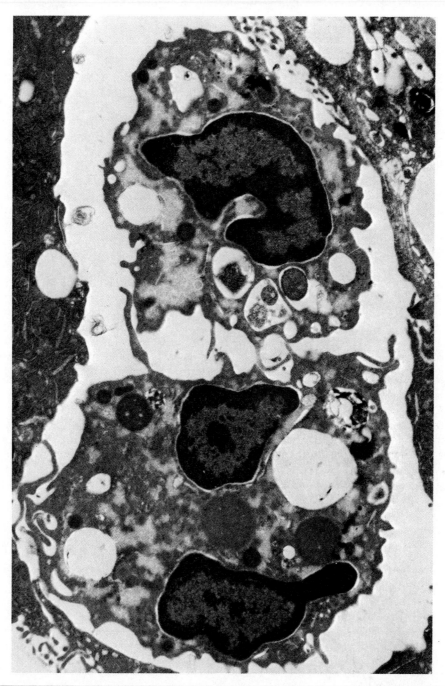

FIGURE 3-9

Two neutrophils seen in an electron-microscopic photograph have depleted their cytoplasmic granules during phagocytosis. The upper cell contains bacteria at different levels of destruction in the phagolysosomes just below its nucleus.

(From Barrett JT: Textbook of immunology, ed 5, St. Louis, 1988, The CV Mosby Co.)

Neutrophils as Mediators of Noninfectious Inflammatory Diseases

Although neutrophils provide the major means of defense against bacterial and fungal infections, they can also be destructive to host tissues. The same oxidative and nonoxidative processes that destroy microorganisms can affect adjacent host tissues. The accumulation of neutrophilic infiltrates and the side effects of phagocytosis can be important as the cause of tissue destruction in a number of noninfectious disease processes (see box below).

ACUTE PHASE PROTEINS
An Overview of Acute Phase Proteins (Reactants)

Plasma concentrations of a group of glycoproteins known as acute phase reactants increase as a specific adaptive response to inflammation. Acute tissue damage and inflammation often result in an initial decrease in the concentration of acute phase proteins, possibly resulting from a loss of protein from the vascular space, followed by an increase. Twenty plasma proteins show acute phase behavior

and most have a definable role in inflammation (see box below). They include inflammatory mediators such as complement proteins (see Chapter 5) and clotting factors, transport proteins such as haptoglobin, and inhibitors such as alpha$_1$-antitrypsin. Acute phase reactants (Table 3-2) constitute the majority of the serum glycoproteins.

Synthesis and Catabolism of Acute Phase Proteins

All of the acute phase proteins are synthesized rapidly in response to tissue injury; however, C-reactive protein (CRP) is synthesized by hepatocytes and is probably under the influence of humoral mediators such as endogenous pyrogen. The rate of change and peak concentration of separate acute phase reactants varies with the component as well as in different clinical situations. In acute inflammation, for example, CRP and alpha$_1$-antichymotrypsin levels become elevated within the first 12 hours. The complement components, C3 and C4, and ceruloplasmin do not rise for some days.

Acute phase proteins do not always change in parallel. This dysynchrony is most commonly due to increased catabolism and elimination from the circulation of certain proteins. Differences may also be caused by discrepancies in rates of synthesis. Most acute phase proteins have half-lives of 2 to 4 days but CRP has a half-life of 5 to 7 hours. For this reason, CRP falls much more rapidly than the other acute phase proteins when the patient recovers.

Noninfectious Diseases in which Signs, Symptoms, and Injury may be Partly Mediated by Neutrophils

> Autoimmune arthritides
> Autoimmune vasculitis
> Dermatopathic disorders
>> Autoimmune bullous dermatoses
>> Behcet's disease
>> Psoriasiform dermatoses
>> Pyoderma gangrenosum
>> Sweet's syndrome
> Glomerulonephritis
> Gout
> Inflammatory bowel disease
> Malignant neoplasms at the site of chronic inflammation
> Myocardial infarction
> Respiratory disorders
>> Adult respiratory distress syndrome (ARDS)
>> Asthma and allergic asthma
>> Emphysema

Major Applications of Acute Phase Protein Measurements

> Monitoring the progress of diagnosed disease activity
> Assessing response to therapy in inflammatory diseases, e.g., rheumatoid arthritis, juvenile chronic arthritis, ankylosing spondylitis, Reiter's syndrome, psoriatic arthropathy, vasculitis, and rheumatic fever
> Detection of complications of a known disease, e.g., immune complex deposition, postsurgical infection

---

TABLE 3-2

Examples of Clinically Useful Acute Phase Proteins

Protein	Normal concentration (g/L)	Concentration in acute inflammation (g/L)	Response time (hours)
C-reactive protein	0.0008-0.004	0.4	6-10
Alpha$_1$-antichymotrypsin	0.3-0.6	3.0	10
Alpha$_1$-antitrypsin	2.0-4.0	7.0	24
Orosomucoid	0.5-1.4	3.0	24
Haptoglobin	1.0-3.0	6.0	24
Fibrinogen	2.0-4.5	10	24
C3	0.55-1.2	3.0	48-72
C4	0.2-0.5	1.0	48-72
Ceruloplasmin	0.15-0.6	2.0	48-72

C-Reactive Protein

Because CRP demonstrates a large incremental change, with as much as a 100-fold increase in concentration in acute inflammation, and is the fastest responding and most sensitive indicator of acute inflammation, it is the method of choice for screening for inflammatory and malignant organic diseases and in monitoring therapy in inflammatory diseases. Elevations of CRP occur in nearly 70 disease states, including bacterial infections, viral infections, myocardial infarction, malignant tumors, and rheumatic disease. This lack of specificity rules out CRP as a definitive diagnostic tool.

The CRP test (procedure described later in this chapter) has been widely used to detect infection in circumstances where microbial diagnosis is difficult. These conditions include septicemia and meningitis in neonates, infections in immunosuppressed patients, burns complicated by infection, and serious postoperative infections, such as subphrenic abscess or septicemia following major surgery. CRP levels rise following the tissue injury or surgery. In uncomplicated cases the level of CRP peaks about 2 days postoperatively and gradually returns to normal levels within 7 to 10 days. If the CRP level is persistently elevated or returns to an increased level, it can be suggestive of underlying sepsis preceding clinical signs and symptoms and should alert the clinician to postoperative complications.

In rheumatoid arthritis, CRP reflects both short- and long-term disease activity. Monitoring of CRP levels allows for early prediction of response to a particular drug—often several months before clinical and radiologic confirmation is possible. In disorders such as rheumatoid arthritis, CRP can be used to assess the effect of antiinflammatory drugs, e.g., aspirin, and the nature of their action. Aspirin-like drugs do not suppress acute phase proteins in inflammation. This permits a patient to have optimal therapy in the shortest possible time and minimizes ongoing inflammation and joint damage. Assessment of CRP is also valuable in monitoring therapy and disease activity in other arthritides, such as Still's disease, ankylosing spondylitis, Reiter's syndrome, and psoriatic arthropathy. In addition, CRP assessment has been found to enhance the value of traditional enzyme measurements in myocardial infarction. Rheumatic fever and Crohn's disease can also be monitored by CRP.

Evaluation of tissue damage resulting from inflammation can include tests such as the CRP. This procedure detects the presence of a liver-derived serum protein which is normally undetectable. In inflammatory reactions, however, the levels of CRP parallel the course of the inflammatory response and return to lower undetectable levels as the inflammation subsides. The advantages of assessing CRP are that it rises rapidly and it is reliable. The CRP increases faster than ESR in responding to inflammation, while the leukocyte count may remain within normal limits despite infection. An elevated CRP can signal infection many hours before it can be confirmed by culture results; therefore, treatment can be prompt.

In a number of chronic inflammatory diseases, however, CRP is an unreliable indicator. CRP values may be normal when other acute phase proteins are altered in disorders such as systemic lupus erythematosus (SLE), dermatomyositis, and ulcerative colitis. SLE shows little or no CRP response despite apparently active inflammation, but this condition does demonstrate a CRP response to intercurrent infection.

In general, the CRP is advocated as an indicator of bacterial infection in at-risk patients in whom the clinical assessment of infection is difficult to make. It is also helpful in differentiating viral from bacterial meningitis. Quantitative assays of CRP can detect progressive elevations of this serum protein.

❏ CASE STUDY

SIGNS AND SYMPTOMS. A 39-year-old female was admitted for a cholecystectomy (Fig. 3-10). She had a history of chronic cholecysitis; recent x-ray studies revealed a large stone in the biliary duct. During surgery, a large stone was removed from the duct and a cholangiogram was taken in the operating room. It showed no further obstructions of the hepatic or common bile ducts.

The patient became febrile one day after surgery. A 48-hour postoperative complete blood count (CBC) and C-reactive protein (CRP) were ordered. On the seventh postoperative day, she had abdominal pain and began vomiting. A CBC, erythrocyte sedimentation rate (ESR), CRP, and blood culture were ordered at that time. The patient was started on a broad-spectrum antibiotic. She was discharged on the thirteenth hospital day.

LABORATORY DATA. At 48 hours postoperatively, the CBC was within normal limits and the CRP was 11 g/L. A repeat CRP on the sixth day postoperative was 7 g/L.

The results following the episode of abdominal pain demonstrated a normal CBC and ESR and a CRP value of 15 g/L. The blood culture was positive for *Pseudomonas sp.*

QUESTIONS

1. Which test was the most rapid and sensitive indicator of infection?
2. Is the CRP diagnostic?
3. Why was the CRP elevated immediately after surgery?

DISCUSSION

1. The CRP was the most sensitive indicator of infection and was consistent with the patient's febrile state. Neither the white blood count nor the ESR was elevated.
2. No, the CRP is suggestive of inflammation and/or infection, but it is not diagnostic. The growth of *Pseudomonas sp.* in the blood culture was diagnostic of sepsis.
3. The CRP was elevated after surgery because any tissue trauma will cause an elevation. The level of acute phase proteins, such as CRP, should decline within a few days following surgery.

DIAGNOSIS. Postoperative infection

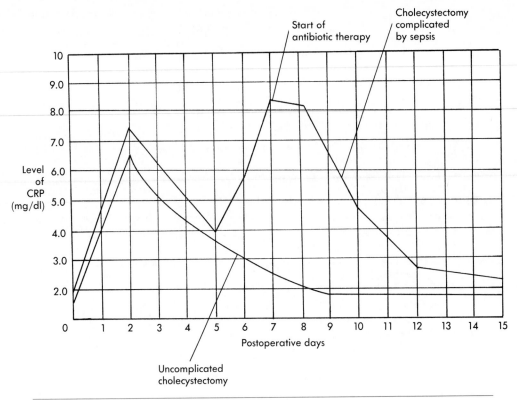

FIGURE 3-10

CRP levels following cholecystectomy.

The Significance of Other Acute Phase Reactants

Alpha$_1$-antitrypsin is an acute phase protein that increases in acute inflammatory reactions. Generalized vasculitis, such as occurs in immune complex disease, may result in inappropriately low levels of alpha$_1$-antitrypsin, probably resulting from increased elimination of complexes with leukocyte lysosomal enzymes.

Defects in the complement components, C3a, C5a, and the opsonin, C3b, result in serious infections. In addition, immune complex disease and gram-negative bacteremia result in low levels of complement components, particularly C3 and C4, because the components are consumed during complement activation. Acute inflammation leads to normal or slightly elevated levels. If both disorders are present, complement consumption may be masked, making it deceptive to use complement measurement as the only index of immune complex deposition in disease. The detection of complement breakdown products is more useful than the measurement of total complement component concentrations. It is more desirable to measure C3 breakdown products than total C3 in conditions such as peritonitis or pancreatitis.

Lymphomas may result in a marked increase in C1 esterase inhibitor with little other change.

Ceruloplasmin, often measured as serum copper, is used to monitor Hodgkin's disease. Increases are considered to be a specific indication of relapse. Although it has not been definitely established, ceruloplasmin monitoring may provide similar information in non-Hodgkin's lymphoma.

NEUTROPHILIC AND ACUTE PHASE REACTANT ASSESSMENT METHODS

Inflammation almost always follows acute tissue damage. Diagnostic categories of acute inflammation can include bacterial causes and nonbacterial causes, such as trauma, chronic inflammation, or viral disease. Many laboratory tests have been advocated for early diagnosis of acute inflammation: total white blood cell count (including the absolute count and the percentage of band and segmented neutrophils as determined by a 100 cell differential count on a peripheral blood smear), acute phase proteins, and the erythrocyte sedimentation rate (ESR).

The ESR, or sedrate, is a nonspecific indicator of disease with increased sedimentation of erythrocytes seen in acute and chronic inflammation and malignancies. Although this procedure is nonspecific, it is one of the most frequently performed laboratory tests.

In addition to these hematologic tests (refer to *Clinical Hematology: Theory and Procedures* for a complete description and the methods of performing these tests) several tests are of direct value in immunologic testing. These procedures include a simple phagocytic cell function test, in which the ability of neutrophils to engulf bacteria can be determined, and the determination of CRP.

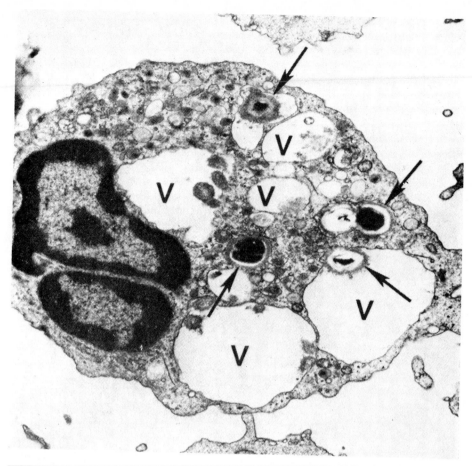

FIGURE 3-11

An electron photomicrograph from a polymorphonuclear leukocyte from a normal control patient incubated with staphlococci for 30 minutes. Many bacteria (see arrows) in various stages of destruction are evident within the cell. Note the cytoplasmic vacuoles (V) around and adjacent to degenerating bacteria.
(From Bauer JD: Clinical laboratory methods, ed 9, St Louis, 1982, The CV Mosby Co.)

❑ PROCEDURE

Screening Test for Phagocytic Engulfment

PRINCIPLE

A mixture of bacteria and phagocytes is incubated and examined for the presence of engulfed bacteria. This simple procedure may be useful in supporting the diagnosis of impaired neutrophilic function in conjunction with clinical signs and symptoms (Fig. 3-11).

SPECIMEN COLLECTION AND PREPARATION

No special preparation of the patient is required before specimen collection. The patient must be positively identified when the specimen is collected. The specimen label should be completed at the bedside and include the patient's full name, the date, the patient's hospital identification number, and the phlebotomist's initials.

Blood should be drawn by an aseptic technique. A minimum of 2 mL of heparin blood (green-top evacuated tube) or 15 to 20 heparinized capillary tubes are required. The specimen should be centrifuged, and the test should be performed promptly.

REAGENTS, SUPPLIES, AND EQUIPMENT

1. Broth culture of *Bacillus subtilis* or *Staphlococcus* coagulase (negative) species
2. Microscope slides
3. Pasteur pipettes and rubber bulb
4. 12 × 75 mm test tubes
5. Wright's stain

QUALITY CONTROL

A fresh, heparinized sample of blood from a healthy volunteer should be tested simultaneously.

PROCEDURE

1. Label two 12 × 75 mm test tubes: patient and control.

2. Add four to eight drops of the buffer coat from either the patient's heparinized blood or the normal control to the respectively labeled test tubes.
3. Add two to three drops of the bacterial broth culture to each tube.
4. Incubate both tubes at room temperature or 37° C for 30 minutes.
5. Place one drop of the incubated specimen on a glass slide and prepare a smear.
6. Air dry the slides and stain with Wright's stain.
   WRIGHT'S STAIN PROCEDURE.
   A. Cover each smear generously with filtered Wright's stain, and allow the stain to remain on the slide for at least 5 minutes.
   B. Slowly add distilled water or buffer to the stain until the buffer begins to overflow the stain. Watch for the appearance of a metallic luster.
   C. Gently blow on the slide to mix the stain and buffer.
   D. Allow the buffer to remain on the slide for at least 5 minutes.
   E. Gently wash the stain and buffer off the slide with distilled water.
   F. Air dry or carefully blot the slide between two sheets of bibulous paper.
7. Place a drop of immersion oil on each smear and examine microscopically with the oil (100X) immersion objective.

REPORTING RESULTS

Positive—demonstration of the engulfment of bacteria
Negative—no engulfment of bacteria

PROCEDURE NOTES

SOURCES OF ERROR. This procedure may produce false negative results if the blood specimen is not fresh or if a coagulase positive *Staphylococcus* specimen is used. It is important to distinguish between granules and cocci. In addition, the bacteria must be intracellular and not extracellular in order for the test to be positive.

CLINICAL APPLICATIONS. The failure of phagocytes to engulf bacteria can support the diagnosis of neutrophilic dysfunction; however, these results must be used in conjunction with patient signs and symptoms.

LIMITATIONS. This is a simple screening procedure for engulfment. The presence of engulfed bacteria does not demonstrate that the bacteria have been destroyed.

☐ PROCEDURE

C-Reactive Protein Rapid Latex Agglutination Test*

PRINCIPLE

The C-reactive protein (CRP) agglutination test is based on the reaction between patient serum containing CRP as the antigen and the corresponding antibody coated to the treated surface of latex particles. The coated particles enhance the detection of an agglutination reaction when antigen is present in the serum being tested. The clinical applications of CRP evaluation include detecting inflammatory diseases, particularly infections. It is also a useful indicator in screening for organic disease, both inflammatory and malignant disease, and in monitoring therapy in inflammatory diseases. Because CRP is more rapidly synthesized than other acute phase proteins, assays of CRP are the measurement of choice in suspected inflammatory conditions.

SPECIMEN COLLECTION AND PREPARATION

No special preparation of the patient is required before specimen collection. The patient must be positively identified when the specimen is collected, and the specimen should be labeled at the bedside. Specimen labels shall include the patient's full name, the date, the patient's hospital identification number, and the phlebotomist's initials.

Blood should be drawn by an aseptic technique. A minimum of 2 mL of clotted blood (red-top evacuated tube) is required. The specimen should be centrifuged promptly and an aliquot of serum removed. Lipemia, hemolysis, or contamination with bacteria renders a specimen unsuitable for testing. Although icteric and turbid specimens have given valid results, fresh non-heat inactivated serum is recommended for use in the test.

If the test cannot be performed immediately, the specimen should be refrigerated (2° to 8° C) for no longer than 72 hours. If additional delay occurs, the serum should be frozen at −18° C or below. Frozen serum should be thawed rapidly at 37° C.

Preliminary specimen preparation. Serum must be at room temperature. Prepare a 1:5 dilution of patient serum by pipetting 0.1 mL of serum into a test tube and adding 0.4 mL of the commercially prepared glycine-saline buffer diluent. Mix the contents thoroughly.

REAGENTS, SUPPLIES AND EQUIPMENT

REAGENTS.
C-RP Latex Reagent with dropper assembly (commercially prepared ICL CRP kit)
One percent suspension of stabilized polystyrene

---

*Adapted from C-Reactive Protein Test (Latex) product insert, ICL Scientific, Fountain Valley, Calif.

latex particles coated with specific antihuman C-RP produced in goats or sheep. **Note:** Store at 2° to 8° C. *Do not freeze C-RP latex reagent.* Properly stored reagent is stable until expiration date indicated on the label. Reagent that does not produce appropriate quality control results should be discarded after verification by repeat testing.

Glycine-saline buffer (pH 8.2 ≤ 0.1) (commercially prepared ICL CRP kit)

Note: Store at 2° to 8° C. Properly stored reagent is stable until expiration date indicated on the label. Reagent that does not produce appropriate quality control results should be discarded after verification by repeat testing. Discard if contaminated, i.e., evidence of cloudiness or particulate material in solution.

Supplies and equipment.

Capillary pipettes (in ICL CRP kit)
Applicator sticks (in ICL CRP kit)
Glass slide (in ICL CRP kit)
Stopwatch or timer
12 × 75 mm test tubes
Serologic pipettes (1 mL graduated) and safety pipetter
Calibrated pipetter (optional)

QUALITY CONTROL

POSITIVE CONTROL SERUM (HUMAN). Prediluted and provided in ICL CRP kit. Store at 2° to 8° C.

Note: Failure to observe a positive reaction with this serum is indicative of deterioration of the latex reagent and/or positive control.

NEGATIVE CONTROL SERUM (HUMAN). Prediluted and provided in ICL CRP kit. Store at 2° to 8° C.

Note: A smooth or slightly granular reaction must be observed with the negative control. If agglutination is exhibited with this control, the test should be repeated. If repeat testing produces the same results, the reagents should be replaced.

A positive and a negative control must be tested with each unknown patient specimen. *Caution:* Because the control sera is derived from human sources, it should be handled in the same manner as clinical serum specimens (see *Universal blood and body fluid precautions* in Chapter 6).

PROCEDURE

Note: All reagents and specimens must be at room temperature before testing.

QUALITATIVE SLIDE TEST.

1. Using one of the capillary pipettes provided in the kit, fill the capillary pipette with undiluted serum to approximately ⅔ of the pipette length. While holding the capillary pipette perpendicular to the slide, deliver one free-falling drop to the center of one of the oval divisions of the slide.

2. Using a clean capillary pipette provided in the kit, fill the capillary pipette with the 1:5 dilution of serum to approximately ⅔ of the pipette length. While holding the capillary pipette perpendicular to the slide, deliver one free-falling drop to the center of one of the oval divisions of the slide.

Note: Capillary pipettes must be held perpendicular to the test slide to deliver correct and consistent amounts of test serum using the free-falling drop method. Do not reuse capillary pipettes or applicator sticks.

If a calibrated pipetter is used instead of a capillary pipette, adjust the pipetter to deliver 0.05 mL (50 uL) of the specimen.

3. Using the squeeze dropper vials provided, add one drop of the prediluted positive control and one drop of the prediluted negative control to separate labeled divisions on the slide.

4. Resuspend the C-RP Latex Reagent by gently mixing until the suspension is homogeneous. Using the dropper provided, add one drop of the C-RP Latex Reagent to each serum specimen and to each control.

5. Using separate applicator sticks, mix each specimen and each control thoroughly. The contents of the mixtures should be spread evenly over the entire area of their respective divisions on the slide.

6. Tilt the slide back and forth, slowly and evenly, for 2 minutes. Place the slide on a flat surface, and observe *immediately* for macroscopic agglutination using a direct light source.

Warning: The latex reagent, controls, and buffer contain 0.1% sodium azide as a preservative. Sodium azide may react with lead and copper plumbing to form highly explosive metal azides. Upon disposal, flush with a large volume of water to prevent azide buildup.

SEMI-QUANTITATIVE SLIDE TEST. If a patient serum exhibits a positive reaction, the serum may be serially diluted with glycine-saline buffer to determine a semi-quantitative estimate of the CRP level. Serial dilutions of the patient serum, beginning with a 1:2 dilution prepared by mixing 0.1 mL of serum and 0.1 mL of glycine-saline buffer can be prepared. After mixing each dilution, 0.05 mL of the dilution is placed on a separate division of the glass slide and tested as described in Steps *4* through *6* above. The titer of CRP is the last dilution that exhibits a positive reaction.

When a titration is performed, a dilution control must be tested simultaneously. The control consists of one drop of the latex reagent and one drop of the glycine-saline buffer. If agglutination/clumping is observed with this control, the titration is invalid and should be repeated.

REPORTING RESULTS

In patients who are free of inflammation and/or tissue necrosis, CRP is absent from the serum or present in concentrations below 0.5 mg/dL. Reference range mean values are 0.01 mg/dL in newborns and <0.05 mg/dL in adult males and non-pregnant females.

POSITIVE REACTION. Agglutination of the latex

suspension is a positive result that indicates the presence of CRP in the specimen at a level equal to or greater than 1.0 ± 0.2 mg/dL. A positive reaction is reported when either the undiluted or 1:5 diluted specimen demonstrates agglutination or when both exhibit agglutination. Agglutination in the 1:5 dilution is indicative of a CRP level >5 mg/dL.

NEGATIVE REACTION. The absence of visible agglutination and the presence of opaque fluid constitutes a negative reaction. A negative reaction is reported *only* when both the undiluted and 1:5 diluted specimen exhibit no visible agglutination.

PROCEDURE NOTES

Specimen collection and handling are important to the quality of the test. Strict adherence must be paid to technique with a special emphasis on drop size, complete mixing, reaction time, and temperature of reagents.

The strength of a positive reaction may be graded as follows:

1+ Very small clumping with an opaque fluid background

2+ Small clumping with slightly opaque fluid in the background

3+ Moderate clumping with fairly clear fluid in the background

4+ Large clumping with a clear fluid background

SOURCES OF ERROR. False positive results may be observed if serum specimens are lipemic, hemolyzed, or heavily contaminated with bacteria. If the reaction time is longer than 2 minutes, a false positive result may also be produced resulting from a drying effect.

False negative results may be observed in undiluted serum specimens because of high levels of CRP (antigen excess). A 1:5 dilution of serum is also tested for this reason.

CLINICAL APPLICATIONS. Usually with the onset of a substantial inflammatory event such as infection, myocardial infarction, or surgery, the CRP level increases very significantly (>tenfold) above the reference range values for healthy individuals. The test is clinically useful in early detection of inflammatory diseases, particularly infections, as an indicator in screening for organic diseases and in monitoring patient progress.

LIMITATIONS. Because the latex slide agglutination test is a qualitative and semi-quantitative procedure, other methods such as nephelometry should be used for quantitative determination of the level of CRP when indicated. The strength of the agglutination reaction is not always indicative of the CRP concentration. Weak reactions may be produced in samples with either elevated or low CRP values. Results may vary depending on the condition of a patient.

This 2-minute slide latex agglutination test has a detection level of 1 ± mg CRP/dL; therefore, patients with CRP values of <1 mg/dL CRP may be undetected. The sensitivity of the procedure has been assessed at 93%.

Chapter Review

HIGHLIGHTS

The entire leukocytic cell system is designed to defend the body against disease. Each cell type, however, has a unique function and behaves both independently and, in many cases, in cooperation with other cell types. Leukocytes can be functionally divided into the general categories of granulocyte, monocyte-macrophage, and lymphocyte-plasma cells. The primary phagocytic cells are the polymorphonuclear neutrophilic (PMN) leukocytes and the mononuclear monocytes-macrophages. Embryonic blood cells, excluding the lymphocyte type of white blood cell, originate from the mesenchymal tissue that arises from the embryonic germ layer, the mesoderm. The sites of hematopoiesis follow a definite sequence in the embryo and fetus: yolk sac, liver and spleen, and bone marrow. The cellular elements of the blood are produced from a common, multipotential, hematopoietic cell, the stem cell. Following stem cell differentiation, blast cells arise for each of the major categories of cell types: erythrocytes, megakaryocytes, granulocytes, monocytes-macrophages, lymphocytes, and plasma cells. Subsequent maturation of these cells will produce the major cellular elements of the circulating blood, the erythrocytes, thrombocytes, and specific types of leukocytes. In normal peripheral or circulating blood, the following types of leukocytes can be found in order of frequency: neutrophils, lymphocytes, monocytes, eosinophils, and basophils.

The importance of the neutrophil to body defenses is illustrated by the fact that patients with quantitative or qualitative defects of neutrophils have a high rate of infection. Leukocyte mobility may be impaired in some diseases, and defective locomotion or leukocyte immobility can also be seen in patients receiving steroids and in "lazy leukocyte syndrome." A marked defect in the cellular response to chemotaxis, an important step in phagocytosis, can be been in patients suffering from diabetes mellitus, Chediak-Higashi anomaly, sepsis, and in patients with high levels of antibody IgE, such as in Job's syndrome. The neutrophilic leukocyte, particularly the PMN, provides an effective host defense against bacterial and fungal infections. Although the monocytes-macrophages and other granulocytes are also phagocytic cells, the neutrophil is the principle leukocyte associated with phagocytosis and a localized inflammatory response. The formation of an inflammatory exudate, which develops rapidly in an inflammatory response, is primarily composed of neutrophils and monocytes. Although eosinophils and basophils are capable of participating in phagocytosis, they possess less phagocytic activity. The ineffectiveness of these cells is due to both the small number of cells in the circulating blood coupled with the lack of powerful digestive enzymes. Both the eosinophils and basophils, however, are functionally important in body defense.

In the past the mononuclear monocyte-macrophage was known only as a scavenger cell. Only recently has its role as a complex cell of the immune system in the host defense against infection been recognized. The macrophage and its precursors are widely distributed throughout the body. These cells are considered to constitute a physiologic system, the mononuclear-phagocyte system, which includes promonocytes and their precursors in the bone marrow, monocytes in the circulating blood, and macrophages in tissues. Functionally, the most important step in the maturation of macrophages is the lymphokine-drive conversion of the normal resting macrophage to the activated macrophage. Macrophages can be activated during infection by the release of macrophage-activating lymphokines from T lymphocytes specifically sensitized to antigens from the infecting microorganisms. This interaction constitutes the basis of cell-mediated immunity. Functionally, monocytes-macrophages have phagocytosis as their major role. These cells, however, perform at least three distinct but interrelated functions in host defense: phagocytosis, antigen presentation and induction of the immune response, and secretion of biologically active molecules. Macrophages carry out the fundamental function of ingesting and killing invading microorganisms. The phagocytic property of the macrophage is particularly important in the processing of antigens as part of the immune response. Macrophages are believed to process antigens and physically present this biochemically modified and more reactive form of antigen to lymphocytes (particularly T-helper cells) as an initial step in the immune response. Recognition of antigen on the macrophage surface by T-lymphocytes, however, requires an additional match of the surface class II gene product of the major histocompatibility complex. This gene product is the Ia product in the mouse and D gene region product in humans. With proper recognition, the macrophage secretes a lymphocyte-activating factor (interleukin-1), lymphocyte proliferation ensues, and the immune response (T- and/or B-cell response) is facilitated. Qualitative disorders of monocytes-macrophages reflect themselves as lipid storage diseases including a number of rare autosomal recessive disorders. In these conditions the expression in macrophages of a systemic enzymatic defect permits the accumulation of cell debris that is normally cleared by macrophages. The macrophages are particularly prone to accummulate undegraded lipid products. Resistance to infection can be impaired, at least partially, because of an impairment in macrophage function. Disorders of this type include Gaucher's disease and Niemann-Pick disease.

Tissue damage results in inflammation, a series of biochemical and cellular changes that facilitate the phagocytosis of invading microorganisms or damaged cells. If inflammation is sufficiently extensive, it is accompanied by an increase in the plasma concentration of acute phase reactants. Because acute phase protein changes are sensitive indicators of the presence of inflammatory disease, they are especially useful in monitoring such conditions. They are less valuable, however, as a diagnostic tool.

Phagocytosis can be divided into several stages: movement of cells, engulfment, and digestion. If bacteria are not effectively immobilized, subsequent phagocytic activity may take place. Although neutrophils provide the major means of defense against bacterial and fungal infections, they can also be destructive to host tissues. The same oxidative and nonoxidative processes that destroy microorganisms can affect adjacent host tissues. The accumulation of neutrophilic infiltrates and the side effects of phagocytosis can be important as the cause of tissue destruction in a number of noninfectious disease processes.

Plasma concentrations of a group of glycoproteins known as acute phase reactants increase as a specific adaptive response to inflammation. Acute tissue damage and inflammation often result in an initial decrease in the concentration of acute phase proteins, possibly resulting from a loss of protein from the vascular space, followed by an increase. Twenty plasma proteins show acute phase behavior and most have a definable role in inflammation. They include inflammatory mediators such as complement proteins and clotting factors, transport proteins such as haptoglobin, and inhibitors such as alpha$_1$-antitrypsin. Acute phase reactants constitute the majority of the serum glycoproteins.

REVIEW QUESTIONS

1. The major site of hematopoiesis in the second month of gestation is the:
   A. yolk sac
   B. spleen
   C. liver
   D. bone marrow
   E. lymph nodes
2. The principal type of leukocyte in the process of phagocytosis is the:
   A. eosinophil
   B. basophil
   C. monocyte
   D. neutrophil
   E. mast cell
3. *Chronic Granulomatous Disease (CGD)* represents a defect of:
   A. oxidative metabolism
   B. abnormal granulation of neutrophils
   C. diapedesis
   D. chemotaxis
   E. cell-surface glycoproteins
4. A primary function of the eosinophil is:
   A. phagocytosis
   B. suppression of the inflammatory response
   C. reacting in acute, systemic hypersensitivity reactions
   D. antigen recognition
   E. antibody production

5. The cells of the mononuclear phagocytic system include:
   A. monocytes and promonocytes
   B. monocytes and macrophages
   C. lymphocytes and monocytes
   D. Both A and B
   E. Both A and C
6. The host defense function(s) of monocytes-macrophages include(s):
   A. antigen presentation
   B. phagocytosis
   C. induction of the immune response
   D. secretion of biologically active molecules
   E. all of the above
7. The surface class II gene product is important in:
   A. antigen recognition by T lymphocytes
   B. antigen recognition by B lymphocytes
   C. synthesis of antibody by plasma cells
   D. phagocytosis
   E. interleukin-1 secretion by lymphocytes
8. Which of the following factors can induce fever and synthesis of acute phase reactants?
   A. interleukiin-1 and complement
   B. cachectin and interleukin-1
   C. transferrin and interleukin-1
   D. transferrin and interferon
   E. complement and interferon

Questions 9-13. Match the appropriate monocyte-macrophage abnormality with its respective condition.
9. Defect in phagocytic killing
10. Defective monocyte cytotoxicity
11. Defective release of macrophage-activating factors
12. Depressed migration
13. Impaired phagocytosis
    A. Wiskott-Aldrich syndrome
    B. Burns or diabetes
    C. Systemic lupus erythematosus
    D. Corticosteroid therapy
    E. Intracellular infections

Questions 14-17. Arrange the steps of phagocytosis in the proper sequence.
14. ____
15. ____
16. ____
17. ____
    A. Digestion of bacteria
    B. Increase in chemoattractants at site of tissue damage
    C. Ingestion of bacteria
    D. Movement of phagocytic cells
18. Measurement of acute phase proteins is useful in all of the following conditions except:
    A. Monitoring the progress of diagnosed disease activity
    B. Diagnosing conditions such as myocardial infarction

C. Assessing the response to therapy in inflammatory diseases
D. Detection of complications of a known disease
E. Both B and D

19. The acute phase reactant that responds the fastest and is the most sensitive indicator of acute inflammation is:
    A. complement
    B. ceruloplasmin
    C. C-reactive Protein
    D. haptoglobin
    E. fibrinogen

Answers

1. C 2. D 3. A 4. B 5. D 6. E 7. A 8. B 9. D 10. A 11. E 12. B 13. C 14. B 15. D 16. C 17. A 18. B 19. C

BIBLIOGRAPHY

Barrett J: Textbook of immunology, ed 5, St Louis, 1988, The CV Mosby Co.

Becker GJ, Waldburger M, Hughes GRB, and Pepys MB: Value of serum C-reactive protein measurement in the investigation of fever in systemic lupus erythematosus, Ann Rheum Dis 39:50, 1980.

Bellanti JA: Immunology: basic processes, Philadelphia, 1979, WB Saunders Co.

Busby J and Caranasos GJ: Immune function, autoimmunity, and selective immunoprophylaxis, Med Clin North Am 69(3):465-470, May 1985.

Fischler CL and Gill WV: Acute phase proteins. In Ritzmann EE and Daniels TC, editors: Serum protein abnormalities: diagnostic and clinical aspects, Boston, 1975, Little, Brown & Co Inc.

Gee GK, Kephart RH, Turgeon ML, and others: Body defenses—Part A, Integrated science for the health professions laboratory manual, Corning, New York, 1985: Corning College Press.

ICL Scientific Product Brochure. C-Reactive Protein Test, Fountain Valley, Calif,: ICL Scientific, August 1987.

Jandl JH: Blood, Boston, 1987, Little, Brown & Co Inc.

Johnston RB: Monocytes and macrophages, New Eng J Med 318(12):747-752, March 24, 1988.

Katz P: Clinical and laboratory evaluation of the immune system, Med Clin North Am 69(3):453-459, May 1985.

Malech HL and JI: Neutrophils in human diseases, New Eng J of Med 317(11):687-692 Sept 10, 1987.

Roitt IM: Immunology, London, 1985, Gower Medical Publishing.

Roitt IM: Essential immunology, ed 5, Oxford, 1984, Blackwell Scientific Publications Inc.

Turgeon ML: Clinical hematology, Boston, 1988, Little, Brown & Co Inc.

Turgeon ML: Fundamentals of immunohematology, Philadelphia, 1989, Lea & Febiger.

Van Lente F: Rediscovering C-reactive protein, Diagnostic Medicine, pp. 95-96, May/June 1982.

Whicher JT, Bell AM, and Southall PJ: Inflammation measurements in clinical management, Diagnostic Medicine, pp. 62-80, July/Aug 1981.

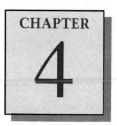

The Cells and Cellular Activities of the Immune System

Lymphocytes and Plasma Cells

Lymphocytes represent the cellular components of the specific system of body defense. These cells function in one of two limbs of the specific immune system: the cell-mediated immune response and humoral immunity. Although the two limbs are not entirely independent and are frequently cooperative, they can be discussed as distinct systems.

THE ANATOMIC ORIGIN AND DEVELOPMENT OF LYMPHOCYTES

In addition to the activities of the granulocytes and monocytes-macrophages, the lymphocytes and plasma cells are the cornerstone of the immune system. Lymphocytes (Fig. 4-1) recognize foreign *antigens* and/or produce *antibodies*; plasma cells produce antibodies.

Sites of Lymphocytic Development

In mammalian immunologic development (Fig. 4-2), the precursors of lymphocytes arise from the pluripotent, precursor stem cells of the yolk sac and liver. Later in fetal development and throughout the life-cycle, the bone marrow becomes the sole provider of undifferentiated stem cells, which can further develop into lymphoblasts. Continued cellular development of the lymphoid precursors and proliferation occurs as the cells travel to the primary and secondary lymphoid tissues. The tissues and organs associated with cellular development and host defense are functionally classified as the immune system.

Primary Lymphoid Tissues

The primary lymphoid organs are the thymus and the *bursa of Fabricius* in birds (Fig. 4-3). In mammals, both the *bone marrow* (and/or fetal liver) and *thymus* are classified as primary or central lymphoid organs (Fig. 4-4). Mammals have no bursa of Fabricius, but the bone marrow and other sites are considered to be the bursal equivalent.

The Thymus

Early in embryonic development, the thymus is derived from the third and fourth pharyngeal pouches. This structure, located in the mediastinum, exercises control over the entire immune system. Stem cells that migrate to the thymus proliferate and differentiate under the influence of the humoral factor, *thymosin*. These lymphocyte precursors with acquired surface membrane antigens are referred to as thymocytes. The reticular structure of the thymus allows a significant number of lymphocytes to pass through it to become fully immunocompetent (able to function in the immune response) thymus-derived T cells. The thymus also regulates immune function by secretion of multiple soluble hormones.

Many cells die in the thymus and are apparently phagocytized, a mechanism to eliminate lympho-

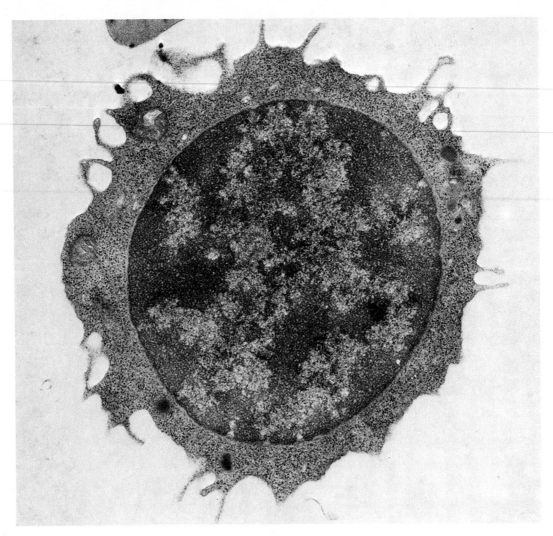

FIGURE 4-1
Electron photomicrograph of a lymphocyte. The lymphocyte tends to lack a well-developed endoplasmic reticulum; biochemically this must be interpreted as a handicap to protein (antibody) synthesis by this cell. Note the cytoplasmic extensions.
(From Barrett JT: Textbook of immunology, ed 5, St Louis, 1988, The CV Mosby Co.)

cyte clones reactive against self-antigens. Viable cells migrate to the secondary tissues. The absence or abnormal development of the thymus results in a T-lymphocyte deficiency. Involution of the thymus is the first age-related change occurring in the human immune system. The thymus gradually loses up to 95% of its mass (Figs. 4-5 and 4-6) during the first 50 years of life. The accompanying functional changes of decreased synthesis of thymic hormones and the loss of ability to differentiate immature lymphocytes are reflected in an increased number of immature lymphocytes both within the thymus and as circulating peripheral blood T cells. Most of the changes in immune function, such as dysfunction of T and B lymphocytes, elevated levels of circulating immune complexes, and increases in autoantibodies and monoclonal gammopathies (see Chapters 23 to 25 for a complete discussion of representative examples of these disorders) are correlated to involution of the thymus. Immune senescence may account for the increased susceptibility of the elderly to infections, autoimmune disease, and neoplasms.

Bone Marrow

The bone marrow is the source of pluripotent stem cells, which differentiate into lymphocytes, granulocytes, erythrocytes, and megakaryocyte populations. In mammals, the bone marrow also supports differentiation of lymphocytes. It is believed that the bone marrow and gut-associated lymphoid tissue (GALT) may also play a role in the differentiation of stem cells into B lymphocyte functions as the bursal equivalent in humans. The B lymphocytes derive their name from the term *bursa*.

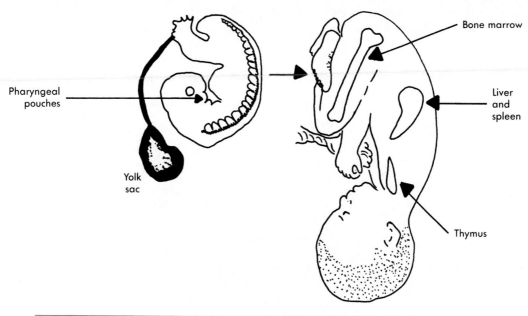

FIGURE 4-2

Development of immunologic organs. The anatomy of the human fetus illustrates the development of the mammalian immune system. Cells of the pharyngeal pouches migrate into the chest and form the thymus. Precursors of lymphocytes originate early in embryonic life in the yolk sac and eventually migrate to the bone marrow via the spleen and liver.

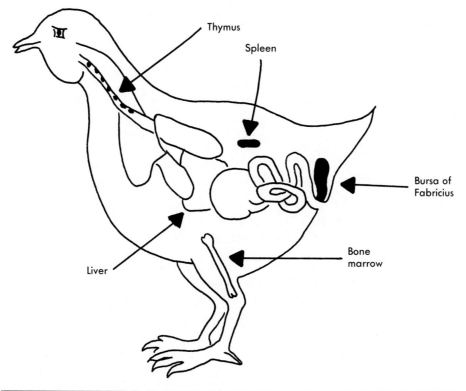

FIGURE 4-3

Avian immunologic organs. The immune system in birds is focused in two organs, the thymus and the bursa of Fabricius.

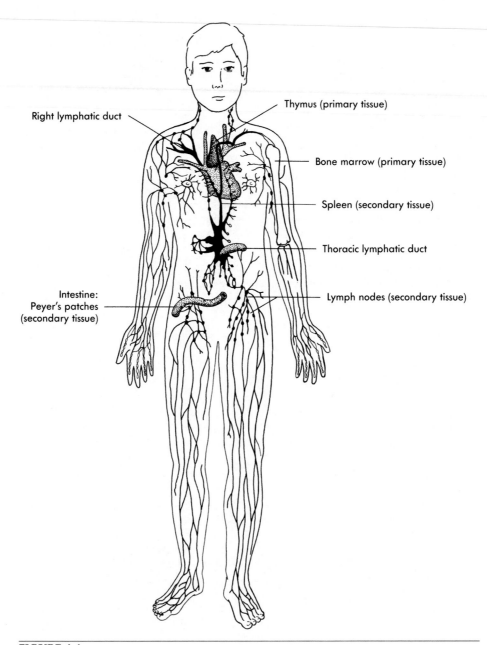

FIGURE 4-4

Human primary and secondary tissues.
(From Turgeon ML: Clinical hematology: theory and procedures, Boston, 1988, Little, Brown and Co.)

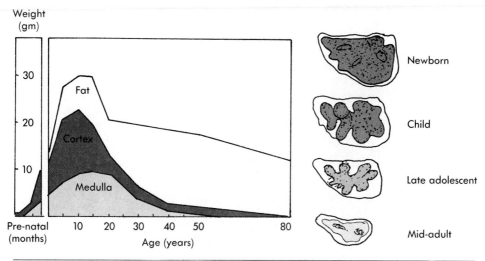

FIGURE 4-5

Thymic development. The histology of the thymus changes with age. The main features of these changes are a loss of cellularity with increasing age.

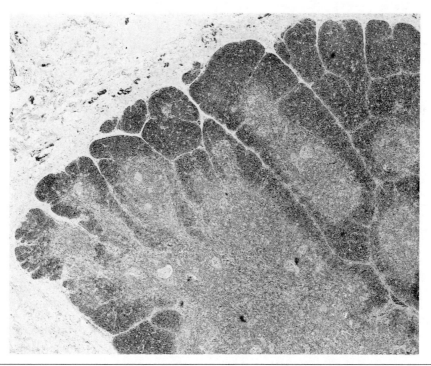

FIGURE 4-6

Normal thymus gland from infant, showing lobulated structure, distinct corticomedullary junction, and prominent Hassall's corpuscles of medulla. (×25.)
(From Kissane JM: Anderson's Pathology, ed 9, St Louis, 1990, The CV Mosby Co.)

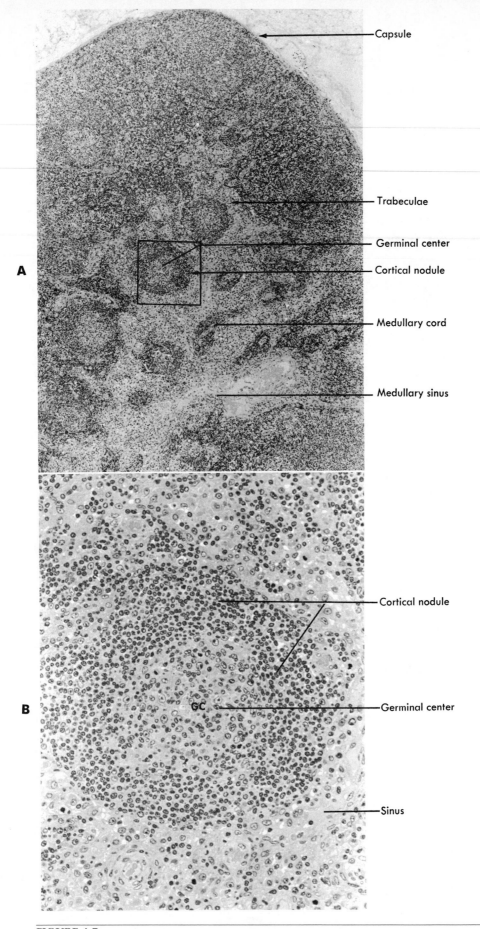

Capsule

Trabeculae

Germinal center

Cortical nodule

Medullary cord

Medullary sinus

A

B

Cortical nodule

GC

Germinal center

Sinus

FIGURE 4-7

A, Lymph node. (x90.) Cortical nodule (enclosed by triangle is enlarged in *B.* **B** Lymph node. (x450.) Enlargement of cortical nodule seen in *A.*
(From Anthony CP and Thibodeau GA: Textbook of anatomy and physiology, ed 12, St Louis, 1987, The CV Mosby Co.)

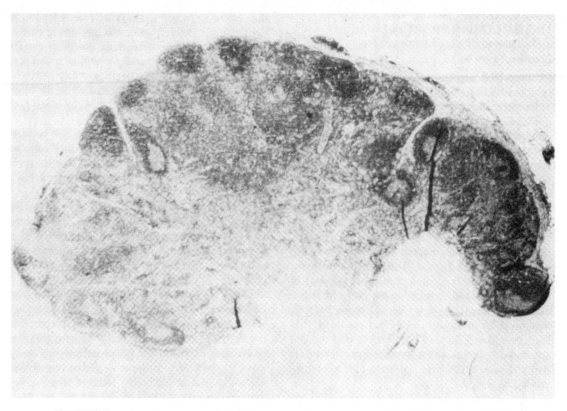

FIGURE 4-8
Normal lymph node of a child, showing germinal centers, deep cortical areas, and medullary cords. T cells are located in the deep cortical areas, whereas B cells are located in germinal centers and medullary cords.
(Courtesy Dr. Richard O'Reilly, New York, NY)

Secondary Lymphoid Tissues

The secondary lymphoid tissues include the *lymph nodes*, (Fig. 4-7) *spleen*, and *Peyer's patches* in the intestine. Proliferation of the T and B lymphocytes in the secondary or peripheral lymphoid tissues is primarily dependent on antigenic stimulation. The T lymphocytes, or T cells (Fig. 4-8), populate the following:

1. Perifollicular and paracortical regions of the lymph node
2. Medullary cords of the lymph nodes
3. Periarteriolar regions of the spleen
4. Thoracic duct of the circulatory system.

The B lymphocytes or B cells multiply and populate the following:

1. Follicular and medullary (germinal centers) of the lymph nodes
2. Primary follicles and red pulp of the spleen
3. Follicular regions of gut-associated lymphoid tissue (GALT)
4. Medullary cords of the lymph nodes.

Lymphocyte Physiology

The mature T lymphocyte survives for several months or years, while the average life span of the B lymphocyte is only a few days. Lymphocytes move freely between the blood and lymphoid tissues. This activity, referred to as *lymphocyte recirculation*, enables lymphocytes to come in contact with processed foreign antigens and to disseminate antigen-sensitized *memory* cells throughout the lymphoid system. Recirculation of lymphocytes back to the blood is via the major lymphatic ducts.

Lymphocytes enter the lymph node (Fig. 4-9) from the blood circulation via arterioles and capillaries to reach the specialized postcapillary venules. From the venule, the lymphocytes enter the node and will either remain there or pass through and return to the circulating blood. Lymphatic fluid, lymphocytes, and antigens from certain body sites enter the lymph node through the *afferent* lymphatic duct and exit the lymph node through the *efferent* lymphatic duct.

THE CATEGORIES AND MEMBRANE CHARACTERISTICS OF LYMPHOCYTES
Major Lymphocyte Functions

Lymphocytes display a great diversity of biologic and chemical properties such as size, density, charge, surface structure, and function. Several major categories of lymphocytes are recognized by the

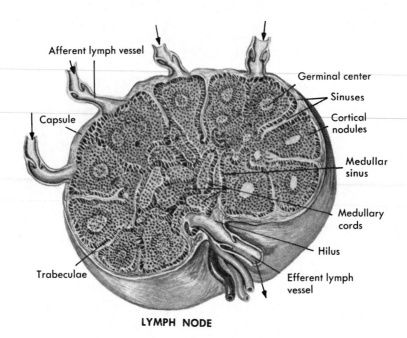

LYMPH NODE

FIGURE 4-9

Structure of a lymph node. Several afferent valved lymphatics bring lymph to the node. An efferent lymphatic leaves the node at the hilus. Note that the artery and vein enter and leave at the hilus.

(From Anthony CP and Thibodeau GA: Textbook of Anatomy and physiology, ed 12, St Louis, 1987, The CV Mosby Co.)

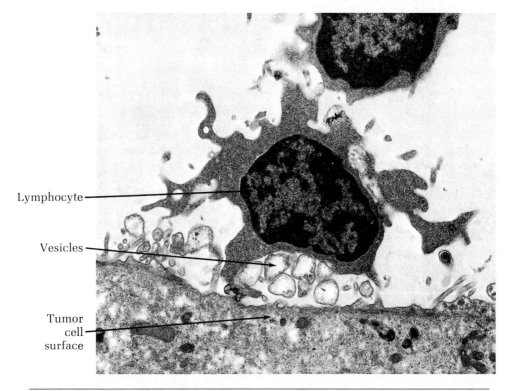

FIGURE 4-10, A

Transmission electron photomicrograph demonstrating the initial stages of the attack of a cytotoxic lymphocyte on a tumor cell, only a portion of which is seen. Notice the vesicles and blebs of cytoplasm that are being shed by the lymphocyte.

(From Barrett JT: Textbook of immunology, ed 5, St. Louis, 1988, The CV Mosby Co.)

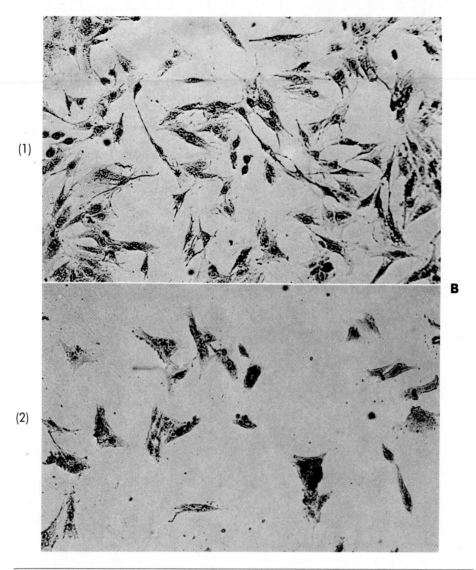

FIGURE 4-10, B
The effects of cytotoxic lymphocytes on tumor cells. (1) The tumor cells prior to contact with the immune lymphocytes. (2) The tumor cells after this contact. Note that many cells have detached from the surface, some cells are swollen, and few cells exhibit the morphology of normal cells.
From Barrett JT: Textbook of immunology, ed 5, St. Louis, 1988, The CV Mosby Co.)

presence of cell surface membrane markers. These categories are the *T cells, B cells,* and the *natural killer (NK)* and *K-type* lymphocytes.

T Lymphocytes

Of the total circulating lymphocytes 60% to 80% are cells derived from the stem cells that mature in the thymus gland under the influence of thymic hormones, T cells. T cells are responsible for cellular immune responses and are involved in the regulation of antibody reactions either by helping or suppressing the activation of B lymphocytes.

The major normal functions of T cells include:

1. Mediated delayed hypersensitivity reactions such as contact hypersensitivity. This func-

tion is primarily accomplished by the release of mediating substances termed *lymphokines.* Migration inhibition factor (MIF) is an example of such a mediator that participates in delayed hypersensitivity by limiting the egress of macrophages from a site of inflammation.

2. Mediated cytolytic reactions. Cytotoxic T cells have the capacity to kill other cells. This process is demonstrated by the immune response to virus-infected cells or tumor cells (Figs. 4-10 A and B).

3. Regulation of the immune response. The regulatory functions of T cells can be either beneficial or harmful. T-helper cells in cooperation with macrophages cooperate with B cells

or other T cells in the initiation of a normal immune response. T-suppressor cells are capable of suppressing a variety of T cell functions, such as contact sensitivity and the T-cytotoxic response, and B cell responses, such as suppression of T-helper cells or antibody synthesis by plasma cells. Because it is clear that T-regulatory cells play a critical role in the immune system, evaluation of the quantities and ratios of helper and suppressor cells has proved to be a valuable tool in the diagnosis or monitoring of immune disorders.

Interleukin-2 (IL-2), also known as the T cell growth factor, plays an important role in cell-mediated immunity. Following antigen stimulation, IL-2 promotes the growth of T cell clones, helper T cells, and cytolytic T cells. Specific receptors are present on helper T cells and on cytolytic T cells that allow for binding of IL-2 to these cells. The molecular weight and structure of IL-2 are defined; and, depending on the species involved, IL-2 is a protein of 15,000-30,000 daltons. IL-2 is used to allow long-term growth of T cells, a technique that has facilitated the study of T cell immunity. Because of this important role, it also offers clinical applicability, e.g., tumor immunity.

Sensitized T cells protect the human body against infection by mediating intracellular pathogens that are viral, bacterial, fungal, or protozoan. In addition, T cells are responsible for chronic rejection in organ transplantation. It is accepted that antigen binds to T cells to initiate a cellular immune response. A specific antigen-binding protein consisting of two chains linked by disulfide bonds has been demonstrated on the surface of cells. The concensus is that antigen-binding receptors, not conventional surface immunoglobulin as is found on B cells, are responsible for the various functions of T cells.

Soluble mediators *(lymphokines)* (Table 4-1) are secreted by monocytes, lymphocytes or neutrophils providing the language for cell-to-cell communication. Some of the most important lymphokines follow:

1. *Migration inhibition factor (MIF)*—affects macrophage migration during delayed hypersensitivity reactions.
2. *Interleukin-2 (T cell growth factor)*—major factor stimulating T cell proliferation.
3. *Chemotactic factors*—attract granulocytes to affected areas.
4. *Interleukin-1*—released by macrophages and activates T-helper cells.

B Lymphocytes

B cells, which represent less than 15% of the circulating lymphocytes, are derived from stem cells through an antigen-independent maturation process occurring in the bone marrow and GALT. These cells serve as the primary source of cells responsible for humoral (antibody) response, which is

TABLE 4-1

Soluble Products of Lymphocytes (Lyphokines)

Product	Action
Blastogenic factor	Proliferation of lymphocytes
Bone-resorbing factor	Decalcification of bone
Chemotactic factor	Chemotaxis of various leukocytes
Interferon	Interference with viral reproduction
Interleukin-2 (IL-2), or T cell growth factor	Stimulation of growth of helper and cytolytic T cells
Leukocyte migration inhibition factor	Inhibition of polymorphonuclear leukocyte migration
Lymphotoxin	Inhibition of cell growth
Macrophage-activating factor	Activation of macrophages, with increase in their metabolism
Macrophage aggregation factor	Aggregation of macrophages
Migration inhibitor factor (MIF)	Inhibition of the migration of macrophages
Skin-reactive factor	Mononuclear inflammation caused by intradermal injection
Transfer factor	Transfer of delayed hypersensitivity to a nonsensitized recipient

a primary host defense against microorganisms. The condition of hyperacute rejection of transplanted organs is also mediated by B cells.

B cells, however, are not generally antibody-secreting cells. Participation of B cells in the humoral immune response is accomplished by their maturation into plasma cells with subsequent synthesis and secretion of immunoglobulins after antigenic stimulation. Stimulation of B cells to produce antibodies is a complex process usually requiring interactions between *macrophages* (that phagocytize, process, and present antigens to T cells), *T cells*, and *B cells*.

Natural Killer and K-Type Lymphocytes

A subpopulation of circulating lymphocytes (5% to 10%), lacking most of the recognizable surface membrane markers of mature T or B cells, include the *natural killer (NK)* and *K-type* lymphocytes. NK cells are classified as a population of effector lymphocytes that produce such mediators as *interferon* and *interleukin-2*. These cells have been previously termed *null cells*, and a number of different cell lines are probably included in this term.

The NK and K cells destroy target cells through an extracellular nonphagocytic mechanism referred to as a *cytotoxic reaction*. NK cells are able to bind and lyse antibody-coated nucleated cells through a membrane Fc receptor, which can recognize a part of the heavy chain of immunoglobulins. Target cells include tumor cells, some cells of the embryo, cells of the normal bone marrow and thymus, and microbial agents. Increasing evidence suggests that a considerable number of NK cells may be present in other tissues, particularly in the lungs and liver, where they may play important roles in inflammatory reactions and in host defense, including defense against certain viruses such as cytomegalovirus (CMV) and hepatitis. NK cells are stimulated by *interferon* (an antiviral substance) and will actively kill the virally infected target cell. If this is completed before the virus has time to replicate, they will combat viral infection.

The term *large granular lymphocyte (LGL)* can synonymously refer to the NK cell. Up to about 75% of LGLs function as NK cells, and LGLs appear to account fully for the NK activity in mixed cell populations. As a group, LGLs represent a small subpopulation in the blood or spleen (about 5% of mononuclear cells).

K-type cells exhibit a different kind of cytotoxic mechanism than NK cells. The target cell must be coated with low concentrations of IgG antibody; this is referred to as an *antibody-dependent cell-mediated cytotoxicity (ADCC) reaction.* An ADCC reaction may be exhibited by both K cells and phagocytic and nonphagocytic myelogenous-type leukocytes. K cells are capable of lysing tumor cells. Although morphologically similar to a small lymphocyte, the precise lineage of the K cell is uncertain.

Changes in Lymphocyte Subpopulations with Aging

Except for inconsistent values seen in extremely elderly persons, the total number of T cells in the peripheral blood is relatively stable throughout adult life. There is, however, a change in the distribution of T cell subpopulations. A decrease in the number of suppressor cells and an increase in the helper cell population is demonstrated in the elderly.

The effect of aging on the immune response is highly variable, but the ability to respond immunologically to disease is age-related. It has been suggested that faulty immunologic reactions such as aberrant functioning of immunoregulatory cells, effector T cells, and antibody-producing B cells contribute to poor immunity in the aged. Functional deficits of T lymphocytes with aging have been identified that cause impairment of cell-mediated immunity. In addition, skin testing has revealed decreases in the intensity of delayed hypersensitivity. The proliferative response of T lymphocytes to mitogens or antigens such as *Mycobacterium tuberculosis* or *varicella zoster* virus is impaired.

A decrease in T-helper cells is the primary cause of impaired humoral response seen in elderly sub-

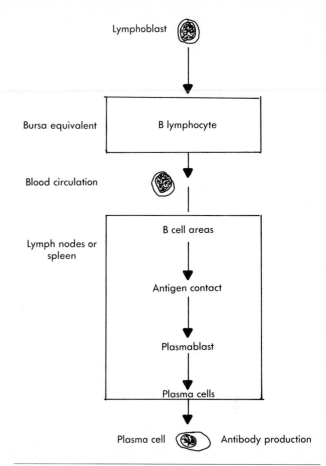

FIGURE 4-11

Plasma cell development from B lymphocytes.
(From Turgeon ML: Clinical hematology: theory and procedures, Boston, 1988, Little, Brown and Co.)

jects. Although the total number of B cells and total concentration of immunoglobulin produced remains unchanged, the serum concentration of IgM is decreased. Concentrations of IgA and IgG have been demonstrated to be increased.

Plasma Cells

The function of plasma cells is the synthesis and excretion of immunoglobulins. Plasma cells are not normally found in the circulating blood but in the bone marrow in concentrations that do not normally exceed 2%. Two well-established pathways of plasma cell development have been documented. Some plasma cells arise from immature plasma cells; others arise as the end stage of B cell differentiation into a large, activated plasma cell.

Plasma Cell Development

The pathway from the B lymphocyte to the antibody-synthesizing plasma cell (Fig. 4-11) occurs when the B cell is antigenically stimulated and undergoes *blast transformation*. The immune antibody response begins when individual B lymphocytes encounter an antigen that binds to their specific immunoglobulin surface receptors. After receiving an appropriate "second signal" provided by interaction with helper T cells, these antigen-binding B cells undergo blast cell transformation and proliferation to generate a clone of mature plasma cells that secrete a specific type of antibody.

An increase in plasma cells can be seen in a variety of nonmalignant disorders such as viral disorders, e.g., *rubella* and *infectious mononucleosis,* allergic conditions, chronic infections, and collagen diseases. In plasma cell dyscrasias, the plasma cells can be extremely increased or completely infiltrate the bone marrow, e.g., *multiple myeloma* or *Waldenstrom's macroglobulinemia.*

Antibody molecules secreted by plasma cells consist of four chains (two light chains and two heavy chains, based on molecular weight) and can be enzymatically cleaved into Fab and Fc fragments. The Fab portion of the molecule binds antigen and contains the light chains and their antigenic markers (kappa, lambda). The Fc fragment, which readily crystallizes after enzymation, (c represents crystallizability) contains the markers that distinguish the different classes of antibody (M, G,A,D,E). It also contains sites that will bind and activate complement and bind to Fc receptors on cells. The amino acid sequence for most of the antibody protein is constant, except for the antigen-binding portion of the molecule that has a hypervariable region and accounts for the various antigenic specificities that the antibody is programmed to recognize.

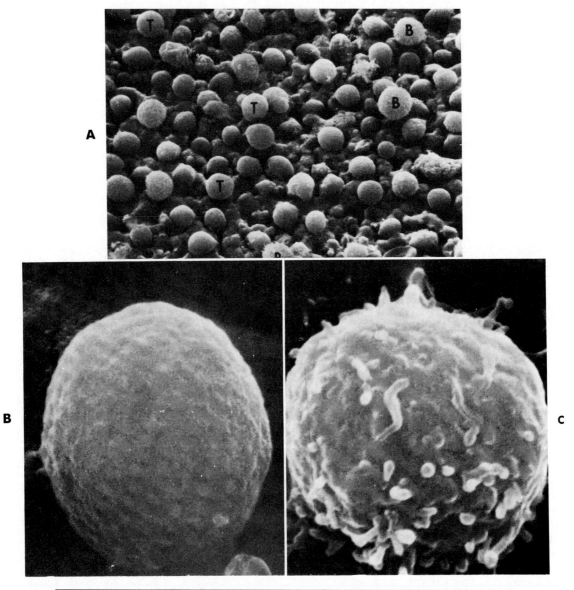

FIGURE 4-12
Scanning electron photomicrograph of T and B lymphocyte cell surface membranes.

Membrane Markers and Associated Functions

Cells of the immune system have specialized receptors on their membrane surfaces for eliciting an immune response. Before 1979 human lymphocytes could be classified as B cells, which produced antibodies, and T cells, which regulated antibody production and directly killed target cells. Observation of these cells with an electron microscope (Fig. 4-12) revealed that T lymphocytes have a relatively smooth surface compared with the rough pattern of the B lymphocytes.

The introduction of monoclonal antibody testing led to the present identification of surface membrane markers (Table 4-2). Monoclonal antibodies to cell surface antigens now provide a method for classifying and identifying specific cellular membrane characteristics. This technology is one application of flow-cell technology (see Chapter 11). In practical terms, surface markers are used to identify and enumerate various lymphocyte subsets. The evaluation of surface membrane markers is useful for establishing lymphocyte maturity, identifying imbalances of lymphocyte subsets, classifying leukemias, and monitoring patients receiving immunosuppressive therapy.

T Cells

Separate subsets of T cells have been recognized with monoclonal antibodies. T cells are divided into two subsets: the *suppressor/cytotoxic* subset and the *helper/inducer* subset. During T cell development, associated membrane antigens vary.

Some antigens appear early in development and remain on mature T cells. Others appear on early cells and are lost as cells mature. Some antigens appear at an intermediate stage and are lost before maturity, while others remain in the mature cell. The naming of the surface membrane antigen varies with the monoclonal antibody used to identify it. The relationship between lymphocyte phenotype and the subset is found in Table 4-2. Each manufacturer of monoclonal antibodies has a separate nomenclature.

T cell differentiation begins during the fetal and early neonatal period when the lymphocyte precursors migrate to the thymus. In the thymus they are processed, acquire T cell surface antigens, and become functionally competent. This pathway has been well documented with monoclonal antibodies in the following sequence (Fig. 4-13). The early thymocyte is initially OKT9+ and OKT10+. It then loses OKT9 and acquires the OKT6 surface marker as well as the OKT4 and OKT8. This *common thymocyte* further differentiates by losing OKT6 and acquiring the mature T cell antigens, OKT3 and OKT1 and T1. Concurrently with this step, two subpopulations are formed by the segregation of thymocytes into OKT4+ and OKT8+ subsets. These cells then lose OKT10 and gain functional maturity with their entry into the peripheral blood as either OKT1+, OKT3+, and OKT4+, or OKT1+, OKT3+, and OKT8+ cells.

All mature T cells express T_3 antigen as well as the pan T cell antigens, OKT1 and OKT12. Markers present on all T cells are used to evaluate total T cell number including OKT1, OKT3, and OKT11.

Subsets of T lymphocytes. The OKT4 subset has been initially described as representing the helper-inducer T cell; it accounts for 55% to 70% of the peripheral T cells. The OKT8+ subset has been initially described as representing the suppressor-cytotoxic T cells, and it accounts for 25% to 40% of the peripheral T cells. T helper-inducer cells are identified by OKT4, while T suppressor-cytotoxic cells are identified by the OKT8 surface marker. The complexity of the T-regulator systems has increased with recent documented reports describing subpopulations of the cells. In the suppressor (Ts) system, T cell circuits activate an induced cell (Ts_1), which induces a Ts_2 suppressor, which in turn activates a Ts_3 effector cell.

Identification of surface markers and the defini-

TABLE 4-2

Examples of Normal T Lymphocyte Membrane Markers

Cell type detected	Designation	Monoclonal antibody source	Cells in peripheral blood
All or most T lymphocytes	Leu 4	Becton-Dickinson	80%-95%
	OKT 3	Ortho	95%
	T11	Coulter	95%
	Anti-CD5	Sigma	>90%
T cell subsets			
Helper/inducer	Leu 3	Becton-Dickinson	40%-60%
	OKT 4	Ortho	65%
	T4	Coulter	60%
	Anti-CD4	Sigma	30%-50%
Suppressor/cytotoxic	Leu 2	Becton-Dickinson	20%-40%
	OKT 8	Ortho	35%
	T8	Coulter	35%
	Anti-CD8	Sigma	20%-45%

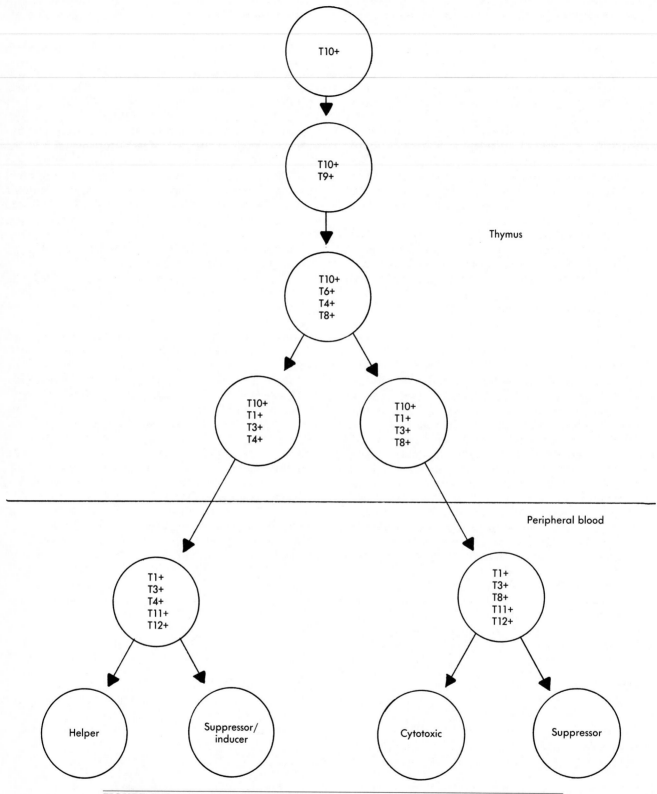

FIGURE 4-13

T cell membrane marker development.

tion of cellular phenotype are frequently associated with cellular function. An *absolute correlation*, however, between phenotype (expressed surface membrane marker) and a particular function does *not* exist. T cells bearing the OKT4 antigen recognize class II products of the MHC gene (IaHLA-D, SB, or DC), while T cells bearing the OKT8 antigen recognize class I products of the MHC gene (HLA-A, B, or C) of target cells. Thus, cytotoxic T cells express either OKT4 or OKT8 depending on the major histocompatibility antigen restriction that governs their antigen recognition, i.e., class I or class II antigens.

OKT4. Functionally, the helper T cells signal B cells to generate antibodies, control production and switching of types of antibodies formed, and activate suppressor cells. Suppressor cells are relatively increased in clinical conditions such as AIDS.

OKT4 cells recognize foreign antigens or markers on infected cells and help to activate B cells. These cells also orchestrate cell-mediated immunity, the killing of infected cells by cytotoxic cells such as OKT8 and natural killer cells. OKT4 cells influence the activity of another group of cells, the mobile scavenger known as macrophage-monocyte. Activated monocytes secrete a variety of cytokines, highly potent proteins that modulate the activity of many cell types. The loss of OKT4 cells impairs the body's ability to fight most invaders, but it has a particularly severe impact on the defenses against viruses, fungi, parasites, and certain bacteria, including mycobacteria.

Some observations suggest the OKT4 subset is heterogeneous. Naturally occurring anti-T-cell antibodies found in the serum of some patients with active juvenile rheumatoid arthritis (JRA) have been used to subdivide OKT4+ into a helper-inducer subpopulation (OKT4+JRA−) and an inducer of suppressor subpopulation (OKT4+JRA+) for pokeweed mitogen and antigen-driven immunoglobulin production.

OKT8. The suppressor-cytotoxic lymphocytes control and inhibit antibody production either by suppressing helper cells or by turning off B cell differentiation. The majority of cytotoxic T cells reside in the OKT8 subset. Cytotoxic T cells, however, can also express OKT4 surface membrane marker.

OKT3. The OKT3 molecules are a trimolecular complex of three polypeptide chains (gamma, delta, and epsilon). This molecule is closely associated with the T cell antigen receptor and is expressed on the surface of all mature T cells. Expression of OKT3 antigen is coordinantly linked with that of the T cell antigen receptor. The T cell antigen receptor is a 90,000 molecular weight heterodimer consisting of an alpha and a beta chain. Each of the two chains contains a variable portion and a constant portion analogous to immunoglobulin heavy and light chains. The T cell receptor and genes thus far show almost as close a familial relationship with immunoglobulin (Ig) genes as that between Ig light (L) and heavy (H) chain genes themselves.

T cell activation. The OKT11 antigen is the sheep erythrocyte receptor found on all peripheral mature T cells. It is a 50,000 mw glycoprotein that appears to be involved under certain conditions in the T cell activation-recognition unit. The T cell activation-recognition unit is recognized by the T cell in association with MHC gene products that are expressed on the surface of accessory cells such as monocytes.

When the T cell receptor binds to antigen presented by accessory cells, T cell activation begins following activation by either pathway. T cells express new surface markers, including receptors for interleukin 2, IaHLA-DR antigens, and transferrin recognized by the monoclonal antibody OKT9. With T cell proliferation, a number of lymphokines is secreted including T cell growth factor, B cell growth factor, B cell differentiation, and gamma interferon. It is through these soluble T cell factors that the T cell regulation influences the action of other T cells, accessory cells, and nonimmune constituents.

T cell control of nonimmune cells. Helper T cells secrete soluble factors that can regulate nonimmune cells. Interleukin 3 and other colony-stimulating factors can drive maturation of hematopoeitic cells, such as monocyte, megakaryocytes, and mast cells. Gamma interferon can induce Ia antigen on fibroblasts, endothelial cells, Langerhans cells, melanocytes, and astrocytes. These Ia+ cells, like monocytes and B cells, can in turn function as antigen-presenting cells and increase T cell activation, which further increases gamma interferon. In this manner, a cascading inflammatory response can be generated and perpetuated.

Alterations in lymphocyte subsets. The normal functioning of *helper cells* and *suppressor cells* in the immune response can be reversed under certain conditions. Functionally, the helper-inducer subset cells signal B cells to generate antibodies, control production and switching of types of antibodies formed, and activate suppressor cells. The suppressor-cytotoxic lymphocytes control and inhibit antibody production either by suppressing helper cells or by turning off B cell differentiation. The normal ratio of *helper cells* and *suppressor cells* (approximately 2:1) can be reversed under certain conditions. Imbalances in the normal distribution of T cell subsets (Table 4-3), with an excess or deficiency of helper or suppressor subsets, can be displayed in a variety of disorders and may lead to abnormalities in B cell immunoglobulin production.

B Cells

B cells are lymphocytes that can synthesize and secrete immunoglobulins after a specific antigenic challenge. Monoclonal antibodies specific for B cells can demonstrate the presence of characteristic surface membrane markers. These markers, how-

TABLE 4-3

Diseases with Imbalances of Regulatory T Cells

Major immunoregulatory T cell defect	Disease	Remarks
Decreased T cell (helper)	Transient hypogammaglobulinemia of infancy	Decrease in number and function of OKT4 helper cells
	Acquired hypogammaglobulinemia	
	Acquired immunodeficiency syndrome	
Increased T cell (helper)	Kawasaki's disease	Circulating activated Ia OKT4 cells; increased spontaneous Ig synthesis
Decreased T cell (suppressor)	Acute graft-vs-host disease	Decreased numbers of suppressor OKT8 cells; hypergammaglobulinemia autoantibody production
	Juvenile rheumatoid arthritis	
	Systemic lupus erythematosus	
	Severe atopic dermatitis	
Increased T cell (suppressor)	Common variable agammaglobulinemia	Increased activity of OKT8 suppressor cells; decreased immunoglobulin production and T cell response to antigens; anergy
	Chronic graft-vs-host disease	
	Systemic viral infections, measles, infectious mononucleosis, cytomegalovirus	

ever, exhibit less specificity than those for T cell markers.

In humans, there is evidence of the existence of four types of B cell markers, including the following:

1. Immunoglobulin (Ig) receptor. Surface Ig (sIg) is usually determined in conjunction with monoclonal testing. B cells have sIg (except for very immature lymphocytes and mature plasma cells), which are normally polyclonal, i.e., kappa and lambda light chains are present on the cytoplasmic membrane of B cells. Mu and delta heavy chains are usually found with either the kappa or lambda chains on any one cell surface. Gamma and alpha are rarely found on the surface of properly prepared normal lymphocytes.

2. An Fc receptor that specifically binds the Fc portion of IgG antibody. The function of this receptor may be to aid B cells in binding to antigen already bound to antibody.

3. Receptors that bind fragments of the cleaved complement component C3 have been reported on the surface of approximately 75% of B cells. This receptor binds C3b, iC3b (inactivated C3b) and C3d, but the function of these receptors is not totally understood.

4. B cell surface antigens coded by the class II genes of the major histocompatibility complex (MHC). It has been suggested that these surface proteins are critical to the cooperation of T and B cells in B cell differentiation and antibody synthesis.

The best studied B cell surface marker is the Ig receptor. This receptor is actually an antibody molecule with antigenic specificity. According to the clonal selection theory, B cells exist in the body with Ig receptors specific for antigen before exposure to the antigenic substances. When specific antigen exposure does occur, the antigen will select the B cell having an Ig receptor with the best fit. Following binding and cooperative interaction with T-regulatory cells (helper or suppressor cells), B cells transform into plasma cells. The secreted antibody in turn has the same specificity as the Ig receptor on the B cell. Virtually all of the antibody produced by plasma cells is secreted (plasma cells have few Ig receptors), but 90% of the antibody produced by B cells is expressed as surface Ig receptors.

In addition, antigenic stimulation prompts B cells to multiply. The specific antibodies produced are able to bind to infected cells and to free organisms bearing the antigen, inactivate those cells or organisms, and destroy them. Some antigens such as lipopolysaccharides from some gram negative organisms can bind to the Ig receptor and also stimulate an antibody response independent of T cell cooperation (T-independent antigens). This type of response, however, is generally of low intensity and is class-restricted to the production of IgM antibody.

NK Cells

Although these cells have long been classified as null cells, monoclonal antibodies demonstrate that NK cells share a variety of surface membrane markers with T cells. Some surface membrane markers are associated with monocytes, granulocytes, or B cells.

EVALUATION OF SUSPECTED DEFECTS
Evaluation of Suspected Defects: Cell-Mediated Immune System

Deficiencies of cell-mediated immunity (discussed in detail later in this chapter) are often suspected in individuals with recurrent viral, fungal, parasitic, and protozoan infections. Patients with AIDS (see Chapter 22) exhibit some of the most severe manifestations of cell-mediated immunity.

One avenue of testing involves delayed hypersensitivity skin testing to determine the integrity of the patient's cell-mediated immune response. Over 90% of normal adults will react to one of the following antigens within 48 hours after antigen exposure: *Candida albicans*, trichophyton, tetanus toxoid, mumps, and streptokinase-streptodornase (SKSD). Reactivity to histoplasmin or purified protein derivative (PPD) is positive in patients with active infection or previous exposure to histoplasmosis or tuberculosis, respectively; therefore, they are not useful in the assessment of anergy.

Hematologic testing can include determination of the absolute number of lymphocytes. The absolute number of lymphocytes (see box below) is the total number of lymphocytes compared to the total number of leukocytes.

The number of T lymphocytes, the primary effector cell in cell-mediated reactions, can be determined by a number of different techniques. The "gold standard" has previously been the E (erythrocyte rosette formation) technique. Development of monoclonal antibodies, however, has permitted a quick and specific method for determining the number of T cells. The method of testing is by use of immunofluorescent techniques in which the fluorescent microscope or fluorescence-activated cell sorter (FACS) is used. Additional testing can include functional testing or the measurement of biologic response modifiers, such as Interleukin 2 (T cell growth factor) using bioassay and radioimmunoassay.

Evaluation of Suspected Defects: Humoral System

The humoral system can be screened for abnormalities by quantitating the concentration of IgM, IgG, and IgA. Serum protein electrophoresis, however, may not be sensitive enough to detect selective Ig class deficiencies. IgD and IgE are not useful in the determination of a suspected humoral deficiency.

The number of B lymphocytes in the peripheral blood and lymphoid organs can be determined by several different techniques. The most common procedure involves the detection of surface Ig (sIg). Most B cells bear IgM and/or IgD. Flouresceinated antihuman Ig antibody can be added to isolated cells in suspension and the percent of B cells determined. Normally, 5% to 15% of peripheral blood lymphocytes are B cells and 40% of splenic and lymph node lymphocytes are surface Ig-bearing. Although surface Ig is the only membrane characteristic unique to B cells, other markers such as Fc receptors, C3 receptors, and gene production of the HLA-Dr region are present. B cell function such as proliferation and antibody production can be assessed in vitro. These techniques generally use mitogens or antigens to detect polyclonal antigen-specific responses.

Testing of Lymphocytes

In functional testing, phenotypes are enumerated in proportional relationship to one another. Functional assays evaluate the response of lymphocytes to nonspecific mitogens. In the case of T lymphocytes, mitogens such as pokeweed mitogen (PWM), or specific antigens such as purified protein derivative (PPD) are used. Functional testing of B lymphocytes is confined to determining the response to pure B cell mitogen such as *Staphlococcus aureus*-Cowan strain and antibody production. These substances provoke DNA synthesis and mitosis or production of antibodies that can determine which cells are functioning abnormally. A patient may have a normal proportion of phenotypically defined suppressor cells, but functional tests might show that those cells are impaired.

Before the introduction of highly specific fluorescent monoclonal antibody tests, several other tests were used to distinguish T and B cells (see box). T lymphocytes were defined by their ability to form rosettes with sheep erythrocytes (Fig. 4-14) and further subclassified by their ability to rosette with immunoglobin or *complement* (a soluble blood protein consisting of nine components, C1-C9, which, if activated, can lead to rupture of the cellular membrane) coated with bovine erythrocytes. This test demonstrated that the surface membrane of T cells had receptors for attachment to normal sheep erythrocytes. B cells had membrane-bound antibody and receptors including the complement (C3) receptor. The presence of the C3 receptor could be demonstrated by the ability of B cells to bind erythrocytes with complement to form the erythrocyte-antibody-complement (EAC) rosettes. B lymphocytes were indisputably characterized by their surface membrane immunoglobulin markers. Using these techniques, a population of non-B, non-T (atypical T cells) known as NK (Null) cells could also be demonstrated.

Absolute Lymphocyte Count

An example of a determination of the absolute number of lymphocytes is as follows:

Absolute number=	Total leukocyte count × % of lymphocytes
Total leukocyte count=	25.0×10^9/L
Relative number percentage (%) of lymphocytes =	76%
Absolute number =	19.0×10^9/L

Techniques for Identification of Lymphocyte Types in Blood or Bone Marrow

Rosette formation

1. Sheep erythrocytes incubated with lymphocytes for T cell identification.
2. Bovine erythrocytes coated with antibody (IgG or IgM) or complement (C3) for the Fc portion of the IgG or IgM antibodies or complement (C3) receptor-bearing cells.
3. Mouse erythrocytes for pre-B cell indentification.

Membrane immunofluorescence

1. Manual methods of direct and indirect binding of fluorescent dyes coupled to antibodies for the detection of surface (antigen) markers.
2. Laser flow cytometry methods.

Techniques for markers of B lymphocytes

1. Surface immunoglobulins (sIg)
2. Receptor sites for activated C3 component complement
3. Receptor sites for aggregated immunoglobuin (Fc receptor)
4. Receptor sites for Fc portion of IgG
5. Receptor sites for complement: erythrocytes coated with antibody and complement (EAC) rosette formation
6. Receptor sites for mouse red cells

Techniques for selected markers of T lymphocytes

1. E receptors for sheep red cells (nonimmune E rosettes)
2. Mitogen-induced lymphocyte transformation
3. Migration inhibition factor (MIF) assay
4. Cytotoxicity assay (complement dependent)
5. Receptor sites for ox red cell coated with IgG antibody
6. Receptor sites for ox red cell coated with IgM antibody

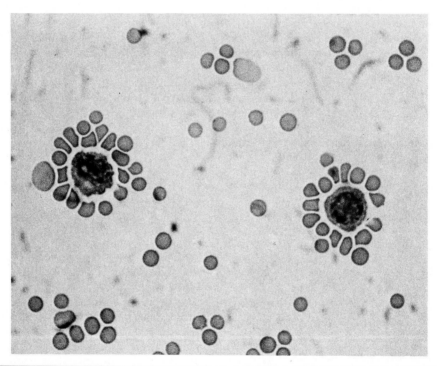

FIGURE 4-14

A rosette in Giemsa-stained cytocentrifuge preparation from a normal adult peripheral blood sample.
(From JD Bauer: Clinical laboratory methods, ed 9, St Louis, 1982, The CV Mosby Co.)

PROCEDURE

Sheep Erythrocyte (E) Rosette for T Lymphocytes

PRINCIPLE

The rosette technique exposes identical receptors (E receptors) on test cells (lymphocytes) and on "signal" cells (sheep red cells). Human thymus derived (T lymphocytes) form spontaneous nonimmunoglobulin-mediated rosettes with sheep red cells. (Attachment of sheep erythrocytes to specific receptors on the cell membrane-technique is known as *rosetting*.) A rosette-forming T cell is defined as a lymphocyte that has three or more red cells adhering to its surface.

SPECIMEN COLLECTION AND PREPARATION

No special preparation of the patient is required before specimen collection. The patient must be positively identified when the specimen is collected. The specimen should be labeled at the bedside and include the patient's full name, the date, and the patient's hospital identification number. The phlebotomist's initials should also appear on the label.

Blood should be drawn by an aseptic technique. The required specimen is three full heparinized tubes, if both T and B cells are to be quantitated and an EDTA anticoagulated blood specimen taken for performance of complete blood and differential count. Keep the heparinized blood at room temperature, and use within 4 hours of collection.

REAGENTS, SUPPLIES, AND EQUIPMENT

1. Phosphate buffered saline (PBS)
2. Sheep red cells. Anticoagulated, fresh cells (less than 3 weeks old) should be used. Pipette 2 mL of cell into a test tube and add 8 mL of PBS
3. Centrifuge at 200 × g for 5 minutes
4. Remove supernatant and top layer of sheep red cell (to remove any sheep white cells), and resuspend the button of red cells to a 5% suspension with PBS (0.5 mL packed volume of cells to 10 mL of solution)
5. Repeat washing and centrifugation two times
6. Resuspend cell in 1 mL of Hank's 10% FCS absorbed
7. Titrate by diluting 1:10³ (100 lambda to 9.9 mL mix or 100 lambda to 0.9 mL mix)
8. In hemocytometer count number of cells in 16 squares × 10⁷, which is equal to the number of cells/mL
9. Adjust to 4 × 10⁸ cell in 1 mL by using the following equation:

$$\text{Vol of cells} = \frac{4 \times 10^8}{\text{SRBC titer}}$$

10. Adjust to final volume of 1.0 with Hank's 10% FCS absorbed.
11. Mix and transfer 0.1 mL to 0.9 mL of PBS to yield 4×10^7 cells/mL for active E rosettes

QUALITY CONTROL

A normal control specimen should be tested simultaneously.

PROCEDURE

Mononuclear layer separation (Ficoll-Hypaque cell separation technique—Boyum's method)

EQUIPMENT AND SUPPLIES

1. Lymphocyte separation medium (LSM, Ficoll-Hypaque, Bionetics Laboratory); specific gravity 1.076 ± .001; store at 2° to 8°C. May be used until expiration date on label.
2. Pasteur pipettes.
3. Conical, glass centrifuge tubes of volume sufficient to contain three times the blood volume drawn.
4. Hanks' balanced salt solution (HBSS, 1 × Grand Island Biological); store at room temperature. May be used indefinitely unless contamination occurs.
5. WBC pipettes and hemacytometer.

PROCEDURE

1. Measure LSM into each of two centrifuge tubes to a volume equal to ½ the collected blood volume. Place in 37°C water for several minutes.
2. Remove from the bath and bring to room temperature. Allow about 30 minutes for complete warming.
3. Dilute the blood samples with an equal volume of HBSS.
4. Overlay the LSM in each tube with the diluted blood sample, taking care not to disturb the surface of LSM. If disturbance does occur, discard tube and replace with a new tube of LSM at room temperature.
5. Centrifuge tubes for approximately 30 minutes at 400 × g.
6. Immediately remove the tubes from the centrifuge.
7. Carefully remove the interface layer and place it in a graduated centrifuge tube.
8. Add HBSS to wash. Centrifuge at 200 × g for 15 minutes. Decant the supernate and repeat.
9. Resuspend the cell button in 1 mL of HBSS.
10. Calculate the expected number of mononuclear cells by using the CBC and differential count results and the following equation: number of WBC × % mononuclear cells= absolute number of mononuclear cells/mL.
11. Using a white cell pipette and hemacytometer, count the cells in the four corner square of the chamber and multiply by 20 for total mononuclear cells harvested per mL.

12. Compare the total cell yield per mL to the calculated absolute number of mononuclear cells. A yield of at least 70% is expected with LSM techniques. A smaller yield may result in irregular numbers of various cell types.

JONDAL ASSAY.

1. Adjust the mononuclear cell suspensions to 12 × 10⁶ cells/mL using HBSS. Most commonly, adjustment in cell concentration is performed by adding an appropriate amount of the indicated diluent. However, if suspensions need to be more concentrated, the packed cells may be centrifuged and resuspended in a smaller amount of diluent.

2. Pipette 0.2 mL of the 12×10^6 cell/mL suspension in a test tube. Add 0.4 mL of HBSS. Mix and transfer 0.25 mL to a conical centrifuge tube.

3. Wash approximately 3 mL of sheep red blood cells three times in 0.9% saline, 0.5% suspensions, to a total volume of 5 mL.

4. Mix sheep red blood cells and mononuclear cell suspension. Add 0.25 mL 0.5% sheep red blood cells to the 0.25 mL of 4×10^6 mononuclear cells/mL.

5. Incubate for 5 minutes at 37°C.

6. Centrifuge each tube for 5 minutes at 200 × g.

7. Refrigerate on ice for 1 to 2 hours.

8. Discard approximately half the supernate from the tube. Gently suspend the cells in the remaining fluid and fill a counting chamber. Read using a high dry lens, counting a total of 200 cells, and record the percent of cells rosetting. Three or more red blood cells attached to a mononuclear cell is considered a rosette-forming cell (RFC).

CALCULATIONS

$$\text{T cells (\%)} = \frac{\text{no. in rosettes}}{\text{no. in rosettes} + \text{no. not in rosettes}}$$

REPORTING RESULTS

Adult normal range= 52%-81%

PROCEDURE NOTES

SOURCES OF ERROR. Cold reacting antilymphocyte antibodies, e.g., rheumatoid arthritis, systemic lupus erythematosus, Sjogren's syndrome, and infectious mononucleosis are known to cause inaccurate readings in the E rosette assay, notably inhibition of rosetting during the short (1-hour) incubation.

CLINICAL APPLICATIONS. The procedure is useful in the identification and quantitation of mature T lymphocytes.

LIMITATIONS. Sheep erythrocyte rosette assay labels virtually all of the T lymphocytes in a mononuclear layer and almost no other cells. A <10% variation of E rosettes should be seen. With the Jondal method rosetting occurs only with active cells.

DISORDERS WITH IMMUNOLOGIC ORIGINS

A breakdown in any part of the immune mechanism can lead to disease. These disorders can involve stem cells, phagocytosis (see Chapter 3), T cells, B cells, or complement (see Chapter 5). Immunologic disorders can be divided into primary (dysfunction in the immune organ itself) and acquired or secondary (disease or therapy causing an immune defect) processes. A third category, diseases mediated through immune mechanisms, can also be included. In this section examples and general characteristics of immunodeficiency disorders are discussed. Because of its complexity and contemporary importance, the acquired immunodeficiency syndrome, AIDS, is discussed in detail in a separate chapter (see Chapter 22). Other immune disorders such as immunoproliferative and autoimmune disorders are presented in detail in later chapters of this book.

Immune Disorders

Immune deficiency disorders may be caused by defects in the quality (defects) or quantity (deficiencies) of lymphocytes and may be congenital or acquired. These conditions may be combined disorders or either T or B cell disorders (Table 4-4).

TABLE 4-4

Examples of T and B Cell Disorders

T cell disorder	B cell disorder
Congenital	
Thymic hypoplasia (DiGeorge's syndrome)	Bruton's agammaglobulinemia
Acquired	
Acquired immune deficiency syndrome (AIDS)	Autoimmune disorders
Hodgkin's disease	Multiple myeloma
Chronic lymphocytic leukemia	
Systemic lupus erythematosus	

Primary Immune Disorders

Diseases associated with a primary defect (Table 4-5) in the immune response are composed of 40% T cell disorders, 50% B cell disorders, 6% phagocytic abnormalities, and 4% complement alterations (Fig. 4-15). The most common T cell deficiency states are those associated with a concurrent B cell abnormality. Primary immunodeficiency disorders are predominantly seen (75%) in children under 5 years.

Severe Combined Immunodeficiency (SCID)

Etiology

SCID is caused by inappropriate development of stem cells into lymphocyte precursors. This hereditary and invariably fatal disorder in infants results from the lack of both T and B cells and the consequent inability to synthesize antibody. Two modes of inheritance are known: autosomal and X-linked recessive, which accounts for the 3:1 ratio of males to females with the disorder.

Half the patients with autosomal SCID have a concomitant deficiency of adenosine deaminase, an aminylhydrolase that converts adenosine to inosine. Analysis by cDNA probe has revealed that the deficiency results from a hereditable point mutation in the adenosine deaminase gene. Another variant with a severe deficiency in T cell immunity but normal B cell concentrations is associated with purine nucleotiside phosphorylase deficiency.

A less common cause of SCID is *bare lymphocyte syndrome.* This is a variable disorder in which class I HLA antigens and sometimes class II antigens are not expressed on lymphocyte surfaces, and patient lymphocytes cannot be typed by standard serologic cytotoxicity tests.

Signs and Symptoms

No important differences in signs and symptoms exist between the two major genetic types of SCID. Initial manifestations of SCID are repeated debilitating infections beginning the first 6 months of life. These infections are dominated by bacterial, viral, and fungal infections of the respiratory and intestinal systems and skin. Infants with SCID usually die within 2 years of birth from lung abscesses, pneumocystis pneumonitis, or a common viral disorder such as chickenpox or measles.

Immunologic Manifestations

The bone marrow is devoid of lymphoblasts, lymphocytes, and plasma cells. Lymphocytes are also absent from lymphoid tissues such as the spleen, tonsils, appendix, and intestinal tract. Lymphocytopenia is detectable early in infancy. The circulating blood contains no OKT4, OKT8, or OKT3 cells.

Three major phenotypes of severe combined immunodeficient disease have been recognized:

1. Patients with lymphocytes that mature to the level of early thymocyte antigen expression

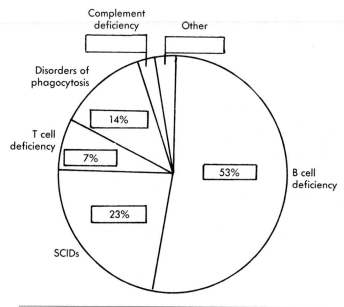

FIGURE 4-15
Distribution of immunodeficiencies.

TABLE 4-5

Primary Immunodeficiency Disease

T cells	B cells
Combined immunodeficiency	***Selective IgA deficiency associated with***
Thymic alymphophasia	Normal state
Swiss type	Allergy
Adenosine deaminase deficiency	Autoimmune disease
Nezelof syndrome	CNS disease
DiGeorge's syndrome (thymic hypoplasia)	GI disorders
Wiskott-Aldrich syndrome	Malignancy
Chronic mucocutaneous candidiasis	Pulmonary infections
Immunodeficiency associated with nucleoside phosphorylase deficiency	X-linked infantile agammaglobulinemia
Short-limbed dwarfism	X-linked immunodeficiency with hyper-IgM
Ataxia telangiectasia	Common variable hypogammaglobulinemia
Thymoma	Selective IgM deficiency
	IgG subclass deficiency

From Graziano FM and Bell CL: The normal immune response and what can go wrong. Corman LC and Katz P, editors: The medical clinics of North America, Symposium on Clinical Immunology I 69(3):445, May 1985, Philadelphia, WB Saunders Co.

(OKT10 antigen exclusively). This type of case would be described as the classic Swiss-type, severe combined immunodeficiency disease.

2. Patients who have both OKT9 and OKT10 on the surface of their peripheral blood lymphocytes.
3. Patients in the third type have more advanced thymocyte development with expression of the more mature OKT3, OKT4, OKT5, OKT8, and OKT10 surface antigens. This group would be considered as having impaired maturation at the stage III level of primary development.

Primary T Cell Deficiencies
DiGeorge's Syndrome

Etiology. DiGeorge's syndrome is a nongenetic, congenital anomaly that represents faulty embryogenesis of the endodermal derivation of the third and fourth pharyngeal pouches, which results in aplasia of the parathyroid and thymus glands. Upon autopsy, parathyroid and a vestigial thymus may be found in ectopic locations. The newborn infant may exhibit an assortment of facial and vascular anomalies. These combined abnormalities are collectively referred to as *pharyngeal pouch syndrome*. In addition to the established embryonic cause of the disorder, a question of a nutrient (zinc) deficiency in utero has been suggested as a cause.

Signs and symptoms. DiGeorge's syndrome is present at birth. Initial manifestations can include hypocalcemic tetany, unusual facies, and congenital heart defects. An increased susceptibility to viral, fungal, and disseminated bacterial infections such as acid-fast bacilli, *Listeria monocytogenes*, and *P. carinii* from the defect of T cells that is normally controlled by cell-mediated immunity. Infants usually die of sepsis during their first year.

Immunologic manifestations. Peripheral lymphoid tissue appears to be normal except for depletion of T cells in the thymus-dependent zones such as the subcortical region of the lymph nodes and the perifollicular and periartereolar lymphoid sheaths of the spleen.

In the circulating blood, lymphopenia is generally present. In some cases, however, the concentration of lymphocytes is normal. The total number of OKT10 cells is usually normal; however, an abnormally high OKT4:OKT8 ratio is due to a decrease in OKT8 cells. Most patients with DiGeorge's syndrome have a decreased percentage of cells expressing the OKT3 (mature T cell) antigen. Because patients do demonstrate lymphocytes that are capable of differentiating to the more mature surface markers, such as T4, a small rudimentary thymus is believed to be present in these patients. Blood lymphocytes, however, do not grow in vitro culture, and they are unresponsive to antigenic and mitogenic stimulation.

Serum immunoglobulin concentrations are normal. Antibody response to primary antigenic stimulation, therefore, may be unimpaired. Cell-mediated immune reactions, however, such as delayed hypersensitivity and skin allograft rejection are absent or feeble.

Hereditary Ataxis Telangiectasia

Etiology. Hereditary ataxis telangiectasia is an autosomal recessive disorder that apparently results from the coexistence of a T cell deficiency with a defect in DNA repair, which leads to extreme nonrandom chromosome instability.

Signs and symptoms. Ataxis telangiectasia is characterized by ataxis and choreoathetosis in infancy. Multiple telangiectasia appears on exposed oculocutaneous surfaces during childhood. A high incidence of malignancy, such as lymphoma, is also displayed. Children with this disorder eventually die of respiratory insufficiency and sepsis.

Immunologic manifestations. The thymus is hypoplastic or dysplastic, and the thymus-dependent zones of the lymph nodes are void of cells. About 80% of patients lack serum and secretory IgA, and some develop IgG antibodies to injections of IgA. The signs and symptoms of the disease appear to result from a concomitant T cell deficiency, a deficiency of DNA repair, and disordered IgG synthesis.

Chronic Mucocutaneous Candidiasis (CMC)

Etiology. This disorder results from a primary defect in cell-mediated immunity. T cells specifically fail to recognize only the *Candida* antigen.

Signs and symptoms. Patients with CMC usually survive to adulthood. The manifestation of the disorder is *Candida* infection of mucous membranes and the scalp, skin, and nails. Endocrine abnormalities, often polyendocrinopathies, are frequently associated with fungal manifestation. Sudden death from adrenal insufficiency has been reported in patients with CMC.

Immunologic manifestations. Patients suffering from this disorder demonstrate normal skin reactions to testing to all antigens except *Candida*.

Primary B Cell Deficiencies

Because the primary function of B cells is to produce antibody, the major clinical manifestation of a B cell deficiency is an increased susceptibility to severe bacterial infections. Selective IgA deficiency is the most common B cell disorder occurring in 1 of every 400 to 800 persons. Because IgA is the primary immunoglobulin in secretions, a lack of it contributes to pulmonary infections, gastrointestinal disorders, and allergic respiratory disorders. The majority (50%) of reported cases are associated with immunoglobulin deficiencies and are autoimmune in nature, such as rheumatoid arthritis, SLE, thyroiditis, and pernicious anemia.

Bruton's X-Linked Agammaglobulinemia

Etiology. Although it has been questioned whether a functional T cell defect may have been responsible for the lack of B cell development in Bruton's X-linked agammaglobulinemia, the cause is generally believed to result from an isolated B cell deficiency that reflects a failure to translocate the V_H region in gene production during early B cell differentiation. The defective LSA gene has been mapped to the Xq21.3-Xq22 location. This disorder occurs primarily in young boys, but scattered occasional cases have been identified in girls.

Signs and symptoms. Manifestations of this disorder begin in the first or second year of life. Hypersusceptibility to infection does not develop until 9 to 12 months after birth because of passive protection by residual maternal immunoglobulin. This disorder is characterized by sinopulmonary and central nervous system infectious episodes and severe septicemia, but patients are not abnormally susceptible to common viral infection, excluding fulminant hepatitis or to enterocci or most gram-negative organisms. An autoimmune phenomenon, especially a juvenile rheumatoid arthritis-type disease, has also been associated with X-linked agammaglobulinemia. In addition, patients are highly vulnerable to a malignant form of dermatomyositis that eventually involves destructive T cell infiltration surrounding the small vessels of the central nervous system. In addition to infections and connective tissue disorders, agammaglobulinemic patients also suffer from hemolytic anemia, drug eruptions, atopic eczema, allergic rhinitis, and asthma.

Immunologic manifestations. B cells are virtually absent from bone marrow and lymphoid tissues. A deficiency or absence of peripheral blood B lymphocytes is usually noted in this disorder. If B cells are present, they are unresponsive to T cells and incapable of antibody synthesis or secretion. Patients do, however, have normal numbers of OKT3 and OKT8 cells, and many have normal OKT4 cells. Surface immunoglobulins (sIg) however are absent. Male children possess normal T cell function, therefore, homograft rejection mechanisms are intact, and delayed hypersensitivity reaction for both tuberculin and skin contact types can be elicited.

Common Variable Hypogammaglobulinemia

Etiology. Common variable hypogammaglobulinemia is a form of primary acquired agammaglobulinemia occurring equally in males and females. The etiology of this disease seems to be heterogeneous, with abnormalities of B cell maturation, antibody production, antibody secretion, or T cell regulation involved. There is a lack of evidence of genetic transmission, although family clusters have been reported in which relatives have a high incidence of hyperimmune disorders such as systemic lupus erythematosus.

Signs and symptoms. This disorder usually manifests itself in the second or third decade of life. The signs and symptoms include frequent sinopulmonary infections, diarrhea, endocrine and autoimmune disorders, and malabsorption difficulties such as malabsorption of vitamin B_{12}. Intestinal giardiasis is also prevalent.

Immunologic manifestations. Although both the concentration and function of antibodies are usually compromised and some patients with an isolated IgG subclass deficiency have been observed, the number of B cells is usually normal or mildly depressed. The primary defect in immunoglobulin synthesis is caused by the absence or dysfunction of OKT4 cells or by increased OKT8 suppressor cell activity. Therefore, cellular immunity and immunoglobulin production are both markedly impaired by the interaction between helper and suppressor T cell subsets. Lymph nodes lack plasma cells, but these nodes may show striking follicular hyperplasia.

The total IgG level may be normal but a subclass of the immunoglobulin (usually IgG_2 or IgG_3) is deficient. Both IgA and IgM may be detectable, but IgM levels may be elevated.

In addition, some patients may suffer from thymoma and refractory anemia.

Wiskott-Aldrich Syndrome

Etiology. The primary defect in this uncommon pediatric disease stems from a specific inability to respond to polysaccharide antigens. An immunodeficiency and poor humoral immune response to bacterial polysaccharide antigen result.

Signs and symptoms. Wiskott-Aldrich syndrome is characterized by the triad of megakaryocytic thrombocytopenic purpura, increased susceptibility to infection, and eczema. Afflicted boys rarely survive past 10 years. Thrombocytopenia and bleeding are common. Death usually results from sepsis, hemorrhage, or malignancy.

Immunologic manifestations. In this disorder, a progressive deterioration of the thymus leading to a defect in cellular immunity and the attrition of T cell populations from the lymph nodes and spleen takes place. Decreased numbers of T cells and alteration in the normal T4:T8 ratio of lymphocytes are manifested. Serum levels of IgM are low, but IgG concentration is usually normal. IgA levels are normal or elevated, and IgE levels are usually elevated.

Secondary Immunodeficiencies

A secondary immunodeficiency can result from a disease process (see box) that causes a defect in normal immune function, which leads to a temporary or permanent impairment of one or multiple components of immunity in the host. Patients with secondary immunodeficiencies, which are much more common than primary deficiencies, have an increased susceptibility to infections, as is seen in the primary immunodeficiencies.

Immunosuppressive agents and burns are major causes of secondary immunodeficiencies. Immunosuppressive agents have been demonstrated to affect, in varying degrees, every component of the

Secondary Immunodeficiencies

Hematologic lymphoproliferative disorders

Hodgkin's disease and lymphoma
Leukemia
Myeloma, macroglobulinemia
Agranulocytosis and aplastic anemia
Sickle cell disease

Other systemic processes and metabolic disorders

Nephrotic syndrome
Protein-losing enteropathy
Diabetes mellitus
Malnutrition
Hepatic disease
Uremia
Aging

Viral infections

Acquired immunodeficiency syndrome (AIDS)

Surgical procedures and trauma

Splenectomy
Burns

Immunosuppressive agents

Antimetabolites
Corticosteroids
Radiation

From Graziano FM and Bell CL: The normal immune response and what can go wrong. Corman LC and Katz P, editors: The medical clinics of North America, Symposium on Clinical Immunology I 69(3):449, May 1985, Philadelphia, WB Saunders Co.

immune response. In burn patients, septicemia is a common complication in those who survive the initial period of hemodynamic shock. The mechanism that seems most critical in thermal injury is disruption of the skin; however, interference with phagocytosis and deficiencies of serum immunoglobulin and complement levels have also been observed.

Immune-Mediated Disease

The immune system is normally efficient in eliminating foreign antigens. The nature of the antigen or the genetic makeup of the host, however, can cause alterations of the immune response that can be injurious and lead to immune-mediated disease (see box above, right). In these disorders, the immune response is normal but the reactivity is heightened, prolonged or inappropriate.

Of major concern are allergic reactions (see Chapter 23), characterized by an immediate response upon exposure to an offending antigen and the release of mediators, e.g., histamine, leukotrienes, and prostaglandins capable of initiating signs and symptoms. Although allergic reactions are associated with IgE, not all allergic reactions are IgE-mediated. Complement activation by immune

Immune-Mediated Diseases

Allergic hypersensitivity:	Foods
	Drugs
	Aeroallergens (dust, pollens, molds)
	Stinging insects
Contact hypersensitivity:	Poison ivy
	Nickel
	Cosmetics
Transfusion reactions	
Autoimmune disease:	Systemic lupus erythematosus
	Rheumatoid arthritis
	Vasculitis syndromes
	Hemolytic anemia
	Idiopathic thrombocytopenia
	Pernicious anemia
	Goodpasture's disease
	Myasthenia gravis
	Graves' disease

complexes or via the alternative complement pathway has been shown to release complement C3a and C5a anaphylatoxins capable of producing similar reactions.

Autoimmune disease (see Chapter 25) is thought to be caused by antibody or T cell sensitization with autologous "self" antigens. Several of the postulated mechanisms of this process include:

1. Altered antigen or neoantigen. Such antigens may be created by chemical, physical, or biologic processes. Hemolytic anemia caused by a drug interaction is an example of this process occurring in red blood cells.
2. Shared or cross-reactive antigens. Evidence suggests that poststreptococcal disease occurs through this mechanism.

Chapter Review

HIGHLIGHTS

Lymphocytes represent the cellular components of the specific system of body defense. These cells function in either cell-mediated immunity or humoral immunity. Although cell-mediated and humoral immunity are not entirely independent and are frequently cooperative, they can be discussed as distinct systems.

The primary lymphoid organs in mammals are the bone marrow (and/or fetal liver) and thymus. Stem cells that migrate to the thymus proliferate and differentiate under the influence of the humoral factor, thymosin. These lymphocyte precursors with acquired surface membrane antigens are referred to as thymocytes. It is believed that the bone marrow and gut-associated lymphoid tissue (GALT) may also play a role in the differentiation of stem cells into B lymphocyte functions as the bursal equivalent in humans. The secondary lymphoid tissues include the lymph nodes, spleen, and Peyer's patches in the intestine. Proliferation of the T and B lymphocytes in the secondary or peripheral lymphoid tissues is primarily dependent on antigenic stimulation. Lymphocytes display a great diversity of biologic and chemical properties such as size, density, charge, surface structure, and function. Several major categories of lymphocytes are recognized by the presence of cell surface membrane markers. These categories are the T cells, B cells, the natural killer (NK) and K-type lymphocytes. Soluble mediators are secreted by monocytes, lymphocytes, or neutrophils providing the language for cell-to-cell communication. Some of the most important soluble mediators are migration inhibition factor, interleukin 2 (T cell growth factor), chemotactic factors, and interleukin 1. Except for inconsistent values seen in extremely elderly persons, the total number of T cells in the peripheral blood is relatively stable throughout adult life. There is, however, a change in the distribution of T-cell subpopulations. A decrease in the number of suppressor cells and an increase in the helper cell population are demonstrated in the elderly. The effect of aging on the immune response is highly variable but the ability to respond immunologically to disease is age-related.

The function of plasma cells is the synthesis and excretion of immunoglobulins. Plasma cells are not normally found in the circulating blood but in the bone marrow in concentrations not normally exceeding 2%. Two well-established pathways of plasma cell development have been documented. Some plasma cells arise from immature plasma cells; others arise as the end stage of B cell differentiation into a large, activated plasma cell.

The introduction of monoclonal antibody testing led to the present identification of surface membrane markers. Monoclonal antibodies to cell surface antigens now provide a method for classifying and identifying specific cellular membrane characteristics. Separate subsets of T cells have been recognized with monoclonal antibodies. T cells are divided into two subsets: the suppressor/cytotoxic subset and the helper/inducer subset. During T cell development, associated membrane antigens vary. In humans, there is evidence of the existence of four types of B cell markers: immunoglobulin (Ig) receptor; an Fc receptor; receptors that bind fragments of the cleaved complement component, C3; and B cell surface antigens coded by the class II genes of the major histocompatibility complex (MHC). The best studied B cell surface marker is the immunoglobulin (Ig) receptor. This receptor is actually an antibody molecule with antigenic specificity. Although NK cells have long been classified as null cells, monoclonal antibodies demonstrate that NK cells share a variety of surface membrane markers with T cells. Some surface membrane markers that are associated with monocytes, granulocytes, or B cells, are also demonstrable.

T cells respond to antigen by dividing and are responsible for delayed hypersensitivity, graft rejection, bacterial and viral killing, and elimination by direct cytotoxic effects or by release of soluble mediators. Deficiencies of cell-mediated immunity are often suspected in individuals with recurrent viral, fungal, parasitic, and protozoan infections. Patients with AIDS exhibit some of the most severe manifestations of cell-mediated immunity. The number of T lymphocytes, the primary effector cell in cell-mediated reactions, can be determined by a number of different techniques. The "gold standard" has previously been the E rosette technique. Development of monoclonal antibodies, however, has permitted a quick and specific method for determining the number of T cells. The method of testing is by use of immunofluorescent techniques in which the fluorescent microscope or fluorescence-activated cell sorter (FACS) is used. Additional testing can include functional testing or the measurement of biologic response modifiers, such as interleukin 2 using bioassay and radioimmunoassay.

The humoral system can be screened for abnormalities by quantitating the concentration of IgM, IgG, and IgA. Serum protein electrophoresis, however, may not be sensitive enough to detect selective Ig class deficiencies. IgD and IgE are not useful in the determination of a suspected humoral deficiency. The number of B lymphocytes in the peripheral blood and lymphoid organs can be determined by several different techniques. The most common procedure involves the detection of surface Ig (sIg).

A breakdown in any part of the immune mechanism can lead to disease. These disorders can involve stem cells, phagocytosis, T cells, B cells, or complement. Immunologic disorders can be divided into primary acquired, and those mediated through immune mechanisms. Immune deficiency disorders may be caused by defects in the quality or quantity of lymphocytes and may be congenital or acquired. These conditions may be combined disorders or either T or B cell disorders. Diseases associated with a primary defect in the immune response are composed of 40% T cell disorders, 50% B cell disorders, 6% phagocytic abnormalities, and 4% complement alterations. The most common T cell deficiency states are those associated with a concurrent B cell abnormality. Primary immunodeficiency disorders are predominantly seen in children under the age of 5. Primary immune disorders include severe combined immunodeficiency hereditary ataxis telangiectasia, chronic mucocutaneous candidiasis, Bruton's X-linked agammaglobulinemia, common variable hypogammaglobulinemia, and Wiskott-Aldrich syndrome.

REVIEW QUESTIONS

1. A function of the cell-mediated immune response that is not associated with humoral immunity is:
   A. Defense against viral and bacterial infection
   B. Initiation of rejection of foreign tissues and tumors
   C. Defense against fungal and bacterial infection
   D. Antibody production
   E. Both B and C

2. The primary or central lymphoid organs in humans are the:
   A. Bursa of Fabricius and thymus
   B. lymph nodes and thymus
   C. bone marrow and thymus
   D. lymph nodes and spleen
   E. lymph nodes and Peyer's patches

3. All of the following are a function of T cells except:
   A. mediation of delayed hypersensitivity reactions
   B. mediation of cytolytic reactions
   C. regulation of the immune response
   D. synthesis of antibody
   E. defense against intracellular pathogens

Questions 4-7.
Match the type of lymphocyte with its function (use an answer only once).
4. T cells
5. B cells
6. K-type lymphocytes
7. natural killer (NK)
   A. antibody dependent cell-mediated cytotoxicity reaction (ADCC)
   B. cellular immune response
   C. cytotoxic reaction
   D. humoral response
   E. phagocytosis

Questions 8-10.
Match the surface membrane marker with the appropriate normal T cell type.
8. CD 4
9. CD 8
10. CD3
    A. All or most T lymphocytes
    B. Helper-inducer T cells
    C. Suppressor-cytotoxic T cells

Questions 11-14.
11. Decreased helper cells
12. Increased helper cells
13. Decreased suppressor cells
14. Increased suppressor cells
    A. Kawasaki's disease
    B. Infectious mononucleosis
    C. Acquired immunodeficiency syndrome
    D. Acute graft versus host disease

15. All of the following are B cell surface membrane markers except:
    A. sIg
    B. Fc receptor
    C. C3 receptor
    D. CD 4
    E. antigens coded by class II genes

Questions 16-19.
Match the following techniques with the appropriate type of lymphocyte identified.
16. Rosette formation with E receptors with sheep erythrocytes

17. Rosette formation with bovine erythrocytes
18. Detection of receptor sites for the FC portion of IgG
19. Detection of receptor sites for complement

Questions 20-25.
Match the following congenital or acquired disorders with the major type of lymphocyte affected.
20. Thymic hypoplasia
21. AIDS
22. Chronic lymphocytic leukemia
23. Systemic lupus erythematosus
24. Multiple myeloma
25. Bruton's agammaglobulinemia
    A. Congenital T cell disorder
    B. Congenital B cell disorder
    C. Acquired T cell disorder
    D. Acquired B cell disorder

26. The majority of diseases associated with a primary defect are _____ disorders.
    A. T cell
    B. B cell
    C. complement
    D. phagocytic
    E. T cell disorders associated with a concurrent B cell abnormality

27. Severe combined immunodeficiency is caused by:
    A. T cell depletion
    B. B cell depletion
    C. inappropriate development of stem cells
    D. phagocytic dysfunction
    E. complement deficiency

28. DiGeorge's syndrome is caused by:
    A. faulty embryogenesis
    B. deficiency of calcium *in utero*
    C. inappropriate stem cell development
    D. an autosomal recessive disorder
    E. a sex-linked chromosomal disorder

29. The major clinical manifestation of a B cell deficiency is:
    A. impaired phagocytosis
    B. diminished complement levels
    C. increased susceptibility to bacterial infections
    D. increased susceptibility to parasitic infections
    E. lymphadenopathy

30. Bruton's agammaglobulinemia is:
    A. an acquired disorder
    B. an autosomal genetic disorder
    C. a sex-linked genetic disorder
    D. a disorder occurring primarily in young females
    E. Both C and D

31. Which of the following disorders does not result in a secondary immunodeficiency?
    A. Sickle cell disease
    B. Uremia
    C. AIDS
    D. Poison-ivy hypersensitivity
    E. Corticosteroid or antimetabolite therapy

Answers

1. B 2. C 3. D 4. B 5. D 6. A 7. C 8. B 9. C 10. A
11. C 12. A 13. D 14. B 15. D 16. A 17. B 18. B 19. B
20. A 21. C 22. C 23. C 24. D 25. B 26. B 27. C 28. A
29. C 30. C 31. D

BIBLIOGRAPHY

Barrett J: Textbook of immunology, St Louis, 1988, The CV Mosby Co.

Bellanti JA: Immunology: basic processes, Philadelphia, 1979, WB Saunders Co.

Busby J and Caranasos GJ: Immune function, autoimmunity, and selective immunoprophylaxis, Med Clin of North Amer 69(3):465-470, May 1985.

Cooper MD and Lawton AR: The development of the immune System, Scientific American, pp 59-70, Nov 1974.

Graziano FM and Bell CL: The normal immune response and what can go wrong. In Corman LC and Katz P, editors: The medical clinics of North America, Symposium on Clinical Immunology I 69(3):449, May 1985, Philadelphia, WB Saunders Co.

Henry JB, editor: Clinical diagnosis and management, 1982, Philadelphia, WB Saunders Co.

Jandl JA: Lymphocytes and plasma cells. In Blood, pp 540-548, Boston, 1988, Little, Brown & Co.

Katz P: Clinical and laboratory evaluation of the immune system, Med Clin North Am 69(3):453-459, May 1985.

Lawlor GJ and Fischer TJ: Manual of allergy and immunology, ed 2, p 9, Boston, 1988, Little, Brown & Co.

Lovett EJ and others: Applications of flow cytometry to diagnostic pathology, Lab Invest 50(2):115-140, 1984.

Peacock JA and Tomar RH: Manual of laboratory immunology, Philadelphia 1980, Lea & Febiger.

Turgeon ML: Clinical hematology, Boston 1988, Little, Brown & Co.

Turgeon ML: Fundamentals of immunohematology, Philadelphia, 1989, Lea & Febiger.

Young M and Raif SG: Human regulatory T-cell subsets, Ann Rev Med 37:165-72, 1986.

The Complement System

The complement system is a heat-labile series of 18 plasma proteins, many of which are enzymes or *proteinases.* Collectively these proteins are a major fraction of the beta 1 and beta 2 globulins. Complement plays a major role in the immune system as a potent mediator of inflammation. It is composed of two interrelated enzyme cascades, the *classic* and *alternative pathways.* Proteins of the classic activation pathway and the terminal sequence are called *components* and are symbolized by the letter *C* followed by a number, for example, *C4.* Proteins of the alternative activation pathway are called *factors* and are symbolized by letters such as *B.* Control proteins include the inhibitor of C1 (C1 INH), the C4b/C3b inactivator (now called factor I), and (beta) 1H globulin (now called factor H).

ACTIVATION OF COMPLEMENT

Normally, complement components are present in the circulation in an inactive form. In addition, the control proteins C1 INH, factor I, factor H, and C4-bp (C4 binding protein) are normally present to inhibit uncontrolled complement activation.

The classic pathway (Fig. 5-1) is initiated by the complexing of antigen to its specific antibody, either IgG or IgM, and is the primary amplifier of the biologic effects of humoral immunity. The alternative pathway is activated by contact with a foreign surface, such as the polysaccharide coating of a microorganism, and amplifies nonimmune defense against microbial infection and other biologic alterations. It is probable that under normal physiologic conditions, the activation of one pathway also leads to the activation of the other. Either of the two routes leads to a common final pathway. Both pathways convert C3 to C3b, the central event of the common final pathway, which in turn leads to the activation of the lytic complement sequence, C5-C9, and cell destruction. A third set of plasma proteins that function as membrane attack complexes becomes assembled into the structures responsible for lytic lesions in the lipid bilayer of the cell membrane and disrupts membrane integrity.

Once complement is initially activated, each enzyme precursor is activated by the previous complement component or complex, which is a highly specialized proteinase. This converts the enzyme precursor to its catalytically active form by limited proteolysis. During this activation process, a small peptide fragment is cleaved, a membrane binding site is exposed, and the major fragment binds. As a consequence, the next active enzyme of the sequence is formed. Because each enzyme can activate many enzyme precursors, each step is amplified; therefore, the whole system forms an *amplifying cascade.*

COMPLEMENT RECEPTORS

A variety of cell types express surface membrane glycoproteins that react with one or more of the fragments of C3 produced during complement activation and degradation. The functions of these receptors (Table 5-1) depend on the type of cell manifesting them and are, in many instances, incompletely understood. The complement receptor 1

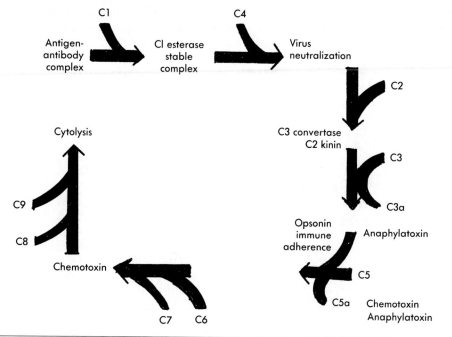

FIGURE 5-1

Complement activation sequence.
(With permission from Turgeon ML: Fundamentals of immunohematology, Philadelphia, 1989, Lea & Febiger.)

TABLE 5-1

Receptors for C_3 Fragments

Receptor name	Specificity	Cellular Distribution
CR1	C3b, (1C3b)	Erythrocytes, granulocytes, monocytes, B cells, glomerular visceral epithelial cells, dendritic cells
CR2	C3dg, (C3d)	B cells
CR3	1C3b	Monocytes, granulocytes, natural killer cells

From Stein J: Internal medicine, ed 2, Boston, 1987, Little, Brown & Co.

(CR1) is important in enhancing phagocytosis. CR1 is the only receptor on human erythrocytes and serves as a cofactor in the cleavage of C3b to iC3b by factor I. CR2 may have an effect on lymphocytes in their response to mitogens or antigen stimulation. CR3 is known to be important in host defense mechanisms such as phagocytosis.

EFFECTS OF COMPLEMENT ACTIVATION

The activation of complement and the products formed during the complement cascade have a variety of physiologic and cellular consequences. Physiologic consequences include blood vessel dilation and increased vascular permeability. The cellular consequences include:

1. Cell activation, such as the production of inflammatory mediators.
2. Cytolysis or hemolysis, if the cells are erythrocytes. The most important biologic role of complement in blood group serology is the production of cell membrane lysis of antibody-coated targets.
3. Opsonization, which renders cells vulnerable to phagocytosis.

In addition to complement's function as a major effector of antigen-antibody interaction, physiologic concentrations of complement have been found to induce profound alteration in the molecular weight, composition, and solubility of immune complexes.

The activation of complement may also play a role in mediating hypersensitivity reactions. This process may occur either from direct alternative pathway activation by IgE-antigen complexes or through a sequence initiated by the activated Hageman coagulation factor that causes the generation of plasmin, which subsequently activates the classic pathway. In either case, activation of complement components from C3 onward leads to the generation of the anaphylatoxins in an immediate hypersensitivity reaction.

CLASSIC PATHWAY

The principal components of the classic pathway are C1 through C9. The sequence of component activation does not follow the expected numerical order. The sequence is C1, 4, 2, 3, 5, 6, 7, 8, and 9.

C3 is present in the plasma in the largest quantities; fixation of C3 is the major quantitative reaction of the complement cascade. Although the principal source of synthesis of complement in vivo is debatable, the majority of the plasma complement components are made in *hepatic parenchymal* cells, except for C1 (a calcium-dependent complex of three glycoproteins C1q, C1r, and C1s), which is primarily synthesized in the epithelium of the gastrointestinal and urogenital tracts.

The classic pathway is composed of three stages:
1. Recognition
2. Enzymatic activation
3. Membrane attack leading to cellular destruction

Fixation of the C_1 Complex

The recognition unit of the complement system is the C_1 complex: C_{1q}, C_{1r}, and C_{1s}, an interlocking enzyme system. The C_1 complex is a unique feature of the classic pathway leading to C_3 conversion. C_1 fixation occurs when the C_{1q} subcomponent binds directly to an immunoglobulin molecule. The other two subcomponents, C_{1r} and C_{1s}, do not bind to the immunoglobulin but are involved in subsequent activation of the classic pathway. Whether or not C_1 fixation occurs depends on a number of factors. These conditions include:
1. Subclass of immunoglobulin. Only certain subclasses of immunoglobulin, such as IgM, and most of the IgG subclasses, can fix C_1 even under optimal conditions.
2. Spatial or configurational constraints.

A single IgM molecule is potentially able to fix C_1, but at least a pair of IgG molecules is required for this purpose. The amount of C_1 fixed is directly proportional to the concentration of IgM antibodies; however, this is not true of IgG molecules.

The C_{1q} molecule is potentially multivalent for attachment to the complement fixation sites of immunoglobulin. The structures of C1q peptide chains are formed into three subunits of six chains each. Each subunit consists of a Y-shaped pair of triple helices joined at the stem and ending in a globular head. The globular ends are assumed to be the sites for multivalent attachment to the complement-fixing sites in immune complexed immunoglobulin. The sites on the IgG molecules are on the C_H2 domains and probably on the C_H4 domain of IgM. The complement-fixing site may become exposed following complexing of the immunoglobulin, or the sites may always be available but need multiple attachments by C_{1q} with critical geometry to achieve the necessary avidity.

C_{1r} and C_{1s} are chemically similar; however, C_{1r} forms dimers, whereas C_{1s} binds monovalently to C_{1r}. C_{1r} and C_{1s} form a tetrad complex that binds to C_{1q} in the presence of Ca^{++} ion. The mechanism of C1r by C1q is unknown because C1q is not known to have enzymatic activity. However, it is known that C1r and C1s activate in sequence still attached to C1q and that both proteins become typical *serine-histidine esterases* on activation. C1s is the only substrate for C1r. C1s will activate C4 and C2, the next components in the classic complement sequence, but C1r will not.

Fixation and Activation of C_4 by the C1qrs Complex

C_{1s} splits a peptide C_{4a} from the N-terminal part of the alpha chain of the C4 component, leaving a large fragment, C4b. This reaction occurs in the fluid phase of the plasma around the C_{1s} catalytic site and a reactive internal thioester bond is revealed on C_{4b}. The stable binding of C4b molecules to membranes has less than 10% efficiency. Binding occurs in proximity to the site of activation, either to the C1qrs complex or to the adjacent erythrocyte membrane. C4b molecules that fail to bind become inactive and decay.

C_{1s} is weakly proteolytic for free intact C_2 but highly active against C2 that has complexed with C4b molecules in the presence of Mg^{++} ions. This reaction will only occur if the C4bC2 complex forms close to the C1s. The resultant C2b fragment joins with C4b to form the new C4b2b enzyme, the classic pathway C3 *convertase*. The catalytic site of the C4b2b complex is probably in the C2b peptide. A smaller, C_{2a} fragment from the C2 component is lost to the surrounding environment. The C4b2b enzyme is unstable and decays with a half-life of 5 minutes at 37° C due to the release and decay of C_{2b}.

There are two chief constraints on the activities of C1s on C4 and C2 and on the stable formation of the C4b2b complex:
1. The action of the proteinase inhibitor, C1 esterase
2. The effect of C_{3b} inactivator

C_1 esterase inhibitor binds to C_{1s} and C_{1r}. This activity may not be important in restraining the action of C1s at a local membrane site, but it is extremely important in preventing the excessive action of free C_1 on C_4 and C_2 in the fluid phase.

C3b inactivator has the ability to disintegrate membrane-bound C4b. This action destroys the acceptor site for C2, which prevents the formation of C4b2b convertase.

Action of C_{4b2b} Complex on C_3

The complement cascade reaches its full amplitude at the C3 stage, which represents the heart of the system. The C4b2b complex, referred to as classic pathway C3 convertase, activates C3 molecules by splitting the peptide, *C3 anaphylatoxin*, from the N-terminal end of the peptide of C3. This exposes a reactive binding site on the larger fragment, C3b.

Consequently, clusters of C3b molecules are activated and bound near the C4b2b complex. Each catalytic site can bind several hundred C3b molecules, even though the reaction is very inefficient because C3 is present in high concentration. Only one C3b molecule combines with C4b2b to form the final proteolytic complex of the complement cascade.

Action of C_{3b} on C5

C_{3b} splits C_{5a} from the alpha chain of C5, to initate C5b fixation and the beginning of the membrane attack complex. No further proteinases are generated in the classic complement sequence. Other bound C_{3b} molecules not involved in the C_{4b2b3b} complex form an opsonic macromolecular coat on the erythrocyte or other target, which renders it susceptible to immune adherence by C_{3b} receptors on phagocytic cells.

C_{5-9} Membrane Attack Complex

Fixation of C5b to biologic membrane is followed by the sequential addition of C6, C7, C8, and C9. When fully assembled in the correct proportions, they form the membrane attack complex. The C5bC6 complex is *hydrophilic*, but with the addition of C7 to the C567 complex, the complex has additional *detergent* and *phospholipid* binding properties as well. This occurrence of both hydrophobic and hydrophilic groups within the same complex may account for its tendency to polymerize and form small protein *micelles* (a packet of chain molecules in parallel arrangement). In free solution, uncombined C567 has a half-life of about 0.1 second. It can attach to any lipid bilayer within its effective diffusion radius, which produces the phenomenon of *reactive lysis* on innocent "bystander" cells. Once membrane bound, C567 is relatively stable and can interact with C8 and C9.

C5-8 polymerizes C9 to form a tubule, known as the *membrane attack complex*, which bridges the membrane. By complexing with C9, the cytolytic reaction is accelerated. This tubule is a hollow cylinder that has one end inserted into the lipid bilayer and the other end projecting from the membrane. Although the micellar arrangement of the membrane insertion region has not been positively established, a structure of this form can be assumed to disturb the lipid bilayer sufficiently to allow the free exchange of ions as well as water molecules across the membrane. The consequence in a living cell is that the influx of Na^+ and H_2O leads to disruption of osmotic balance, which produces cell lysis.

ALTERNATE PATHWAY

The alternate pathway shows points of similarity with the classic sequence. Both pathways generate a C3 convertase that activates C3 to provide the pivotal event in the final common pathway of both systems. However, in contrast to the classic pathway, which is initiated by the formation of antigen-antibody reactions, the alternate complement pathway is predominantly a non-antibody-initiated pathway.

Microbial and mammalian cell surfaces can activate the alternate pathway in the absence of specific antigen-antibody complexes. Factors capable of activating the alternate pathway include inulin, zymosan, a polysaccharide complex from the surface of yeast cells, bacterial polysaccharides and endotoxins, and the aggregated immunoglobulins IgG_2, IgA, and IgE. In paroxysmal nocturnal hemoglobinuria (PNH), the patient's erythrocytes act as an activator and result in the excessive lysis of the patient's erythrocytes. This nonspecific activation is a major physiologic advantage because host protection can be generated before the induction of a humoral immune response.

A key feature of the alternate pathway is that the first three proteins of the classic activation pathway—C_1, C_4, and C_2—do *not* participate in the cascade sequence. The C3A component is considered to be the counterpart of C2a in the classic pathway. C2 of the classic pathway structurally resembles factor B of the alternate pathway. The omission of C1, C4, and C2 is possible because activators of the alternate pathway catalyze the conversion of another series of normal serum proteins that lead to the activation of C3. It was previously believed that *properdin*, a normal protein of human serum, was the first protein to function in the alternate pathway; thus, the pathway was originally named after this protein.

The uptake of factor B onto C3b occurs when C3b is bound to an activator surface. However, C3b in the fluid phase or attached to a nonactivator surface will preferentially bind to factor H and so prevent C3b, B formation. C3b and factor B combine to form C3b,B, which is converted into an active C3 convertase, C3b,Bb. This results from the loss of a small fragment, Ba (a glycine-rich alpha$_2$ globulin believed to be physiologically inert), through the action of the enzyme, factor D. The C3b,Bb complex is able to convert more C3 to C3b, which binds more factor B. And so the feedback cycle continues.

The major controlling event of this pathway is factor H, which prevents the association between C3b and factor B. Factor H blocks the formation of C3b,Bb, the catalytically active C3 convertase of the feedback loop. Factor H (previously called beta$_1$H) competes with factor B for its combining site on C3b, eventually leading to C3 inactivations. Factors B and H apparently occupy a common site on C3b. The factor that is preferentially bound to C3b depends on the nature of the surface to which C3b is attached. Polysaccharides are called *activator surfaces* and favor the uptake of factor B on the chain of C3b, with the corresponding displacement of factor H. In this situation, binding of factor H is inhibited, and consequently factor B will replace H at the common binding site. When factor H is ex-

TABLE 5-2

Complement Deficiency in Humans

Complement deficiency	Associated diseases
C1q	SLE*-like syndrome; decreased secondary to agammaglobulinemia
C1r	SLE–like syndrome, dermatomyositis, vasculitis, recurrent infections and chronic glomerulonephritis, necrotizing skin lesions, arthritis
C1s	SLE, SLE–like syndrome
C1 INH	Hereditary angioedema, lupus nephritis
C2	Recurrent pyogenic infections, SLE, SLE–like syndrome, discoid lupus, membranoproliferative glomerulonephritis, dermatomyositis, synovitis, purpura, Henoch-Schönlein purpura, hypertension, Hodgkin's disease, chronic lymphocytic leukemia, dermatitis herpetiformis, polymyositis
C3	Recurrent pyogenic infections, SLE–like syndrome, arthralgias, skin rash
C3b inactivator	Recurrent pyogenic infections, urticaria
C4	SLE–like syndrome, SLE, dermatomyositis–like syndrome, vasculitis
C5	*Neisseria* infections, SLE
C5 dysfunction	Leiner's disease, gram–negative skin and bowel infection
C6	*Neisseria* infections, SLE, Raynaud's phenomenon, scleroderma–like syndrome, vasculitis
C7	*Neisseria* infections, SLE, Raynaud's phenomenon, scleroderma–like syndrome, vasculitis
C8	*Neisseria* infections, xeroderma pigmentosa, SLE-like syndrome

SLE, systemic lupus erythematosus
Adapted from Cassidy JT and Petty RE: Immunodeficiency and arthritis. In Cassidy JT ed: Textbook of pediatric rheumatology, New York, 1982, John Wiley & Sons, Inc.; Wedgewood RJ, Rosen FS, and Paul NW: Primary immunodeficiency disease, Birth Defects 19:345, 1983; and Pahwa R et al: Treatment of the immunodeficiency diseases, Springer Semin Immunopathol 1:355, 1978.

cluded, C3b is thought to be formed continuously in small amounts. Another controlling point in the amplification loop depends on the stability of the C3b,Bb convertase. Ordinarily, C3b,Bb decays due to the loss of Bb with a half-life of approximately 5 minutes. However, if properdin (P) binds to C3b,Bb, forming C3b,BbP, the half-life is extended to 30 minutes.

Diseases Associated with Hypocomplementemia

Rheumatic diseases with immune complexes
Systemic lupus erythematosus
Rheumatoid arthritis (with extraarticular disease)
Systemic vaculitis
Essential mixed cryoglobulinemia

Glomerulonephritis
Poststreptococcal
Membranoproliferative

Infectious diseases
Subacute bacterial endocarditis
Infected atrioventricular shunts
Pneumococcal sepsis
Gram-negative sepsis
Viremias, e.g., hepatitis B surface antigenemia, measles
Parasitic infections, e.g., malaria

Deficiency of control proteins
C1 inhibitor deficiency: hereditary angioedema
Factor I deficiency
Factor H deficiency

The association of numerous C3b units, factor Bb, and properdin on the surface of an aggregate of protein or the surface of a microorganism has potent activity as a C5 convertase. With the cleavage of C5, the remainder of the complement cascade continues as in the classic pathway.

ALTERATIONS IN COMPLEMENT LEVELS
Complement levels may be abnormal in certain disease states, such as rheumatoid arthritis or systemic lupus erythematous, and in some genetic disorders.

Elevated Complement Levels
Complement can be elevated in many inflammatory conditions. Increased complement levels are often associated with inflammatory conditions, trauma, or acute illness such as myocardial infarction because separate complement components, e.g., C3, are acute-phase proteins. These elevations, however, are common and nonspecific. Therefore increased levels are of limited clinical significance.

Decreased Complement Levels
Deficiencies of complement account for a small percent of primary immunodeficiencies (<2%), but depression of complement levels frequently coexists with SLE and other disorders associated with an immunopathologic process (Fig. 5-2 and the above box).

Hypocomplementemia can result from the complexing of IgG or IgM antibodies capable of activating complement. Depressed values of complement are associated with diseases that give rise to circulating immune complexes. Because of the rapid

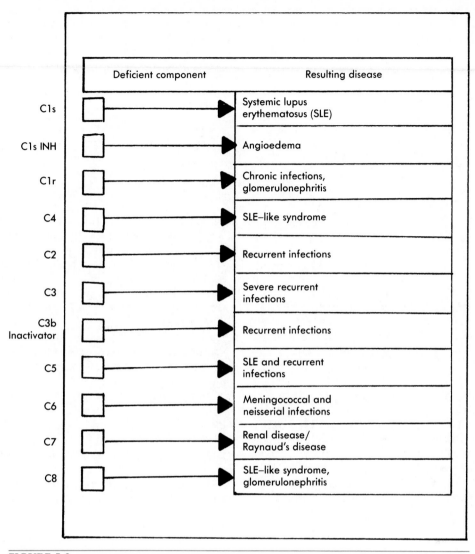

Deficient component	Resulting disease
C1s	Systemic lupus erythematosus (SLE)
C1s INH	Angioedema
C1r	Chronic infections, glomerulonephritis
C4	SLE–like syndrome
C2	Recurrent infections
C3	Severe recurrent infections
C3b Inactivator	Recurrent infections
C5	SLE and recurrent infections
C6	Meningococcal and neisserial infections
C7	Renal disease/ Raynaud's disease
C8	SLE–like syndrome, glomerulonephritis

FIGURE 5-2
Complement deficiencies.

normal turnover of the complement proteins, within 1 or 2 days of the cessation of complement activation by immune complexes, complement levels return to normal rapidly. Low levels, however, suggest the following consequences:

1. Complement has been excessively activated recently.
2. Complement is currently being consumed.
3. A single complement component is absent due to a genetic defect.

Specific component deficiencies (Table 5-2) are associated with a variety of disorders.

DIAGNOSTIC EVALUATION

During immune complex reactions, certain complement proteins become physically bound to the tissue in which the immunologic reaction is occurring. These proteins can be demonstrated in tissue by appropriate immunopathologic stains. The most frequent evaluation of complement, however, is by serum/plasma assay (Table 5-3). Complement can be assessed either by its activity in immune hemolysis or by quantitative immunoassay, i.e., radial immunoassay. These assays are useful in diagnosis and monitoring of patients.

Assessment of Complement

Procedures that can be used in diagnostic immunology include the following:

C1 Esterase Inhibitor (C1 Inhibitor)

C1 measures the activity and/or concentration of C1 inhibitor in serum. A deficiency of this protein is characteristic of hereditary angioedema (HAE). Some patients demonstrate catalytically inactive protein.

C1r, C1s, C2, C3, C4, C5, C6, C7, C8

Homozygous deficiencies predispose a patient to autoimmune disease (especially SLE) and to arthri-

TABLE 5-3

Interpretation of Complement Activation by Individual Components

Complement determination	Classic pathway	Alternative pathway	Improper specimen*	Inflammation
CH_{50}	Decreased	Decreased, normal	Decreased	Increased
C3	Decreased	Decreased	Normal	Increased
C4	Decreased	Normal	Decreased	Increased

*Results if specimen is improperly stored or too old.

tis, chronic glomerulonephritis, infections, and vasculitis. The CH_{50} assay is a good screening tool for these deficiencies.

C1q

The complement component, C1q, is evaluated in serum. Decreased levels can be demonstrated in patients suffering from hypocomplementemic urticarial vasculitis, severe combined immunodeficiency, or X-linked hypogammaglobulinemia.

C1q Binding

This procedure measures the binding of immune complexes containing IgG_1, IgG_2, or IgG_3, and/or IgM to the complement component, C1q. High values of C1q binding are associated with the presence of circulating immune complexes of the type that interact with the classic pathway of complement activation. This test can be useful as a prognostic tool at diagnosis and during remission of acute myelogenous leukemia.

C2

An extremely low level of C2 component is suggestive of a lupus-like disease that may be caused by a genetic deficiency associated with HLA-A25, B18, or DR2. Approximately half of the individuals with decreased levels of C2 have autoimmune disease; the other half are apparently normal but have an increased susceptibility to bacterial infection.

C3

Extremely decreased levels are seen in patients with poststreptococcal glomerulonephritis and in patients with inherited (C3) complement deficiency. This component is also decreased in cases of severe liver disease and in systemic lupus erythematosus patients with renal disease.

C3b Inhibitor (C3b Inactivator)

The C3b component of complement causes low complement C3 levels, the absence of C3PA in serum, and high C3b levels. A deficiency of C3b inhibitor is associated with an increased predisposition to infection.

C3PA (C3 proactivator, Properdin Factor B)

The factor B component is consumed by activation of the alternative complement pathway. As-

sessment of C3PA indicates whether a decreased level of C3 results from the classic or alternate pathways of complement activation. Decreased levels of C3 and C4 demonstrate activation of the classic pathway. Decreased levels of C3 and C3PA with a normal level of C4 indicates complement activation via the alternative pathway.

Activation of the classic pathway (and sometimes with accompanying alternative pathway activation) is associated with disorders such as immune complex diseases, various forms of vasculitis, and acute glomerulonephritis. Activation of the alternative pathway is associated with many disorders, including chronic hypocomplementemic glomerulonephritis, diffuse intravascular coagulation, septicemia, subacute bacterial endocarditis, paroxysmal nocturnal hemoglobinuria (PNH), and sickle cell anemia.

In systemic lupus erythematosus, both the classic and alternative pathways are activated.

C4

A decreased C4 level with elevated anti–DNA and ANA titers confirm the diagnosis of systemic lupus erythematosus (SLE) in a patient. In these cases of SLE, the periodic assessment of C4 can be useful in monitoring the progress of the disorder. Patients with extremely low C4 and CH_{50} levels in the presence of normal levels of the C3 component may be demonstrating the effects of a genetic deficiency of either C1 inhibitor or C4.

C4 Allotypes

The antigenically distinct forms of C4A and C4B are located on the sixth chromosome in the major histocompatibility complex. Identification of C4 allotypes in conjunction with specific HLA antigens are markers for disease susceptibility.

C5

A genetic deficiency of the C5 component is associated with increased susceptibility to bacterial infection and is expressed as an autoimmune disorder, e.g., systemic lupus erythematosus. In the case of dysfunction of C5 (Leiner's disease), the patient is predisposed to infections of the skin and bowel characterized by eczema. In these patients, the level of C5 is normal, but the C5 component fails to promote phagocytosis.

C6

A decreased quantity of C6 predisposes an individual to significant *Neisseria* (bacteria) infections.

C7

A decreased level of C7 is associated with severe bacterial infections caused by *Neisseria* species, Raynaud's phenomenon, sclerodactyly, and telangiectasia.

C8

A decreased quantity of C8 is associated with systemic lupus erythematosus. A C8 deficiency makes patients highly susceptible to *Neisseria* infections.

CH_{50}

This test assesses the hemolytic activity of the complement system, a natural protein found in the blood. Monitoring CH_{50} is useful in following the course of immune complex disease, in screening for genetic deficiencies of the complement system, and in diagnosing hereditary angioneurotic edema. Low levels confirm complement activation or in vitro degradation.

Complement decay rate. A decrease of CH_{50} activity in plasma at 37° C causes 10%-20% decay. A decay rate greater than 50% is abnormal and is consistent with but not diagnostic of C1 esterase inhibitor deficiency.

A traditional method for determination of functional complement activity is the total hemolytic (CH_{50}) assay. This assay measures the ability of a test sample to lyse 50% of a standardized suspension of sheep erythrocytes coated with anti-erythrocyte antibody. Both the classic activation pathway and the terminal complement components are measured during this reaction. Total complement activity is usually abnormal if any component is defective. Individual component abnormalities or abnormalities in the alternative pathway, however, can exist despite a normal CH_{50} value.

Acquired complement deficiencies are frequently encountered in active systemic lupus erythematosus and other autoimmune diseases, a variety of kidney and liver diseases, subacute bacterial endocarditis, cryoglobulinemia, and allograft rejection. Assaying and monitoring specific components, especially C3, C4, and C3 activator for the classic and alternate pathways, provide a valuable guide to the management of such patients. The C4 level often provides the most sensitive indicator of disease activity. C4 is destroyed only when the classic pathway is activated. Although C3 lies at the junction of the two pathways, it is much more severely depressed when activation occurs via the alternative pathway. Reduction of C3 and C4 components implies that activation of the classic pathway has been initiated.

☐ PROCEDURE

CH_{50} Total Hemolytic Complement[*]

PRINCIPLE

The CH_{50} total hemolytic complement assay measures the ability of a test sample to lyse 50% of a standardized suspension of sheep erythrocytes coated with anti-erythrocyte antibody. Antibody-coated erythrocytes are incubated with the test specimen. Activation of complement results in cell lysis and release of hemoglobin. The degree of hemolysis is proportional to the total hemolytic complement activity.

Both the classical activation pathway and the terminal complement components are measured during this reaction. Low levels of complement confirm complement activation (or degradation in vitro). Assessment of CH_{50} is useful in screening for genetic deficiencies of the complement system, in diagnosing hereditary angioneurotic edema, and in monitoring the progress of patients with immune complex disease.

SPECIMEN COLLECTION AND PREPARATION

No special preparation of the patient is required before specimen collection. The patient must be positively identified when the specimen is collected and the specimen is labeled at the bedside. Specimen labels must include the patient's full name, the date the specimen is collected, the patient's hospital identification number, and the phlebotomist's initials.

Blood should be drawn using an aseptic technique. A minimum of 2 mL of clotted blood (red top evacuated tube) is required. The specimen should be allowed to clot at room temperature and the serum should be separated by centrifugation at 4° C. The serum should be removed from the clot and kept at 4° C. Testing should be conducted *immediately* following collection and separation or the serum should be frozen at −70° C until the time of testing. Hemolysis renders a specimen unsuitable for testing.

REAGENTS, SUPPLIES, AND EQUIPMENT

The following components are supplied in the CH_{50} assay kit commercially available from Sigma Diagnostics, St. Louis, Mo.
1. Sensitized sheep red blood cells

   A standardized concentration of sheep erythrocytes coated with antisheep erythrocytes suspended in buffer, pH 7.3 with stabilizer. Sodium azide 0.02% is added as a preservative. It is stored under refrigeration (2° to 6° C). The cells are stable until the expiration date shown.

---

[*]Sigma Diagnostics Product Brochure, 1988, Sigma Chemical Co, St. Louis, Mo.

2. Reference standard CH_{50}

This is a lyophilized human serum containing a known CH_{50} value. The total hemolytic complement activity (unit/mL) is indicated on the label. Dry vials are stored in the freezer ($-20°$ C). Vial label bears expiration date.

Immediately before use, the contents of the vial are reconstituted by adding 0.3 mL deionized water and mixed gently until dissolution is complete. Within 30 minutes of reconstitution, aliquot and store any remaining solution at $-70°$ C or in liquid nitrogen. If such storage means are not available, discard contents of the vial.

Warning: Sodium azide may react with lead and copper plumbing to form highly explosive metal azides. Upon disposal, flush with a large volume of water to prevent azide buildup. Sodium azide is also toxic. Care should be taken to avoid ingestion.

ADDITIONAL REQUIRED EQUIPMENT AND SUPPLIES

1. Refrigerated centrifuge
2. Spectrophotometer and cuvettes
3. Pipetting device capable of accurately delivering 0.005 mL (5 μL)
4. Timer

QUALITY CONTROL

CH_{50} low activity control and CH_{50} high activity control (Sigma Diagnostics) should be tested with the patient specimen.

Immediately before use, reconstitute the contents of each vial by adding 0.3 mL deionized water. Mix gently until dissolution is complete. Within 30 minutes of reconstitution, aliquot and store any remaining solutions at $-70°$ C or in liquid nitrogen. If such storage means are not available, discard contents of the vials.

The reconstituted controls should be treated in the exact manner as a test specimen. The total hemolytic complement activity should be within ± 10% of the value indicated on the vials.

Caution: Because the reference standard and control sera are derived from human sources, they should be handled in the same manner as clinical serum specimens (see "Universal blood and body fluid precautions," Chapter 6).

PROCEDURE

Preliminary preparation: Allow the sensitized sheep red blood cells to warm to room temperature before use. Immediately before use, resuspend the cells by repeated inversions. Reconstitute or defrost the reference standard and controls.

1. For each test sample and control, label one tube of sheep cells. Label one tube for the reference standard and one tube "Lysis Control" (spontaneous lysis).
2. Remove the tube caps and pipette 0.005 mL (5 μL) of test sample, controls, or reference standard to the appropriately labeled tube. No sample is added to the lysis control.

3. Replace caps and mix immediately by inverting each tube two or three times.
4. Incubate the tubes at room temperature (18°-26° C) for 60 ± 5 minutes.
5. Mix the contents of all tubes again by inverting two or three times.
6. Centrifuge all tubes at approximately 600 × g for 10 minutes.
7. Transfer the supernatant fluid to a cuvette.
8. Read absorbance of the supernatants at 415 nm within 15 minutes after centrifugation. Zero the instrument using a water blank. Read and record the absorbance of the Lysis Control ($A_{control}$). Zero the instrument using the Lysis Control as a blank. Read and record the absorbance value of the Reference Standard ($A_{standard}$) and of each test specimen and the controls ($A_{specimen}$).

CALCULATIONS

The CH_{50} value of each specimen or control is calculated as follows:

$$CH_{50} \text{ value of a specimen} = \frac{A_{specimen}}{A_{standard}} \times$$

$$CH_{50} \text{ value of standard.}$$

Example:
Stated CH_{50} value of the standard = 192 units/mL
Absorbance value of $A_{specimen}$ = 1.104
Absorbance value of $A_{standard}$ = 0.901

$$CH_{50} \text{ value of a specimen} = \frac{1.104}{0.901} \times 192$$

$$= 235 \text{ units/mL}$$

REPORTING RESULTS

The reference CH_{50} titer is about 200 CH_{50} units/mL.

PROCEDURE NOTES

The concentration of sensitized cells has been adjusted to yield 50% hemolysis in the presence of 5 μL of normal human serum, i.e., 1 CH_{50} unit.

Because the assay is nearly linear over a broad range, a single point can be used for calibration of this method.

The absorbance value of the lysis control when read against water at 415 nm should be less than 0.15 using a spectrophotometer with a 1 cm lightpath. If the $A_{control}$ exceeds 0.15, the assay results will not be valid and the assay must be repeated with new sensitized sheep cells.

SOURCES OF ERROR. Only serum, not plasma, should be used in the assay. Proper collection, handling, and storage of the serum are essential to accuracy.

CLINICAL APPLICATIONS. Increases in complement levels occur because of increased synthesis. An increased rate of complement is part of the acute-phase reactant response. Elevations in total hemolytic activity can be associated with:

1. Acute inflammatory conditions
2. Leukemia
3. Hodgkin's disease
4. Sarcoma
5. Behçet's disease

Decreases in complement levels, hyposynthesis, can be caused by a variety of conditions. These conditions include:

1. Congenital defects
2. Liver disease
3. Nutritional imbalance
4. Hypocatabolism

In addition, complement fixation can result from the presence of tissue or cell-bound immune complexes, or when circulating immune complexes are displayed. Bound immune complexes can be associated with chronic glomerulonephritis, rheumatoid arthritis, hemolytic anemia, and graft rejection. Circulating immune complexes are characteristically associated with systemic lupus erythematosus, acute glomerulonephritis, subacute bacterial endocarditis, and cryoglobulinemia.

Limitations

The limitations of this procedure should be noted:

1. Results of the CH_{50} assay, which are a quantitative value, represent the functional total hemolytic complement activity. Values achieved with this method can be used to determine the presence of abnormal whole complement levels but *cannot* identify the abnormal component. In cases of abnormal values, the serum must be assayed for the value of each of the individual (C1-C9) components.
2. The measurement of total CH_{50} hemolytic activity cannot exclude all acquired or congenital abnormalities of individual components.
3. The procedure has been developed to aid in diagnosis but is not diagnostic in itself.

Chapter Review

HIGHLIGHTS

The complement system is a heat–labile series of 18 plasma proteins, many of which are enzymes, or *proteinases.* Collectively, these proteins are a major fraction of the beta 1 and beta 2 globulins. Complement plays a major role in the immune system as a potent mediator of inflammation. Normally, complement components are present in the circulation in an inactive form.

Complement is composed of two interrelated enzyme cascades, the classic and alternative pathways. The classic pathway is initiated by the complexing of antigen to its specific antibody, either IgG or IgM, and is the primary amplifier of the biologic effects of humoral immunity. The alternative pathway is activated by contact with a foreign surface, such as the polysaccharide coating of a microorganism, and amplifies nonimmune defense

against microbial infection and other biologic alterations. It is probable that under normal physiologic conditions, the activation of one pathway also leads to the activation of the other. Either of the two routes leads to a common final pathway. Both pathways convert C3 to C3b, the central event of the common final pathway that in turn leads to the activation of the lytic complement sequence, C5-C9, and cell destruction. A third set of plasma proteins that function as membrane attack complexes becomes assembled into the structures responsible for lytic lesions in the lipid bilayer of the cell membrane and disrupts membrane integrity.

A variety of cell types express surface membrane glycoproteins that react with one or more of the fragments of C3 produced during complement activation and degradation. The functions of these receptors depend on the type of cell manifesting them and are, in many instances, incompletely understood. The complement receptor 1 (CR1) is important in enhancing phagocytosis. The activation of complement and the products formed during the complement cascade have a variety of physiologic and cellular consequences. Physiologic consequences include blood vessel dilation and increased vascular permeability. The cellular consequences include cell activation, cytolysis, or hemolysis and if the cells are erythrocytes, opsonization occurs which renders cells vulnerable to phagocytosis. In addition to complement's function as a major effector of antigen-antibody interaction, it has been found that physiologic concentrations of complement can induce profound alteration in the molecular weight, composition, and solubility of immune complexes. The activation of complement may also play a role in mediating hypersensitivity reactions. This process may occur either from direct alternative pathway activation by IgE-antigen complexes or through a sequence initiated by the activated Hageman coagulation factor that causes the generation of plasmin, which subsequently activates the classic pathway. In either case, activation of complement components from C3 onward leads to the generation of the anaphlatoxins in an immediate hypersensitivity reaction.

Complement levels may be abnormal in certain disease states. Increased complement levels are often associated with inflammatory conditions, trauma, or acute illness such as myocardial infarction because separate complement components, e.g., C3, are acute–phase proteins. These elevations, however, are common and nonspecific. Therefore increased levels are of limited clinical significance. In contrast, deficiencies of complement account for a small percentage of primary immunodeficiencies, but depression of complement levels frequently coexists with SLE and other disorders associated with an immunopathologic process.

Hypocomplementemia can result from the complexing of IgG or IgM antibodies that are capable of activating complement. Depressed values of complement are associated with diseases that give rise to circulating immune complexes. The most frequent evaluation of complement is by serum/plasma assay. Complement can be assessed either by its activity in immune hemolysis or by quantitative immunoassay, i.e., radial immunoassay. These assays are useful in diagnosis and monitoring of patients. A traditional method for determination of functional complement activity is the total hemolytic (CH_{50}) assay. This assay measures the ability of a test sample to lyse 50% of a standardized suspension of sheep erythrocytes coated with anti-erythrocyte antibody. Both the classic activation pathway and the terminal complement components are measured during this reaction.

REVIEW QUESTIONS

1. The complement system is:
   A. a heat stable series of plasma proteins
   B. a heat labile series of plasma proteins
   C. composed of many proteinases
   D. composed of two interrelated pathways
   E. all of the above except A

2. All of the below are complement-controlling proteins except:
   A. C1 (INH)
   B. factor I
   C. factor H
   D. C3
   E. C4-bp

3. A variety of cell types express surface membrane glycoproteins that react with one or more of the fragments of ___ produced during complement activation and degradation.
   A. C1
   B. C3
   C. C5
   D. C8
   E. C9

4. All of the following result from complement activation except:
   A. decreased cell susceptibility to phagocytosis
   B. blood vessel dilation and increased vascular permeability
   C. production of inflammatory mediators
   D. cytolysis or hemolysis
   E. opsonization

Questions 5-8.
Complete the following activation sequence of the classic complement pathway:
C1-C_(5)_ _-C_(6)_ _-C3- C_(7)_ _-C6-C7- C_(8)_ _-C9
   A. 2
   B. 4
   C. 5
   D. 8
   E. 10

9. Which complement component is present in the greatest quantity in plasma?
   A. 2
   B. 3
   C. 4
   D. 8
   E. 9

Questions 10-12.
Arrange the three stages of the classic complement pathway in their correct sequence.
10. ___
11. ___
12. ___
   A. enzymatic activation
   B. membrane attack
   C. recognition

13. Fixation of the C1 complement component is related to each of the following factors except:
   A. molecular weight of the antibody
   B. the presence of IgM antibody
   C. the presence of most IgG subclasses
   D. spatial constraints
   E. configurational constraints

14. At which stage does the complement system reach its full amplitude?
   A. C1q, C1r, C1s complex
   B. C2
   C. C3
   D. C4
   E. C9

15. Which of the following is not a component of the membrane attack complex?
   A. C3b
   B. C6
   C. C7
   D. C8
   E. C9

Questions 16-19.
Select the appropriate pathway response.
16. activated by antigen-antibody complexes
17. generates a C3 convertase
18. activated by microbial and mammalian cell surfaces
19. terminates in a membrane attack complex
   A. classic pathway
   B. alternate pathway
   C. both A and B

20. Which of the following conditions can be associated with hypercomplementemia?
   A. myocardial infarction
   B. systemic lupus erythematosus
   C. glomerulonephritis
   D. subacute bacterial endocarditis
   E. hereditary angioedema

Questions 21-25.
Match the following complement deficiency states in humans with their respective deficient components. (Use an answer only once.)
21. C2
22. C5
23. C6
24. C7
   A. Neisseria infections
   B. Leiner's disease
   C. Raynaud's phenomenon
   D. recurrent pyogenic infections

25. If the test result in the CH_{50} assay is low or below normal, the following many be the cause:
   A. in vitro degradation
   B. complement activation
   C. inflammation
   D. Both A and B
   E. Both B and C

Answers

1. E 2. D 3. A 4. A 5. B 6 A 7. C 8. D 9. B 10. C
11. A 12. B 13. A 14. C 15. A 16. A 17. C 18. B 19. C
20. A 21. D 22. B 23. A 24. C 25. D

BIBLIOGRAPHY

Alper CA and Rosen FS: Clinical applications of complement assays. In Stollerman GH, ed: Advances in internal medicine, vol 20, Chicago, 1975, Year Book Medical Publishers.

Ashman RF: Rheumatic diseases. In Lawlor GJ and Fischer TJ, eds: Manual of allergy and immunology, ed 2, Boston, 1988, Little, Brown & Co.

Carpentier NA, et al: Circulating immune complexes and the prognosis of acute myeloid leukemia, N Engl J Med 307:1174-1180, 1982.

Fearon DT and Austen KF: Current concepts in immunology: the alternative pathway of complement-A system for host resistance to microbial infection, N Engl J Med 303:259-263, 1980.

Frank MM: Complement in the pathophysiology of human disease, N Engl J Med 316:1525, 1987.

Knutsen AP and Fischer TJ: Immunodeficiency diseases. In Lawlor GJ and Fischer TJ, eds: Manual of allergy and immunology, ed 2, Boston, 1988, Little, Brown & Co.

Larchmann PJ and Rosen FS: Genetic defects of complement in man, Springer Semin Immunopathol 1:339-353, 1978.

Muller-Eberhardt HJ: Complement abnormalities in human disease, Hosp Pract 13(12):65-76, 1978.

Peter JB: The use and interpretation of tests in medical laboratory immunology, ed 5, Los Angeles, 1986, Specialty Laboratories, Inc.

Ruddy S: Complement. In Stein J ed: Internal medicine, ed 2, Boston, Little, Brown & Co.

Ruddy S: Complement measurement. In Stein J ed: Internal medicine, ed 2, 1987, Boston, Little, Brown & Co.

Ruddy S: Complement. In Rose NR, Friedman H, and Fahey JL, eds: Manual of clinical laboratory immunology, ed 3, Washington, DC, 1986, Am Soc of Microbiology.

Tizmann, SE and Daniels JC, eds: Serum protein abnormalities, 1975, Boston, Little, Brown & Co.

Turgeon ML: Fundamentals of immunohematology, Philadelphia, 1989, Lea & Febiger.

Zeiss CR, et al: An hypocomplementemic vasculitic urticarial syndrome, Am J Med 68:867-875, 1980.

PART II

The Theory of Immunologic and Serologic Procedures

CHAPTER

6

Safety and Basic Techniques in the Immunology-Serology Laboratory

In the immunology-serology laboratory, precautions must be taken to prevent accidental exposure to infectious disease. In addition, laboratories using radioactive test protocols must adhere to strict safety standards.

UNIVERSAL BLOOD AND BODY FLUID PRECAUTIONS

The rapid increase in the number of patients identified with human immunodeficiency virus (HIV) was partially responsible for a change in the initial recommendations issued in 1983 by the Centers for Disease Control (CDC) in regard to the handling of blood and body fluids from patients suspected of or known to be infected with a blood-borne pathogen. Current safety guidelines for the control of infectious disease are based on the CDC publication, "Recommendations for Prevention of HIV Transmission in Health-Care Settings" (MMWR, Sup. 2S, 1987). In addition, safety practices should conform to the guidelines described in "Protection of Laboratory Workers from Infectious Disease Transmitted by Blood and Tissue" by the National Committee for Clinical Laboratory Standards (NCCLS Document M29-P, 1987) and the 1988 CDC clarifications of the original guidelines (MMWR, vol. 37, no. 24, June, 1988). Laboratory personnel should also remain alert to further updates of these policies.

Universal blood and body fluid precautions or *universal precautions* have been instituted in clinical laboratories to prevent parenteral, mucous membrane, and nonintact skin exposures of health-care workers to blood-borne pathogens, such as HIV and hepatitis B virus (HBV). Universal precautions state that the blood and certain body fluids (Table 6-1) of *all* patients should be treated as potentially infectious.

Although HIV has been isolated from blood, semen, vaginal secretions, saliva, tears, breast milk, cerebrospinal fluid (CSF), amniotic fluid, and urine, *only* blood, semen, vaginal secretions, and breast milk have been implicated in transmission of HIV to date. Evidence for the role of saliva in the transmission of virus is unclear; however, universal precautions do not apply to saliva uncontaminated with blood.

TABLE 6-1

Potentially Infectious Body Fluids

Potentially infectious	Questionable	Noninfectious*
Amniotic Fluid	Colostrum	Nasal
Blood		secretions
Bloody fluids		Saliva
Cerebrospinal fluid		Sputum
Pericardial fluid		Stool
Peritoneal fluid		Sweat
Pleural fluid		Tears
Pus and purulent		Urine
discharge		
Semen		
Synovial fluid		
Vaginal secretions		

*If not contaminated with blood.

OCCUPATIONAL TRANSMISSION OF HBV AND HIV

Medical personnel should be aware of the fact that HBV and HIV are totally different diseases caused by completely unrelated viruses. The most feared hazard of all, the transmission of HIV through occupational exposure, is among the least likely to occur if proper safety practices are followed. Exposure to HIV is uncommon, but cases of occupational transmission to health-care personnel with no other known high-risk factors have been documented (Table 6-2). The transmission of hepatitis B, which can also be fatal, is more probable than transmission of HIV.

Blood is the single most important source of HIV, HBV, and other blood-borne pathogens in the occupational setting. HBV can be present in extraordinarily high concentrations in blood, but HIV is usually found in lower concentrations. HBV may be stable in dried blood and blood products at 25° C for up to 7 days. HIV retains infectivity for more than 3 days in dried specimens at room temperature and for more than a week in an aqueous environment at room temperature. The likelihood of infection after exposure to blood infected with HBV or HIV depends on a variety of factors including:

1. The concentration of HBV or HIV of virus. Viral concentration is higher for HBV than for HIV
2. The duration of the contact
3. The presence or skin lesions or abrasions on the hands or exposed skin of the health-care worker

TABLE 6-2

Risk of Occupationally Transmitted HIV Infection To Health-Care Workers

Institution	Route of exposure			
	Parenteral	Contami-nation	Total	Infected
Centers for Disease Control (CDC)	901	169	1070	4
National Institutes of Health (NIH)	103	691	794	0

Adapted from Update: Acquired immunodeficiency syndrome and HIV infection among health care workers, MMWR 37:229, April 22, 1988.

TABLE 6-3

HIV Portals of Entry and Estimates of Risk

Portal of entry	Type of risk	Risk of getting to site	Risk of viral entry	Risk of inoculation
Blood				
Blood products*	Medically required	High	High	High
Shared needles†	Choice	High	High	Very high
Needle injury†	Accidental	Low	High	Low
Traumatic wound	Accidental	Moderate	High	High
Conjunctiva	Accidental	Moderate	Moderate	Very low
Nasal mucosa	Accidental	Low	Low	Very low
Oral mucosa	Accidental/choice	Moderate	Moderate	Low
Perinatal	Accidental	High	High	High
Respiratory (lower)	Accidental	Very low	Very low	Very low
Sexual				
Anus	Choice	Very high	Very high	Very high
Penis	Choice	High	Low	Low
Ulcers	Choice	High	High	Very high
Vagina	Choice	Low	Low	Medium
Skin				
Intact	Accidental	Very low	Very low	Very low
Broken	Accidental	Low	High	High

*Unscreened donors and/or untreated products.
†If the needles are contaminated with virus-infected blood.
Data from recommendations for prevention of HIV transmission in health-care settings, MMWR 36:3S, August 21, 1987; Update: universal precautions for prevention of transmission of HIV, hepatitis B virus, and other blood borne pathogens in the health care setting. MMWR 37:377, June 24, 1988.

4. The immune status of the health-care worker for HBV

HBV and HIV may be *directly* transmitted by various portals of entry (Table 6-3). In the occupational setting, however, the following list of situations may lead to infection:

1. Percutaneous (parenteral) inoculation of blood, plasma, serum, or certain other body fluids from accidental needlesticks, etc.
2. Contamination of the skin with blood or certain body fluids without overt puncture, because of scratches, abrasions, burns, weeping, or exudative skin lesions.
3. Exposure of mucous membranes (oral, nasal, or conjunctiva) to blood or certain body fluids, as the direct result of pipetting by mouth, splashes, or spattering.
4. Centrifuge accidents or the improper removal of rubber stoppers from test tubes that produces droplets. If these aerosol products are infectious and come in direct contact with mucous membranes or nonintact skin, direct transmission of virus can potentially result.

HBV and HIV may be *indirectly* transmitted. Viral transmission can result from contact with inanimate objects such as work surfaces or equipment contaminated with infected blood or certain body fluids. If the virus is transferred to the skin or mucous membranes by hand contact between a contaminated surface and non-intact skin or mucous membranes, it can produce viral exposure.

PROTECTIVE TECHNIQUES FOR INFECTION CONTROL

Universal precautions are intended to supplement rather than replace recommendations such as handwashing for routine infection control. Infection control efforts for HIV, HBV, and other blood-borne pathogens must focus on prevention of exposure to blood. It is a possible and wise preventative measure to be vaccinated against HBV. The risk of nosocomial transmission of HBV, HIV, and other blood-borne pathogens can be minimized if laboratory personnel are aware of and adhere to essential safety guidelines.

Selection and Use of Gloves

Gloves for medical use are either sterile surgical or nonsterile examination gloves made of vinyl or latex. There are no reported differences in barrier effectiveness between intact latex and intact vinyl gloves. Tactile differences have been observed between the two types of gloves with latex gloves providing more tactile sensitivity; however, either type is usually satisfactory for phlebotomy and as a protective barrier when performing technical procedures. Rubber household gloves may be used for cleaning procedures.

The general guidelines related to the selection and general use of gloves include:

1. Use sterile gloves for procedures involving contact with normally sterile areas of the body or during procedures where sterility has been established and must be maintained. Use nonsterile examination gloves for procedures that do not require the use of sterile gloves.
2. Wear gloves when processing blood specimens, reagents, or blood products. Gloves should be changed frequently and immediately if they become visibly contaminated with blood or certain body fluids or if physical damage occurs.
3. Do not wash or disinfect latex or vinyl gloves for reuse. Washing with detergents may cause increased penetration of liquids through undetected holes in the gloves. Rubber gloves may be decontaminated and reused, but disinfectants may cause deterioration. Rubber gloves should be discarded if they have punctures, tears, or evidence of deterioration or if they peel, crack, or become discolored.

Gloves as a Barrier Protection During Testing

Vinyl gloves should be worn when:

1. Handling blood, serum, plasma, or certain body fluids.
2. Handling blood or potentially infectious blood products, such as antiserums of human origin.
3. Testing human serum or plasma.
4. Using items potentially contaminated with blood or certain body fluids, e.g., specimen containers, laboratory instruments, or counter tops.

Care must be taken to avoid indirect contamination of work surfaces or objects in the work area. Gloves should be properly removed or covered with an uncontaminated glove or paper towel before answering the telephone, handling laboratory equipment, or touching door knobs.

Facial Barrier Protection and Occlusive Bandages

Facial barrier protection should be used if there is a potential for splashing or spraying of blood or certain body fluids. Masks and/or facial protection should be worn if mucous membrane contact with blood or certain body fluid is anticipated. All disruptions of exposed skin should be covered with a water-impermeable occlusive bandage. This includes defects on the arms, face, and neck.

Laboratory Coats or Gowns as Barrier Protection

A color-coded, two-laboratory coat or equivalent system should be used whenever laboratory personnel are working with potentially infectious specimens. The garment worn in the laboratory must be changed or covered with an uncontaminated coat when leaving the immediate work area. Garments should be changed immediately if grossly contaminated with blood or body fluids to prevent seepage through to street clothes or skin. Contaminated coats or gowns should be placed in an appropriately designated biohazard bag for laundering. Disposable plastic aprons are recommended if there is a significant possibility that blood or certain body fluids may be splashed. Aprons should be discarded into a biohazard container.

Important Safety Practices
Hand Washing

Frequent hand washing is an important safety precaution. It should be performed after contact with patients and laboratory specimens. Hands should be washed with soap and water:

1. After completing laboratory work and before leaving the laboratory.
2. After removing gloves.
3. Before eating, drinking, applying make up, and changing contact lenses, and before and after using the lavatory.
4. Before all activities that involve hand contact with mucous membranes or breaks in the skin.
5. Immediately after accidental skin contact with blood, body fluids, or tissues. If the contact occurs through breaks in gloves, the gloves should be removed immediately and the hands thoroughly washed. If accidental contamination occurs to an exposed area of the skin or because of a break in gloves, one must wash first with a liquid soap, rinse well with water, and apply a 1:10 dilution of bleach or 50% isopropyl or ethyl alcohol. The bleach or alcohol is left on skin for at least 1 minute before final washing with liquid soap and water.

Decontamination of Work Surfaces, Equipment, and Spills

All work surfaces should be cleaned and sanitized at the beginning and end of the shift with a 1:10 dilution of household bleach (see box below). Instruments such as scissors or centrifuge carriages should be sanitized daily with a dilute solution of bleach. Diluted household bleach prepared *daily* inactivates HBV in 10 minutes and HIV in 2 minutes. Disposable materials contaminated with blood must be placed in containers marked *Biohazard* and properly discarded.

All blood spills should be treated as *potentially* hazardous. In the event of a blood spill, this procedure for cleaning up the spill should be used:

1. Wear gloves and a laboratory coat.
2. Absorb the blood with disposable towels. Bleach solutions are less effective in the presence of high concentrations of protein. Remove as much liquid blood or serum as possible before decontamination.
3. Using a diluted bleach solution, clean the spill site of all visible blood.

4. Wipe down the spill site with paper towels soaked with diluted bleach.
5. Place all disposable materials used for decontamination into a biohazard container.

Needle Precautions

To prevent needlestick injuries, one should *never* recap needles, separate them from syringes, or otherwise manipulate them by hand. Used needles should be placed intact into specifically designated red, puncture-proof, biohazard containers. The same criteria should be applied to used scalpel blades and any other sharp device that may be contaminated with blood. The container should be located as close as possible to the work area. Phlebotomists should carry red, puncture-resistant containers in their collection trays. Needles should not project from the top of the container. To discard the container, close it and place it in the biohazard waste. An accidental needlestick must be reported to the appropriate individual.

Other Safety Precautions

A variety of other safety practices should be adhered to in order to reduce the risk of inadvertent contamination with blood or certain body fluids. These practices include:

1. Food and drink should not be consumed in work areas or stored in the same area as specimens. Containers, refrigerators, or freezers used for specimens should be marked as containing a biohazard.
2. Specimens needing centrifugation should be capped and placed into a centrifuge with a sealed dome.
3. Rubber-stoppered test tubes should be slowly and carefully opened with a 2×2 gauze square placed over the stopper to minimize aerosal production (the introduction of substances into the air).
4. Safety bulbs should be used for pipetting. Pipetting *by mouth* of any clinical material must be strictly forbidden.

Compliance with Universal Precautions

In addition to a clear policy on the institutionally required universal precautions previously discussed, compliance with the enforcement of universal precautions also requires that categories of risk classifications for all routine and reasonably anticipated job-related tasks and personal protective equipment be included with the departmental procedures manual. Risk classification is divided into three categories:

Category I

Tasks that involve exposure to blood, body fluids, or tissues. All procedures or job-related tasks that involve an inherent potential for mucous membrane or skin contact with blood, body fluids, or tissues or a potential for spills or splashes of them are Category I tasks.

Preparation of Diluted Household Bleach

Vol. of bleach	Vol. of H$_2$O	Ratio	% Sodium hypochlorite
1 mL	9 mL	1:10	0.5

Category II

Tasks that generally involve no exposure to blood, body fluids, or tissues, but may require performing unplanned Category I tasks. The normal work responsibilities involve no exposure to blood, body fluids, or tissues, but exposure or potential exposure may be required as a condition of employment.

Category III

Tasks that involve no exposure to blood, body fluids, or tissues, and Category I tasks are not a condition of employment. A person in this category does not perform and is not expected to perform tasks that can lead to potential exposure. Activities such as answering the telephone or the use of shared bathroom facilities with workers in other categories are not considered to be a risk.

HAZARDOUS MATERIAL AND WASTE MANAGEMENT

The control of infectious, chemical, and radioactive waste is regulated by a variety of government agencies, including the Occupational Safety and Health Administration (OSHA) and the Food and Drug Administration (FDA). Legislation and regulations that affect laboratories include the Resource Recovery and Conservation Act (RCRA), the Toxic Substances Control Act (TOSCA), clean air and water laws, "Right to Know" laws, and HAZCOM (chemical hazard communication). Laboratories should implement applicable federal, state, and local laws that pertain to hazardous material and waste management by establishing safety policies. Laboratories with multiple agencies should follow the guidelines of the most stringent agency. Safety policies should be reviewed and signed annually or whenever a change is instituted. Employers are responsible for ensuring that personnel follow the safety policies.

Infectious Waste

Infectious waste, such as contaminated gauze squares and test tubes, must be discarded into proper biohazard containers. These containers should be:
1. Conspicuously marked *Biohazard* and bear the universal biohazard symbol.
2. The universal color: orange, or orange and black, or red.
3. Rigid, leakproof, and puncture resistant. Cardboard boxes lined with a leakproof plastic bag are available.
4. Used for blood and certain body fluids* and dis-

posable materials contaminated with them.

If the primary infectious waste containers are red plastic bags, they should be kept in secondary metal or plastic cans. Extreme care should be taken not to contaminate the exterior of these bags. If they do become contaminated on the outside, the entire bag must be placed into another red plastic bag. Secondary plastic or metal cans should be decontaminated regularly and immediately after any grossly visible contamination, using an agent such as a 1:10 solution of household bleach.

Sharps, i.e., needles, blades, glass, or pressurized cans that can explode, must be carefully disposed. Needles should never be recapped but should be placed directly into disposable containers that are marked *Biohazard*. These containers should be impervious to disruption by the sharps. The container must be made of material that is compatible with the method of decontamination. For example, if the container is incinerated, it must be of material that will incinerate completely. If the container is to be autoclaved, it must be made of material that will not melt. If it is to be hauled away, material must be acceptable to the disposal service.

If any of the sharps are taken to a landfill they must be decontaminated first. Terminal disposal of infectious waste should be by incineration; however, an alternate method of terminal sterilization is autoclaving. If incineration is not done in the health-care facility or by an outside contractor, all contaminated disposables should be autoclaved before leaving the facility for disposal with routine waste. Pressurized cans should be punctured under controlled conditions before sending to a landfill or incinerating.

Glass should be placed into specifically marked containers at the point of use. Glass can be incinerated in a Class VI incinerator. A Class VI incinerator is one that produces heat of 1800° F or more and will incinerate human tissue. Some lower class incinerators will render the glass harmless, but the glass may coat the sides of the incinerator and harm it by lowering the achievable temperature.

Chemical Hazards

OSHA recommends that all chemically hazardous material be properly labeled with the hazardous contents and severity of the material, as well as bearing a hazard symbol. Guidelines for chemical hazards can be found in the National Fire Prevention Association's document, NFPA 704.

Chemical hazard precautions legislation, such as state "right to know" laws and OSHA document 29 CFR 1910, sets the standards for chemical hazard communication (HAZCOM) and determines the types of documents that must be on file in a laboratory. For example, a yearly physical inventory of all hazardous chemicals must be performed and material safety data sheets (MSDs) should be available in each department of use. Each institution should also have at least one centralized area where all MSDs are stored.

---

*Some local health codes currently permit blood and body fluids to be disposed of by pouring them down the sink into the sanitary sewage system. If disposal by this method is used, care must be taken to prevent splashing. Water should not be running in the sink, and facial protection and a plastic apron should be worn in addition to gloves and a laboratory coat. *Sinks used for hazardous waste disposal should not be used for hand washing.*

Many toxic chemicals now have limits that must met within the laboratory, specifically *threshold limit values* (TLVs) and *permissible exposure limit* (PEL). TLVs are the maximum safe exposure limits as set down by the federal government. PEL is the personal allowable limit per time.

Radioactive Waste

The Nuclear Regulatory Commission (NRC) regulates the methods of disposal of radioactive waste. Radioactive waste associated with the radioimmunoassay (RIA) laboratory must be disposed of with special caution. In general, low-level RIA radioactive waste can be discharged in small amounts into the sewer with copious amounts of water. This will probably be illegal in the future; therefore, the best method of disposal is to store the used material in a locked, marked room until the background count is down to 10 half-lives for I^{125}. It can then be disposed of with other refuse. Meticulous records are required to document the amounts and method of disposal.

BASIC SEROLOGIC PROCEDURES
Accuracy in Testing

In order to eliminate the *most* frequent source of pretesting error, a patient must be positively identified when a blood specimen is obtained. This specimen must be properly collected and labeled. In general, hemolyzed specimens should not be used for serologic testing.

Inaccuracies in testing can be systematic or sporadic. Systematic errors can be eliminated by a continuing quality assurance program that monitors equipment, reagents, etc. Reagents should be checked for turbidity or an abnormal appearance at each time of use. Contaminated reagents can produce erroneous results. Tests protocols must be strictly followed. Techniques must be exact.

Sporadic or isolated errors in technique can produce false positive and/or false negative results. Depending on the technique used for testing, possible causes of technical errors include:

Possible causes of false-positive errors:
1. Addition of the wrong reagent to a test tube
2. Overcentrifugation of a serum-cell mixture
3. Dirty glassware
4. Hemolyzed patient serum
5. Inadequate dispersal of centrifuged serum-cell mixture
6. Extended incubation

Possible causes of false-negative errors:
1. Omitting patient serum from the test mixture
2. Omitting reagent from the test mixture
3. Undercentrifugation of a serum-cell mixture
4. Vigorous shaking of a centrifuged serum-cell mixture

Possible causes of false-positive or false-negative errors:
1. Incorrect labeling of test tubes
2. Addition of the wrong reagent

3. Erroneously reading or interpreting results
4. Inaccurately recording results
5. Expired or improperly stored reagents

Blood Specimen Preparation

After blood has been obtained from a patient, it should be allowed to clot and the serum should be promptly removed for testing. Clotting and clot retraction should take place at room temperature or in the refrigerator, depending on the protocol for the specific procedure. Complete clot retraction normally takes about an hour. Following clot retraction, the clot should be loosened from the sides of the test tube with an applicator stick and centrifuged for 10 minutes at a moderate speed. After centrifugation, serum can be transferred to a labeled tube with a Pasteur pipette and rubber bulb. If the serum is contaminated with erythrocytes, it should be recentrifuged. The serum-containing tube should be sealed. Testing should be promptly conducted or the serum should be frozen at $-20°$ C. *Universal precautions* must be followed when handling blood specimens.

Inactivation of Complement

Some procedures require the use of inactivated serum. Inactivation is the process that destroys complement activity. Complement is known to interfere with the reactions of certain syphilis tests and complement components, such as C1q. It can agglutinate latex particles and cause a false positive reaction in latex passive agglutination assays. Complement may also cause lysis of the indicator cells in hemagglutination assays.

Complement in body fluids can be inactivated by heating to 56° C for 30 minutes. When more than 4 hours has elapsed since inactivation, a specimen can be reinactivated by heating it to 56° C for 10 minutes.

Pipettes

Pipettes are used in the immunology-serology laboratory for the quantitative transfer of reagents and the preparations of serial dilution of specimens such as serum. Although semiautomated micropipettes have largely replaced traditional glass pipettes in the laboratory, there are occasions where traditional methods may be needed.

The type of pipette used in manual procedures is the *serologic* pipette. It is recognized by a frosted ring at the noncalibrated end with calibrations extending to the tip. The letters *T.D.* (to deliver) appear on the pipette, and for quick recognition, each size of pipette has an imprinted color-coded band that indicates the volume. The serologic pipette is usually allowed to empty by gravity. Depending on the calibration, the remaining drop needs to be expelled in order to deliver the full volume.

Each serologic pipette is marked with identifying numerals, e.g., 10 in 1/10. The first of these numbers represents the total capacity of the pipette.

TABLE 6-4

An Example of the Preparation of a Serial Dilution

Tube	1	2	3	4	5	6	7	8	9	10
Saline (mL)	1	1	1	1	1	1	1	1	1	1
Patient serum or preceding dilution (mL)	1	1 of 1:2	1 of 1:4	1 of 1:8	1 of 1:16	1 of 1:32	1 of 1:64	1 of 1:128	1 of 1:256	1 of 1:512
Final dilution	1:2	1:4	1:8	1:16	1:32	1:64	1:128	1:256	1:512	1:1024

The second number represents the smallest gradation into which the pipette is divided. In the example cited, therefore, the total pipette volume is 10 mL. Markings then divide it into 1-mL sections and each mL is further divided into tenths. Sizes of serologic pipettes most frequently used are: 10 mL in 1/10, 5 mL in 1/10, 2 mL in 1/10, 2 mL in 1/100, 1 mL in 1/10, and 1 mL in 1/100. For greatest accuracy, the smallest pipette that will hold the desired volume should be used.

Before use, glass pipettes should be inspected for broken or chipped ends or contamination. A safety bulb must be used to aspirate liquid into the pipette as well as dispense it. Liquid should be aspirated to about 1 inch above the top (zero) line of the pipette. After aspirating a liquid, the pipette should be raised vertically to avoid the introduction of air bubbles, and the exterior surface must be wiped off with a clean gauze or tissue square. Working at eye level, the liquid should be slowly lowered so to that the *meniscus* is at zero. The contents of the pipette can then be aspirated into the appropriate test tube or vessel. Gloves should be worn during pipetting procedures in compliance with universal precautions.

PRINCIPLES OF IMMUNOLOGIC-SEROLOGIC TESTING

Procedures used in immunology apply many techniques that are common to other scientific disciplines, such as chemistry and immunohematology. In the field of immunology, however, many serologic techniques are used to detect the interaction of antigens with antibodies. These methods are suitable for the detection and quantitation of antibodies to infectious agents (see Section III) as well as microbial and nonmicrobial antigens.

Antibodies can be detected in various ways. The purpose of Section II is to present the various methods of antibody or antigen detection. In some cases, antibodies to an agent may be detected in more than one way, but different procedures may not detect the same antibody.

Serum for detection of antibodies should be drawn during the *acute* phase of illness or when first discovered and again during convalescent period, usually 2 weeks later. A difference in antibody titer may be noted when the acute and convalescent specimens are tested concurrently. Some infections, however, such as Legionnaires' disease or hepatitis, may not manifest a rise in titer until months after the acute infection.

A central concept of serologic testing is the manifestation of a rise in titer. The titer or concentration of an antibody is the reciprocal of the highest dilution of the patient's serum in which the antibody is detectable. Therefore a high titer indicates that a considerable amount of antibody is present in the serum.

Determination of the concentration of antibody (titer) for a specific antigen involves two steps:
1. Preparing a serial dilution of the antibody containing solution, e.g., serum.
2. Adding an equal volume of antigen suspension to each dilution.

A serial dilution represents progressive and regular increments of serum. Most commonly, serial dilutions are "two fold"; that is, each dilution is half as concentrated as the preceding one (Table 6-4). The total volume in each tube is the same. The generation of normal reference ranges is established for each type of test. Titers are usually reported as the reciprocal of the last dilution demonstrating the desired results, such as a color change or agglutination.

For most pathogens, an increase in the patient's titer of two doubling dilutions, for example, from a positive result of 1:8 to a positive result of 1:32 over several weeks, is considered to be diagnostic of a current infection. This is called a *fourfold rise* in titer.

Chapter Review

HIGHLIGHTS

In the immunology-serology laboratory, precautions must be taken to prevent accidental exposure to infectious disease. In addition, laboratories using radioactive test protocols must adhere to strict safety standards. The rapid increase in the number of patients identified with human immunodeficiency virus (HIV) was partially responsible for a change in the initial recommendations issued in 1983 by the Centers for Disease Control (CDC) in regard to the handling of blood and body fluids from patients suspected of or known to be infected with a blood-borne pathogen. Universal blood and body fluid precautions, or *universal precautions,* have been instituted in clinical laboratories to prevent parenteral, mucous membrane, and nonintact skin exposures of health-care workers to blood-borne pathogens such as HIV and hepatitis B virus (HBV). Universal precautions state that the blood and certain body fluids of all patients should be treated as potentially infectious.

Although HIV has been isolated from blood, semen, vaginal secretions, saliva, tears, breast milk, cerebrospinal fluid (CSF), amniotic fluid, and urine, *only* blood, semen, vaginal secretions, and possibly breast milk have been implicated in transmission of HIV to date. Medical personnel should be aware of the fact that HBV and HIV are totally different diseases caused by totally unrelated viruses. The most feared hazard of all, the transmission of HIV through occupational exposure, is among the least likely to occur if proper safety practices are followed. Although exposure to HIV is uncommon, a few cases of occupational transmission to health-care personnel with no other known high-risk factors have been documented. HBV and HIV may be *indirectly* transmitted. Viral transmission can result from contact with inanimate objects such as work surfaces or equipment contaminated with infected blood or certain body fluids, if the virus is transferred to nonintact skin or mucous membranes by hand contact. Universal precautions are intended to supplement rather than replace recommendations for routine infection control, such as handwashing. Infection control efforts for HIV, HBV, and other blood-borne pathogens must focus on prevention of exposure to blood. It is a possible and wise preventative measure to be vaccinated against HBV. The risk of nosocomial transmission of HBV, HIV, and other blood-borne pathogens can be minimized if laboratory personnel are aware of and adhere to essential safety guidelines.

In addition to a clear policy on the institutionally required universal precautions previously discussed, compliance with the enforcement of universal precautions also requires that categories of risk classifications for all routine and reasonably anticipated job-related tasks and personal protective equipment be included with the departmental procedures manual. The control of infectious, chemical, and radioactive waste is regulated by a variety of government agencies, including the Occupational Safety and Health Administration (OSHA) and the Food and Drug Administration (FDA).

In order to eliminate the most frequent source of pretesting error, a patient must be positively identified when a blood specimen is obtained. This specimen must be properly collected and labeled. Inaccuracies in testing can be systematic or sporadic. Systematic errors can be eliminated by a continuing quality assurance program that monitors equipment, reagents, etc. Reagents should be checked for turbidity or an abnormal appearance at each time of use. Contaminated reagents can produce erroneous results. Test protocols must be strictly followed. Techniques must be exact. Sporadic or isolated errors in technique can produce false-positive and/or false-negative results, depending upon the technique that is used for testing. Procedures used in immunology apply many techniques that are common to other scientific disciplines, such as chemistry and immunohematology. In the field of immunology, however, many serologic techniques are used to detect the interaction of antigens with antibodies. These methods are suitable for the detection and quantitation of antibodies to infectious agents, as well as microbial and nonmicrobial antigens.

Antibodies can be detected in various ways. In some cases, antibodies to an agent may be detected in more than one way, but different procedures may not detect the same antibody. Serum for detection of antibodies should be drawn during the acute phase of illness or when first discovered and again during the convalescent period, usually 2 weeks later. A central concept of serologic testing is the manifestation of a rise in titer. The titer, or concentration, of an antibody is the reciprocal of the highest dilution of the patient's serum in which the antibody is detectable. Therefore a high titer indicates that a considerable amount of antibody is present in the serum.

REVIEW QUESTIONS

1. Which of the following body fluids is considered to be noninfectious?
   A. amniotic fluid
   B. urine
   C. bloody fluids
   D. pleural fluid
   E. vaginal secretions
2. Which of the following body fluids in addition to blood has been implicated in the transmission of HIV?
   A. saliva
   B. taers
   C. semen
   D. cerebrospinal fluid
   E. amniotic fluid
3. HBV may be stable in dried blood specimens at room temperature for up to:
   A. 24 hours
   B. 48 hours
   C. 3 days
   D. 5 days
   E. 7 days
4. HIV retains infectivity for:
   A. 24 hours
   B. 48 hours
   C. 3 days
   D. 5 days
   E. 7 days
5. The likelihood of infection after exposure to HBV or HIV infected blood or body fluids depends on all of the following factors except:

A. the source (anatomical site) of the blood or fluid
B. the concentration of the virus
C. the duration of the contact
D. the presence of non-intact skin
E. the immune status of the health care worker

6. HBV and HIV may be directly transmitted in the occupational setting by all of the following except:
   A. parenteral inoculation with contamianteed blood
   B. exposure of skin to contaminated blood or certain body fluids
   C. exposure of mucous membranes to contaminated blood or certain body fluids
   D. improper removal of rubber stoppers
   E. sharing bathroom facilities to an HIV positive person

Questions 7-11 True or False.
   F. A= true
   G. B= false

7. sterile gloves should be worn when processing specimens
8. latex or vinyl gloves can be washed or disinfected for reuse
9. gloves should be worn when handling blood, serum, plasma or certain body fluids
10. gloves should be worn when handling antisera of human origin
11. your hands should be washed after removing gloves
12. Diluted household bleach prepared daily inactivates HBV in ___(12)__minutes and HIV in __(13)__minutes.

12.
   A. 1 minute
   B. 2 minutes
   C. 5 minutes
   D. 7 minutes
   E. 10 minutes

13.
   A. 1 minute
   B. 2 minutes
   C. 5 minutes
   D. 7 minutes
   E. 10 minutes

14. Diluted bleach for disinfecting work surfaces, equipment, and spills should be prepared daily by preparing a ___(14)__ dilution of household bleach. This dilution requires __(15) mL of bleach per 100 mL of H_2O.

14.
   A. 1:5
   B. 1:10
   C. 1:20
   D. 1:100
   E. 1:1000

15.
   A. 1
   B. 10
   C. 25
   D. 50
   E. 75

16. Infectious waste must be discarded into containers with all of the following characteristics except:

A. marked "Biohazard"
B. bear the universal biohazard symbol
C. be orange, orange and black or red in color
D. manufactured of sturdy cardboard for landfill disposal
E. be rigid, leakproof, and puncture-resistant

Questions 17-21.
Select the appropriate answer for each of the following questions.
   F. A= false positive
   G. B= false negative
   H. C= false positive or false negative

17. Omiting patient serum or reagent from the test mixture
18. Dirty glassware
19. Addition of the wrong reagent
20. Inaccurately recording results
21. Hemolyzed patient serum
22. Complement can be inactivated in human serum by heating to_ _(22)__ 'C for __(23)__ minutes.

22.
   A. 25
   B. 37
   C. 45
   D. 56
   E. 100

23.
   A. 5
   B. 10
   C. 15
   D. 30
   E. 60

24. A specimen should be reinactivated when more than ____hour(s) has/have elapsed since inactivation.
   A. 1
   B. 2
   C. 4
   D. 8
   E. 24

25. If a serial dilution is prepared in two dilutions, the final dilution in tube 6 is:
   A. 1:25
   B. 1:32
   C. 1:64
   D. 1:256
   E. 1:512

Answers

1. B 2. C 3. E. 4. C 5. A 6. E 7. B 8. B 9. A 10. A 11. A 12. E 13. B 14. B 15. B 16. D 17. B 18. A 19. C 20. C 21. A 22. D 23. D 24. C 25. C

BIBLIOGRAPHY

Baron EJ and Finegold SM: Bailey and Scott's diagnostic microbiology, ed 8, St Louis, 1990, The CV Mosby Co.

Peacock JE and Tomar RH: Manual of laboratory immunology, Philadelphia, 1980, Lea & Febiger.

Turgeon ML: Fundamentals of immunohematology, Philadelphia, 1989, Lea & Febiger.

Turgeon ML: Clinical hematology, Boston, 1988, Little, Brown & Co.

CHAPTER 7 Agglutination Methods

CHAPTER 7

Agglutination Methods

PRINCIPLES OF AGGLUTINATION

Precipitation and agglutination are the visible expression of the aggregation of antigens and antibodies through the formation of a framework in which antigen particles or molecules alternate with antibody molecules (Fig. 7-1). *Precipitation* is the term applied to aggregation of soluble test antigens. *Agglutination* is the term used to describe the aggregation of particulate test antigens.

Agglutination of particles to which soluble antigen has been adsorbed produces a serum method of demonstrating precipitins. Examples of artificial carriers include latex particles and colloidal charcoal. Cells unrelated to the antigen, such as erythrocytes coated with antigen in a constant amount, can be used as biologic carriers. Whole bacterial cells can contain an antigen that will bind with antibodies produced in response to that antigen when it was introduced into the host.

The quality of test results depends on a variety of factors. These factors include the following:
1. Time of incubation with the antibody source, i.e., patient serum
2. Amount and *avidity* of an antigen conjugated to the carrier
3. Conditions of the test environment, e.g., pH and protein concentration

Agglutination tests are easy to perform and in some cases are the most sensitive tests currently available. These tests have a wide range of applications in the clinical diagnosis of noninfectious immune disorders and infectious diseases.

LATEX AGGLUTINATION

In latex agglutination procedures (see box), antibody molecules can be bound to the surface of latex beads. Many antibody molecules can be bound to

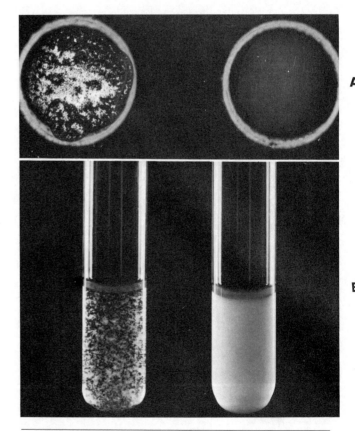

FIGURE 7-1

Agglutination patterns. **A,** Slide agglutination of bacteria with known antisera or known bacteria. A positive reaction is demonstrated by the specimen on the left, a negative reaction by the specimen on the right. **B,** Tube agglutination. A positive reaction is demonstrated by the specimen on the left, a negative reaction by the specimen on the right.
(From Barrett JT: Textbook of immunology, ed 5, St. Louis, 1988, The CV Mosby Co.)

Examples of Immunologic Assays Performed
by Latex Particle Agglutination

C-Reactive Protein (CRP)
IgG rheumatoid factors
IgM rheumatoid factors
Rubella antibody

each latex particle, increasing the potential number of exposed antigen-binding sites. If an antigen is present in a test specimen, such as the C-reactive protein, the antigen will bind to the combining sites of the antibody exposed on the surface of the latex beads, forming visible cross-linked aggregates of latex beads and antigen (Fig. 7-2). In some test systems, such as rubella antibody testing, latex particles can be coated with antigen. In the presence of serum antibodies, these particles agglutinate into large, visible clumps.

Procedures based on latex agglutination must be performed under standardized conditions. The amount of antigen-antibody binding is influenced by factors such as pH, osmolarity, and ionic concentration of the solution.

Coagglutination and *liposome-enhanced* latex agglutination are variations of latex agglutination (Fig. 7-3). Coagglutination employs antibodies bound to a particle to enhance the visibility of agglutination. It is a highly specific method but may not be as sensitive as latex agglutination for detecting small quantities of antigen.

FLOCCULATION TESTS

Flocculation tests for antibody detection are based on the interaction of soluble antigen with antibody

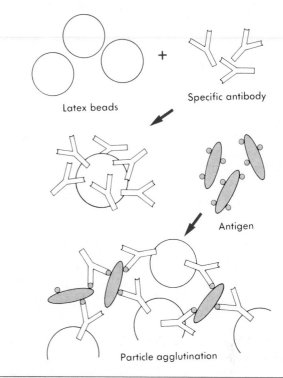

FIGURE 7-2

Alignment of antibody molecules bound to the surface of a latex particle and latex agglutination reaction.
(From Baron EJ and Finegold SM: Bailey and Scott's Diagnostic microbiology, ed 8, St. Louis, 1990, The CV Mosby Co.)

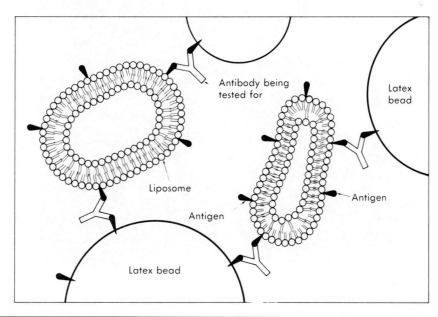

FIGURE 7-3

Diagram of liposome-latex agglutination reaction.
(From Baron EJ and Finegold SM: Bailey and Scott's Diagnostic microbiology, ed 8, St. Louis, 1990, The CV Mosby Co.)

that results in the formation of a precipitate of fine particles. These particles are macroscopically or microscopically visible only because the precipitated product is forced to remain in a confined space.

Two variations of flocculation testing can be used in syphilis serologic testing (see Chapter 16). These tests are the Venereal Disease Research Laboratory (VDRL) and the rapid plasma reagin (RPR) tests. In the VDRL test an antibody-like protein, *reagin*, binds to the test antigen, cardiolipid-lecithin–coated cholesterol particles, and produces the particles that flocculate. In the RPR test, the antigen, cardiolipid-lecithin–coated cholesterol with choline chloride, also contains charcoal particles that allow for macroscopically visible flocculation.

DIRECT BACTERIAL AGGLUTINATION

Direct whole pathogens can be used to detect antibodies directed against pathogens. The most basic tests are those that measure the antibody produced by the host to determinants on the surface of a bacterial agent in response to infection with that bacterial. In a thick suspension of the bacteria, the binding of specific antibodies to surface antigens of the bacteria causes the bacteria to clump together in visible aggregates. This type of agglutination is called *bacterial agglutination.* Febrile agglutinin tests (see Chapter 14) use this principle of testing (Fig. 7-4).

The formation of aggregates in solution is influenced by electrostatic and other forces; therefore, certain conditions are usually necessary for satisfactory results. The use of sterile physiologic saline with free positive ions in the agglutination procedure enhances the aggregation of bacteria because most bacterial surfaces exhibit a negative charge that causes them to repel each other. Because tube testing allows more time for antigen-antibody reaction, it is considered to be more sensitive than slide testing. The small volume of liquid used in slide testing requires rapid reading before the liquid evaporates.

INDIRECT OR PASSIVE HEMAGGLUTINATION

Hemagglutination, agglutination of red blood cells, tests for antibody detection. In the indirect or *passive hemagglutination* technique, erythrocytes are coated with substances such as extracts of bacterial cells, rickettsiae, pathogenic fungi, or protozoa or with purified polysaccharides or proteins. Erythrocytes of animals such as sheep or rabbits, or from group *O* humans, function as carriers for detecting and *titrating* the corresponding antibodies by agglutination. This technique is called *indirect hemagglutination* or *passive hemagglutination* (PHA) *testing* because it is not the antigen of the erythrocytes themselves but the passively attached antigens that are bound by antibody. In passive hemagglutination techniques, such as some rubella antibody procedures, erythrocytes are coated with rubella antigen. In the presence of antibody,

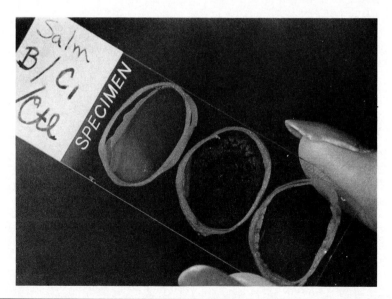

FIGURE 7-4

Slide agglutination test for febrile agglutinins. An organism biochemically resembling a *Salmonella* species is emulsified in several drops of saline on a slide. Drops of antiserum prepared against specific *Salmonella* serotypes are added to the suspension. The organism agglutinates in the presence of homologous antiserum *(center circle). (From Baron EJ and Finegold SM: Bailey and Scott's Diagnostic microbiology, ed 8, St Louis, 1990, The CV Mosby Co.)*

agglutination occurs. Control specimens are necessary to ensure that positive results are caused by antibodies against the adsorbed antigen rather than by natural antierythrocyte antibodies.

HEMAGGLUTINATION

The hemagglutination method of testing detects antibodies to erythrocyte antigens. The antibody-containing specimen can be serially diluted and a suspension of red cells added to the dilutions. If a sufficient concentration of antibody is present, the erythrocytes are crosslinked and agglutinated. If non-reacting antibody or an insufficient quantity of antibody is present, the erythrocytes will fail to agglutinate.

By binding different antigens to the red cell surface in indirect hemagglutination or passive hemagglutination, the hemagglutination technique can be extended to detect antibodies to antigens other than those present on the cells (see box). Chemicals such as chromic chloride, tannic acid, and glutaraldehyde can be used to crosslink antigens to the cells.

Some antibodies (e.g., IgG) do not directly agglutinate erythrocytes. This incomplete or blocking type of antibody may be detected by using an enhancement medium such as antihuman globulin reagent. If antihuman globulin reagent is added, this second antibody binds to the antibody present on the erythrocytes.

Mechanism of Agglutination

Agglutination is the clumping of particles that have antigens on their surface, such as erythrocytes, by antibody molecules that form bridges between the antigenic determinants. This is the endpoint for most test involving erythrocyte antigens. Agglutination is influenced by a number of factors and is believed to occur in two stages: *sensitization* and *lattice formation.*

Sensitization

The first phase of agglutination, *sensitization*, represents the physical attachment of antibody molecules to antigens on the erythrocytic membrane. In this initial reversible interaction, antibodies combine rapidly with antigenic particles. The amount of antibody that will react is affected by the equilibrium constant, or *affinity constant*, of the antibody. In most cases, the higher the equilibrium constant, the higher the rate of association

Examples of Immunologic Assays Performed by Indirect Hemagglutination

> Antinuclear ribonucleoprotein (Anti-nRNP)
> Anti-Sm
> Antithyroglobulin and antithyroid microsome
> Rubella antibodies
> Sheep cell agglutination titer (SCAT)

and the slower the rate of dissociation of antibody molecules. The degree of association of antigen with antibody is affected by a variety of factors and can be altered in some cases in vitro by altering some of these factors. The factors influencing antigen-antibody association include:
1. The antigen-antibody ratio, or the number of antibody molecules in relation to the number of antigen sites per cell
2. Physical conditions such as pH, temperature, and length of time of incubation, ionic strength, and steric hindrance

Decreased Antigen-Antibody Ratio

Under conditions of antibody excess, a surplus of molecular antigen-combining sites that are not bound to antigenic determinants exists. The outcome of excessive antibody concentration is known as the *prozone phenomenon*, which can result in false-negative reaction. This phenomenon can be overcome by serially diluting the antibody-containing serum until optimum amounts of antigen and antibody are present in the test system.

pH

Although the optimum pH for all reactions has not been determined, a pH of 7.0 is used for routine laboratory testing. It is known that some antibodies react best at a lower pH.

Temperature and Length of Incubation

The optimum temperature needed to reach equilibrium in an antibody-antigen reaction differs for different antibodies. IgM antibodies are cold-reacting (thermal range 4° to 22° C) and IgG antibodies are warm-reacting, with an optimum temperature of reaction at 37° C. The length of time of incubation required to achieve maximum results depends on the rate of association and dissociation of each specific antibody. In laboratory testing, incubation times range from 15 to 60 minutes. The optimum time of incubation varies, depending on the class of immunoglobulin and how tightly an antibody attaches to its specific antigen.

Ionic Strength

The concentration of salt in the reaction medium has an effect on antibody uptake by the membrane-bound erythrocyte antigens. Sodium (Na^+) and chloride (Cl^-) ions in a solution have a shielding effect. These ions cluster around and partially neutralize the opposite charges on antigen and antibody molecules, which hinders the association of antibody with antigen. By reducing or lowering the ionic strength of a reaction medium such as low ionic strength saline (LISS) or Polybrene, antibody uptake is enhanced.

Steric Hindrance

Steric hindrance is an important physiochemical effect that influences antibody uptake by cell surface antigens. If dissimilar antibodies with approximately the same binding constant are directed against antigenic determinants located close to each other, they will compete for space in reaching their specific receptor sites. The effect of this competition can be mutual blocking, *steric hindrance,* and neither antibody type will be bound to its respective antigenic determinant. Steric hindrance can occur whenever a conformational change in the relationship of an antigenic receptor site to the outside surface occurs. In addition to antibody competition, competition with bound complement, other protein molecules, or the action of agents that interfere with the structural integrity of the cell surface can produce steric hindrance.

The combination of antigen and antibody is a reversible chemical reaction. Altering the physical conditions can result in the release of antibody from the antigen-binding site. When physical conditions are purposely manipulated in order to break the antigen-antibody complex, with subsequent release of the antibody into the surrounding medium, the procedure is referred to as an *elution procedure.*

Lattice Formation

Lattice formation, or the establishment of cross-links between sensitized particles (e.g., erythrocytes) and antibodies resulting in aggregation (clumping), is a much slower process than the sensitization phase. The formation of chemical bonds and resultant lattice formation depends on the ability of a cell with attached antibody on its surface to come close enough to another cell to permit the antibody molecules to bridge the gap and combine with the antigen receptor site on the second cell. Cross-linking is influenced by factors such as the *zeta potential.*

Methods of Enhancing Agglutination

Several techniques can be used to enhance agglutination. These techniques include the following:
1. Centrifugation
2. Treatment with proteolytic enzymes
3. The use of colloids
4. Antihuman globulin (AHG) testing

Treatment with proteolytic enzymes and the use of colloids or AHG techniques are commonly used techniques in blood banking. These methods, however, can also be applied in the immunology laboratory. Centrifugation attempts to overcome the problem of distance by subjecting sensitized cells to a high gravitational force that counteracts the repulsive effect and physically forces the cells together. Enzyme treatment alters the zeta potential or dielectric constant to enhance the chances of demonstrable agglutination. Mild proteolytic enzyme treatment can strip off some of the negative charges on the cell membrane by removing surface sialic acid (cleaving sialoglycoproteins from the cell surface) residues, which reduces the surface charge of cells, lowers the zeta potential, and permits cells to come closer together for chemical linking by specific antibody molecules. Some IgG antibodies will

agglutinate if the zeta potential is carefully adjusted by the addition of colloids and salts. In some cases antigens may be so deeply embedded in the membrane surface that the previously described techniques will not bring the antigens and antibodies close enough to cross-link. The antihuman globulin test is frequently incorporated into the protocol of many laboratory techniques to facilitate agglutination. The direct antiglobulin test can be used to detect disorders such as hemolytic disease of the newborn, transfusion reactions, and differentiation of immunoglobulin from complement coating of erythrocytes.

Graded Agglutination Reactions

Observation of agglutination is initially made by gently shaking the test tube containing the serum and cells and viewing the lower portion, the *button,* with a magnifying glass as it is dispersed. Because agglutination is a reversible reaction, the test tube must be treated delicately and hard shaking must be avoided; however, all of the cells in the button must be resuspended before an accurate observation can be determined. Attention should also be given to observing whether or not discoloration of the fluid above the cells, the *supernatant,* is present. If the erythrocytes have been ruptured or hemolyzed, this is as important a finding as agglutination.

The strength of agglutination (Table 7-1), called *grading,* uses a scale of 0 or negative (no agglutination) to 4+ (all of the erythrocytes are clumped).

Pseudoagglutination, or false appearance of clumping, may rarely occur because of the presence of *rouleaux formation.* Rouleaux formation can be

---

TABLE 7-1

Grading Agglutination Reactions

Grade	Description
Negative	No aggregates.
Mixed field (MF)	Few isolated aggregates, mostly free-floating cells, supernatant appears red.
Weak (+/−)	Tiny aggregates that are barely visible macroscopically, many free erythrocytes, turbid and reddish supernatant.
1+	A few small aggregates just visible macroscopically, many free erythrocytes, turbid and reddish supernatant.
2+	Medium-sized aggregates, some free erythrocytes, clear supernatant.
3+	Several large aggregates, some free erythrocytes, clear supernatant.
4+	All erythrocytes are combined into one solid aggregate, clear supernatant.

encountered in patients with high or abnormal types of globulins in their blood, such as in multiple myeloma, or after receiving dextran as a plasma expander. If this condition is present, upon microscopic examination the erythrocytes will appear as rolls resembling stacks of coins. To disperse the pseudoagglutination, a few drops of physiologic sodium chloride (saline) can be added to the reaction tube, remixed, and reexamined. This procedure, *saline replacement,* should be performed carefully after pseudoagglutination is suspected. It should never be done before the initial testing protocol is followed, for a false-negative result may occur from the dilutional effect of the saline.

Microplate Agglutination Reactions

Serologic testing has usually been performed by slide or test tube techniques, but the increased emphasis on cost containment has stimulated interest in microtechniques as an alternative to conventional methods. Capillary tubes and microplates have been used in some laboratories for a long time. Microtesting for typing lymphocytes was introduced 20 years ago. This method has been adopted internationally and is basically the only method used today for typing lymphocytes. Micromethods for red cell antigen and antibody testing are either hemagglutination or solid-phase adherence assays. These methods are also considered to be simpler to perform. Use of microplates allows for the performance of a large number of tests on a single plate, which eliminates time-consuming steps, such as labeling test tubes.

A microplate is a compact plate of rigid or flexible plastic with multiple wells. The wells may be U-shaped or V-shaped or have a flat bottom configuration. The U-shaped well has been the most commonly used in immunohematology. The volume capacity of each well is approximately 0.2 mL, which prevents spilling during mixing. Samples and reagents are dispensed with small-bore Pasteur pipettes. These pipettes are recommended because they deliver 0.025 mL, which prevents splashing. After the specimens and reagents are added to the wells, they are mixed by gentle agitation of the plates. The microplate is then centrifuged for an immediate reading. Countertop or floor model centrifuges are suitable, if they are equipped with special rotors that can accommodate microplate centrifuge carriers and are capable of speeds between 400 and 2000 rpm. Smaller plates can be centrifuged in serologic centrifuges with an appropriate adapter.

After centrifugation, the cell buttons are resuspended either by gently tapping the microplate or by using a flat-topped mechanical shaker. A shaker provides a more consistent and standard resuspension of the cells than manual tapping. After the cells are resuspended, the wells are examined with an optical aid or over a well-lit surface. A positive reaction will settle in a diffuse, uneven button; negative reactions are manifested by a smooth, compact button. Detection of weakly positive reactions is enhanced by allowing the red cells to settle.

HEMAGGLUTINATION-INHIBITION TECHNIQUE

Many human viruses have the ability to bind to surface structures on erythrocytes from different species. The rubella virus, for example, can bind to human group O, goose, or chicken red blood cells and cause agglutination of these cells. For the detection of some viral antibodies, *hemagglutination-inhibition* (HAI) is the standard against which other screening and diagnostic tests are measured.

Serologic tests for the presence of viral antibodies, such as rubella, exploit the agglutinating properties of the virus particles. Serum suspected of containing disease-causing virus is pretreated with a substance such as kaolin to remove nonspecific inhibitors such as beta lipoproteins, (of red cell agglutination and nonspecific antibodies to the red cells). A known quantity of rubella viral antigen is mixed with dilutions of the patient's serum, to which red blood cells are added. If the serum lacks antibody, the virus will spontaneously attach to the red cells, link together, and agglutinate. If antibodies to the virus are present, all of the virus particles will be bound by antibody, which prevents or inhibits hemagglutination. The serum is therefore positive for hemagglutination-inhibition antibodies. The highest dilution of serum that totally inhibits agglutination of red cells determines the antibody titer of the serum.

The HAI detects a combination of IgG and IgM class antibodies. If IgG antibodies are separated from IgM antibodies by techniques such as sucrose density gradient fractionation or protein absorption, HAI can be used to test for IgM antibodies.

Disadvantages of this technique include the time-consuming nature of the procedure with the requirement of pretreatment of the serum, the fact that the method is highly technique-dependent for accuracy, and the need for visual interpretation of results. Subjective interpretation can influence results, and this type of variability may lead to a finding of seroconversion when none has occurred.

Negative results do not always indicate the absence of antibody. In some cases, false-negative results can result from a low titer of antibody or the removal of antibody by the pretreatment process. False-positive results can be caused by nonspecific inhibitors. The lack of a procedural control removes the assurance that all nonspecific inhibitors have been removed.

Chapter Review

HIGHLIGHTS

Agglutination of particles to which soluble antigen has been adsorbed produces a serum method of demonstrating precipitins. Examples of artificial carriers include latex particles and colloidal charcoal. Cells unrelated to the antigen, such as erythrocytes coated with antigen in a constant amount, can be used as biologic carriers. Whole bacterial cells can contain an antigen that will bind with antibody produced in response to that antigen when it was introduced into the host.

In latex agglutination procedures, antibody molecules can be bound to the surface of latex beads. Many antibody molecules can be bound to each latex particle, which increases the potential number of exposed antigen-binding sites. If an antigen is present in a test specimen, the antigen will bind to the combining sites of the antibody exposed on the surface of the latex beads, forming visible cross-linked aggregates of latex beads and antigen. In some test systems, latex particles can be coated with antigen. In the presence of serum antibody, these particles agglutinate into large, visible clumps. Procedures based on latex agglutination must be performed under standardized conditions. The amount of antigen-antibody binding is influenced by factors such as pH, osmolarity, and ionic concentration of the solution.

Flocculation tests for antibody detection are based on the interaction of soluble antigen with antibody that results in the formation of a precipitate of fine particles. These particles are macroscopically or microscopically visible only because the precipitated product is forced to remain in a confined space. Two variations of flocculation testing can be used in syphilis serologic testing. These are the Venereal Disease Research Laboratory (VDRL) and the rapid plasma reagin (RPR) tests.

Direct whole pathogens can be used to detect antibodies directed against pathogens. The most basic methods are those that measure the antibody produced by the host to determinants on the surface of a bacterial agent in response to infection with that bacteria. In a thick suspension of the bacteria, the binding of specific antibodies to surface antigens of the bacteria causes the bacteria to clump together in visible aggregates. This type of agglutination is called bacterial agglutination. Febrile agglutinin tests use this principle of testing.

In the indirect or passive hemagglutination technique, erythrocytes are coated with substances such as extracts of bacterial cells, rickettsiae, pathogenic fungi, or protozoa or with purified polysaccharides or proteins. Erythrocytes of animals such as sheep or rabbits, or from group O humans, function as carriers for detecting and titrating the corresponding antibodies by agglutination.

This technique is called indirect hemagglutination or passive hemagglutination (PHA) testing, because it is not the antigen of the erythrocytes themselves but the passively attached antigens that are bound by antibody. For the detection of some viral antibodies, hemagglutination-inhibition (HAI) is the standard against which other screening and diagnostic tests are measured.

REVIEW QUESTIONS

1. The quality of test results in an agglutination reaction depends on all of the following except:
   A. length of incubation
   B. amount of antigen conjugated to the carrier
   C. avidity of antigen conjugated to the carrier
   D. whether the carrier is artificial or biologic
   E. the pH of the test system
2. Flocculation procedures differ from latex agglutination procedures because:
   A. antigen is bound to a carrier
   B. antibody is bound to a carrier
   C. soluble antigen reacts with antibody
   D. they are only qualitative procedures
   E. they are only quantitative procedures
3. Indirect hemagglutination is:
   A. also referred to as passive hemagglutination
   B. a system that uses passively attached antibody
   C. a system that uses passively attached antigen
   D. a system that detects whole pathogens to detect antibodies
   E. both A and C
4. In the hemagglutination technique antihuman globulin is used as an enhancement medium to detect _ _ _ _ _type antibodies.
   A. IgM
   B. IgG
   C. IgD
   D. IgE
   E. IgA
5. The prozone phenomenon can result in a (an)_ _ _ _ _ _ _ _
   A. false-positive
   B. false-negative
   C. enhanced agglutination
   D. diminished antigen response
   E. abnormally elevated
6. The effect of competing antibodies seeking to attach to antigen sites is called:
   A. prozone phenomenon
   B. ionic strength
   C. steric hindrance
   D. sensitization
   E. lattice formation
7. All of the following are methods that can be used to enhance agglutination of IgG type antibodies except:
   A. centrifugation
   B. treatment with proteolytic enzymes
   C. acidifying the mixture
   D. using colloids
   E. using antihuman globulin (AHG) testing

Questions 8-11.
Match the following grades of agglutination with the appropriate description.
 8. Mixed field
 9. 1+
10. 2+
11. 4+
  A. all of the erythrocytes are combined into one solid aggregate, clear supernatant
  B. few isolated aggregates, supernatant appears red
  C. medium-sized aggregates, clear supernatant
  D. a few small aggregates, turbid and reddish supernatant
  E. several large aggregates, clear supernatant
12. A classic technique for the detection of viral antibodies is:
  A. passive hemagglutination
  B. indirect hemagglutination
  C. hemagglutination inhibition
  D. latex particle agglutination
  E. biologic carrier agglutination

Answers

1. D 2. C 3. E 4. B 5. B 6. C 7. C 8. B 9. D 10. C 11. A 12. C

BIBLIOGRAPHY

Aloisi RM: Principles of immunology and immunodiagnostics, Philadelphia, 1988, Lea & Febiger.

Baron EJ and Finegold SM: Bailey and Scott's diagnostic microbiology, ed 8, St Louis, 1990, The CV Mosby Co.

Barrett J: Textbook of immunology, St Louis, 1988, The CV Mosby Co.

Henry JB ed: Clinical diagnosis and management, Philadelphia, 1982, WB Saunders.

Peacock JE and Tomar RH: Manual of laboratory immunology, Philadelphia, 1980, Lea & Febiger.

Turgeon ML: Fundamentals of immunohematology, Philadelphia, 1989, Lea & Febiger.

CHAPTER 8

Precipitation Methods

PRECIPITATION REACTIONS

Precipitins can be produced against most proteins and some carbohydrates and carbohydrate-lipid complexes. One of the earliest observations of antigen-antibody reactions was their ability to precipitate when combined in proportions at or near equivalence (Fig. 8-1). Gel diffusion precipitation methods permit the easy identification of soluble antigenic components in a mixture and are useful in the study of the homogeneity and identity of antibodies in a natural material, e.g., serum. This method has been extended to the examination of the relationship between different antigens.

A variety of systems are available in which precipitation tests are performed in semisolid media, such as agar or agarose, or non-gel support medium, such as cellulose acetate. Agar, which is extracted from seaweed, has been found to interfere with the migration of charged particles and has been largely replaced as an immunodiffusion medium by agarose. Agarose is a transparent, colorless, neutral gel.

Antigens and antibodies can diffuse toward one another in gel. If they cross-react, they bind to one another to form a visible precipitate in a band or line when they meet in or near optimal proportions. The antigens and antibodies, however, must be in agar cuts of identical size and shape. The shape of the precipitation band depends in part on the relative molecular weights of both the antigen and antibody. If both are of the same molecular weight, the band is usually straight; if not, the band tends to be concave toward the constituent of higher molecular weight. In general the diffusion rate and the location and density of the precipitation band are influenced by the molecular weights and amount of reactants.

In the clinical laboratory, several applications of the precipitin reaction are used. These methods include the following:
1. Double immunodiffusion
2. Electroimmunodiffusion
3. Immunoelectrophoresis
4. Countercurrent electrophoresis

DOUBLE IMMUNODIFFUSION

Single and double diffusion procedures can be of either the single or double diffusion type. The double diffusion technique, also referred to as the Ouchterlony method, may be used to determine the relationship between antigens and antibodies.

Principle

Antibody dilutions and specific soluble antigens are placed in adjacent wells. If the well size and shape, distance between wells, temperature, and incubation time are optimal, these solutions diffuse out, bind to each other, crosslink and form a visible precipitate at the point of equivalence perpendicular to the axis line between the wells. The patient's spec-

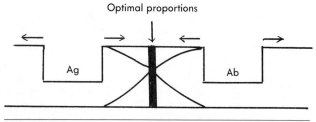

FIGURE 8-1
Gel diffusion.

imen is examined for precipitation bands and compared with a standard antigen, which has reacted with a known concentration of specific antibody in a comparison test. The precise location of the band depends on the concentration and rate of diffusion of antigen and antibody. In a condition of antibody excess, the band will be located nearer the antigen well. If two antigens are present in the solution that can be recognized by the antibody, two precipitin bands form independently (Fig. 8-2, *A*). Antibodies associated with autoimmune disorders such as rheumatoid arthritis and systemic lupus erythematosus can be identified by double diffusion (see box below).

Double Immunodiffusion Technique
Specimen Collection and Preparation
No special preparation of the patient is required before specimen collection. The patient must be positively identified when the specimen is collected. The specimen shall be labeled at the bedside and include the patient's full name, the date, and the patient's hospital identification number. The phlebotomist's initials should also appear on the label.

Blood should be drawn by an aseptic technique. A minimum of 2 mL of clotted blood (red-top evacuated tube) is required. The blood should be centrifuged and the serum should be removed. Hemolysis makes the specimen unsuitable for testing.

Reagents, Supplies, and Equipment
1. Immunodiffusion plates (about 3 × 9 cm in diameter and 1.5 mm thick filled with 1% agarose) with pre-cut wells (available commercially) or slides (prepared by pouring 1% to 2% agar in buffer at pH 7.0 to 8.5 on them and allowing them to set before punching wells into the gel).
2. Liquid antigen
3. Specific antisera (commercially available) for known control antiserum dilutions and known antigen controls. The dilutions of the antisera varies from 1:1 to 1:640.
4. Micropipettes

Examples of Immunologic Assays Performed by Double Diffusion

> Anti-Rheumatoid Arthritis Nuclear Antigen (Anti-RANA)
> Antinuclear Ribonucleoprotein (Anti-nRNP)
> Anti-Scl or Anti-Scl-70
> Anti-Sm
> Anti-SS-A (SS-A Precipitin, Anti-Ro)
> Anti-SS-B (SS-B Precipitin, Anti-La)
> Jo-1 Antibody
> Ku Antibody
> Mi-1-Antibody
> PM-1 Antibody

Quality Control
Antisera containing known soluble antigens and a known control of diluted antiserum must be tested concurrently with patient specimens.

Procedure
1. Remove the commercial immunodiffusion plate from the plastic envelope. Open the plate and allow it to stand open for about 5 minutes so that any excess moisture in the wells has a chance to evaporate.
2. Number the wells on the bottom of the plate with a permanent marker.
3. Prepare a reference card to identify sera, antigens, and controls.
4. Fill the appropriate wells almost to the brim with antiserum, and fill the peripheral wells with antigen, e.g., homologous, related, and unrelated.
5. Close the lid of the plate; put it back in the plastic envelope and seal.
6. Incubate for 18 to 48 hours or longer at 37° C for for 2 to 3 days at room temperature.
7. If the test has been performed on a slide, the gel is washed from the slide and stained with a protein stain, such as Coomassie Blue.

Reporting Results
Three basic reaction patterns result from the relationship of antigens and antibodies. These patterns are identity, non-identity, and partial identity.

Identity
An identity reaction is indicated when the precipitin band forms a single smooth arc. This precipitin arc formed between the antibody and the two test antigens fuse (Fig. 8-2, *A*), indicating that the antibody is precipitating identical antigen specificities in each preparation. This does not mean that the antigens are necessarily identical, they are only identical as far as the antibody can distinguish the difference.

Non-identity
A non-identity pattern (Fig. 8-2, *B*) is expressed when the precipitation lines cross each other. They intersect or cross because the samples contain no antigenic determinants in common.

Partial Identity
In a partial identity pattern (Fig. 8-2, *C*), the precipitation lines merge with spur formation. This merger indicates that the antigens are nonidentical but possess common determinants.

Procedure Notes
Sources of error. Excessive condensation in the wells may alter the diffusion pattern. Filling the wells improperly can also contribute to error. Failure to identify the wells properly can lead to confu-

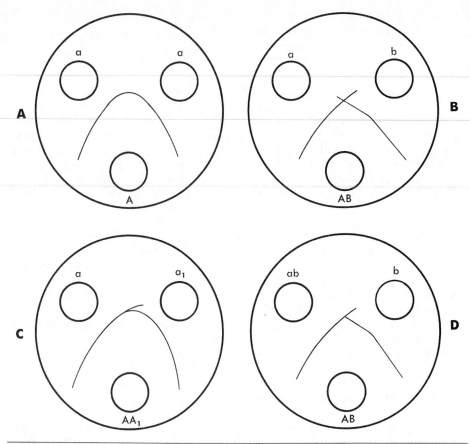

FIGURE 8-2

Precipitation pattern of Ouchterlony type of immunodiffusion. **A,** Type I: reaction of identity. The antiserum cannot distinguish one antigen from the other. **B,** Type II: reaction of nonidentity. The two antigens react with different antibodies. **C,** Type III: reaction of partial identity. One antigen cross-reacts with the other antigen to which it is serologically related but not identical. **D,** Type IV: reaction of inhibition. The antigens carry unrelated determinants, and the antibody contains separate antibody components.
(From Bauer JD: Clinical laboratory methods, ed 9, St Louis, 1982, The CV Mosby Co.)

sion. Insufficient incubation can produce a false negative result.

Clinical applications. Antibodies associated with autoimmune disorders such as rheumatoid arthritis, systemic lupus erythematosus (SLE), systemic sclerosis, Sjogren's syndrome, and vasculitis can be identified by double diffusion. The clinical applications of these tests can be found in Appendix B.)

Limitations. Although the thickness of a band suggests the increased or decreased levels of an antibody, the double diffusion method is only semiquantitative.

RADIAL IMMUNODIFFUSION (RID)

Gel techniques only identify antigens and antibodies qualitatively; however, by further modification and the use of single radial immunodiffusion (RID) they can become quantitative. The RID is a simple

and specific method for identification and quantitation of a number of proteins found in human serum and other body fluids (see box below). This technique may be used when the nature of a protein is not readily differentiated by standard electrophoretic procedures.

Examples of Immunologic Assays Performed by Radial Immunodiffusion

Alpha-1-Acid Glycoprotein
Alpha-1-Antitrypsin
Haptoglobin
Transferrin
C3
C4
C5
C-Reactive Protein
Immunoglobulins (IgM, IgG, IgA, and IgD)

Principle

The quantitation of proteins by gel diffusion using antibody incorporated in agar was reported in 1957. In the last several decades a wide selection of specific antisera has become available, which allows for the quantitation of their corresponding antigen.

Radial immunodiffusion is based on a technique using a precipitin reaction in which the internal reactants, i.e., specific antibody, is added to a buffered agarose medium. Serum containing standard volumes of the protein, i.e., test antigen, are placed in a well centered in the agarose. When this immunodiffusion system has an unlimited amount of antibody available and no undue restrictions placed on free diffusion of the antigen, the diameter of the resulting precipitin zone is related to the concentration of antigen placed in the well. While the precipitin ring is enlarging, the log of the antigen concentration is approximately proportional to the diameter of the endpoint, and the area (square of the diameter) varies directly with the concentration.

Methods

Two principal RID methods have been developed: the Fahey method and the Mancini method. The difference between the two techniques is that the Fahey method is a kinetic approach in which the ring diameter is read at a specified time. The Mancini method is an endpoint method in which the ring diameter is read after diffusion is completed. In the Mancini method the quantitative determination of proteins is after 24 hours of diffusion.

After antibody is added to the well cut in the agar gel and fixed volumes of test antigen of different concentrations are put into the wells, the gel plate is allowed to incubate for 18 to 24 hours (Mancini method) for the antigen to diffuse out from the wells. Antigen continues to diffuse and bind more antibody until an equivalence point is reached and the soluble complexes precipitate in a ring. If the antibody concentration and gel thickness are uniform and constant, the area within the precipitin ring (measured as the ring diameter squared) is proportional to the antigen concentration. When the diameter of the ring (D^2) is plotted against the antigen concentration, a straight line results based on the equation:

$$D^2 = K(Cag) + So$$

K = constant; Cag = concentration of antigen; and So = intercept (function of antigen well diameter and of antigen volume)

The concentration of protein in an unknown specimen is derived by interpolation from a standard curve. The whole process may be reversed to determine the concentrations of unknown antibody.

Advantages and Disadvantages

RID requires no special equipment and can be performed in many clinical laboratories. The procedure is considered to be sensitive, rapid, and accurate. In addition, for many smaller laboratories, it is an economical and practical method of performing quantitative studies.

Some of the limitations of procedure include the fact that it is limited by the assay ranges of the plate. The precision of the assay as expressed by the coefficient of variation is about 10%. In addition, idiotypically related differences in the immunologic reactivity to IgG, IgA, or IgM may result in differences in the quantitative values obtained with the RID method. Multiple myeloma or other disorders involving monoclonal gammopathies may yield values either higher or lower than those reported with other methods.

RID Protocol
Principle

A qualitative relationship exists between the concentration of a protein deposited in a well, cut into a thin agarose layer containing the corresponding monospecific antiserum. The wells are filled with unknown serum or a suitable standard and incubated in a moist environment at room temperature. After the optimal point of diffusion has been reached, the diameters of the precipitin rings are measured. The diameter of the ring is related to the concentration of the constituent, e.g., immunoglobulin (Fig. 8-3). RID is intended for the quantification of specific proteins such as IgM, IgG, IgA, alpha$_1$ antitrypsin, transferrin, and complement components, e.g., C3.

Specimen Collection and Preparation

No special preparation of the patient is required before specimen collection. The patient must be positively identified when the specimen is collected, and the specimen should be labeled at the bedside. Specimen labels should include the patient's full name, the date, the patient's hospital identification number, and the phlebotomist's initials.

Blood should be drawn by an aseptic technique. A minimum of 2 mL of clotted blood (red-top evacuated tube) is required. The specimen should be centrifuged promptly and an aliquot of serum removed. Lipemia, hemolysis, or contamination with bacteria renders a specimen unsuitable for testing. Although icteric and turbid specimens have given valid results, fresh nonheat inactivated serum is *recommended* for use in the test.

If the test cannot be performed immediately, the specimen should be refrigerated (2° to 8° C) for no longer than 72 hours. If additional delay occurs, the serum should be frozen at −18° C or below. Frozen serum should be thawed rapidly at 37° C.

Reagents, Supplies, and Equipment
1. RID plates (available commercially)
2. Three standard serum dilutions
3. Microliter dispenser
4. Semi-log and linear graph paper
5. Ruler

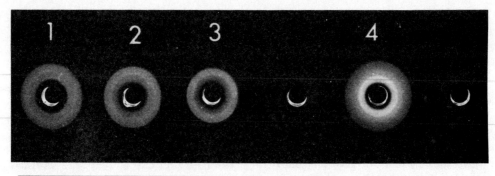

FIGURE 8-3

Quantitation of IgG by radial immunodiffusion. Increasing diameters of precipitin rings reflect increasingly larger protein concentrations. Wells *1* through *3* are known IgG standards; well *4* is an unknown serum.
(From Bauer JD: Clinical laboratory methods, ed 9, St Louis, 1982, The CV Mosby Co.)

Quality Control

Reference sera with known values should be tested simultaneously. **Caution:** Because the control sera is derived from human sources, it should be handled in the same manner as clinical serum specimens (see *Universal blood and body fluid precautions* in Chapter 6).

Procedure

1. Remove plate from envelope and allow to stand open for about 5 minutes to allow any moisture to evaporate.
2. Label the wells on the outer margin of the plate and on a card to identify sera and controls to be deposited into the wells.
3. Fill three wells with 2 to 20 μL (in accordance with manufacturer's instruction) with the standards supplied.
4. Fill the remaining groups of two or three wells with diluted or undiluted patient's sera (follow manufacturer's instruction).
5. Tightly close plate and place into envelope that is sealed with tape to prevent loss of moisture.
6. Store the plate in a horizontal position at room temperature for a minimum of 6 to 12 hours (Fahey-McKelvey technique) or for about 50 hours (Mancini technique) depending on the type of immunoglobulin assayed.
7. After the appropriate time (see below) measure the diameter (D) of the precipitin ring (in millimeters) of the unknown and standards to an accuracy of 0.1 mm using a calibrated magnifier and a light source beneath the plate.

Calculations

Square the diameter reading (D^2) and construct a standard curve. Two methods are available for the construction of the standard curve and the calculation of patient values.

Fahey-McKelvey method. The early readout method of Fahey measures the precipitin rings (unknown and standards) before they reach maximal size, after about 6 to 12 hours. In this method the logarithm of the antigen concentration is proportional to the area of the precipitin ring (D^2). Plot the squared diameter (D^2) of the precipitin rings obtained from three standards on the ordinate of semilog graph paper, and enter the corresponding concentrations of the standards (in milligrams/deciliter) on the abscissa. Because the concentrations are plotted on semilog paper, a straight line is obtained.

Mancini method. Based on fact that after a certain time, depending on the concentration and the molecule weight of the protein, a precipitin ring reaches a maximal value and further incubation fails to increase its size. The area of the precipitin ring (square of its diameter) is linearly proportional to the antigen concentration in the well. Plotting these values on linear graph paper produces a straight line. The maximal ring diameter is obtained in about 24 hours by IgG in normal concentration and in about 50 hours by IgM of normal concentration. The linear relationship between the area (in square millimeters) and concentration is not established until the rings (standard and unknown) reach their maximal size. The endpoint method has a high degree of accuracy, reproducibility, and sensitivity but requires time.

1. Plot the squared diameter (D^2) of the precipitin rings obtained from the three standards on ordinate of linear graph paper, and enter the corresponding concentrations of the standards (in milligrams/deciliter) on the abscissa. Connecting the three reference points should result in a straight line. The patient's value is obtained by reference to this calibration curve.
2. If diluted patient's serum is used, multiply the concentration by the dilution factor to obtain the value for whole serum.

Reporting Results

Method is sensitive (10 to 20 mg protein/dL, depending on the protein).

Procedure Notes

Sources of error. Sources of technical error include the following:

1. Specimen contamination
2. Spilling of the antigen
3. Inadequate filling of the wells
4. Damaged or out-of-date gel

Clinical applications. If the procedure is used for immunoglobulin assay, hypogammaglobulinemia or hypergammaglobulinemia may be detected.

Limitations. The procedure is limited by the assay ranges of the plate and the precision of the immunoglobulin assay (cv) is about 10%.

ELECTROIMMUNODIFFUSION (EID)

EID is a variation of the double immunodiffusion reaction in a support medium such as cellulose acetate or agarose through the use of an electric current that enhances the mobility of reactants and increases their movement toward each other. The technique is similar to double immunodiffusion, but it combines the speed of electrophoresis with the accuracy and sensitivity of immunodiffusion.

Antibody is placed in the well favoring its migration in the direction of the cathode; antigens that tend to be more negatively charged are placed in the well that favors migration to the anode.

Precipitin bands form at a point of equivalence in a shorter period of time. These bands flank the lateral borders of the moving antigen until the exhaustion of antigen as a result of precipitation causes the precipitin bands to converge. They finally meet in the middle of the leading edge of the antigen path when all the antigen is precipitate. The precipitin pattern resembles the outline of a rocket.

EID allows quantitation of proteins (see box) having a negative charge that differs from that of the antibody. Immunoglobulins must be modified by special alkaline buffers to increase their negative charge and thus their anodic migration. The method is not suitable for quantitation of M proteins of monoclonal gammopathies, since their variations are responsible for abnormal electrophoretic mobilities that may stop short of the expected endpoint.

EID methods, like immunodiffusion procedures, are classified into one- or two-dimensional, single, or double diffusion. By applying a voltage across the gels to move the antigens and antibodies together immuno-double diffusion becomes counter-current immunoelectrophoresis (CIE); radial immunodiffusion (RID) become electroimmunoassay (EIA), or rocket electrophoresis.

Countercurrent Immunoelectrophoresis

Counterimmunoelectrophoresis (CIE) is a variation of the classic precipitin procedure; it merely adds an electrical current to help antigens and antibodies move toward each other more quickly than in simple diffusion (Fig. 8-4). The procedure takes advantage of the net electric charge of the antigens and antibodies being tested in a particular test buffer. All variables such as type of gel, amount of current, amounts and concentrations of antigen and antibody, must be carefully controlled for maximum reactivity.

Principle

Countercurrent immunoelectrophoresis is performed in agar gels where the pH is chosen so that the antibodies are positively charged and the antigens are negatively charged. Solutions of antibody and specimens to be tested are placed in small wells cut into agarose on a glass surface. Because several wells can be cut in one agarose slab, small portions of a specimen can be tested against several different antibodies. A paper or fiber wick is used to connect the opposite sides of the agarose to troughs of buffer.

When an electric current is applied through the buffer, the negatively charged antigen molecules (if they are present) migrate toward the positive electrode, which is also toward the wells on the other side of the agarose. The neutrally charged antibodies are carried toward the negative electrode by the flow of the slightly alkaline buffer. When a zone of equivalence is reached, the antigen-antibody complexes form a visible precipitin band. The entire procedure usually takes about 1 hour.

The agarose gel may require overnight washing in distilled water to remove nonspecific precipitin reactions. Testing positive and negative controls is especially critical because antisera may contain nonspecifically reacting agents that form nonstable complexes in the gel.

Advantages and Disadvantages

The sensitivity of CIE is 10 to 20 times greater (detecting approximately 0.01 to 0.05 mg antigen per mL) than in immuno-double diffusion. These techniques operate in the range 20 µg/mL to 2 mg/mL of antigen or antibody. If the specimen contains only minute amounts of antigen or the molecule is too small to yield a visible precipitin band, a more sensitive immunoassay is needed.

Any antigens for which antisera are available (see box) can be tested by CIE. Precipitin bands, however, are often difficult to see. Although the

---

Examples of Immunologic Assays Performed by Electroimmunodiffusion

$C1_q$
$C2$
Immunoglobulin G (IgG) subclasses

Examples of Immunologic Assays Performed by Counterimmunoelectrophoresis

Antinuclear Ribonucleoprotein (Anti-nRNP)
Anti-Sm
Radioimmunoprecipitation

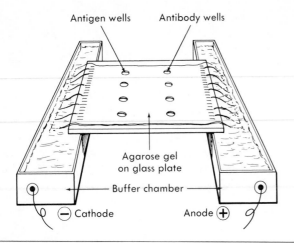

FIGURE 8-4

Apparatus for performing counterimmunoelectrophoresis.

(From Baron EJ and Finegold SM: Bailey and Scott's Diagnostic microbiology, ed 8, St Louis, 1990, The CV Mosby Co.)

technique is specific, it is time consuming to perform. CIE is more expensive than other techniques, such as immunodiffusion, because of initial capital outlay and the large quantities of antigen and antibody that must be used to produce a visible reaction.

Rocket Electrophoresis

By applying a voltage across a gel to move the antigens and antibodies together, radial immunodiffusion (RID) becomes electroimmunoassay or rocket electrophoresis. This technique combines the speed of electrophoresis with the accuracy and sensitivity of RID.

Principles

Antigens may be quantitated by electrophoresing them in an antibody-containing gel in rocket electrophoresis. This technique relies on antigens and antibodies having different charges at the selected pH, which is true of most antigens because antibodies have a relatively high isoelectric point; i.e., they are neutrally charged at a more alkaline pH than most antigens. Immunoglobulins must be modified using a special alkaline buffer to increase their negative charge and thus their anode migration. Rocket electrophoresis can be reversed to estimate antibody concentration, if a suitable pH that will immobilize the antigen (without damaging it or preventing an antigen-antibody reaction) can be found.

Immunoglobulin-specific antibodies are added to agarose and the pH is adjusted to inhibit antibody migration. With this method, antigen samples are applied to wells in an antibody-containing agarose gel. The support medium contains 16 application

sites. Two dilutions of the patient serum are applied to two sites, and three or four increasing dilutions of the protein standard are applied to the other sites. The pH of the gel is chosen so that the antibodies remain immobile and the negatively charged antigens migrate. Precipitin bands of antigen-antibody complexes aggregating in a thin visible line flank the lateral borders of the migrating antigen until the concentration of antigen is exhausted. These bands converge and finally meet in the middle of the leading edge of the antigen path when all the antigen is precipitated. The precipitin pattern resembles a shooting rocket. The height of the rocket is proportional to the antigen concentration. Quantitation of the unknown specimen is possible by constructing a standard curve using a calibrator and plotting the concentration values versus migration length (height of the rocket) on a graph.

Advantages and Disadvantages

In rocket electrophoresis, antigen levels can be determined in less than 4 hours instead of the 48 to 72 hours needed for an RID procedure. The calibrators are human sera with known immunoglobulin levels. This procedure, however, is not suitable for quantitation of M protein of monoclonal gammopathies because their variations are responsible for abnormal electrophoretic mobilities that may stop short of the expected endpoint.

Chapter Review

HIGHLIGHTS

Precipitation is the term applied to aggregation of a soluble test antigen. Precipitins can be produced against most proteins and some carbohydrates and carbohydrate-lipid complexes. A variety of systems is available in which precipitation tests are performed in semisolid media, such as agar or agarose, or non-gel support medium, such as cellulose acetate. Antigens and antibodies can diffuse toward one another in gel. If they cross-react, they bind to one another to form a visible precipitate in a band or line when they meet in or near optimal proportions. The antigens and antibodies, however, must be in agar cuts of identical size and shape. The shape of the precipitation band depends in part on the relative molecular weights of both the antigen and antibody. If both are of the same molecular weight, the band is usually straight; if not, the band tends to be concave toward the constituent of higher molecular weight. In general the diffusion rate and the location and density of the precipitation band are influenced by the molecular weights and amount of reactants. In the clinical laboratory, several applications of the precipitin reaction are used. These methods include double immunodiffusion, electroimmunodiffusion (counter immunoelectrophoresis), immunoelectrophoresis (IEP), and countercurrent electrophoresis.

Single and double diffusion procedures can be of either the single or double diffusion type. The double diffusion technique, (also referred to as the Ouchterlony method) may be used to determine the relationship between antigens and antibodies. An identity reaction is indicated when the precipitin band forms a single smooth arc. In this type of reaction the precipitin arc formed between the antibody and the two test antigens fuse indicating that the antibody is precipitating identical antigen specificities in each preparation. This does not mean that the antigens are necessarily identical; they are only identical as far as the antibody can distinguish the difference. A nonidentity pattern is expressed when the precipitation lines cross each other. They intersect or cross because the samples contain no antigenic determinants in common. In a partial identity pattern, the precipitation lines merge with spur formation. This indicates that the antigens are nonidentical but possess common determinants. Antibodies associated with autoimmune disorders such as rheumatoid arthritis, systemic lupus erythematosus (SLE), systemic sclerosis, Sjogren's syndrome, and vasculitis can be identified by double diffusion.

Gel techniques only identify antigens and antibodies qualitatively, but by further modification and using single radial immunodiffusion they can become quantitative. The radial immunodiffusion technique (RID) is a simple and specific method for identification and quantitation of a number of proteins found in human serum and other body fluids. This technique may be used when the nature of a protein is not readily differentiated by standard electorphoretic procedures. RID is based on a technique using a precipitin reaction in which the internal reactants, i.e., specific antibody, is added to a buffered agarose medium. Serum containing standard volumes of the protein, i.e., test antigen, are placed in a well centered in the agarose. When this immunodiffusion system has an unlimited amount of antibody available and no undue restrictions placed on free diffusion of the antigen, the diameter of the resulting precipitin zone is related to the concentration of antigen placed in the well. While the precipitin ring is enlarging, the log of the antigen concentration is approximately proportional to the diameter of the endpoint, and the area (square of the diameter) varies directly with the concentration.

Electroimmunodiffusion (EID) is a variation of the double immunodiffusion technique. EID merely adds an electrical current to accelerate the diffusion of antigen and antibody toward each other. Antigens are first separated in the gel by placing an electrical charge across it. The pH of the media is chosen so that positively charged proteins move to the negative electrode and negatively charged proteins move to the positive electrode. EID allows quantitation of proteins that have a negative charge that differs from that of the antibody. Immunoglobulins must be modified by special alkaline buffers to increase their negative charge and thus their anodic migration. The method is not suitable for quantitation of M proteins of monoclonal gammopathies, since their variations are responsible for abnormal electrophoretic mobilities that may stop short of the expected endpoint. EID methods, like immunodiffusion procedures, are classified into one- or two-dimensional, single, or double diffusion. By applying a voltage across the gels to move the antigens and antibodies together, immuno-double diffusion becomes countercurrent immunoelectrophoresis (CIE); radial immunodiffusion (RID) becomes electroimmunoassay (EIA), or rocket electrophoresis.

Counterimmunoelectrophoresis (CIE) is a variation of the classic precipitin procedure, it merely adds an electrical current to help antigens and antibodies move toward each other more quickly than in simple diffusion. The procedure takes advantage of the net electric charge of the antigens and antibodies being tested in a particular test buffer. All variables such as type of gel, amount of current, amounts and concentrations of antigen and antibody, must be carefully controlled for maximum reactivity. The sensitivity of CIE is 10 to 20 times greater than in immuno-double diffusion.

By applying a voltage across a gel to move the antigens and antibodies together, RID become electroimmunoassay, or rocket electrophoresis. This technique combines the speed of electrophoresis with the accuracy and sensitivity of RID. It relies on antigens and antibodies having different charges at the selected pH, which is true of most antigens because antibodies have a relatively high isoelectric point, i.e., they are neutrally charged at a more alkaline pH than most antigens. Immunoglobulins must be modified using a special alkaline buffer to increase their negative charge and thus their anode migration. Rocket electrophoresis can be reversed to estimate antibody concentration, if a suitable pH that will immobilize the antigen (without damaging it or preventing an antigen-antibody reaction) can be found. In rocket electrophoresis, antigen levels can be determined in less than 4 hours instead of the 48 to 72 hours needed for an RID procedure. This procedure, however, is not suitable for quantitation of M protein of monoclonal gammopathies because their variations are responsible for abnormal electrophoretic mobilities that may stop short of the expected endpoint.

REVIEW QUESTIONS

Questions 1 and 2.

Match the term and its respective definition.

1. Precipitation
2. Agglutination
   A. Aggregation of a soluble test antigen
   B. Aggregation of a particulate antigen
3. Applications of the precipitin reaction are used in all of the following laboratory methods except:
   A. Double immunodiffusion
   B. Electroimmunodiffusion
   C. Immunoelectrophoresis
   D. Hemagglutination
   E. Countercurrent electrophoresis

Questions 4-6.

Match the following terms and their respective definitions.

4. Identity
5. Non-identity
6. Partial identity
   A. Precipitation lines merge with a spur formation
   B. Precipitin band forms a single smooth arc
   C. Precipitin lines remain parallel to each other
   D. Precipitin lines cross each other
   E. Precipitin lines move away from each other
7. The difference between the Fahey and Mancini methods of radial immunodiffusion is that in the _____method the endpoint is read after diffusion is complete.
   A. Fahey
   B. Mancini
8. Which of the following applications is *not* suitable for quantitation by the electroimmunodiffusion technique?
   A. Ciq
   B. C2

C. IgG$_1$
D. IgG$_2$
E. M proteins

Questions 9 and 10. True or False.

A = True,
B = False.

9. The sensitivity of counterimmunoelectrophoresis is 10 to 20 times greater than immunodiffusion.
10. Rocket electrophoresis is slower than radial immunodiffusion.

Answers

1. B 2. A 3. D 4. B 5. D 6. A 7. B 8. E 9. A 10. B

BIBLIOGRAPHY

Aloisi RM: Principles of immunology and immunodiagnostics, Philadelphia, 1988, Lea & Febiger.

Barrett J: Textbook of immunology, St. Louis, 1988, The CV Mosby Co.

Fahey JL and McKelvey EM: Quantitative determination of serum immunoglobulin in antibody-agar plate, J Immunol 94:84-94, 1965.

Feinbert JG: Identification, discrimination and quantification in Ouchterlony gel plates, Int Arch Allergy 11:129-152, 1957.

Henry JB, editor: Clinical diagnosis and management, Philadelphia, 1982, WB Saunders Co.

Mancini G, Carbonara AO, and Heremans JF: Immunochemical quantitation of antigens by single radial immunodiffusion, Immunochem 2:235-254, 1965.

Ouchterlony O: Handbook of immunodiffusion and immunoelectrophoresis, Ann Arbor, Mich., Ann Arbor Sci Publ, 1968.

Peacock JA and Tomar RH: Manual of laboratory immunology, Philadelphia, 1980, Lea & Febiger.

Tizmann SE and Danields JC, editors: Serum protein abnormalities, Boston, 1975, Little, Brown & Co.

CHAPTER 9

Electrophoresis Techniques

IMMUNOELECTROPHORESIS (IEP)

Serum electrophoresis results in the separation of proteins into five fractions on cellulose acetate. This separation is based on the rate of migration of these individual components in an electrical field. By comparison, immunoelectrophoresis (IEP) involves the electrophoresis of serum or urine followed by immunodiffusion. The size and position of precipitin bands provide the same type of information regarding equivalence or antibody excess as the double immunodiffusion method. Proteins, however, are differentiated not only by their electrophoretic mobility but also by their diffusion coefficient and antibody specificity.

While double-diffusion produces a separate precipitation band for each antigen-antibody system in a mixture, it is often difficult to determine all of the components in a very complex mixture. IEP separates the antigen mixture by electrophoresis before performing immunodiffusion.

Principle

IEP is a combination of the techniques of electrophoresis and double immunodiffusion. IEP consists of two phases: electrophoresis and diffusion. In the first phase, serum is placed in an appropriate medium, e.g., cellulose acetate or agarose, and then electrophoresed to separate its constituents according to electrophoretic mobilites: albumin, alpha$_1$, alpha$_2$, beta, and gammaglobulin fractions. In the second phase following electrophoresis, the fractions are allowed to act as antigens and to interact with their corresponding antibodies. Antiserum, polyvalent or monovalent, is deposited in a trough cut into the gel to one side and parallel to this line of separated proteins. Incubation allows double immunodiffusion of these antigens and antibodies toward each other to take place. Each antiserum diffuses outward, perpendicular to the trough, and each serum protein diffuses outward from its point of electrophoresis. When a favorable antigen-to-antibody ratio exists (equivalence point), the antigen-antibody complex becomes visible as precipitin lines or bands. Diffusion is halted by rinsing the plate in 0.85% saline. Unbound protein is washed from the agarose with saline, and the antigen-antibody precipitin arcs are stained with a protein sensitive stain.

Each line represents one specific protein. Proteins are thus differentiated not only by their electrophoretic mobility but also by their diffusion coefficient and antibody specificity. Antibody diffuses as a uniform band parallel to the antibody trough. If the proteins are homogeneous, the antigen diffuses in a circle and the antigen-antibody precipitation line resembles a segment or arc of a circle. If the antigen is heterogeneous, the antigen-antibody line assumes an elliptical shape.

One arc of precipitation forms for each constituent in the antigen mixture. This technique can be used to resolve the protein of normal serum into 25 to 40 distinct precipitation bands. The exact number depends on the strength and specificity of the antiserum used.

Normal Appearance of Precipitin Bands

Immunoprecipitation bands should be of normal curvature, symmetry, length, position, intensity, and distance from the antigen well and antibody trough (Fig. 9-1). In normal serum, IgG, IgA, and IgM are present in sufficient concentrations of 10mg/mL, 2 mg/mL, and 1mg/mL, respectively, to produce precipitin lines. The normal concentrations of IgD and IgE are too low to be detected by IEP.

A normal IgG precipitin band is elongated, ellip-

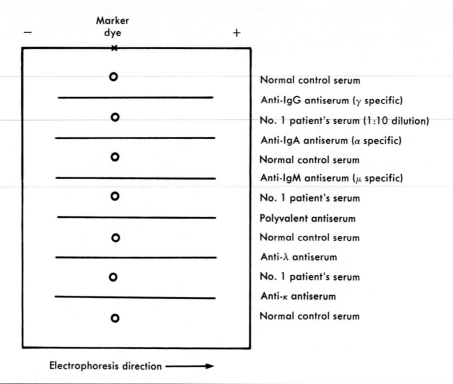

FIGURE 9-1

Suggested sequence of antigen-antiserum combinations employed in immunoelectrophoresis (IEP).

(From Bauer JD: Clinical laboratory methods, ed 9, St. Louis, 1982, The CV Mosby Co.)

tical, slightly curved, and clearly visible in undiluted and in 1:10 diluted serum. An IgG band is located cathodic to the antigen well in the alpha area of the electrophoretogram, if monospecific serum is used, it is fused with a thin precipitin line positioned midway between the antigen well and antibody trough and extending into the beta area. The IgM and IgA bands are visible in undiluted serum but disappear at a 1:10 dilution of serum. The IgA band is a flattened thin arc, slightly cathodic to the well in the alpha-beta position. The IgM line is a barely visible, thin line, slightly cathodic to the antigen well.

Clinical Applications of IEP

IEP is a reliable and accurate method for detecting both structural abnormalities and concentration changes in proteins. It is possible to identify the absence of a normal serum protein, such as a congenital deficiency of some complement components or alterations in serum proteins. This method can be used for screening for circulating immune complexes, characterization of cryoglobulinemia and pyroglobulinemia, recognition and characterization of antibody syndromes, and recognition and characterization of the various forms of dysgammaglobulinemias.

The most common application of IEP is in the diagnosis of a *monoclonal gammopathy*, a condition in which a single clone of plasma cells produces elevated levels of a single class and type of immunoglobulin. The elevated immunoglobulin is referred to as a *monoclonal protein, M-protein,* or *paraprotein.* Monoclonal gammopathies may indicate a malignancy such as multiple myeloma or macroglobulinemia. Anti-kappa and anti-lambda antisera are necessary for complete typing of the immunoglobulin in the evaluation of the ratio and for the diagnosis of monoclonal M proteins. The class (heavy [H] chain) and type (light [L] chain) must be established because a patient's prognosis and treatment may differ depending on the immunoglobulin identified. Differentiation must also be made between monoclonal and *polyclonal gammopathies.* A polyclonal gammopathy is a secondary condition caused by disorders such as liver disease, collagen disorders, rheumatoid arthritis, and chronic infection. It is characterized by elevation of two or more (often all) immunoglobulins by several clones of plasma cells. Polyclonal increases of proteins are usually twice the normal levels.

The most important application of IEP of urine is the demonstration of *Bence Jones* (BJ) protein. IEP detects very low concentrations of BJ protein (about 1 to 2 mg/dL). If BJ protein is present in a urine specimen, precipitin lines will form with either kappa or lambda anti-light chain antisera because BJ protein is composed of homogeneous light chains of a single antigen type, either kappa or lambda. Normal light chains are heterogeneous and include equal concentrations of kappa and lambda.

Abnormal Appearance of Precipitin Bands

The size and position of precipitin bands provide the same type of information regarding equivalence or antigen-antibody excess as double immunodiffusion systems. The position and shape of precipitin bands in the IEP assay of serum are relatively stable and reproducible. Virtually any deviation is abnormal. These abnormalities can be detected by evaluating the following features of the precipitin bands:

1. The position of the band in relationship to electrophoretically identified protein fractions
2. The position of the band between the antigen well and the antibody trough
3. Distortion of the curvature or arc formation
4. Thickening (density) and elongation of a band
5. Shortening (inhibition), thinning, or doubling

Position of the Band

The precipitin band may be displaced compared to its normal position in the control serum because molecular charges in the abnormal protein may affect its speed of migration in the electrophoresis phase of IEP. A precipitin band may form a line of fusion or partial fusion with another protein, indicating the presence of proteins immunologically similar but electrophoretically distinct. A distinct abnormality in the position of the band is seen in cases of monoclonal IgA gammopathy. The monoclonal IgA band is closer to the antibody trough than normal IgA.

Distortion of curvature or arc

An abnormal curvature of the precipitin band can be observed with M proteins because of an antigen excess. The monoclonal IgG band shows an arc of a circle rather than the elongated, elliptical shape of a normal band. This distortion of IgG reflects the homogeneous nature and limited electrophoretic mobility of the abnormal protein.

Normal IgM and IgD bands are hardly visible, but the monoclonal IgM or IgD bands are skewed arcs of a circle.

Thickening and elongation

Thickening and elongation can be seen in the presence of M proteins because excess antigen diffuses a greater distance. Monoclonal IgM, IgG, IgD, and IgA all demonstrate denser than normal bands. In addition, monoclonal IgG touches the antisera trough.

Shortening, thinning, or doubling

A band may be shortened and incomplete because of inhibition of a segment due to the antibody reacting only with a portion of the abnormal protein. Monoclonal IgE elevation leads to a short, thick arc in the antigen well area extending to the anodal side.

Polyvalent and Monovalent Antisera

Polyvalent antiserum confirms the presence or absence of major protein fractions. Monospecific antisera for specific individual immunoglobulins identify only the corresponding proteins. If the nonspecific antisera have combining sites for H and L chains, the combining sites will react with L chains of other immunoglobulins or with the free L chains of Bence Jones protein. H chain-specific sera do not cross-react with other proteins.

Procedural Protocol

Procedure

Immunoelectrophoresis (IEP).

Principle

The patient specimen, e.g., serum, is placed on an appropriate medium and electrophoresed to separate its constituents according to electrophoretic mobilities. Following electrophoresis, antiserum, polyvalent or monovalent, is deposited in a trough cut into the gel to one side and parallel to the line of separated proteins. Incubation allows double immunodiffusion of these antigens and antibodies toward each other to take place. When an equivalence point is reached, bands become visible as precipitin lines. Diffusion is halted, unbound protein is washed away, and the antigen-antibody precipitin arcs are stained with a protein sensitive stain. This technique can be used to identify the protein of normal serum into 25 to 40 distinct precipitation bands.

Specimen Collection and Preparation

Fresh human serum or urine is the specimen of choice. No special preparation of the patient is required before specimen collection. The patient must be positively identified when the specimen is collected, and the specimen should be labeled at the bedside. Specimen labels should include the patient's full name, the date, the patient's hospital identification number, and the phlebotomist's initials.

Blood should be drawn by an aseptic technique. A minimum of 2 mL of clotted blood (red-top evacuated tube) is required. The specimen should be centrifuged promptly and an aliquot of serum removed. Hemolysis or contamination with bacteria renders a specimen unsuitable for testing.

Urine specimens should be tested in both unconcentrated and concentrated ($10\times$ to $50\times$) forms because of the wide range of light chain concentrations.

Serum and urine samples for assay should be fresh. If the test cannot be performed immediately, the specimen can be refrigerated ($2°$ to $8°$ C) for up to 5 days after collection.

Reagents, Supplies, and Equipment

Reagents and supplies for gel electrophoresis are commercially available from Helena Laboratories, Beaumont, Texas.

1. 0.85% saline solution.
2. Barbital buffer (sodium barbital, pH 8.3 to 8.7). Packaged, dry buffer should be stored at room temperature (15° to 30° C) and is stable until the expiration date on the package. Discard packaged buffer if the material shows signs of dampness or discoloration.

   Prepare the buffer by transferring one prepackaged packette to a 1 L volumetric flask and dilute to the calibration mark with purified water. The buffer is ready for use when it is completely dissolved. Transfer the reconstituted buffer to a clean storage bottle. Label the bottle with the appropriate identification, warning, and date of preparation. Reconstituted buffer solution is stable for 6 months at 15° to 30° C. Discard buffer solution if it becomes turbid. *Caution:* Barbital can be toxic if ingested.
3. Destaining solution. Prepare by measuring and adding 675 mL of 95% ethanol (denatured with either methanol or isopropanol) and 675 mL of purified water to a 1 L volumetric flask. Mix. *Note:* Wear safety glasses and perform the next step under a hood. Measure and add 150 mL of glacial acidic acid. Mix thoroughly and transfer to a clean, labeled bottle with a cap.
4. IEP stain (Coomassie brilliant blue). Dry stain should be stored at room temperature (15° to 30° C) and is stable until the expiration date indicated on the package.

   Prepare by adding one packette of stain to a 1 L volumetric flask. Measure and add 450 mL of 95% ethanol (denatured with either methanol or isopropanol). Mix thoroughly to dissolve all of the stain. Add 450 mL of purified water and mix. *Note:* Wear safety glasses and perform the next step under a hood. Measure and add 100 mL of glacial acidic acid. Mix thoroughly and transfer to a clean, labeled bottle with a cap.

   Stain solution is stable for 6 months when stored at room temperature (15° to 30° C) in a tightly closed container. The stain can be returned to the bottle and reused. If the stain shows signs of deterioration, i.e., evidence of precipitate, it should be discarded.
5. Albumin marker. Albumin marker is 0.5% bromphenol blue in aqueous solution. The bromphenol blue binds with the albumin in the control. The tagged albumin allows for verification of protein mobility. The solution should be stored at 15° to 30° C and is stable until the expiration date indicated on the vial. Discard if the solution color changes from yellow to brown.
6. IEP normal human serum control contains pooled normal human serum with 0.1% sodium azide as a preservative. It is in liquid form and ready for use as packaged. Before using, add two drops of albumin marker to the control vial. Store at 2° to 6° C. The solution is stable until the expiration date indicated on the vial. Stability is not affected by the addition of albumin marker. Control should be light yellow and slightly hazy before the addition of the marker.

   Caution: Because the control sera is derived from human sources, it should be handled in the same manner as clinical serum specimens (see *Universal blood and body fluid precautions* in Chapter 6).

   Warning: Sodium azide is used as a preservative. To prevent the formation of toxic vapors, do not mix with acidic solutions. Sodium azide may react with lead and copper plumbing to form highly explosive metal azides. Upon disposal, flush with a large volume of water to prevent azide buildup. In addition to purging pipes with water, plumbing should occasionally be decontaminated with 10% NaOH.
7. Gel plates. Titan gel IEP plates containing 1% agarose (w/v) in barbital-sodium barbital buffer with 0.1% sodium azide as a preservative. They are ready to use as packaged and should be stored flat at 2° to 6° C in the protective packaging in which they are shipped. **Caution:** Do not freeze the plates or expose them to excessive heat.

   The plates are stable until the expiration date indicated on the label unless signs of deterioration are apparent. If the plates do not have a smooth, clear agarose surface, deterioration has occurred. Discard plates that are cloudy, exhibit bacterial growth, or have been exposed to freezing (a cracked or bubbled surface) or excessive heat (a dried, thin surface).
8. Antiserum for assay (commercially prepared). Depending on the desired assay, one of the following should be used:

   An antiserum to human IgG, IgM, IgA, IgD or IgE Trivalent antiserum to human immunoglobulins (heavy chain specific for IgG, Ig, IgM) Antiserum to human kappa or lambda light chain

   Antisera, supplied in liquid form, are prepared in horse, sheep, goat, donkey, or rabbit. Each vial contains 0.1% sodium azide as a preservative. The antisera should be stored at 2° to 6° C and are stable until the expiration date indicated on the vial and should be colorless to light yellow in color.
9. Gel blotter C
10. Gel blotter E
11. Serologic rotator
12. Gel staining set
13. Humidity chamber
14. Microdispenser tubes (1 to 10μL) or (1 to 25 μL)
15. Gel chamber
16. Sponge wicks
17. Digital power supply
18. Incubator/dryer
19. Development weight

20. Viewbox (optional)
21. Immunocamera (optional)

Quality Control

The normal human serum control with albumin marker added should be used as a control for each antiserum specificity used. It should be tested with each test run.

Procedure

Preparation of gel chamber

A. Measure 200 mL of barbital buffer in a graduated cylinder. (The buffer may be reused one time by reversing the polarity of the chamber. The plates must then be placed with the wells on the left side [formerly the anodic side].) Add 100 L of the buffer to each outer section of the chamber.

B. Place a long IEP sponge wick in each buffer-filled compartment. Allow the sponges to become saturated with buffer. Place the sponges against the chamber walls.

C. Cover the chamber until ready to use.

Sample application

A. Remove the gel plates from the refrigerator, and allow the plates to come to room temperature while still in the protective packaging.

B. Remove the needed number of plates from the protective packaging and save the plastic holder for later use in the incubation chamber.

C. Apply 2 μL of the control to the wells labeled "C" using a microdispenser. The sample should be applied with care in order not to damage the wells during sample application.

D. Apply 2 μL of the patient sample to wells labeled "P" using a microdispenser. The sample should be applied with care in order not to damage the wells during sample application.

Electrophoresis

A. Quickly put the plate(s) in the electrophoresis chamber, agarose side down, with the wells toward the cathode (−). Make sure that the agarose is in good contact with the sponge wicks. Two plates may be electrophoresed in one chamber.

B. Put the cover on the electrophoresis chamber and wait 30 to 60 seconds before applying current. This allows the plate(s) to equilibrate with the buffer.

C. Electrophorese the plate(s) at 100 volts for a migration distance of 35 mm or greater. This requires approximately 40 to 50 minutes. Migration distance can be verified by observing the position of the albumin marker.

Antisera application

A. Remove the plate(s) from the chamber and put them on a flat surface, agarose side up.

B. Apply 25 μL of the appropriate antiserum to each trough in the plate. Fill the troughs by placing the tip of a microdispenser in the end of the trough farthest from the sample well. Holding the microdispenser in place, slowly depress the plunger and dispense the antiserum into the trough. The antiserum will flow down the trough by capillary action. The troughs easily hold 25 μL of antiserum without overflowing. Severe overfilling may cause antisera to contaminate other troughs, yielding erroneous results.

C. Before moving the plates, allow the antisera to absorb for approximately 3 to 5 minutes.

D. Put each plate in the protective packaging that was previously removed from the gel plate.

E. Stack the plates (within the holders) in a humidity chamber containing a moist paper wick.

F. Incubate the plate(s) at room temperature (15° to 30° C) for 18 to 24 hours. The minimum incubation time is 18 hours. Optimum precipitation will occur between 2 μL of sample and at least 25 μL of antiserum following 18 to 24 hours. If less than 25 μL of antiserum is used, diffuse precipitin arcs will result, interfering with pattern interpretation.

Washing and staining the gel plate(s)

A. At the end of the incubation period, remove the plate(s) from the plastic packaging, and put it in 0.85% saline. The saline stops the diffusion reaction and washes out unbound protein.

B. Wash and press-dry the plate using a quick wash (described below), 6-hour wash, or overnight wash.

Quick Wash

Press dry the plate for 5 minutes using the following procedure.

A. Lay the plate on a flat surface, agarose side up. Place one blotter C directly on the plate, followed by 2 blotter E's. Then place a development weight on top of the plate and blotters for 5 minutes.

B. Remove the weight and discard the blotters.

C. Wash the plate in 0.85% saline for 5 to 10 minutes.

D. Repeat the press and wash steps two more times. After the third wash, press again.

Completion of procedure

A. After washing and pressing, place the plate on a blotter, agarose side up, in a drying oven at 60° to 75° C for 3 to 5 minutes or until dry. The plate must be completely dry to stain and destain it properly.

B. Fill a staining chamber with staining solution.

C. Fill three destaining chambers with destaining solution.

D. Place the dried plate(s) in a staining rack and lower into the staining chamber. Stain the plate(s) for 4 minutes.

E. Remove the staining rack containing the plate(s), and put it on a paper towel to drain off surplus stain.

F. Raise and lower the rack 4 times in the first destaining chamber to further remove excess stain.

G. In the second destaining chamber, raise and

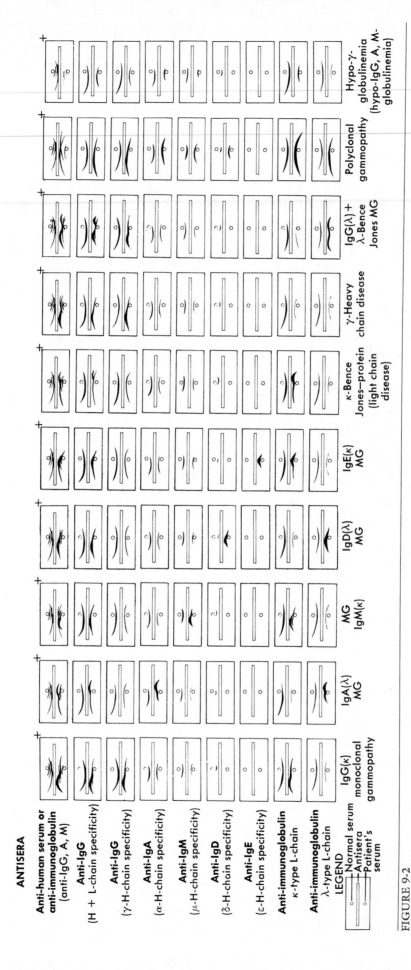

(From Ritzman SE and Daniels JC: Laboratory notes—serum proteins, No. 3, Somerville, NJ, 1973, Behring Diagnostics/Hoechst Pharmaceuticals Inc.)

FIGURE 9-2

Abnormal immunoglobulin pattern (IEP).

lower the rack 4 times to further remove excess stain. The background should be clear after this wash, if not, put the plate(s) in the third destaining chamber until the background is clear, no more than 2 to 3 minutes. Do not destain further if the stain in the IgM arc will be lost. Plates can be restained if necessary.

H. Remove the plate(s) from the rack, and put each plate on a blotter agarose side up.

I. Dry the plate(s) in a laboratory drying oven at 60° to 70° C for 3 to 5 minutes or until dry. A stained and dried gel plate is stable for an indefinite period.

Reporting Results

The formation of a precipitin arc between a well containing a test specimen and a trough containing antiserum indicates the presence of the protein specific to the antisera. The lack of a precipitin arc indicates that a detectable amount of the protein is not present in the test specimen. The size, location, and shape of the precipitin arc, as compared to the control, are indications of the amount of protein in the test specimen.

When protein concentrations are below normal, precipitin arcs are shortened and located farther from the antiserum trough compared to the corresponding arc in the control. When protein concentrations are above normal, precipitant arcs are thicker and located closer to the antiserum trough compared to the control. Fig. 9-2 is a sample immunoglobulin profile. The pattern of precipitin arcs are interpreted comparing the patient sample to the control. In the figure, the patient serum forms a dense, bowed arc against IgG antiserum. There appears to be a diminished IgA level and virtually no IgM in the patient serum when compared to the IgA and IgM in the control. The abnormal IgG band is also visible against both human and univaleny antisera. The patient specimen reveals a bowed, abnormal kappa arc and a decreased lambda arc. This composite is indicative of an IgG monoclonal gammopathy, kappa type.

Reference ranges to be considered include patient age, sex, history, and clinical presentation, which will affect immunoglobulin levels.

Procedure Notes

Interpretation of IgM light chain reactions is often difficult because of the umbrella effect of IgG. IgM (19S) can be depolymerized with 2-mercaptoethanol into single molecular (7S) units, which diffuse through the agarose more rapidly. In rare instances, this may be necessary for IgA typing.

Sources of error. Prozone is an incomplete precipitin reaction caused by antigen excess (too high an antigen-antibody ratio). Prozoning should be suspected if a precipitin arc appears to "run" into a trough, if a light chain appears fuzzy when a heavy chain is increased, or if an arc appears to be incomplete.

Clinical applications. IEP is a reliable and accurate method for detecting both structural abnormalities and concentration changes in proteins. The most common application of IEP is in the diagnosis of monoclonal gammopathies.

Limitations. IEP is a semiquantitative technique.

IMMUNOFIXATION ELECTROPHORESIS (IFE)

Immunofixation electrophoresis (IFE) is a two-stage procedure using agarose gel protein electrophoresis in the first stage and immunoprecipitation in the second. The test specimen may be serum, urine, cerebrospinal fluid, or other body fluids. The primary use of IFE in clinical laboratories is for the characterization of monoclonal immunoglobulins.

Applications

Although IFE was first described in 1964, it was introduced as a procedure for the study of immunoglobulins in 1976. Immunoelectrophoresis (IEP) and immunofixation electrophoresis (IFE) are complementary techniques best used in the workup of a patient with a suspected monoclonal gammopathy. The laboratory protocol for ruling out monoclonal gammopathy should include high-resolution electrophoresis, immunoelectrophoresis of both serum and urine, and a quantitative immunoglobulin assay. These procedures are usually sufficient to detect and characterize monoclonal proteins with a serum concentration of 1 g or more.

Three variables of protein can be determined using IFE:

1. Antigenic specificity
2. Electrophoretic mobility
3. Quantity or ratio of the test and control proteins

Procedural Protocol

In the first step of the IFE procedure, a single specimen is applied to six different positions on an agarose plate and the proteins are separated according to their net charge by electrophoresis. In the second phase, monospecific antisera are applied to five of the electrophoresis patterns: IgG, IgA, IgM, and kappa and lamda antisera. A protein fixative solution is applied to the sixth pattern to produce a complete protein reference pattern. The plate is incubated for 10 minutes.

If complementary antigen is present in the proper proportions in the test sample, antigen-antibody complexes form and precipitate. The formation of a stable antigen-antibody precipitate fixes the protein in the gel. After fixation, the gel is washed in deproteination solution, e.g., dilute sodium chloride, and nonprecipitated proteins are washed out of the agarose leaving only the antigen-antibody complex. The protein reference pattern and the antigen-antibody precipitation bands are stained with a protein sensitive stain, e.g., Amido black.

Comparison of IEP and IFE

IEP is technically simpler and less subject to antigen excess phenomenon than IFE. In IFE high concentrations of monoclonal protein give no visible reactions. IEP is considered to be a better technique for typing large monoclonal gammopathies. IFE, however, can be optimized to give both greater sensitivity and resolution than IEP. IFE should be reserved for anomalous proteins, which are difficult to characterize by IEP. These include small bands such as those exhibited in the early stages of monoclonal gammopathies or light chain disease, and any multiple, closely spaced bands. IFE is easier to interpret than IEP because interpretation is based on examination of a precipitate pattern directly analogous to routine electrophoresis; it does not depend on detecting slight deviations in the shape of a precipitin arc.

Chapter Review

HIGHLIGHTS

Serum electrophoresis results in the separation of proteins into five fractions on cellulose acetate. This separation is based on the rate of migration of these individual components in an electrical field. By comparison, immunoelectrophoresis (IEP) involves the electrophoresis of serum or urine followed by immunodiffusion. The size and position of precipitation bands provide the same type of information regarding equivalence or antibody excess as the double immunodiffusion method. IEP is a combination of the techniques of electrophoresis and double immunodiffusion. IEP consists of two phases: electrophoresis and diffusion. Proteins are thus differentiated not only by their electrophoretic mobility, but also by their diffusion coefficient and antibody specifity. Antibody diffuses as a uniform band parallel to the antibody trough. If the proteins are homogeneous, the antigen diffuses in a circle and the antigen-antibody precipitation line resembles a segment or arc of a circle. If the antigen is heterogeneous, the antigen-antibody line assumes an elliptical shape. One arc of precipitation forms for each constituent in the antigen mixture. This technique can be used to resolve the protein of normal serum into 25 to 40 distinct precipitation bands.

The most common application of IEP is in the diagnosis of monoclonal gammopathies. A monoclonal gammopathy is a condition in which a single clone of plasma cells produces elevated levels of a single class and type of immunoglobulin. Differentiation can also be made between monoclonal and polyclonal gammopathies. A polyclonal gammopathy is a secondary condition caused by disorders such as liver disease, collagen disorders, rheumatoid arthritis, and chronic infection. It is characterized by elevation of two or more (often all) immunoglobulins by several clones of plasma cells. Polyclonal increases of proteins are usually twice the normal levels. The most important application of IEP of urine is the demonstration of Bence Jones (BJ) protein.

Immunofixation electrophoresis (IFE) is a two-stage procedure using agarose gel protein electrophoresis in the first stage and immunoprecipitation in the second. The test specimen may be serum, urine, cerebrospinal fluid, or other body fluids. The primary use of IFE in clinical laboratories is for the characterization of monoclonal immunoglobulins. Antigenic specificity, electrophoretic mobility, and the quantity or ratio of the test and control proteins can be determined using IFE. IEP is technically simpler and less subject to antigen excess phenomenon than IFE. In IFE high concentrations of monoclonal protein give no visible reactions. IEP is considered to be a better technique for typing large monoclonal gammopathies. IFE, however, can be optimized to give both greater sensitivity and resolution than IEP. IFE should be reserved for anomalous proteins, which are difficult to characterize by IEP.

REVIEW QUESTIONS

1. Which of the following is the most common application of immunoelectrophoresis (IEP)?
   A. identification of the absence of a normal serum protein
   B. structural abnormalities of proteins
   C. screening for circulating immune complexes
   D. diagnosis of monoclonal gammopathies
   E. demonstration of Bence-Jones protein in urine
2. Abnormalities of precipitin bands in an IEP assay can be evaluated by all of the following features except:
   A. position of the band between antigen well and antibody trough
   B. position of the band in relationship to electrophoretically identified protein fractions
   C. general location of the band
   D. distortion of the arc formation
   E. density of the band
3. Immunofixation electrophoresis is best used in:
   A. the workup of a polyclonal gammopathy
   B. the workup of a monoclonal gammopathy
   C. screening for circulating immune complexes
   D. identification of hypercomplementemia
   E. identification of hypocomplementemia

Questions 4-8.
   F. True or False.
   G. A=True B=False
4. IEP is technically simpler and less subject to antigen excess phenomenon than IFE.
5. IFE is considered to be a better technique than IEP for typing large monoclonal gammopathies.
6. IFE can be optimized to give both greater sensitivity and resolution than IEP.
7. IFE should be reserved for anomalous proteins that are difficult to characterize by IEP.
8. IEP is easier to interpret than IFE.

Answers

1. D 2. C 3. B 4. A 5. B 6. a 7. A 8. B

BIBLIOGRAPHY

Killingsworth LM and Warren BM: Immunofixation for the identification of monoclonal gammopathies, Beaumont, Tex, 1986, Helena Laboratories.

Ritzmann EE: Immunoglobulin abnormalities. In Ritzman S, editor: Serum protein abnormalities, diagnostic and clinical aspects, Boston, 1976, Little, Brown & Co Inc.

Sun T: Immunofixation electrophoresis procedures. In Protein abnormalities, vol 1, Physiology of immunoglobulins: diagnostic and clinical aspects, New York, 1982, Alan R Liss Inc.

Labeling Techniques in Immunoassay

The original technique of using antigen-coated cells or particles in agglutination techniques may be considered the earliest method for labeling components in immunoassays. Ideal characteristics of a label include the quality of being measurable by several methods, including visual inspection. The properties of a label used in an immunoassay determine the ways in which detection is possible. For example, coated latex particles can be detected by various methods: visual inspection, light scattering (nephelometry), and particle counting. The conversion of a colorless substrate into a colored product in enzyme immunoassay (EIA) allows for two methods of detection, colorimetry, and visual inspection.

TYPES OF LABELS

The use of a radioactive label, the radioimmunoassay (RIA) method, that could identify an immunocomponent at very low concentrations was developed by Yalow and Berson in 1959. In the 1960s, researchers began to search for a substitute for the successful RIA method because of the inherent drawbacks of using radioactive isotopes as labels, e.g., radioactive waste and short-shelf life. Since that time, techniques that use nonradioactive substances as labels, such as enzymes and fluorescent molecules, have also been developed. The principles and applications of radioisotopes, enzymes, and fluorescent substances as labels are presented in this chapter.

RADIOIMMUNOASSAY (RIA)

The RIA method continues to be widely used in immunologic assays (see box, right). Radioisotopes can be used to measure the concentration of antigen or antibody in serum samples. The basis of the RIA procedure relies on the principle of competitive binding (Fig. 10-1).

Examples of Immunologic Assays that Can Be Performed by Radioimmunoassay

Acetylcholine receptor (AchR) binding antibody
Acetylcholine receptor (AcHR) blocking antibodies
Anti-DNA antibodies
Antiglomerular basement membrane antibodies
Antiintrinsic factor
Antimyelin
Antisperm
Beta$_2$-microglobulin
C1q binding
Carcinoembryonic antigen (CEA)
Conglutinin solid phase (Kg SP) assay for immune complexes
Diphtheria antibodies
Ferritin
Hepatitis A IgM antibody
Hepatitis A antigen
Hepatitis Delta virus IgM antibody
Immunoglobulin E (IgE)
Immunoglobulin G (IgG) rheumatoid factors
Immunoglobulin G (IgG) subclasses
Myelin basic protein
Platelet-associated IgG (PAIgG)
Platelet antibody
Pneumococcal antibodies
Radio Allergo Sorbent Test (RAST)
Raji cell assay
Thyroid-Stimulating Immunoglobulin (TSI)

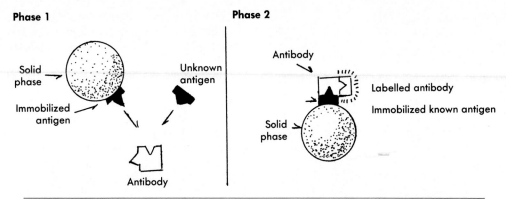

FIGURE 10-1

RAST inhibition assay represents a competitive inhibition of binding technique. In the first phase, a known quantity of antibody is allowed to react in a competitive reaction between antigen immobilized on a solid phase and the unknown antigen to be measured. In the second phase, the bound antibody is measured in a standard noncompetitive (direct) RIA technique that allows the quantitation of the unknown antigen.

If antibody concentration is being measured, the principle of the procedure is that radioactive-labeled antibody competes with patient unlabeled antibody for binding sites on a known amount of antigen. When all three components are present in the system, an equilibrium exists.

A typical RIA procedure begins with antigen in saline being incubated on a microplate or in a test tube. Small quantities of the antigen become absorbed onto the plastic surface. Following incubation, free antigen is washed away. The plate may then be blocked with an excess amount of an irrelevant protein that prevents any subsequent binding of proteins.

Test antibody is then added, which binds to the antigen. Unbound proteins are washed away, and the antibody is detected by a radiolabeled *ligand*. The ligand may be a molecule, such as staphylococcal protein A (which binds to the Fc region of IgG), or more often another antibody specific to the test antibody. Unbound ligand is washed away, and the radioactivity of the plate or tube is counted on a gamma counter.

As the amount of test antibody increases, the counts per minute (CPM) rise from a background level through a linear range to a plateau. Antibody titers can only be detected correctly within the linear range. Typically the plateau binding rate is 20 to 100 times the background count. A reduction in radioactivity of the antigen-antibody complex compared to the radioactive counts measured in the control test with no antibody is used to quantitate the amount of patient antibody bound to the antigen.

The main advantage of the RIA method is the extreme sensitivity and ability to detect trace amounts of antigen or antibody. In addition, a large number of tests can be performed in a relatively short time period. The disadvantages, as previously cited, are the hazard and instability of isotopes.

RADIOALLERGOSORBENT TEST (RAST)

This test measures antigen-specific IgE in a radioimmunoassay where the ligand is a labeled anti-IgE antibody. The steps are identical to the standard radioimmunoassay except that the antigen (allergen) is covalently bound to a cellulose disc rather than non-covalently to a radioimmunoassay plate. By having much more antigen available on the disc, this permits the high sensitivity necessary to bind the small quantities of IgE present in serum.

RADIOIMMUNOSORBENT TEST (RIST)

This a competition radioimmunoassay for total serum IgE. The plate is sensitized with anti-IgE and increasing amounts of labeled IgE are added to the plate to determine the maximum amount of IgE that the plate can bind. A quantity of labeled IgE equivalent to approximately 80% of the plateau binding is chosen. In the test experiment, this amount of labeled IgE is mixed with the serum containing the IgE to be tested. The test IgE competes with the labeled IgE. Therefore, the more IgE that is present in the test serum the less the amount of labeled IgE that binds.

ENZYME IMMUNOASSAY (EIA)

The EIA method uses a nonisotopic label, which offers the advantage of safety, and shares the specificity, sensitivity, and rapidity of RIA. Like the RIA method, EIA is usually an objective measurement that provides numerical results. Some EIA procedures provide diagnostic information as well as measuring immune status, e.g., detection of either total antibody, IgM or IgG.

An enzyme-labeled antibody or enzyme-labeled antigen conjugate is used in immunologic assays (see box, p. 134) for a variety of antigens or antibodies, respectively. The enzyme with its substrate detects the presence and quantity of antigen or anti-

Examples of Enzyme Immunoassays

Borrelia burgdorferi (IgG and IgM)
Cytomegalovirus (IgG and IgM Ab)
Cytomegalovirus (Ag)
Hepatitis A (Total Ab)
Hepatitis B:
   anti-HBs
   anti-HBc
   anti-HBe
   anti-HBc (IgM)
   HBs Ag
   HBe Ag
Hepatitis Delta virus (total Ab)
Hepatitis non-A, non-B
HIV Ab
HIV Ag
HTLV-I Ab
HTLV-II AB
Human B lymphotropic virus Ab
Rubella virus (IgG and IgM Ab)
Toxoplasma gondii (IgG and IgM Ab)

TABLE 10-1

Enzymes Used in Enzyme Immunoassay

Enzyme	Source
Acetylcholinesterase	*Electrophorous electicus*
Alkaline phosphatase	*Escherichia coli*
(B)-Galactosidase	*Escherichia coli*
Glucose oxidase	*Asperqillis niqer*
Glucose 6-phosphate Dehydrogenase (G 6-PD)	*Leuconostoc mesenteroides*
Lysozyme	Egg white
Malate dehydrogenase	Pig heart
Peroxidase	Horseradish

body in a patient specimen. In some tissues, an enzyme-labeled antibody can identify antigenic locations.

A variety of enzymes (Table 10-1) are employed in enzyme immunoassay. The most commonly used enzymes are peroxidase and alkaline phosphatase. To be used in EIA, an enzyme must fulfill a number of criteria, including:
1. A high amount of stability
2. Extreme specificity
3. Absence from the antigen or antibody
4. No alteration by inhibitor with the system

In a representative EIA test (Fig. 10-2), a plastic bead or plastic plate is coated with antigen, e.g., virus. The antigen reacts with antibody in the patient serum. The bead or plate is then incubated with an enzyme-labeled antibody conjugate. If antibody is present, the conjugate reacts with the antigen-antibody complex on the bead or plate. The enzyme activity is measured spectrophotometrically after the addition of the specific chromogenic substrate. For example, peroxidase cleaves its substrate, o-dianisidine, causing a color change. In some cases, the test can be read subjectively. The results of a typical test are calculated by comparing the spectophotometric reading of patient serum to that of a control or reference serum. The advantage of an objective enzyme test is that results are not dependent on a technician's interpretations. In general, the EIA procedure is faster and requires less laboratory work than comparable methods.

IMMUNOFLUORESCENT TECHNIQUES

Fluorescent labeling is another method of demonstrating the complexing of antigens and antibodies (Fig. 10-3). Fluorescent molecules are used as substitutes for radioisotope or enzyme labels. The fluorescent antibody technique consists of labeling antibody with fluorescein isothiocyanate (FITC), a fluorescent compound that has an affinity for proteins, to form a complex *(conjugate)*. This conjugate is able to react with antibody-specific antigen.

Fluorescent techniques are extremely specific and sensitive. Antibodies may be conjugated to other markers in addition to fluorescent dyes; these markers are called *colorimetric immunologic probe detection.* The use of enzyme-substrate marker systems has been expanded. Horseradish peroxidase, alkaline phosphatase, and avidin-biotin conjugated enzyme labels have all been used as visual tags for the presence of antibody. These reagents have the advantage of requiring only a standard light microscope.

Fluorescent conjugates are used in the following basic methods:
1. Direct immunofluorescent assay
2. Inhibition immunofluorescent assay
3. Indirect immunofluorescent assay

Direct Immunofluorescent Assay

In the direct technique, a conjugated antibody is used to detect antigen-antibody reactions at a microscopic level (Fig. 10-4). This technique can be applied to tissue sections or in smears for microorganisms. Fluorescein-conjugated antibodies bound to the flurochrome fluorescein isothiocyanate (FITC) are used to visualize many bacteria in direct specimens. Peroxidase conjugated to antibody, the immunoperoxidase stain, can be used to detect cytomegalovirus (CMV), other viruses, or nucleic acids in cells. In biotin-avidin enzyme-conjugated methods, single stranded nucleic acid probes, antimicrobial antibodies, or antibiotin antibodies can be bound to the small molecule, biotin. These molecules have a strong affinity for the protein avidin, which has four binding sites. Biotin bound to avidin or antibody can be complexed to fluorescent dyes or to color-producing enzymes to form specific detector systems. This system can be applied to the detection of nucleic acids in organisms such as

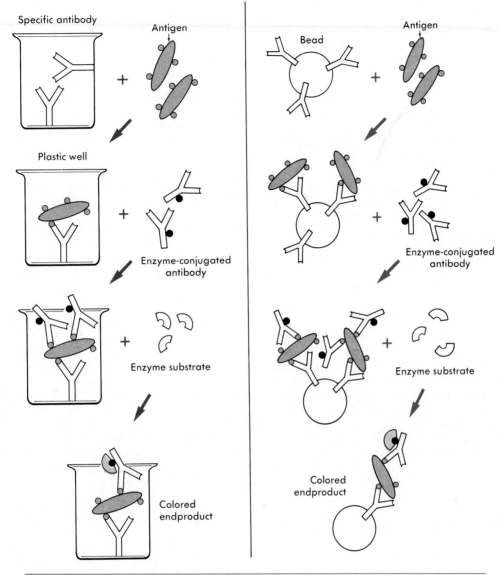

FIGURE 10-2
Principle of solid-phase enzyme immunosorbent assay.
(From Baron EJ and Finegold SM: Bailey and Scott's Diagnostic microbiology, ed 8, St Louis, 1990, The CV Mosby Co.)

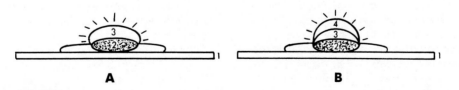

FIGURE 10-3
Principles of direct and indirect fluorescent techniques. **A,** Direct fluorescence. **B,** Indirect fluorescence. Key: *1*=microscopic slide, *2*=cell (cytoplasm and nucleus), *3*=antiserum, conjugate in **A** and unconjugate in **B**, *4*=conjugated antiglobulin serum.

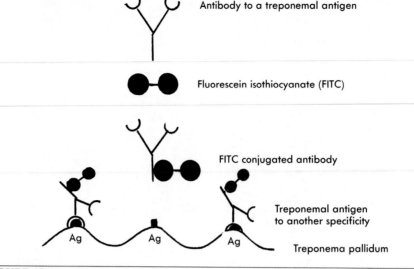

FIGURE 10-4

Direct fluorescent antibody (DFA) technique. After labeling a specific antibody with FITC, it can be reacted with its antigen and identified microscopically.

CMV, hepatitis B virus, Epstein-Barr virus, and Chlamydia.

The chemical manipulation in labeling antibodies with fluorescent dyes to permit detection by direct microscopic examination does not seriously impair antibody activity i.e. the ability of the fluorescent antibody conjugate to react specifically with its homologous antigen. Monoclonal antibodies have also been successfully conjugated to fluorescein for the detection of chlamydiae, rabies virus, and other pathogens in directly stained specimens.

A fluorescent substance is one upon which when absorbing light of one wavelength, emits light of another (longer) wavelength. In fluoresent antibody microscopy, the incident or exciting light is often blue-green to ultraviolet. The light is provided by a high pressure mercury arc lamp with a primary, e.g., blue-violet filter, between the lamp and the object that passes only fluorescein-exciting wavelengths. The color of the emitted light depends on the nature of the substance. Fluorescein gives off yellow-green light, and the rhodamines fluoresce in the red portion of the spectrum. The color observed in the fluorescent microscope depends on the secondary or barrier filter used in the eyepiece. A yellow filter absorbs the green fluorescence of fluorescein and transmits only yellow. Fluorescein fluoresces an intense apple green color when excited.

Inhibition Immunofluorescent Assay

The inhibition immunofluorescent assay is a blocking test in which an antigen is first exposed to unlabeled antibody, then to labeled antibody, and is finally washed and examined. If the unlabeled and labeled antibodies are both homologous to the antigen, there should be no fluorescence. This result confirms the specificity of the fluorescent antibody technique. Antibody in an unknown serum can also be detected and identified by the inhibition test.

Indirect Immunofluorescent Assay (IFA)

The indirect method is based on the fact that antibodies (immunoglobulins) not only react with homologous antigens but can also act as antigens and react with antiimmunoglobulins (Table 10-2).

The serologic method most widely used for the detection of diverse antibodies is the indirect fluorescent antibody assay (IFA). Immunofluorescence is used extensively in the detection of autoantibodies and antibodies to tissue and cellular antigens. For example, antinuclear antibodies (ANAs) a heterogenous group of circulating immunoglobulins that react with the whole nucleus or nuclear components such as nuclear proteins, deoxyribonucleic acid [DNA], or histones in host tissues, are frequently assayed by indirect fluorescence. By using tissue sections, which contain a large number of antigens, it is possible to identify antibodies to several different antigens in a single test. The antigens are differentiated according to their different staining patterns.

Immunofluorescence can also be used to identify specific antigens on live cells in suspension, i.e., flow-cell cytometry. When a live stained cell suspension is put through a fluorescent active cell sorter (FACS), which measures its fluorescent intensity, the cells are separated according to their particular fluorescent brightness. This technique permits the isolation of different cell populations with different surface antigens, e.g., OKT4 and OKT8 lymphocytes (see Chapter 11).

In the indirect immunofluorescent assay, the an-

TABLE 10-2

Examples of Immunologic Assays Performed by Indirect Fluorescence Antibody Technique

Antiadrenal antibodies
Anticentriole antibodies
Anticentromere antibodies
Antiglomerular basement membrane antibodies
Antiislet-cell antibodies
Anti-LKM
Antimitochondrial
Antimyelin
Antimyocardial
Antinuclear antibody
Antiparietal Cell
Antiplatelet
Antireticulin
Antiribosome
Anti-skin (dermal-epidermal)
Anti-skin (inter-epithelial)
Antismooth muscle
Antistriational
Cytomegalovirus (IgM antibody)
Histone reactive antinuclear
Human immunodeficiency virus (HIV) total and
   IgM antibody
Antibody (HRANA)
IgM antibodies (antigen specific)
Lymphocyte typing
Rubella virus antibody
Toxoplasma gondii antibody

tigen source, such as a whole Toxoplasma microorganism or virus in infected tissue culture cells, to the specific antibody being tested is affixed to the surface of a microscope slide. The patient's serum is diluted and place on the slide to cover the antigen source. If antibody is present in the serum, it will bind to its specific antigen. Unbound antibody is then removed by washing the slide. In the second phase of the procedure, antihuman globulin (directed specifically against IgM or IgG) conjugated to a fluorescent substance that will fluoresce when exposed to ultraviolet light is placed on the slide. This conjugated marker for human antibody will bind to the antibody already bound to the antigen on the slide and will serve as a marker for the antibody when viewed under a fluorescent microscope.

SOL PARTICLE IMMUNOASSAY (SPIA)
A *sol* is a dispersion of colloidal particles in a liquid, hence the name *sol particle immunoassay (SPIA)*. The use of colloidal particles consisting of a metal or an insoluble metal compound as a label in immunoassay was introduced in 1980.

Types
Various colloidal particles, such as silver, gold, silver iodide, and barium sulfate, can be used as labels in immunoassay. This type of labeled antibody can be used in both *heterogeneous* and *homogeneous* immunoassays.

In heterogeneous immunoassays a separation of the free and bound fractions of the labeled immunocomponent is required. The sandwich and sandwich inhibition SPIA techniques are in this category. If two different labels, e.g., silver and gold, are used, it is possible to develop simultaneous sandwich immunoassays for two noncross-reacting antigens with this method. The limits of detection depend on the method used but ranges from 0.02 pmol/L to 170 pmol/L. If incubated for less than overnight, the procedure is not as sensitive.

Homogeneous SPIAs are based on agglutination or agglutination inhibition of antibody coated with gold particles. In the homogeneous method, separation of bound and free-labeled immunocomponents is not necessary. This same type of immunochemical reaction is comparable to hemagglutination inhibition and latex agglutination inhibition immunoassays. Various methods of detection can be used in combination with inhibition of agglutination SPIAs. One application of inhibition agglutination SPIA is in the detection of specific antibodies.

Advantages
The following are the main advantages of SPIA:
1. A nonisotopic label can be used
2. Better stability than enzymes
3. No need for an extra chemical reaction
4. Allows the possibility of using various methods of detection, including visual inspection

Homogeneous SPIA involves a simple test procedure. Applications can include qualitative tests appropriate for home and laboratory testing, e.g., pregnancy testing.

Chapter Review

HIGHLIGHTS
The original technique of using antigen-coated cells or particles in agglutination techniques may be considered the earliest method for labeling components in immunoassays. Ideal characteristics of a label include the quality of being measurable by several methods, including visual inspection. The properties of a label determine the ways in which detection is possible. The conversion of a colorless substrate into a colored product in enzyme immunoassay (EIA) allows for two methods of detection, colorimetry and visual inspection.

Radioisotopes can be used to measure the concentration of antigen or antibody in serum samples. The basis of the RIA procedure relies on the principle of competitive binding. If antibody concentration is being measured, the principle of the procedure is that radioactive-labeled antibody competes with patient unlabeled antibody for binding sites on a known amount of antigen. When all three components are present in the system, an equilibrium exists.

The EIA method uses a nonisotopic label, which offers the advantage of safety, and shares the specificity, sensitivity, and rapidity of RIA. Like the RIA method, EIA is usually an objective measurement that provides numerical results. Some EIA procedures provide diagnostic information as well as measuring immune status, e.g., detection of either total antibody, IgM or IgG. A variety of enzymes are employed in enzyme immunoassay. The most commonly used enzymes are peroxidase and alkaline phosphatase. To be used in EIA, an enzyme must fulfill a number of criteria, including a high amount of stability, extreme specificity, absence from the antigen or antibody, and no alteration by inhibitor with the system. In the enzyme-linked immunosorbent assay (ELISA) method, enzyme-bound antibodies remain able to catalyze a reaction that yields a visual endpoint. The antibody binding sites, however, remain free to react with their specific antigen. If the method is intended to detect antibodies, the antigen in question is firmly fixed to a solid matrix such as the inside of the microplate well or the outside of a bead. Such a system is called *solid phase immunosorbent assay.*

Fluorescent labeling (direct and indirect) is another method of demonstrating the complexing of antigens and antibodies. Fluorescent molecules are used as substitutes for radioisotope or enzyme labels. The fluorescent antibody technique consists of labeling antibody with fluorescein isothiocyanate (FITC), a fluorescent compound that has an affinity for proteins, to form a conjugate. This conjugate is able to react with antibody-specific antigen. Fluorescent techniques are extremely specific and sensitive. Antibodies may be conjugated to other markers in addition to fluorescent dyes; these

markers are called *colorimetric immunologic probe detection.* The use of enzyme-substrate marker systems has been expanded. Horseradish peroxidase, alkaline phosphatase, and avidin-biotin, conjugated enzyme labels have all been used as visual tags for the presence of antibody. These reagents have the advantage of requiring only a standard light microscope.

Fluorescent conjugates are used in the basic methods of direct immunofluorescent assay, inhibition immunofluorescent assay, and indirect immunofluorescent assay. In the direct technique, a conjugated antibody is used to detect antigen-antibody reactions at a microscopic level. This technique can be applied to tissue sections or in smears for microorganisms. A fluorescent substance is one upon which when absorbing light of one wavelength, emits light of another (longer) wavelength. The indirect method is based on the fact that antibodies (immunoglobulins) not only react with homologuos antigens but can also act as antigens and react with antiimmunoglobuins. The serologic method most widely used for the detection of diverse antibodies is the indirect fluorescent antibody assay (IFA). Immunofluorescence is used extensively in the detection of autoantibodies and antibodies to tissue and cellular antigens. Immunofluorescence can also be used to identify specific antigens on live cells in suspension, i.e., Flow-cell cytometry. When a live stained cell suspension is put through a fluorescent active cell sorter (FACS), which measures the fluorescent intensity of each cell, the cells are separated according to their particular fluorescent brightness. This technique permits the isolation of different cell populations with different surface antigens, e.g., OKT4 and OKT8 lymphocytes.

Sol particle immunoassay is another labeling method analysis. A sol is a dispersion of colloidal particles in a liquid, hence the name *sol particle immunoassay (SPIA)*. The use of colloidal particles consisting of a metal or an insoluble metal compound as a label in immunoassay was introduced in 1980. Various colloidal particles, such as silver, gold, silver iodide, and barium sulfate, can be used as labels in immunoassay. This type of labeled antibody can be used in both heterogeneous and homogeneous immunoassays. In heterogeneous immunoassays a separation of the free and bound fractions of the labeled immunocomponent is required. Homogeneous SPIAs are based on agglutination or agglutination inhibition of antibody coated with gold particles. The main advantages of SPIA are that a nonisotopic label can be used, it has better stability than enzymes, there is no need for an extra chemical reaction, and it allows the possibility of using various methods of detection, including visual inspection.

REVIEW QUESTIONS

Questions 1-4.
Match the following.
1. Radioimmunoassay (RIA)
2. Enzymeimmunoassay (EIA)
3. Immunofluorescent technique
4. Sol particle immunoassay
   A=uses a nonisotopic label
   B=if antibody concentration is being measured, radioactive labeled antibody competes with patient unlabeled antibody for binding sites on a known amount of antigen
   C=uses antibody labeled with fluorescein isothiocyanate (FITC)
   D=uses a colloidal particle consisting of a metal or an insoluble metal compound

5. In the RIA procedure, a reduction in radioactivity in the test specimen compared to the radioactive counts measured in the control test with _____is used to quantitate the amount of patient antibody bound to the antigen.
   A. a labeled amount of antibody
   B. a labeled amount of antigen
   C. no antibody
   D. no antigen
   E. a trace amount of antigen or antibody
6. The main advantage of the RIA method is:
   A. procedural safety
   B. isotope stability
   C. extreme sensitivity
   D. ability to detect trace amounts of antigen or antibody
   E. Both C and D
Questions 7-9.
Match the following.
7. Direct immunofluorescent assay
8. Inhibition immunofluorescent assay
9. Indirect immunofluorescent assay
   A. Based on the fact that antibodies can act as antigens and react with anti-immunoglobulins
   B. Uses conjugated antibody to detect antigen-antibody reactions
   C. Antigen first exposed to unlabeled antibody, then labeled antibody

Answers

1. B 2. A 3. C 4. D 5. C 6. E 7. B 8. C 9. A

BIBLIOGRAPHY

Leuvering JH: SPIA: a new immunological technique, American Clinical Products Review, Sept 1986.

Automated Procedures

NEPHELOMETRY

The quantity of cloudiness or **turbidity** in a solution can be measured photometrically. When specific antigen-coated latex particles acting as reaction intensifiers are agglutinated by their corresponding antibody, the increased light scatter of a solution can be measured by *nephelometry* as the macromolecular complexes form. The use of polyethylene glycol (PEG) enhances and stabilizes the precipitates, thus increasing the speed and sensitivity of the technique by controlling the particle size for optimal light angle deflection. The kinetics of this change can be determined when the photometric results are analyzed by computer. In immunology, nephelometry is used to measure complement components, immune complexes, and the presence of a variety of antibodies (see box).

Principle

Formation of an macromolecular complex is a fundamental prerequisite for nephelometric protein quantitation. The procedure is based on the reaction between the protein being assayed and a specific antisera. Protein in a patient specimen reacts with specific nephelometric antisera to human proteins and forms insoluble complexes. When light is passed through such a suspension, the resulting complexes of insoluble precipitants scatter incident light in solutions. The scattered light can be detected with a photodiode. The amount of scattered light is proportional to the number of insoluble complexes and can be quantitated by comparing the unknown patient values with standards of known protein concentration.

The relationship between the quantity of antigen and the measuring signal at a constant antibody concentration is given by the Heidelberger curve. If antibodies are present to excess, a proportional relationship exits between the antigen and the resulting signal. If the antigen overwhelms the quantity of antibody, the measured signal drops.

By optimizing the reaction conditions, the typical antigen-antibody reactions as characterized by the Heidelberger curve are effectively shifted in the direction of high concentration. This ensures that these high concentrations will be measured on the ascending portion of the curve. At concentrations higher than the reference curve, the instrument will transmit an out-of-range warning.

Examples of Immunologic Assays Performed by Nephelometry

Acid α_1-glycoprotein
Albumin
α_1-Antitrypsin
α_2-Macroglobulin
C1 Esterase inhibitor (C1 inhibitor)
C3
C3b Inhibitor (C3b inactivator)
C3PA (C3 ProActivator, Properdin factor B)
C4
C6
C7
C8
Ceruloplasmin
Complement components (C1r, C1s, C2, C3, C4, C5, C6, C7, C8)
C Reactive protein (CRP)
Cryofibrinogen
Cryoglobulins
Haptoglobin
Hemopexin
Immunoglobulins
Properdin factor B
Transferrin

Physical Basis

Nephelometry is based on the principle of light scattering particles; the scattered light is measured in the forward direction (MIE). The physical basis of measurement in nephelometry is based on MIE light scatter; MIE scattering occurs with larger particles.

Optical System

In the nephelometric method, an infrared high-performance LED is used as the light source. Because an entire solid angle is measured after convergence of this light via a lens system, an intense measuring signal is available when the primary beam is blocked off. In connection with the lens system, this produces a light beam of high collinearity. The wavelength is 840 nm. Light scattered in the forward direction in a solid angle to the primary beam ranges between 13 and 24 feet and is measured by a silicon photodiode with an integrated amplifier. The electrical signals generated are digitalized, compared with reference curves, and converted into protein concentrations.

Measuring Methods

A fixed-time method is used routinely for precipitation reactions. Ten seconds after all reaction components have been mixed, a cuvette, an initial blank measurement is taken. Six minutes later a second measurement is taken, and after subtraction of the original 1-second blanking value, a final answer is calculated against the multiple-point or single-point calibration in the computerized program memory for the assay.

Advantages and Disadvantages of Nephelometry

Nephelometry is both rapid and highly reproducible. It has many applications in the immunology laboratory. However, interfering substances, such as microbial contamination, may cause protein denaturation and erroneous test results. Intrinsic specimen turbidity or lipemia may exceed the preset limits. In these cases, a clearing agent may be needed before an accurate assay can be performed.

FLOW CELL CYTOMETRY
The Fundamentals of Laser Technology

In 1917 Einstein speculated that under certain conditions atoms or molecules could absorb light or other radiation and then be stimulated to shed this gained energy. Today, lasers have been developed that have numerous medical and industrial applications.

The electromagnetic spectrum ranges from long radio waves to short, powerful gamma rays (Fig. 11-1). Within this spectrum is a narrow band of visible or white light, which is composed of red, orange, yellow, green, blue, and violet light. Laser (*Light Amplified Stimulated Emitted Radiation*) light ranges from the ultraviolet and infrared spectrum through all of the colors of the rainbow. In contrast to other diffuse forms of radiation, laser light is concentrated. It is almost exclusively of one wavelength or color, and its parallel waves travel in one direction. Through the use of fluorescent dyes, laser light can occur in numerous wavelengths. The types of laser include glass-filled tubes of helium and neon lasers, the most common; YAG-type (Yttrium-Aluminum-Garnet), which is an imitation diamond; argon; and krypton.

Lasers sort the energy in atoms and molecules, concentrate it, and release it in powerful waves. In most lasers a medium of gas, liquid, or crystal is energized by high-intensity light, an electrical discharge, or even nuclear radiation. When an atom extends beyond the orbits of its electrons or when a molecule vibrates or changes its shape, they instantly snap back, shedding energy in the form of a photon (Fig. 11-2). The *photon* is the basic unit of all radiation. When a photon reaches an atom of the

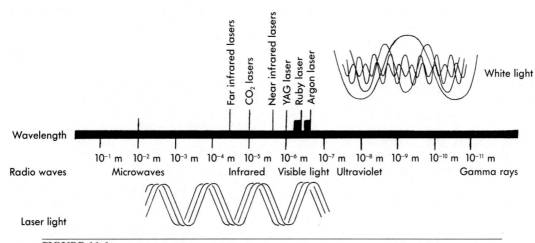

FIGURE 11-1

The electromagnetic spectrum. YAG = yttrium, aluminum, and garnet.
(From Turgeon ML: Clinical hematology:theory and procedures, Boston, 1988, Little, Brown & Co Inc.)

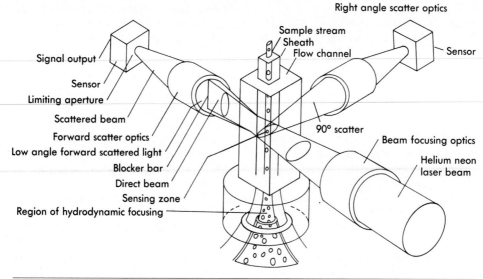

FIGURE 11-2

Laser flow cytometry.

(From Turgeon ML: Clinical hematology:theory and procedures, Boston, 1988, Little, Brown & Co Inc.)

medium, the energy exchange stimulates the emission of another photon in the same wavelength and direction. This process continues until a cascade of growing energy sweeps through the medium.

Photons travel the length of the laser and bounce off mirrors. First a few and eventually countless photons synchronize themselves, until an avalanche of light streaks between the mirrors. In some gas lasers, transparent disks referred to as Brewster windows, are slanted at a precise angle that polarizes the laser's light. The photons, which are reflected back and forth, finally gain so much energy that they exit as a powerful beam. The power of lasers to pass on energy and information is rated in watts.

Principles of Cell Cytometry

The principle of flow cytometry is based on the fact that cells are stained in suspension with an appropriate fluorochrome, which may be either an immunologic reagent, a dye that stains a specific component, or some other marker with specified reactivity. Fluorescent dyes used in flow cytometry must bind or react specifically with the cellular component of interest, such as reticulocytes, peroxidase enzyme, or DNA content. Fluorescent dyes include acridine orange, thioflavin T, pyronin Y, fluorescein isothiocyanate (FITC), and phycoerythrin (PE). FITC and PE are used when dual color analysis is desired.

Laser light is the most common light source used in flow cytometers because of its properties of intensity, stability, and monochromaticity. Argon is preferred for fluorescein isothiocyanate (FITC) labeling. Krypton is often used as a second laser in dual analysis systems and serves as a better light source for compounds labeled by tetramethyl-

rhodamine isothiocyanate (TRITC) and tetra-m cyclopropylrhodamine isothiocyanate (XRITC).

A suspension of stained cells is pressurized using gas and transported through plastic tubing to a flow chamber within the instrument. In the flow chamber, the specimen is injected through a needle into a stream of physiologic saline called the sheath. The sheath and specimen both exit the flow chamber through a 75 micron orifice. This laminar flow design confines the cells to the very center of the saline sheath with the cells moving in single file.

The stained cells next pass through the laser beam. The laser activates the dye and the cell fluoresces. Although the fluorescence is emitted throughout a 360-degree circle, it is usually collected via optical sensors located at 90 degrees relative to the laser beam. The fluorescence information is then transmitted to a computer. Flow cytometry performs fluorescence analysis on single cells at rates up to 50,000 cells per minute.

The computer is the heart of the instrument; it controls all decisions regarding data collection, analysis, and cell sorting. The major applications of this technology are as follows:
1. Identification of cells
2. Cell sorting before further analysis

Cell Sorting

Using flow cytometry, cells can be sorted from the main cellular population into subpopulations for further analysis (Fig. 11-3). Sorting is accomplished using stored computer information.

When the laser strikes a stained cell, the dye creates distinctive colored light that the cytometer recognizes. This fluorescent intensity is recorded and analyzed by the computer, and cells are sorted according to a preprogrammed selection. If the par-

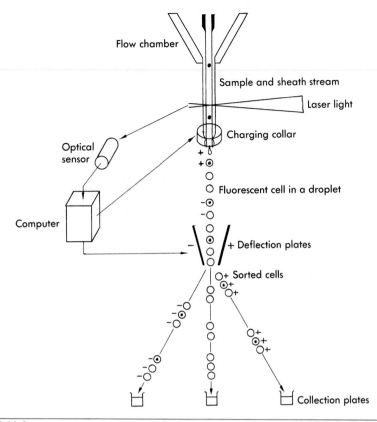

FIGURE 11-3

Laser and cell sorting schematic.

ticular cell in the laser beam is of interest, the computer waits an appropriate length of time for the cell to reach the droplet break-off point within the charging collar. At that point, the computer signals the charging collar to administer either an electrostatically positive or negative charge to the stream containing the target cell. A droplet containing this cell is then removed from the main stream before the charge has time to redistribute.

This action produces the cell of interest within a liquid drop that has on its surface an electrostatic charge (only the droplet is charged). The droplet falls between a set of deflection plates that creates an electrical field. The charged droplets are deflected either to the left or right, depending on their polarity, and collected for further analysis.

Chapter Review

HIGHLIGHTS

The quantity of turbidity in a solution can be measured photometrically. When specific antigen-coated latex particles acting as reaction intensifiers are agglutinated by their corresponding antibody, the increased light scatter of a solution can be measured by nephelometry as the macromolecular complexes form. In immunology, nephelometry is used to measure complement components, immune complexes, and the presence of a variety of antibodies. The procedure is based on the reaction between the protein being assayed and a specific antisera. Protein in a patient specimen reacts with specific nephelometric antisera to human proteins and forms insoluble complexes. When light is passed through such a suspension, the resulting complexes of insoluble precipitants scatter incident light in solutions that can be measured. Nephelometry is a rapid and highly reproducible automated method.

Within the electromagnetic spectrum is a narrow band of visible or white light, which is composed of red, orange, yellow, green, blue, and violet light. Laser (Light Amplified Stimulated Emitted Radiation) light ranges from the ultraviolet and infrared spectrum through all of the colors of the rainbow. Laser light is almost exclusively of one wavelength or color and its parallel waves travel in one direction. Through the use of fluorescent dyes, laser light can occur in numerous wavelengths. The principle of flow cytometry is based on the fact that cells are stained in suspension with an appropriate fluorochrome, which may be either an immunologic reagent, a dye that stains a specific component, or some other marker with specified reactivity. Laser light is the most common light source used in flow cytometers because of the properties of intensity, stability, and being monochromaticity. The stained cells pass through the laser beam. The laser activates the dye and the cell fluoresces. The major applications of this technology are identification of cells and cell sorting before further analysis.

REVIEW QUESTIONS

1. Nephelometry measures the light scatter of:
   A. ions
   B. macromolecules
   C. antibodies
   D. soluble antigens
   E. both C and D
2. LASER is an acronym for:
   A. Light Amplified Stimulated Emitted Radiation
   B. Light Augmented Stimulated Emitted Radiation
   C. Light Amplified Stimulated Energy Radiation
   D. Large Angle Stimulated Emitted Radiation
   E. Large Angle Spurious Emitted Radiation
3. All of the following are descriptive characteristics of laser light except:
   A. intensity
   B. stability
   C. polychromatic
   D. monochromatic
   E. a form of electromagnetic energy

Answers

1. B 2. A 3. C

BIBLIOGRAPHY

Behring nephelometer system folder, Branchburg, NJ, 1987, Behring Diagnostics, Inc.
Hoffman EG: Laboratory evaluation of monoclonal gammopathies, Can J Med Tech 49(2):99-115, 1987.
Lovett EJ and others: Application of flow cytometry to diagnostic pathology, Lab Invest 50(2):115-140, 1984.
Turgeon ML: Clinical hematology, Boston, 1988, Little, Brown & Co Inc.

CHAPTER 12

Miscellaneous Techniques

COMPLEMENT FIXATION

Complement fixation (CF) is a classic method for demonstrating the presence of antibody, e.g., anti-streptolysin O, in serum; however, more sensitive and less demanding systems for the detection of antibodies have replaced the complement fixation procedure.

The CF method consists of two components. The first component is an indicator system consisting of a combination of sheep red blood cells, complement-fixing antibody (IgG) produced against the sheep red cells in another animal, and an exogenous source of complement, usually guinea pig serum. When these three components are combined in an optimum concentration, the anti-sheep cell antibody, *hemolysin*, can bind to the surface of the red cells. Complement can subsequently bind to this antigen-antibody complex and cause cell lysis. The second component consists of a known antigen and patient serum. The known antigen and patient serum are added to a suspension of sheep erythrocytes, hemolysin, and a complement.

The two components of the complement fixation procedure are tested in sequence (Fig. 12-1). Patient serum is first added to the known antigen and complement is added to the solution. If the serum contains antibody to the antigen, the resulting antigen-antibody complexes will bind all of the complement. Sheep red cells and hemolysin are then added. If complement has not been bound by an antigen-antibody complex formed from the patient serum and known antigen, it is available to bind to the indicator system of sheep cells and hemolysin.

Lysis of the indicator sheep cells indicates both a lack of antibody and a negative complement-fixation test. If the patient's serum *does* contain a complement-fixing antibody, a positive result will be demonstrated by the lack of hemolysis, intact red cells.

NEUTRALIZATION PROCEDURES

The evaluation of *neutralizing antibodies,* which destroy the infectivity of viruses, can be measured by the neutralization method. In this procedure patient serum is mixed with a suspension of infectious virus particles of the same type as those suspected to be causing disease in the patient. A control suspension of virus is mixed with normal serum. The viral suspension is then inoculated into an appropriate cell culture. If the patient serum contains antibody to the virus, the antibody will bind to the virus particles and prevent them from invading the cells in culture as well as neutralizing the infectivity of the virus. Disadvantages include the fact that this procedure is technically demanding and time consuming. It is restricted to laboratories that routinely perform viral cultures.

CRYOGLOBULINS

Cryoglobulin analysis is frequently requested when patient symptoms such as pain, cyanosis, Raynaud's phenomenon, or skin ulceration upon exposure to cold temperatures are present. Cryoglobulins are proteins that precipitate or gel when cooled to 0° C and dissolve when heated. In most cases, monoclonal cryoglobulins are IgM or IgG. Occasionally, the macroglobulin is both cryoprecipitable and capable of cold-induced anti-i-mediated agglutination of red cells.

Cryoglobulins can have a monoclonal protein component, and when detected, normally prompt a clinical investigation to determine whether an underlying disease exists. Cryoglobulins are classified as:

1. Type I—the cryoprecipitate is a monoclonal IgG, IgA, or IgM.
2. Type II—the cryoprecipitate is mixed containing two classes of immunoglobulins, at least one of which is monoclonal.

145

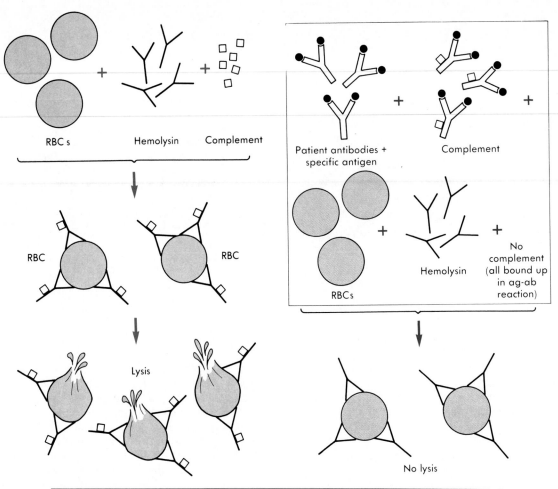

FIGURE 12-1

Complement fixation test.
(From Baron EJ and Finegold SM: Bailey and Scott's Diagnostic microbiology, ed 8, St Louis, 1990, The CV Mosby Co.)

3. Type III—the cryoprecipitate is mixed and no monoclonal protein is found.

To test for the presence of cryoglobulins, blood is collected, placed in warm water, and centrifuged at room temperature. The serum is then put into a graduated centrifuge tube and placed in a 4° C environment for seven days. If a gel or precipitate is observed, the tube is centrifuged, the precipitate washed at 4° C, redissolved at 37° C, and evaluated by double diffusion and immunoelectrophoresis for the content of the cryoglobulin.

Chapter Review

HIGHLIGHTS

Complement fixation is a classic method for demonstrating the presence of antibody. Newer systems, however, have replaced this methodology in many cases. Complement fixation consists of two components: (1) an indicator system and (2) known antigen and patient serum. These two components are tested in sequence. Lysis of the indicator cells indicates hemolysis; the lack of hemolysis is considered to be a positive test.

Neutralization procedures are used to evaluate antibodies that destroy the infectivity of viruses. If a patient's serum contains antibody to the virus, the antibody will bind to the virus particles and prevent them from invading the cell in culture as well as neutralizing the infectivity of the virus.

Cryoglobulin analysis is frequently requested when patient symptoms such as pain or cyanosis develop upon exposure to cold temperatures. Cryoglobulins are proteins that precipitate or gel when cooled to 0° C and dissolve when heated.

REVIEW QUESTIONS

1. In the complement fixation procedure, a negative result is manifested by:
   A. antigen binding
   B. lysis of guinea pig cells
   C. lysis of sheep red blood cells
   D. agglutination of sheep red blood cells
   E. none of the above
2. The neutralization assay is used for:
   A. evaluation of antibodies that destroy infectivity of viruses
   B. evaluation of antibodies that destroy infectivity of bacteria
   C. quantitation of complement
   D. quantitation of immune-complexes
   E. quantitation of virus levels
3. Cryoglobulins are proteins that precipitate or gel when cooled to ° C.
   A. −18° C
   B. 0° C
   C. 4° C
   D. 18° C
   E. 37° C

Match the following types of cryoglobulin with their respective description.

4. Type I
5. Type II
6. Type III
   A. contains two classes of immunoglobulins at least one of which is monoclonal
   B. mixed, no monoclonal protein found
   C. monoclonal IgG, IgA or IgM

Answers

1. C 2. A 3. B 4. C 5. A 6. B

BIBLIOGRAPHY

Finegold SM and Baron EJ: Bailey and Scott's diagnostic microbiology, ed 7, St. Louis, 1986, The CV Mosby Co.
Turgeon ML: Clinical hematology, Boston, 1988, Little, Brown & Co Inc.

PART III

Immunologic Manifestations of Infectious Diseases

CHAPTER 13

The Immune Response in Infectious Diseases

CHARACTERISTICS OF INFECTIOUS DISEASES

The acquisition of an infectious disease, e.g., viral, bacterial, parasitic, or fungal, is influenced by factors related to both the micro-organism and the host. Factors that can influence the exposure to and actual development of an infectious disease include the following:

1. The immune status of an individual, e.g., immunocompromised individuals have a much higher rate of microbial disease
2. Overall incidence of an organism in the population
3. Pathogenicity or virulence of the agent
4. Actual presence of a large enough dose of the agent or organism to produce an infection
5. Appropriate portal of entry

In many cases, the successful dissemination of a micro-organism results from the fact that the micro-organism can be spread over long distances because of insect vectors or rapidly from country to country by travelers in the jet age. Other considerations in microbial disease development include the abilities of some micro-organisms to multiply in an intracellular habitat, such as in macrophages, and some to display antigen variation, which makes it difficult for a normal immune mechanism to control.

Host factors, such as the general health and age of an individual, influence the likelihood of developing an infectious disease and are important determinants of its severity. The very young and the elderly develop infectious diseases more frequently than individuals in other other age groups. In addition, a history of previous exposure to a disease or the harboring of an organism, such as a virus in a dormant condition, is also a determining factor in the development of a variety of diseases.

DEVELOPMENT OF INFECTIOUS DISEASES

In order for an infectious disease to develop in a host, the organism must penetrate the skin or mucuous membrane barrier, the first line of defense, and survive other natural and adaptive body defense mechanisms (see Chapter 1). These mechanisms include phagocytosis, antibody and cell-mediated immunity or complement activation, and associated interacting effector mechanisms. Phagocytosis and complement activation may be initiated within minutes of the invasion of a micro-organism; however, unless primed by previous contact with the same or a similar antigen, antibody and cell-mediated responses do not become activated for several days. It should also be noted that complement and antibodies are the most active constituents against micro-organisms free in the blood or tissues, but cell-mediated responses are most active against those micro-organisms that are cell associated. The mechanism of body defense that is the most effective in a healthy host depends on factors such as an appropriate portal of entry and the characteristics of each individual micro-organism. The routes of infection or portals of entry can include transmission through oral routes, such as food or water-borne contamination; maternal-fetal transmission; insect vectors; sexual transmission; parenteral routes, such as the injection or transfusion of infected blood; and respiratory transmission. Development of infectious disease, therefore, occurs only if a micro-organism can evade, overcome, or inhibit the body defense mechanisms that are normally operational.

IMMUNITY TO INFECTIOUS DISEASES
Bacterial Diseases

The presence of substances such as the natural antibiotic, lysozyme, and phagocytosis represent ma-

151

jor immunologic defense mechanisms against bacteria. A micro-organism, however, is able to survive phagocytosis if it possesses a capsule that impedes attachment, a cell wall which interferes with digestion, and/or the release of exotoxins, which damage phagocytic and other cells. Most capsules and toxins are strongly antigenic, but antibodies can overcome many of their effects, which is the basis of the majority of antibacterial vaccines.

Fungal Diseases

Fungal infections are normally superficial but a few fungi can cause serious systemic disease, usually entering through the respiratory tract in the form of spores. Disease manifestation depends on the degree and type of immune response elicited by the host. Fungi, such as *Candida albicans*, are a common and harmless inhabitant of skin and mucous membranes under normal conditions. In immunocompromised hosts, however, *Candida* and other fungi become opportunistic agents that take advantage of the host's weakened resistance. Manifestations of fungal disease may range from unnoticed respiratory episodes to rapid fatal dissemination of a violent hypersensitivity reaction. Survival mechanisms of fungi that successfully invade the body are similar to bacterial characteristics, such as the presence of an antiphagocytic capsule; resistance to digestion within macrophages; and destruction of phagocytes, such as neutrophils. Some types of yeast activate complement via the alternative pathway, but it is unknown if this activation has any effect on the micro-organism's survival.

Viral, Rickettsial, and Mycoplasmal Diseases

The characteristic process associated with viral infections is cellular replication, which may or may not lead to cell death. Interferon plays a major role in body defenses against viral infections. Antibodies are valuable in preventing entry and bloodborne spread of some viruses; but the ability of other viruses to spread from cell to cell places the burden of adaptive immunity on the T-cell system, which specializes in recognizing altered "self" histocompatibility (HLA) antigens. Macrophages may also play a role in immunity. Some of the most virulent viruses to humans are zoonoses, e.g., rabies. Other viruses, however, can persist for years without symptoms and then be reactivated to cause serious disease, possibly including tumors.

Organisms intermediate between viruses and bacteria are those obligatory intracellular organisms that possess cell walls (Rickettsiae) and those without cell walls but capable of extracellular replication (mycoplasma). Immunologically the former are closer to viruses, the latter to bacteria.

Parasitic Disease

Parasites are relatively large, may have resistant body walls, and may avoid being phagocytized because of their ability to migrate away from an inflamed area. These differences set parasitic infections apart from bacterial and viral infections, to which some forms of natural and adaptive immunity afford protection.

Effectors, however, are present against parasitic disease. These immune responses to parasitic infections include: immunoglobulins, complement, antibody-dependent cell-mediated cytotoxicity, and cellular defenses, such as eosinophils and T cells. Some cestodes, especially in their larval stages, may be eradicated by complement-fixing IgG antibodies. In addition, some antibodies may cross-react with other parasitic antigens. Demonstrating the protective effect of IgA has been difficult. Increased levels of IgE may be noted in many helminth infections. Activation of both the classic and alternate complement pathways may take place in some cases of schistosomiasis, and the alternate pathway of activation may kill larvae in the absence of antibody. Phagocytosis may have some direct activity against parasitic organisms, but the most effective protection in some parasitic infections is provided by antibody-dependent cell-mediated cytotoxicity (ADCC). Macrophages, neutrophils, and eosinophils may demonstrate direct toxicity or phagocytosis toward parasites. The actual attachment of the cytotoxic cells is most frequently mediated by IgG, although IgE may be effective. The role of eosinophils is complex. They may phagocytize immune complexes and act as effector cells in mediating local (type I) reactions, primarily in tissue-stage parasites. T cells are frequently involved in body defenses against parasites. Sequestration of micro-organisms is a classic T-cell–dependent hypersensitivity response. In addition, helper T cells may sensitize B cells to specific parasitic antigens.

Other protective nonspecific factors, such as nonstimulated monocytes are a major protective mechanism against parasites, such as *Giardia*. NK cells also have a direct activity against cancer cells as well as some parasites. Delayed hypersensitivity may be helpful in preventing some parasitic infections but may cause disease in other cases. Deposition of antigen-antibody complexes, demonstrated by Raji cell assays, is responsible for severe pathologic lesions in some parasitic infections. In addition, high levels of circulating IgE may cause hypersensitivity reactions in helminth and cestode infections. Anaphylaxsis is a clear risk in echinococcal infections, especially with spontaneous or surgical rupture of a hydatid cyst.

LABORATORY DETECTION OF IMMUNOLOGIC RESPONSES

Because IgM is usually produced in significant quantities during the first exposure of a patient to an infectious agent, the detection of specific IgM can be of diagnostic significance. This immunologic characteristic is particularly important in diseases that do not manifest decisive clinical signs and symptoms, such as toxoplasmosis, or those conditions in which a rapid therapeutic decision may be required, such as rubella. Procedures that specifically evaluate the presence of IgM are frequently used to detect cytomegalovirus (CMV), herpes viruses, *Toxoplasma gondii*, rubella, or *T. pallidum.* The names of some of the tests for these agents have been grouped together under the acronym TORCH (Toxoplasma, Rubella, Cytomegalovirus, and Herpes). Several methods have been developed to measure only the specific IgM in sera that may also contain specific IgG. In addition to using a labeled antibody specific for only IgM as the marker, immunoglobulins can be separated by physical means, such as high-speed centrifugation through a sucrose gradient. New systems of separation are also available. The advantage of methods such as an IgM separation column is that the rheumatoid factor, which is IgM antibodies produced by some patients against their own IgG, will often bind to the IgG molecules being washed through the column and be removed along with the IgG. This action is advantageous because rheumatoid factors can cause nonspecific and interfering results with many serologic tests.

In many diseases there exists a spectrum of responses from infected individuals. Some patients may develop and manifest antibodies from a subclinical infection or after colonization of an agent without actually developing disease. In these cases, the presence of antibody in a single serum specimen or a comparative titer of antibody in paired specimens may merely indicate past contact with the agent; the presence of antibodies *cannot* be used to accurately diagnose a recent disease. In comparison, some patients may respond to an antigenic stimulus by producing antibodies that can cross-react with other antigens. These antibodies are nonspecific and may lead to misinterpretation of serologic tests.

In most cases, serologic procedures for the diagnosis of recent infection using *acute* and *convalescent* specimens is the method of choice. Except for the detection of IgM or in diseases in which no chance of developing an immune response exists, such as rabies virus or the toxin of botulism, the testing of a single specimen is not usually recommended. In a number of circumstances, however, when only one specimen is tested to determine immune status, antibody to past infection or to immunization can be determined.

Throughout this section, a variety of testing protocols are described for the immunologic detection of representative infectious diseases. These protocols are examples of the types of procedures that are commonly encountered in the serology/immunology laboratory.

Chapter Review

HIGHLIGHTS

The acquisition of an infectious disease is influenced by factors related to both the micro-organism and the host. These factors can influence the exposure to and actual development of an infectious disease. In many cases the successful dissemination of a micro-organism results from the fact that some micro-organisms can be spread over long distances and some are able to multiply in an intracellular habitat or display antigen variation. Host factors such as the general health and age of an individual influence the likelihood of developing an infectious disease; these factors are important determinants of the severity of disease. In addition, a history of previous exposure to a disease or the harboring of an organism is also a determining factor in the development of a variety of diseases.

In order for an infectious disease to develop in a host, the organism must penetrate the skin or mucous membrane barrier and survive other natural and adaptive body defense mechanisms. Phagocytosis and complement activation may be initiated within minutes of the invasion of a micro-organism; however, unless primed by previous contact with the same or a similar antigen, antibody and cell-mediated responses do not become activated for several days. Complement and antibody are the most active constituents against micro-organisms that are free in the blood or tissues, but cell-mediated responses are most active against those micro-organisms that are cell associated. Development of infectious disease, therefore, occurs only if a micro-organism can evade, overcome, or inhibit the body defense mechanisms that are normally operational.

The mechanism of body defense that is the most effective in a healthy host depends on the type of micro-organism. Defenses such as phagocytosis are highly effective in bacterial immunity but are relatively ineffective in the prevention of parasitic disease. T cells, however, are frequently involved in body defenses against parasites. Sequestration of micro-organisms is a classic T-cell−dependent hypersensitivity response.

Because IgM is usually produced in significant quantities during the first exposure of a patient to an infectious agent, the detection of specific IgM can be of diagnostic significance and is a frequently used serologic method in the detection of infectious disease. This immunologic characteristic is particularly important in diseases that do not manifest decisive clinical signs and symptoms or in conditions in which a rapid therapeutic decision may be required. Procedures that specifically evaluate the presence of IgM are frequently used to detect cytomegalovirus (CMV), herpes viruses, *Toxoplasma gondii*, rubella, or *T. pallidum.* The names of some of the tests for these agents have been grouped together with the acronym TORCH (*To*xoplasma, *r*ubella, *c*ytomegalovirus, and *h*erpes). Several methods have been developed to measure only the specific IgM in sera that may also contain specific IgG. This is advantageous because rheumatoid factors can cause nonspecific results that interfere with many serologic tests. In most cases serologic procedures for the diagnosis of recent infection using acute and convalescent specimens is the method of choice. Except for the detection of IgM or in diseases in which no chance of developing an immune response exists, the presence of the testing of a single specimen is not usually recommended. In a number of circumstances, however, when serum is tested only on specimens to determine immune status, antibody to past infection or to immunization can be determined.

REVIEW QUESTIONS

1. Factors that influence the development of an infectious disease include all of the following except the:
   A. immune status of the individual
   B. incidence of an organism in the population
   C. pathogenicity of the agent
   D. sole presence of the agent or micro-organism
   E. general health and age of an individual

Match the appropriate immunologic defense mechanism with the class of micro-organism.

2. Bacteria
3. Fungi
4. Viruses
5. Parasites
   A. Interferon
   B. Lysozymes and phagocytosis
   C. Immunoglobulins, complement, ADCC, and cellular defenses
   D. Phagocytosis

6. The detection of_ _ _ _ _ _ _ _ _can be of diagnostic significance during the first exposure of a patient to an infectious agent.
   A. IgM
   B. IgG
   C. IgA
   D. IgD
   E. IgE

7. Serologic procedures for the diagnosis of recent infection should include:
   A. only an acute specimen
   B. only a convalescent specimen
   C. an acute and convalescent specimen
   D. an acute, convalescent, and 6-month post-infection specimen
   E. only a 6-month post-infection specimen

Answers

1. D 2. B 3. D 4. A 5. D 6. A 7. C

BIBLIOGRAPHY

Davidson RA: Immunology of parasitic infections, Med Clin North Am 69:(4):751-757, July 1985.

Finegold SM and Baron EJ: Bailey and Scott's diagnostic microbiology, ed 7, St Louis, 1986, The CV Mosby Co.

Playfair JHL: Immunology at a glance, Oxford, 1979, Blackwell Scientific Publications Inc.

Turgeon ML: Bloodborne infectious diseases. In Fundamentals of immunohematology, Philadelphia, 1989, Lea & Febiger.

Febrile Diseases

When the human body is invaded by any pathogenic micro-organism, the natural response is the production of antibodies. This immune response is highly individualized. In addition to the host's physiologic status and genetic capabilities, a number of other factors are involved in the production of antibodies, including the antigenicity, dose, and route of the micro-organism and the immune status of the host. The rate of antibody formation, the type and amount of antibodies produced, and the persistence of antibody in the circulation are influenced by the host and microbial factors.

Among the kinds of antibodies that can be produced in response to certain pathogenic micro-organisms are those referred to as the *febrile agglutinins*. The common characteristics of micro-organisms, which elicit the production of febrile agglutinins, are that they can produce persistent fever and are frequently difficult to grow in laboratory cultures. Febrile agglutinin assays, however, are difficult to interpret because of the cross-reactivity of antigens, production of heterologous antibodies, prior immunization of the patient, and prozone reactions.

Febrile antigens include *Salmonella* O antigens of groups A (Paratyphoid A), B (Paratyphoid B), and D (Typhoid O), and flagellar a, b, d (Typhoid H) antigens; *Brucella abortus* antigen; Proteus OX-19, OX-2, and OX-K antigens; and *Francisella tularensis* antigen. Febrile antigen tests are serologic applications of the classic *Widal reaction* devised for the diagnosis of typhoid fever and the *Weil-Felix* reactions where antigens prepared from a *Proteus* organism are used to detect related rickettsial antibodies. Serologic diagnosis of a patient suspected of having infectious diseases characterized by persistent fever is dependent on demonstration of an agglutination reaction between the appropriate antigen and the patient's serum. A rising titer of any specific agglutinin in conjunction with clinical evidence of the corresponding disease gives only presumptive evidence for a diagnosis. Definite diagnosis must be based on accepted methods of microbial isolation or more sensitive and specific antibody methods.

BRUCELLA ABORTUS
Etiology

Brucella abortus (B. abortus) is a gram-negative bacilli. It is the causative micro-organism of brucellosis. The primary virulence factor for *Brucella* seems to be the organism's ability to survive intracellularly. This characteristic as well as granuloma and abscess formation account for the chronic and relapsing nature of this febrile disease.

Epidemiology

B. abortus is a zoonoses that infects humans by accident. The agents of brucellosis, *Brucella* species, are normal flora of the genital and urinary tract of many animals including pigs, cows, and dogs. Most humans acquire brucellosis because of the ingestion of contaminated food products or through occupational exposure. Farmers, veterinarians, and slaughterhouse workers are particularly prone to infection.

Signs and Symptoms

The most frequent signs and symptoms of disease are a gradual onset of nonspecific systemic symptoms including malaise, chills and fever, fatigue, and mental changes. Localized lesions can occur in almost any organ or the skeletal system. Pulmonary, cardiovascular, urogenital, and central nervous systems' localization of infection are also possible complications.

Immunologic Manifestation

Because of the difficulty of isolating this organism by the culturing technique, many cases of brucellosis are diagnosed serologically by identifying the presence of *Brucella* febrile agglutinin. Antibodies appear within 2 to 3 weeks after infection. The maximum time of appearance of serum antibodies is 3 to 5 weeks after infection.

Diagnostic Evaluation

A febrile agglutinin titer of 1:80 to 1:160 strongly suggests infection. The reference range is less than 1:20. In addition to detection of febrile agglutinins by direct agglutination, enzyme immunoassay (EIA) procedures are available for detection of acute disease with specific IgG and IgA antibodies. The reference range of antibodies by EIA is less than 2 standard deviations (SD). Complement fixation is useful because of the prozone effect sometimes encountered with direct agglutination. Antibody detected by complement fixation has a reference range of less than 1:8 for IgM, IgG, and IgA antibodies. EIA, however, is the method of choice for detection of *brucella*-specific IgM and IgG antibodies.

FRANCISELLA TULARENSIS

Etiology

F. tularensis is the causative agent of human and animal tularemia. It is a gram-negative micro-organism possessing a capsule that may be a factor in its virulence. The organism is extremely invasive, being one of only a few infectious agents believed to penetrate intact skin. In addition, it is able to survive in the cells of the mononuclear phagocytic system after a bacteremic phase.

Epidemiology

F. tularensis is a zoonoses and infects humans by accident. It is carried by many species of wild rodents, rabbits, beavers, and muskrats in North America. Humans become infected by handling the carcasses or skins of infected animals; through insect vectors, mainly deerflies and ticks in the United States; by being bitten by carnivores that have themselves eaten infected animals; or by inhalation.

Signs and Symptoms

Patients have high fevers, headache, lymphadenopathy, and ulcerative lesions at the site of inoculation. Pneumonia is a common complication. In addition, granulomatous lesions may develop in various organs (Fig. 14-1).

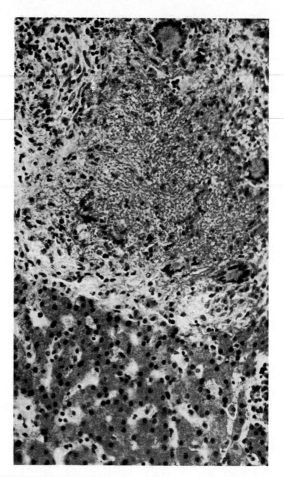

FIGURE 14-1

Ulcerative lesions of *Francisella tularensis*. The granulomatous reaction in the liver closely simulates tuberculosis.

Immunologic Manifestations

Antibody concentration is usually undetectable during the first week of illness but rises to detectable levels within 2 weeks of infection. An agglutination titer of 1:160 or greater is considered to be significant and can be found in 50% to 70% of patients within 2 weeks after infection. An average antibody titer of 1:640 is found 5 weeks after infection. Therefore, fourfold increases in titer between sera taken at 1- to 2-week intervals are strong evidence of infection. Specific IgG, IgM, and IgA antibodies persist for years after infection.

Diagnostic Evaluation

F. tularensis is a slow-growing micro-organism; it is hazardous to handle infectious material. It takes 2 to 4 days for maximum colony formation, but some strains may require up to 2 weeks to develop visible colonies.

Serologic diagnosis, therefore, can be more rapid and safer to perform. In addition to febrile agglutinin detection, a complement fixation or EIA method may be used. In agglutination testing, the reference range is less than 1:20. The reference ranges in complement fixation are less than 1:8; in EIA methodology IgG, IgM, and IgA are not detectable. Cross-reactions with *Brucella* are known to occur but have not been reported with EIA methodology. Therefore, EIA is the method of choice because it is more sensitive than direct agglutination and it is diagnostic with rising levels of *F. tularensis*-specific IgG and elevation of specific IgM. Using EIA methodology, abnormal results may be detected with the initial blood specimen.

SALMONELLA SPECIES

Etiology

Salmonella is a member of the gram-negative bacilli *Enterobacteriaceae*. *S. typhi* is more likely than other species to systemically invade the body, enter the blood circulation, and cause the serious febrile disease, typhoid fever.

Epidemiology

Enterobacteriaceae comprise the major bacteria of the normal flora of the human bowel. These microorganisms are found in natural habitats worldwide, including soil, water, plants, fish, insects, and other animals. *Salmonella* species are the etiologic agents of the majority of food-borne gastroenteritis in the United States. *Salmonella* is naturally found in poultry, but it can be transmitted to food or contaminate water.

Infection is spread by poor hygiene and inadequate sanitary conditions. Fecal contamination of food or water with resultant infection is most serious among the very young, very old, or other compromised individuals.

Domestically acquired typhoid, however, is often transmitted by a chronic carrier of *S. typhi*. After recovering from typhoid fever, some individuals carry the bacteria asymptomatically for extended periods of time. Another group of individuals will be asymptomatic carriers without ever suffering from the disease. These silent carriers contribute to continued episodes of infections.

Signs and Symptoms

The clinical manifestations of salmonella infection are quite varied. Asymptomatic infection is the most common sequela of ingestion of salmonellae. When clinical disease does develop, it usually takes the form of one of the following diseases: enterocolitis, enteric or typhoid fever, bacteremia, localized infection, or a chronic carrier state. These categories are not rigid; some patients exhibit the signs and symptoms of several of the syndromes.

Typhoid or enteric fever is a clinical syndrome characterized by fever, headache, prostration, cough, splenomegaly, and leukopenia. Without antimicrobial therapy, the illness is prolonged and associated with serious complications. The incubation period from the time of exposure until the development of signs and symptoms is 7 to 14 days (the range is from 3 to 60 days). Relapse occurs in 5% to 10% of untreated patients. Symptoms in relapse are usually milder than those of the initial illness and begin about 2 weeks after discontinuation of antimicrobial therapy.

The carrier state is asymptomatic. The chronic intestinal carrier state, defined as documented fecal excretion of *S. typhi* for a minimum of 1 year, is observed in 1% to 3% of typhoid fever patients. The gallbladder is the site of persistent intestinal infection.

Immunologic Manifestation

Salmonella is divided into five distinct serogroups (A, B, C, D, E) on the basis of "O" (somatic, cell wall) antigens. It is further subdivided into more than 1200 serotypes on the basis of "H" (flagellar) antigens. Appearance of serum antibodies begins with the manifestation of antibodies to febrile antigen (group D), which appear 7 to 10 days after infection. Antibody to flagellar D antigen appears later. Antibodies to group D antigen reach their maximum 3 to 5 weeks after infection, and flagellar antibody reaches a maximum concentration later. A *Salmonella*, Group D titer of 1:80 (in early stages) in unvaccinated individuals is suspicious. A titer of 1:160 in unvaccinated individuals is strongly suggestive of infection. Antibody to flagellar D antigen in a titer of 1:40 in unvaccinated individuals is suspicious and 1:160 is strongly suggestive. Antibody titers are much higher in vaccinated individuals.

Diagnostic Evaluation

Diagnosis of typhoid fever should be based on culture of the micro-organism. Testing for antigens comprises the Widal test (see box), *Salmonella* O (Group D), and flagellar D antigens.

The results of the Widal test, a classic procedure, can be difficult to interpret because of factors such as the state of the disease, a higher baseline titer in endemic areas, the effects of previous vaccination, and serologic cross-reactions. For example, *Salmonella* O group D *(S. typhi)* cross-reacts with 98% of the *Salmonella* serotypes. False positive results can be manifested by individuals with various auto-immune diseases. The number of false positives greatly exceeds the number of true positives.

Fourfold or greater increases in antibodies to O (somatic) antigens are typically more helpful than antibodies to H (flagellar) antigen, which are frequently elevated after vaccination. A single titer of

---

Widal Test

| Ab to O Ag Group D (Typhoid O) |
| Ab to H Ag a (Paratyphoid A) |
| Ab to H Ag b (Paratyphoid B) |
| Ab to H Ag d (Typhoid H) |

1:40 or greater to O antigen and 1:80 or greater of H antigen are only suggestive in unvaccinated individuals from non-endemic areas. If febrile agglutinin testing is performed, fastidious quality control and parallel-tested specimens taken over the course of several weeks are mandatory.

Antibodies to the Vi antigen of *S. typhi* (a bacterial antigen characteristic of virulent strains) are sometimes used to screen for typhoid carriers. Antibodies to Vi antigen, however, are only present in about 70% of chronic carriers of *S. typhi*.

Salmonella Paratyphi (S. paratyphi A and S. paratyphi B)

Etiology

The causative agents of paratyphoid fever are *Salmonella paratyphi A*, and *Salmonella paratyphi B*. *Salmonella sedai* is less commonly a cause.

Epidemiology

See preceding discussion.

Signs and Symptoms

Paratyphoid fever is characterized by a prolonged fever and typhoid-like symptoms. See preceding discussion.

Immunologic Manifestation

Demonstration of serum antibodies and the titer of antibodies are similar to *S. typhi*. Low titers, however, may be more significant depending on the prevalence of a particular *Salmonella* species.

Diagnostic Evaluation

Agglutination of antibodies in the patient serum to the febrile antigen *Salmonella* (Groups A or B), and flagellar a and b antigens are diagnostic.

Rickettsial Diseases

Etiology

The rickettsiaceae are the causative agents of the typhus fevers and Rocky Mountain Spotted Fever (RMSF). Some cases of epidemic typhus are caused by *R. prowazekii*-like organisms. The rickettsiaceae are gram negative like coccobacilli.

Epidemiology

Rickettsiaceae infect wild animals; humans are accidental hosts in most cases. The micro-organism is passed between animals by an insect vector, and it multiplies only intracellularly. *R. prowazekii*-like organisms have been isolated from eastern flying squirrels (squirrel-related epidemic typhus). Rocky Mountain spotted fever is the most prevalent rickettsial disease in the United States, followed by murine typhus and Q fever.

Signs and Symptoms

Rocky Mountain spotted fever is a representative model of rickettsial infection and the most important rickettsiosis in the United States. After an incubation period that lasts from 2 to 12 days, the signs and symptoms of disease range from subclinical or mild forms to severe disease with complications.

The three cardinal features of RMSF are fever, rash, and a history of tick bite or exposure. Although all three of these features are present in about 60% of patients, only a small minority of patients will have all three features during the first few days of illness. In addition, gastrointestinal symptoms and central nervous system manifestations are common. As the disease progresses, diffuse edema develops in many patients because of leakage of plasma from damaged blood vessels.

Immunologic Manifestation

Antibodies in typhus fevers and RMSF appear in 7 to 10 days and reach a maximum titer by the fourteenth day after infection. In typhus fevers, a titer of 1:40 to 1:180 (early) is suspicious, and a titer of 1:160 is strongly suggestive of infection. In RMSF antibody titers are usually not above 1:160 to 1:320.

Specific cell-mediated immune responses have been documented in humans and in animal models. These observations indicate that such responses are of major importance in providing immunity to rickettsial diseases. T cells and gamma-interferon are important components of the host response that

---

TABLE 14-1

Weil-Felix Reactions in Rickettsial Diseases

Disease	Antigen		
	Proteus OX-19	*Proteus OX-2*	*Proteus OX-K*
Epidemic typhus	4+	1+	Neg
Murine typhus	4+	1+	Neg
Scrub typhus	Neg	Neg	3+
Spotted fever group	1+ or 4+	1+ or 3+	Neg
Q fever	Neg	Neg	Neg
Rickettsial pox	Neg	Neg	Neg

achieves clearance of rickettsiae and provides long-term immunity in most patients.

Diagnostic Evaluation

Diagnosis of rickettsial disease is primarily accomplished by serologic testing. The least specific but most wisely used test in the United States is the *Weil-Felix* reaction (Table 14-1). This procedure involves testing certain strains of *Proteus vulgaris* with serum from patients with suspected rickettsial disease. Weil-Felix testing is only presumptive; a more specific serologic method such as complement fixation or direct immunofluorescence (IFA) must be used for confirmatory testing.

Latex agglutination testing has demonstrated good sensitivity for the diagnosis of RMSF. Detection of complement fixation antibodies to spotted fever group antigens has good specificity but is less sensitive than IFA. However, it is too insensitive to allow for its exclusive use in the serodiagnosis of Rocky Mountain spotted fever or rickettsial pox.

PROCEDURE

Febrile Agglutinins

PRINCIPLE

Febrile agglutinins are antibodies produced in response to a variety of different pathogenic organisms, which can produce persistent fever and are difficult to grow in culture. Serum containing specific agglutinins in combination with homologous antigens under properly controlled conditions is capable of causing visible agglutination. The degree of agglutination depends on factors such as the concentration of the antigen and antibody.

Sera from normal patients may demonstrate agglutination with febrile antigens because of previous immunization, past infection, or the presence of antibodies to related antigens. In these cases, titers will be low and remain at a constant level. If a patient has an active infection or recent immunization with an organism containing homologous antigens, the serum antibody titer will usually be high and will rise over time.

SPECIMEN COLLECTION AND PREPARATION

No special patient preparation is required before specimen collection. The patient must be positively identified when the specimen is collected; the specimen should be labeled at the bedside and include the patient's full name, the date, the patient's hospital identification number, and the phlebotomist's initials.

Blood should be drawn by an aseptic technique. A minimum of 5 mL of clotted blood (red-top evacuated tube) is required. Allow the blood to clot for 20 to 30 minutes. Loosen the clot from the side of the container with a clean applicator stick, stopper the test tube, and centrifuge. Remove and refrigerate an aliquot of serum at 2° to 8° C until testing, or immediately freeze the serum at −15° C or below if the test is delayed more than 4 hours.

REAGENTS, SUPPLIES, AND EQUIPMENT

1. Febrile antigens. These commercially prepared antigens are nonviable bacterial cells in 0.5% phenolized saline with added crystal violet, brilliant green, and chemical stabilizers. Salmonella flagellar antigens contain 0.5% formaldehyde in place of phenol. Store at 2° to 8° C. Do not open until ready to use.
2. 3″ × 6″ glass slide with circles
3. Pipettes
4. Applicator sticks
5. 0.85% saline ? sterile
6. Waterbath 37° C or 50° C (quantitative method)
7. Refrigerator (4° C)
8. 12 mm × 75 mm test tubes (quantitative method)

QUALITY CONTROL

Control antisera are used in the agglutination tests in conjunction with febrile antigens as positive or negative controls. These preparations consist of lapine antiserum (50%), glycerin (50%), and 1:5,000 thimerosal as a preservative. Control antisera should be stored at 2° to 8° C.

PRELIMINARY PREPARATION OF CONTROL ANTISERA. Dilute the control sera to working strength by adding 3 mL of sterile 0.85% saline. Protect from evaporation and contamination. The expiration date on each vial applies to the product in an intact container stored as directed.

At the time of use, both positive and negative antisera controls must be checked to ensure the accuracy of performance of the antigens, techniques, and methodology. *Note: Francisella tularensis* can aid in the control of both positive results with *Francisella tularensis* antigen and cross-reactions, especially *Brucella abortus* antigen.

Reading controls (Table 14-2) are also useful in determining how the *liquid* portion of the tube test should appear for differing degrees of agglutination. These controls are also useful if autoagglutination of the antigen is suspected. Agglutinated material in any or all of the tubes indicates that the antigen is unstable and should be discarded.

TABLE 14-2

Preparation of Reading Controls

Antigen (mL)	Saline (mL)	Liquid reading
0.5	0.5	Negative
0.25	0.75	2+
0.125	0.875	3+

PROCEDURE

NOTE: Observe aseptic technique and establish precautions against microbial hazards during all procedures. After use, specimen containers, slides, tubes and other contaminated materials must be sterilized by autoclaving. Directions for use should be followed carefully.

SLIDE TEST

1. Dispense the following quantities of serum onto the glass slide with circles:
   - circle 1 0.08 mL
   - circle 2 0.04 mL
   - circle 3 0.02 mL
   - circle 4 0.01 mL
   - circle 5 0.005 mL
2. Invert the bottle containing the antigen several times to mix.
3. Add one drop of antigen to each circle using the dropper supplied with the vial.
4. Using a clean applicator stick for each circle, mix the antigen and serum.
5. Rock the slide for 3 minutes. For *Brucella*, mix on a rotary shaker for 4 minutes at 125 rpm. Observe for agglutination. If agglutination is observed, the strength of agglutination should also be recorded as follows:

   100% (4+), 75% (3+), 50% (2+), 25% (1+)

6. The titer is the reciprocal of the highest final dilution producing a 2+ reaction.

Tube	Serum (mL)	Dilution
1	0.08	1:20
2	0.04	1:40
3	0.02	1:80
4	0.01	1:160
5	0.005	1:320

7. Repeat Steps *1* through *5* for each separate antigen.

TUBE TEST

1. Prepare dilutions of patient serum as follows:
   A. Label eight 12 × 75 mm test tubes (1 to 8).
   B. Pipette 0.5 mL of 0.85% saline into each of the eight test tubes.
   C. Pipette 0.8 mL of saline into a separate tube, and add 0.2 mL of patient serum. Mix well.
   D. With a clean pipette, transfer 0.5 mL of the diluted serum to the first of the eight labeled test tubes in Step B.
   E. Using a clean pipette for each serum dilution, mix and transfer 0.5 mL from tube 1 to tube 2; continue to serially dilute the specimen to tube 7.
   F. Discard 0.5 mL of the diluted serum from tube 7. Tube 8 is the antigen control.

2. Prepare dilutions of the control serum as follows:
   A. Label eight 12 mm × 75 mm test tubes (1 to 8).
   B. Pipette 0.5 mL of 0.85% saline into each of the eight test tubes.
   C. Pipette 0.5 mL of saline into a separate tube, and add 0.5 mL of restored control serum. Mix well.
   D. With a clean pipette, transfer 0.5 mL of the control serum to the first of the eight labeled test tubes in Step B.
   E. Using a clean pipette for each serum dilution, mix and transfer 0.5 mL from tube 1 to tube 2; continue to serially dilute the specimen to tube 7.
   F. Discard 0.5 mL of the diluted serum from tube 7. Tube 8 is the antigen control.

3. Prepare antigen dilutions as follows:
   A. Dilute *Brucella*, *Salmonella* and *Francisella* antigens to one part antigen in 50 parts 0.85% saline (1:50); e.g., 0.25 mL antigen and 12.25 mL saline.
   B. Dilute *Proteus* antigen to one part antigen in 25 parts 0.85% saline (1:25), e.g., 0.25 mL antigen and 6.0 ml saline.

4. Add 0.5 mL of the desired diluted antigen to each test tube.
   NOTE: Each antigen must be tested separately.

5. Shake the test tubes 20 times in a period of 10 seconds.

6. Incubate the test tubes. The length of incubation varies depending on the antigen being tested.

Salmonella O (groups A or B)	18 to 24 hours in a 50° C waterbath
Salmonella O (group D)	16 to 18 hours in a 50° C waterbath
Salmonella flagellar (a, b, or d antigens)	1 hour in a 50° C waterbath
Brucella abortus	48 hours in a 37° C waterbath
Proteus (OX-19, OX-2, OX-K)	2 hours in a 37° C waterbath, followed by overnight refrigeration at 2° to 8° C
Francisella tularensis	20 hours in a 37° C waterbath

7. Very gently agitate each tube and record agglutination as follows:

Negative	Very cloudy with no agglutinins	0
25%	Cloudy	1+
50%	Moderately cloudy	2+
75%	Slightly cloudy	3+
100%	Clear liquid above agglutinins	4+

REPORTING RESULTS

SLIDE TEST

Positive—Agglutination observed

The strength of agglutination can be reported as follows:

100% (4+), 75% (3+), 50% (2+), 25% (1+)

Negative—No agglutination

TUBE TEST

The titer is reported as the highest final dilution producing a 2+ reaction.

Tube	Dilution
1	1:20
2	1:40
3	1:80
4	1:160
5	1:320
6	1:640
7	1:1280

PROCEDURE NOTES

The rapid slide test is used primarily as a screening procedure. The tube technique should be used to confirm positive results obtained by slide testing.

SOURCES OF ERROR. Agglutination results can be altered by a variety of factors. These factors include cross-reactions, previous vaccinations, anamnestic responses, antibiotic therapy, other diseases known or unknown, prozone reaction, and auto-agglutination. Because a prozone reaction is possible, care should be taken to observe agglutination at the highest dilutions if no agglutination is observed in lower dilutions. Cross-reactions may occur between *Brucella* and *Francisella* antigens and antisera. Therefore, parallel tests should be performed with those antigens. Generally a higher titer is obtained with the homologous antigen.

CLINICAL APPLICATIONS. Febrile antigens are used in agglutination tests as an aid in the diagnosis of certain febrile diseases such as salmonellosis, brucellosis, and rickettsial disease. The stage of the patient's disease is important in the manifestation of antibodies. Peak titers may occur during convalescence. During infection, antibodies to salmonella O antigen usually appear earlier and disappear sooner than agglutinins to the H antigen.

It is necessary to evaluate two or more serum samples taken at 3- to 5-day intervals after the onset of the disease. A fourfold rise in antibody titer demonstrable in paired acute and convalescent phase sera collected at approximately 5-day intervals is strongly suggestive of a recent infection or immunization.

Patients occasionally fail to develop any serum antibodies. In certain geographic regions and occupations, typhoid fever, *Salmonella*, and *Brucella* are endemic; therefore, a high level of antibodies may be present because of antigenic stimulation rather than disease.

LIMITATIONS. As in other tests, a single test or determination is not diagnostic. The Weil-Felix reactions may vary widely from case to case of spotted fever; hence, the reaction may be of little help in either detecting the disease or differentiating it from murine typhus.

Agglutination is not intended as a substitute for specimen culture. An appropriate attempt should be made to recover and identify the causative micro-organism.

Chapter Review

HIGHLIGHTS

When the human body is invaded by any pathogenic micro-organism, the natural response is the production of antibodies. Among the kinds of antibodies that can be produced are those referred to as the febrile agglutinins. The common characteristics of the micro-organisms that cause the production of febrile agglutinins are that they can produce persistent fever and they are frequently difficult to grow in laboratory cultures. Febrile antigens include *salmonella* O antigens of groups A (paratyphoid A), B (paratyphoid B), and D (typhoid O), and flagellar a, b, d (typhoid H) antigens; *Brucella abortus antigen*; Proteus OX-19, OX-2 and OX-K antigens; and *Francisella tularensis* antigen. Febrile antigen tests are serologic applications of the classic Widal reaction devised for the diagnosis of typhoid fever and the Weil-Felix reactions where antigens prepared from a species of *Proteus* are used to detect related rickettsial antibodies. Serodiagnosis of a patient suspected of having infectious diseases characterized by persistent fever is dependent on the demonstration of an agglutination reaction between the appropriate antigen and the patient's serum. A rising titer of any specific agglutinin in conjunction with clinical evidence of the corresponding disease gives only presumptive evidence for a diagnosis. Definite diagnosis must be based on accepted methods of microbial isolation or more sensitive and specific antibody methods.

The presence of febrile agglutinins is valuable in the detection of infectious diseases caused by a variety of micro-organisms. These micro-organisms include *Brucella abortus (B. abortus)*, the cause of brucellosis; *Francisella tularensis*, the cause of human and animal tularemia; and *Salmonella typhi (S. typhi)* and *S. paratypi A, B*, and *C* that cause typhoid and paratyphoid fever respectively. *Salmonella sedai* is less commonly a cause of paratyphoid fever. Febrile agglutinin testing is also helpful in establishing a diagnosis of rickettsial diseases. The rickettsiaceae are the causative agents of the typhus fevers and Rocky Mountain spotted fever. Some cases of epidemic typhus can be caused by *R. prowazekii*-like organisms.

REVIEW QUESTIONS

1. The common characteristic of pathogenic micro-organisms that can produce febrile agglutinins is that they:
   A. can produce persistent fever
   B. produce homologous antibodies
   C. are frequently difficult to grow in laboratory culture
   D. are antigen-specific
   E. both A and C

2. Febrile antigens include all of the following except:
   A. Salmonella antigens (groups A, B, D and flagellar a, b, d)
   B. *Brucella abortus*
   C. Proteus OX-19, OX-2, OX-K
   D. Francisella tularensis
   E. Treponema pallidum

3. The classic Widal reaction was devised for the diagnosis of:
   A. tularemia
   B. typhoid fever
   C. syphilis
   D. babesiosis
   E. rickettsial infection

4. In the Weil-Felix reaction antigens prepared from organism are used to detect related rickettsial antibodies.
   A. Salmonella
   B. Proteus
   C. Treponema
   D. Shigella
   E. Rickettsia

Match the following:
5. *Brucella abortus*
6. *Francisella tularensis*
7. *Salmonella sp.*
8. *Rickettsia*
   A. survives intracellularly and forms granulomas or abscesses
   B. divided into five distinct serogroups
   C. an encapsulated gram-negative micro-organism that can penetrate intact skin
   D. causes typhus fever and Rocky Mountain spotted fever

9. The febrile agglutinins procedural results can be altered by all of the following except:
   A. previous vaccinations
   B. the presence of complement in patient sera
   C. antibiotic therapy
   D. cross-reactions or auto-agglutination
   E. stage of the patient's disease

Answers

1. E 2. E 3. B 4. B 5. A 6. C 7. B 8. D 9. B

BIBLIOGRAPHY

Febrile antigens for febrile Antigen agglutination tests (product brochure), Becton-Dickinson Microbiology Systems, Cockeysville, Md, July 1988.

Clements ML, Dumler JS, Fiset P, and others: Serodiagnosis of Rocky Mountain spotted fever: comparison of IgM and IgG enzyme-linked immunosorbent assays and indirect fluorescent antibody test, J Infect Dis 148:876-880, 1983.

DeKlerk E and Anderson R: Comparative evaluation of the enzyme-linked immunosorbent assay in the laboratory diagnosis of brucellosis, J Clin Microbiol 21:381-386, 1985.

Finegold SM and Baron EJ: Bailey and Scott's Diagnostic microbiology, ed 7, St. Louis, The CV Mosby Co, 1986.

Koskela P and Salminen A: Humoral immunity against Francisella tularensis after natural infection, J Clin Microbiol 22:973-979, 1985.

Ormsbee RA: Rickettsiae. In Lennette EH, Balows A, Haulser WJ, and Shadomy HJ, editors: Manual of clinical microbiology, ed 4, Washington DC: Am Soc for Microbiology, 1985.

Sack RB: Serologic tests for the diagnosis of enterobacterial infections. In Rose NR, Friedman H, and Fahey JL, editors: Manual of clinical lab immunology, ed 3, Washington DC: Am Soc for Microbiology, 1986.

Sippel JE, El-Masry NA, and Farid Z: Diagnosis of human brucellosis with ELISA, Lancet 2:19-21, 1982.

Stein J: Internal medicine, ed 2, Boston, Little, Brown & Co Inc.

Viljanenen MK, Nurni T, and Salminen A: Enzyme-linked immunosorbent assay (ELISA) with bacterial sonicate antigen for IgM, IgA, and IgG antibodies to *Francisella tularensis:* comparison with bacterial agglutination tests and ELISA with lipopolysaccharide antigen, J Infec Dis 148:715-720, 1983.

Walker DH, Burday MS, and Folds JD: Laboratory diagnosis of Rocky Mountain spotted fever, So Med J 73:1443-1446, 1980.

Yound EJ: Human brucellosis, Rev Infect Dis 5:821-842, 1983.

Zuerlein TJ and Seth PW: The diagnostic utility of the febrile agglutinin tests, JAMA 254:1211-1214, 1985.

CHAPTER 15

Streptococcus Pyogenes Infections

ETIOLOGY

Most streptococci that contain cell wall antigens of Lancefield group A are known as *streptococcus pyogenes (S. pyogenes)*. Members of this species are almost always β-hemolytic. *S. pyogenes* is the most common causative agent of pharyngitis and its resultant disorder, scarlet fever, and the skin infection, impetigo. In terms of human morbidity and mortality worldwide, however, the role of *S. pyogenes* in the subsequent development of complications such as acute rheumatic fever and poststreptococcal glomerulonephritis is more important. Other *S. pyogenes*-associated infections include otitis media in children, and sinusitis in adults, and osteomyelitis, septic arthritis, neonatal septicemia, and rare cases of pneumonia. Cellulitis, a subcutaneous group A streptococcal infection, can also occur as a secondary pyogenic sequelae after an episode of pharyngitis. Erysipelas, a distinct cellulitis syndrome, can be fatal.

Morphologic Characteristics

S. pyogenes is a gram-positive cocci and the serotype most frequently associated with human infection. Lancefield divided these β-hemolytic streptococci into serogroups A through O on the basis of the immunologic action of the cell wall carbohydrate (Fig. 15-1). Structures called *fimbriae* arise near the plasma membrane and project through the cell wall and capsule. These processes contain important surface components of the streptococcus. Lipotechoic acid found on the fimbriae is important in the adherence of the organism to human epithelium and the initiation of infection. The M and R antigens, which are structurally similar but immunologically distinct, are also found on the fimbriae. R antigen has no known biologic role. M protein, a cell protein found in association with the hyaluronic capsule, is a major virulence factor of *S. pyogenes*. Strains of *S. pyogenes* that lack M protein cannot cause infection. M protein inhibits phagocytosis, and antibody synthesized against M protein provides type-specific immunity to group A streptococci. In addition, M protein is the basis for a subclassification of group A streptococci into over 60 M serotypes.

Extracellular Products

Extracellular products are important in the pathogenesis of disease and in the serologic diagnosis of streptococcal disease. Antibodies produced in response to these substances provide evidence of recent streptococcal infection. Two hemolysins (which have the ability to damage human and animal erythrocytes) polymorphonuclear leukocytes and platelets, are produced by most group A strains. *Streptolysin O*, an oxygen-labile enzyme, binds to sterols in the red cell membrane, causing stearic rearrangement. This rearrangement produces submicroscopic holes in the red cell membrane, and hemoglobin diffuses from the cells. *Streptolysin O* is antigenic; the antibody response to it is the most commonly used serologic indicator of recent streptococcal infection. The other hemolysin, *streptolysin S*, an oxygen-stable enzyme, is responsible for the β(clear appearing)-hemolysis on the surface of a blood agar culture plate. *Streptolysin S* disrupts the selective permeability of the red cell membrane, causing osmotic lysis. It is not antigenic.

Other substances produced by group A streptococci presumably facilitate rapid spread through subcutaneous or deeper soft tissues. These include the following:
1. Hyaluronidase, also called *spreading factor*,

163

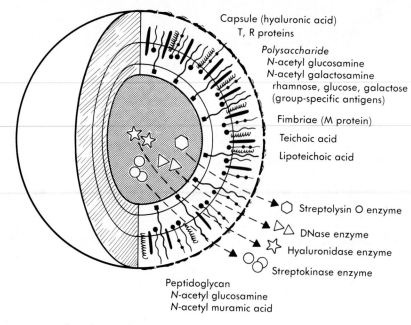

Capsule (hyaluronic acid)
T, R proteins

Polysaccharide
N-acetyl glucosamine
N-acetyl galactosamine
rhamnose, glucose, galactose
(group-specific antigens)

Fimbriae (M protein)

Teichoic acid

Lipoteichoic acid

Streptolysin O enzyme

DNase enzyme

Hyaluronidase enzyme

Streptokinase enzyme

Peptidoglycan
N-acetyl glucosamine
N-acetyl muramic acid

Cytoplasmic membrane

FIGURE 15-1

Streptococcus pyogenes contains many antigenic structural components and produces several antigenic enzymes, each of which may elicit a specific antibody response from the infected host.

(From Baron EJ and Finegold SM: Bailey and Scott's Diagnostic microbiology, ed 8, St Louis, 1990, The CV Mosby Co.)

which breaks down hyaluronic acid found in the host's connective tissue.

2. Four immunologically distinct DNases (A, B, C, D), which degrade deoxyribonucleic acid.

3. Streptokinase, an enzyme that dissolves clots by converting plasminogen to plasmin.

4. Other extracellular products that can elicit an antibody response, such as NADase, proteinase, esterase, and amylase.

5. Erythrogenic toxi, elaborated by scarlet-fever-associated strains, which is responsible for the characteristic rash.

EPIDEMIOLOGY

S. pyogenes is found in the respiratory tract of humans and is always considered a potential pathogen. Upper respiratory infections caused by *S. pyogenes* occur most frequently in school-age children and are uncommon in children under 3 years. No sexual or racial predilection has been described.

Infection is spread by contact with large droplets produced in the upper respiratory tract. Although not as common, food-borne and milk-borne epidemics do occur. Crowding enhances the spread of micro-organisms.

A number of individuals, particularly school-age children, carry *S. pyogenes* without signs of illness. Carriers have positive cultures without serologic evidence of infection. If a person carries the organ-

isms in the pharynx for prolonged periods after untreated infection, the number of organisms carried and their ability to produce M protein decline during carriage. This results in a progressive decline in the likelihood of spreading infection to others.

The incidence of the complication of *S. pyogenes*, rheumatic fever, has decreased in the United States. It occurs primarily in the rural South and in areas of crowding and lower socioeconomic status. The incidence of rheumatic fever is 2% to 3% in epidemics and 0.1% to 1% following sporadic cases of streptococcal infection. The probability of developing rheumatic fever is age-related, with younger patients more likely to develop carditis than older ones.

Rheumatic fever and resultant valvular heart disease, however, are syndromes of major importance among children in developing nations of the world. Patients with a history of rheumatic heart disease, resulting from rheumatic fever, are at a significantly increased risk of developing cardiac malfunction and endocarditis at a later time. The risk of recurrent rheumatic fever depends on factors such as the age of the patient at the time of previous recurrences, the length of time since the last recurrence, and the presence of carditis. In addition, patients who develop streptococcal glomerulonephritis are also at risk of developing later renal failure.

SIGNS AND SYMPTOMS

Manifestations of *S. pyogenes* include upper respiratory infection, scarlet fever, and skin infections.

Upper Respiratory Infection

The clinical manifestations of *S. pyogenes*-associated upper respiratory infection are age-dependent. If the patient is an infant or young child, the infection is characterized by an insidious onset of rhinorrhea, coughing, fever, vomiting, and anorexia. Cervical adenopathy may also be present. Rhinorrhea is sometimes purulent. This syndrome is called *streptococcosis*.

The classic syndrome of streptococcal pharyngitis is seen in children over 3 years. It begins with a sudden onset of sore throat and fever, which rapidly progresses in severity. Pharyngeal erythema with purulent tonsillar exudate and petechiae may be observed on the palate, posterior pharynx, and tonsils. Younger children may have abdominal pain, nausea, and vomiting. Most cases, however, do not manifest the classic syndrome. It is more common for a child with *S. pyogenes* pharyngitis to have a fever, mild sore throat, and pharyngeal erythema without exudate. Viral pharyngitis can produce many of the same symptoms and cannot be reliably differentiated from streptococcal pharyngitis on the basis of clinical examination.

Scarlet Fever

Scarlet fever is the result of pharyngeal infection with a strain of group A streptococcus that produces erythrogenic toxin and is responsible for the characteristic rash. The signs and symptoms of scarlet fever are those of streptococcal pharyngitis with the addition of a rash. The rash usually develops on the second day of illness and results in hyperkeratosis with subsequent peeling similar to the rash of toxic shock syndrome. About 1 week after the onset of illness, the skin of the face begins to peel; peeling progresses over the next 2 weeks. Exposure to erythrogenic toxin confers specific immunity, which limits the number of episodes of scarlet fever in a person to three.

Impetigo and Cellulitis

Impetigo is a skin infection that begins as a papule (Figs. 15-2 and 15-3). The lesion may itch and will eventually crust over and heal. Cellulitis caused by subcutaneous infection with group A streptococci is associated with a warm, red, tender area that may be mildly swollen. Erysipelas, a distinct cellulitis syndrome, usually involves the face and may be associated with pharyngitis. This syndrome is characterized by toxicity and a high fever. If left untreated, erysipelas can be fatal.

Complications of *S. Pyogenes* Infection

Not all infections with *S. pyogenes* lead to complications. Acute rheumatic fever, for example, occurs only after upper respiratory tract infection. In contrast, glomerulonephritis occurs after pharyngitis or

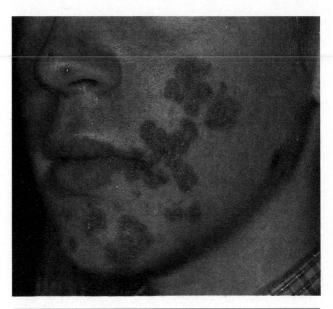

FIGURE 15-2

Vesicular impetigo. A thick, honey-yellow, adherent crust covers the entire eroded surface.
(From Habif TP: Clinical dermatology: a color guide to diagnosis and therapy, St Louis, 1985, The CV Mosby Co.)

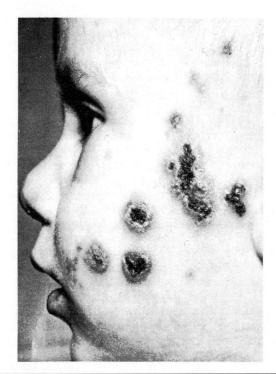

FIGURE 15-3

Impetigo. Older lesions are dark and encrusted.
(From Wehrle PF and Top FH: Communicable and infectious diseases, ed 9, St Louis, 1981, The CV Mosby Co.)

skin infections (pyoderma). Acute rheumatic fever and poststreptococcal glomerulonephritis are considered to be nonsuppurative, because the organs themselves are not directly infected and a purulent inflammatory response is not present in affected organs such as the heart, joints, blood, and kidneys. The pathogenesis of the disease process has not been fully described, but it seems as though an autoimmune phenomenon may be operational. It is believed that cross-reactive antibodies, originally directed against streptococcal cell membranes, bind to myosin in human heart muscle cells. It is further believed that other cross-reactive antibodies bind to components of the glomerular basement membrane and form immune complexes at the affected site. These antigen-antibody complexes attract reactive host cells and enzymes that ultimately cause the cellular damage.

All M serotypes that infect the throat appear to be capable of causing rheumatic fever. A few serotypes, however, have been identified that cause a much lower proportion of cases of rheumatic fever than would be expected from their frequency as a cause of pharyngitis. The incidence of rheumatic fever is directly proportional to the strength of the antibody response to Streptolysin O. Prognosis of rheumatic fever is good when carditis is absent during the initial infection.

Glomerulonephritis may follow an infection of the skin or respiratory tract with one of a limited number of nephritogenic M serotypes. These serotypes are defined by antisera against a protein component of the cell wall, the M protein, which is also associated with virulence. The reason that these serotypes cause glomerulonephritis is unknown.

IMMUNOLOGIC MANIFESTATIONS

S. pyogenes is an example of a pathogen that induces production of several different antibodies. This cocci contains antigenic structural components and produces antigenic enzymes, each of which may elicit a specific antibody response from the infected host. In the course of an infection the extracellular products act as antigens to which the body responds by producing specific antibodies (indications of infection). The majority of infected patients will demonstrate an increase in the concentration of antibody against streptolysin O. The concentration of antibody (titer) begins to rise about 7 days after the onset of infection and reaches a maximum after 4 to 6 weeks. A rise in titer of 50 Todd units in a 1- to 2-week period is of greater diagnostic significance than a single titer. An elevated titer is indicative of a relatively recent infection. Peak titers are seen at the time of acute polyarthritis of acute rheumatic fever, but these titers are no longer at their peak during the carditis of acute rheumatic fever. A patient may demonstrate an elevated antibody titer for up to a year after infection; therefore, the time of infection is not precisely determined by

this technique. Low titers of antistreptolysin O (ASO) can be exhibited by apparently healthy persons because of the frequency of subclinical streptococcal infections, but persistently low titers rule out *S. pyogenes* infection.

Half of the patients with *S. pyogenes*-related acute glomerulonephritis display a normal ASO titer but demonstrate an elevated titer to one of the other streptococcal substances, e.g., DNAase and NADase. Anti-DNase B antibody appears to be the most reliable measure of recent *S. pyogenes* skin infection. Titers of anti-DNase B are elevated in over two thirds of patients with recent streptococcal impetigo. Anti-NADase antibodies are a particularly good marker in patients who develop nephritis following pharyngitis.

DIAGNOSTIC EVALUATION

In addition to cultures such as throat cultures in cases of pharyngitis, antibodies to bacterial toxins and other extracellular products that display measurable activity can be tested. Antistreptolysin O (ASO) and anti-DNase B (ADN-B) are the standard serologic tests.

The ability of a patient's serum to neutralize the erythrocyte-lysing capability of streptolysin O (ASO procedure) has been used for many years as a detection method for previous streptococcal infection. After an infection such as pharyngitis with streptolysin O-producing strains, most patients show a high titer of the antibody ASO. The use of particle agglutination, e.g., latex or indirect hemagglutination, for the presence of antibodies has replaced the use of the classic ASO procedure in many laboratories.

Streptococci produce the enzyme, deoxyribonuclease B (DNase B). A neutralization test that prevents the activity of this enzyme, the anti-DNase B test, is also a standard serologic method for demonstrating recent or previous *S. pyogenes* infection. Antistreptokinase and antihyaluronidase (AHT) have also been used to diagnose streptococcal infection retrospectively.

Serologic testing should compare acute and convalescent sera that have been collected 3 weeks apart. ASO becomes elevated in acute/convalescent paired specimens in 80% to 85% of patients with acute rheumatic fever. ADN-B and AHT levels are elevated in the remaining 15% to 20% of patients. In many cases no acute serum specimen is available; therefore, the antibody titer of the convalescent serum specimen is compared to a reference range value. Reference ranges vary with age, season, and geographic area. False-positive ASO results may be demonstrated because of β-lipoprotein, contamination of the serum specimen by bacterial growth products, or oxidation of ASO. These errors are not encountered with the ADN-B procedure, which is the serologic test of choice for acute rheumatic fever and acute glomerulonephritis after *S. pyogenes* infection.

◻ PROCEDURE

Antistreptolysin O Titer
(Macrotechnique of Rantz and Randall)

PRINCIPLE

Streptolysin O (SLO) is an extracellular toxin with hemolytic properties produced by many strains of streptococci, particularly group A, β-hemolytic streptococci. When released into tissues in the course of infection, streptolysin O antigenically stimulates the production of antistreptolysin O (ASO) antibodies. In the ASO procedure, serial dilutions of patient serum are combined with a constant amount of streptolysin O. If the patient's serum contains antistreptolysin antibody, these antibodies complex with their corresponding antigen and block the hemolytic properties of the antigen in vitro. If the quantity of antibody in the serum is sufficient to neutralize the antigen, no hemolysis will occur when indicator red cells are subsequently added. When the concentration of antigen exceeds the antibody, the excess streptolysin will cause hemolysis. The ASO titer is expressed in Todd units, the reciprocal of the highest dilution of serum showing no hemolysis.

An elevated ASO titer is suggestive of a recent infection with group A (β-hemolytic) streptococci. The consequences of this infectious organism can include rheumatic fever and acute glomerulonephritis.

SPECIMEN COLLECTION AND PREPARATION

No special preparation of the patient is required before specimen collection. The patient must be positively identified when the specimen is collected; the specimen should be labeled at the bedside. Specimen labels should include the patient's full name, the date, the patient's hospital identification number, and the phlebotomist's initials.

Blood should be drawn by an aseptic technique. A minimum of 2 mL of clotted blood (red-top evacuated tube) is required. The specimen should be centrifuged promptly, and an aliquot of serum removed. If the test cannot be performed immediately, serum may be stored for up to 24 hours at 2° to 8° C or up to 2 weeks at −20° C. Lipemia, hemolysis, or contamination with bacteria renders a specimen unsuitable for testing. Inactivation of serum at 56° C for 30 minutes immediately before testing is preferred.

PREPARATION OF TEST SERUM

Prepare serial dilutions of the patient serum as follows:

Tube A (1:10 dilution) = 0.5 mL serum + 4.5 mL SLO buffer

Tube B (1:100 dilution) = 1 mL of 1:10 dilution +9.0 mL SLO buffer

Tube C (1:500 dilution) = 2 mL of 1:100 dilution +8.0 mL SLO buffer

REAGENTS, SUPPLIES, AND EQUIPMENT

1. A 5% suspension of washed human red cells (group O, Rh negative) or rabbit cells. Prepare by suspending 5 mL of washed cells in 95 mL of SLO buffer.
2. SLO reagent. Reconstitute according to manufacturer's directions. Standardize so that 0.% mL will combine with 1 unit of antistreptolysin O. Do not allow the reconstituted reagent to stand for more than 10 minutes before adding to the diluted sera. This reagent is available commercially. **Warning:** The buffer contains sodium azide as a preservative, which may react with lead and copper plumbing to form highly explosive metal azides. Upon disposal, flush with a large volume of water to prevent azide buildup.
3. SLO buffer. Reconstitute according to manufacturer's direction. This solution should be stored at temperatures of 2° to 6° C. **Warning:** The buffer contains the preservative sodium azide, which may react with lead and copper plumbing to form highly explosive metal azides. Upon disposal, flush with a large volume of water to prevent azide buildup.
4. 37° C waterbath or heat block
5. 19 × 150 mm test tubes
6. Serologic pipettes and safety bulb
7. Timer
8. Gauze square or wipes

QUALITY CONTROL

POSITIVE STANDARD. A commercially available lypholized serum standard (166 Todd units) should be used as a control, but this control should be reconstituted according to the manufacturer's directions. Known positive sera with low or high titers can be included as controls. The positive standard must be tested concurrently with patient sera and yield the specified titer.

RED CELL CONTROL. Tube 13 represents a control of the red cell indicator. This control has neither streptolysin O reagent nor serum added (see table below).

STREPTOLYSIN CONTROL. Tube 14 contains buffer, streptolysin O, and indicator red cells. This control must demonstrate marked to complete hemolysis in order for the patient test results to be valid.

Caution: Because the control sera is derived from human sources, it should be handled in the same manner as clinical serum specimens (see *Universal blood and body fluid precautions* in Chapter 6).

PROCEDURE

NOTE: All reagents and specimens must be at room temperature before testing.
1. Label two sets of 13 × 100 mm test tubes (1-14).
2. Pipette the serum dilutions and SLO buffer into the labeled test tubes as follows:

	Serum Dilution						
	1:10			1:100			
Tube No.	1	2	3	4	5	6	7
Diluted serum (mL)	0.8	0.2	1.0	0.8	0.6	0.4	0.3
SLO buffer (mL)	0.2	0.8	—	0.2	0.4	0.6	0.7
		1:500				Red cell control	Streptolysin control
Tube No.	8	9	10	11	12	13	14
Diluted serum (mL)	1.0	0.8	0.6	0.4	0.2	—	—
SLO buffer (mL)	—	0.2	0.4	0.6	0.8	1.5	1.0

3. Shake tubes gently to mix. Add 0.5 mL of SLO reagent to all tubes, *except* tube 13. Gently mix all tubes.
4. Incubate at 37° C for 15 minutes.
5. Add 0.5 mL of the 5% red cell suspension to all tubes. Shake gently to mix.
6. Incubate at 37° C for 15 minutes, shake gently, incubate for an additional 30 minutes at 37° C.
7. Centrifuge for 1 minute at 1000-1500 rpm.
8. Examine for hemolysis. The last tube demonstrating no hemolysis represents the endpoint.
9. The ASO titer, expressed in Todd units,* is the reciprocal of the highest dilution of serum showing *no hemolysis.*

Tube No.   1 2 3 4 5 6 7 8 9 10   11   12
Todd units 12 50 100 125 166 250 333 500 625 833 1250 2500

REPORTING RESULTS

Reference range = less than 166 Todd units. Reference ranges vary with age, season, and geographic area.

PROCEDURE NOTES

The ASO procedure is noted for its good reproducibility. A single titer is difficult to interpret and should be followed by titration of a second specimen obtained 10 to 14 days later.

---

*A Todd unit is the numerical expression of the reciprocal of the quantity of serum times the dilution of the serum in the last tube of the procedure demonstrating no hemolysis. For example, if a serum demonstrates no hemolysis in tubes 1 to 4, a trace of hemolysis in tube 5, and marked-to-complete hemolysis in the remaining tubes, it would be reported as 125 Todd units. Tube 4 represents the endpoint. It contains 0.8 mL of serum diluted 100 times. The reciprocal of 0.8 is 10/8, which when multiplied by 100, yields the value of 125 Todd units.

SOURCES OF ERROR. Erroneous reactions can result from:
1. Oxidation of SLO reagent by shaking or aeration of the vial before testing. Oxidation reduces hemolytic activity.
2. The use of old or leftover reconstituted streptolysin O reagent.
3. Inhibition of a low titer of SLO by lipoprotein cholesterol or bacterial contamination.
4. Incorrect addition of constituents, particularly when irregular amounts are required.
5. Lysis of red cells, if the same pipette is used for dispensing streptolysin solution and red cells.

CLINICAL APPLICATIONS. The signs and symptoms of streptococcal infection often resemble those of other diseases. For example, rheumatic fever can be confused with rheumatoid arthritis at certain stages of the illness. In rheumatoid arthritis, however, the ASO is normal. An elevated titer suggests the presence of group A (β-hemolytic) streptococcal infection. Eighty percent of streptococcal infections are associated with a rise in ASO titer. By repeating the ASO at appropriate intervals, the following can be determined:
1. A rising titer suggests an increase in the severity of the infection.
2. A declining titer suggests a trend toward recovery.
3. A constant (low) titer suggests that a streptococcal infection is not current but that the patient has had a past infection.

LIMITATIONS. Streptococcal skin infections and glomerulonephritis can produce very low titers of ASO. If a streptococcal infection is suspected but the ASO titer does not exceed the reference range, an anti-DNase B (ADN-B) should be performed. The ASO and ADN-B are considered to be the best standard tests.

⬛ PROCEDURE

Rapid Latex Agglutination Antistreptolysin-O Procedure

PRINCIPLE

Group A streptococci produce two hemolytic exotoxins. One of these toxins, streptolysin O, is highly antigenic. Antibodies produced in response to this antigenic stimulation are called streptolysin-O antibodies or antistreptolysin O. If polystyrene latex particles are coated with streptolysin O antigen, visible agglutination will be exhibited in the presence of the corresponding antistreptolysin (ASO) antibody. Group A streptococci can be responsible for postinfection complications such as rheumatic fever and the accompanying cardiac abnormalities, as well as acute glomerulonephritis.

SPECIMEN COLLECTION AND PREPARATION

The patient does not need to be specially prepared before specimen collection. The patient must be positively identified when the specimen is collected; the specimen should be labeled at the bedside. Specimen labels should include the patient's full name, the date, the patient's hospital identification number, and the phlebotomist's initials.

Blood should be drawn by an aseptic technique. A minimum of 2 ml of clotted blood (red-top evacuated tube) is required. The specimen should be centrifuged promptly, and an aliquot of serum removed. If the test cannot be performed immediately, serum may be stored for up to 24 hours at 2° to 8° C or up to 2 weeks at −20° C. Lipemia or contamination with bacteria renders a specimen unsuitable for testing.

REAGENTS, SUPPLIES, AND EQUIPMENT

The ASO Quicktest Kit (Stanbio Laboratory Inc, San Antonio, Texas) contains the following components and positive and negative controls:

1. ASO latex reagent coated with streptolysin-O. Reagent is stable until the expiration date printed on the package when stored at 2° to 8° C. Do not freeze. Mix well before use.
2. 0.9% NaCl solution. A saline solution containing sodium azide as a preservative.
3. Glass slide with 6 cells. Use only the glass slide provided in the kit. It should be rinsed in distilled water and thoroughly dried with a soft cloth or tissue after each use.

Other materials required but not provided in the kit:

1. Applicator sticks
2. Timer
3. 12 × 75 mm test tubes
4. Pasteur pipettes and rubber bulb
5. Serologic pipettes and safety bulb
6. 50 μL disposable pipettes and safety bulb
7. High-intensity direct light

Warning: The latex reagent and controls contain sodium azide as a preservative. Sodium azide may react with lead and copper plumbing to form highly explosive metal azides. Upon disposal, flush with a large volume of water to prevent azide buildup.

QUALITY CONTROL

Positive control serum. A prediluted serum containing at least 200 U/mL of ASO. This control should exhibit visible agglutination (clumping) at the end of the 3-minute test period.

Negative control serum. A prediluted serum containing less than 100 U/mL of ASO. This control should exhibit a smooth or slightly granular appearance at the end of the 3-minute test period.

A positive and negative control should be tested and read concurrently with each group of patient sera.

Caution: Because the control sera is derived from human sources, it should be handled in the same manner as clinical serum specimens (see *Universal blood and body fluid precautions* in Chapter 6).

PROCEDURE

Screening Test

Note: All reagents and specimens must be at room temperature before testing.

1. Label a 12 × 75 mm test tube for each patient serum to be tested.
2. Pipette 1 mL of saline into each test tube.
3. Using a clean Pasteur pipette for each specimen, add one drop of patient serum to each of the appropriately labeled test tubes. Cover the tube and mix the dilution thoroughly by inverting the tube several times.
4. Label one division of the 6 cell slide for the positive control, negative control, and the respective patient sera to be tested.
5. Pipette 50 μL of the controls and patient sera onto the appropriately labeled cells. Use a new pipette for each specimen.
6. Add one drop of latex reagent to each cell.
7. Mix each specimen with a separate, clean applicator stick. Spread the mixture evenly over the cell.
8. Rotate the slide for *exactly* 3 minutes. Examine immediately with a bright source of direct light.

REPORTING RESULTS

Positive—agglutination
Negative—no agglutination

PROCEDURE NOTES

Agglutination demonstrates 200 U/mL or more of ASO. Positive results should be retested quantitatively. In semi-quantitative testing, the U/mL of the highest dilution of serum to produce visible agglutination is the reported value.

Preparation of patient serum should be as follows:

Dilution	U/mL
1:30	300
1:40	400
1:60	600
1:80	800
1:100	1,000

SOURCES OF ERROR. False-positive reactions can result from bacterial contamination of the specimen or if the reaction is observed after 3 minutes. Markedly lipemic serum or plasma may produce nonspecific reactions.

CLINICAL APPLICATIONS. Most of the population will have a detectable ASO titer that varies with age and geographic location. A titer of 200 U/mL or greater may be associated with rheumatic fever or glomerulonephritis. A patient with an elevated titer should be observed over a period of 4 to 6 weeks for an increase in titer.

LIMITATIONS. Because of the subjective reading of results, discrepancies in interpretation may result.

Chapter Review

HIGHLIGHTS

Most streptococci that contain cell wall antigens of Lancefield group A are known as *streptococcus pyogenes (S. pyogenes)*. Members of this species are almost always β-hemolytic. *S. pyogenes* is the most common cause of pharyngitis and its resultant disorder, scarlet fever, and skin infection, impetigo. In terms of human morbidity and mortality worldwide, however, the role of *S. pyogenes* in the subsequent development of complications such as acute rheumatic fever and poststreptococcal glomerulonephritis is more important. Other infections are also associated with *S. pyogenes*. Lancefield divided these β-hemolytic streptococci into serogroups A through O on the basis of the immunologic action of the cell wall carbohydrate. Strains of *S. pyogenes* that lack M protein cannot cause infection.

Extracellular products are important in the pathogenesis of disease and in the serologic diagnosis of streptococcal disease. Antibodies produced in response to these substances provide evidence of recent streptococcal infection. Two hemolysins,

which have the ability to damage human and animal erythrocytes, polymorphonuclear leukocytes and platelets, are produced by most group A strains. Streptolysin O, an oxygen-labile enzyme, binds to sterols in the red cell membrane, causing stearic rearrangement. This rearrangement produces submicroscopic holes in the red cell membrane, and hemoglobin diffuses from the cells. Streptolysin O is antigenic; the antibody response to it is the most commonly used serologic indicator of recent streptococcal infection. Other substances produced by group A streptococci presumably facilitate rapid spread through subcutaneous or deeper soft tissues. These substances include hyaluronidase, four immunologically distinct DNases, streptokinase, other extracellular products that can elicit an antibody response, and erythrogenic toxin. *S. pyogenes* is an example of a pathogen that induces production of several different antibodies. The majority of infected patients will demonstrate an increase in the concentration of antibody against streptolysin O. Half of the patients with *S. pyogenes*-related acute glomerulonephritis display a normal antistreptolysin-O (ASO) titer but demonstrate an elevated titer to one of the other streptococcal substances, e.g., DNAase, NADase. Anti-DNase B (ADN-B) antibody appears to the most reliable measure of recent *S. pyogenes* skin infection. In addition to cultures such as throat cultures in cases of pharyngitis, antibodies to bacterial toxins and other extracellular products that display measurable activity can be tested. ASO and ADN-B are the standard serologic tests.

REVIEW QUESTIONS

1. *Streptococcus pyogenes* is the most common causative agent of all of the following disorders and complications except:
   A. pharyngitis
   B. gastroenteritis
   C. scarlet fever
   D. impetigo
   E. rheumatic fever
2. All of the following characteristics are descriptive of M protein except:
   A. no known biologic role
   B. found in association with the hyaluronic capsule
   C. inhibits phagocytosis
   D. antibody against M protein provides type-specific immunity
   E. is the basis for a subclassification of group A streptococci serotypes

Questions 3 and 4. Match.
3. Streptolysin O
4. Streptolysin S
   A = oxygen labile
   B = oxygen stable

5. Substances produced by *S. pyogenes* include all of the following except:
   A. Hyaluronidase
   B. DNAases (A, B, C, D)
   C. Erythrogenic toxin
   D. Streptokinase
   E. Interferon
6. Laboratory diagnosis of *S. pyogenes* can be made by all of the following except:
   A. culturing of throat or nasal specimens
   B. febrile agglutiniins
   C. ASO procedure
   D. anti-DNase (B)
   E. antibodies to bacterial toxins
7. False ASO results may be due to all of the following except:
   A. room temperature reagents and specimens at the time of testing
   B. the presence of beta lipoprotein
   C. bacterial contamination of the serum specimen
   D. oxidation of ASO reagent due to shaking or aeration of the reagent vial
   E. incorrect addition of constituents

Answers

1. B 2. A 3. B 4. A 5. E 6. B 7. A

BIBLIOGRAPHY

Anthony BF and others: Immunospecificity and quantitation of an enzyme-linked immunosorbent assay for group B streptococcal antibody, J Clin Micro 16:350-354, 1982.

Bisno AL and Ofek I: Serologic diagnosis of streptococcal infection: comparison of a rapid hemagglutination technique with conventional antibody test, Am J Dis Child 127:676-681, 1974.

Dillon JC Jr: Post-streptococcal glomerulonephritis following pyoderma, Rev Infect Dis 1:935-943, 1979.

Finegold SM and Baron EJ: Bailey and Scott's Diagnostic microbiology, ed 7, St Louis, 1986, The CV Mosby Co.

Golubjatnikov R, Koehler JE, and Buccowish J: Comparative study of antistreptolysin O, antideoxyribonuclease B and multi-enzyme tests in streptococcal infections, Health Lab Sci 14:284-290, 1977.

Gotoff SP and others: Human IgG antibody to group B streptococcus type III: comparison of protective levels in a murine model with levels in infected human neonates, J Infect Dis 153:511-519, 1986.

Turner RB and Hendley JO: Streptococcus pyogenes infections. In Internal Medicine, Stein J, editor, Boston, 1987, Little, Brown & Co Inc.

Peacock JA and Tomar RH: Manual of laboratory immunology, Philadelphia, 1980, Lea & Febiger.

Rantz LD, DiCaprio JJ, and Randall E: Am J Med Sci 24, 1952.

Rantz LA and Randall E: Proc Soc Exp Biol Med 59:22, 1945.

Spaun J and others: Bull WHO 24:271, 1961.

Stanbio Product Brochure, Stanbio Laboratory Inc, San Antonio, Texas, 1986.

Todd EW: J Exp Med 55:267, 1932.

Syphilis

The disease *syphilis* was reported in the medical literature as early as 1495. In 1905, it was discovered that syphilis was caused by a spirochete type of bacteria, *Treponema pallidum* (originally called *Spirochaeta pallida*). The first diagnostic blood test, the Wasserman test, was developed in 1906. This classic procedure has subsequently been replaced by a variety of methods. In the treatment of syphilis, heavy metals such as arsenic were replaced by penicillin in the 1940s. Pen-

icillin continues to remain the drug of choice in the treatment of this disease.

ETIOLOGY

Treponema pallidum is a member of the order Spirochaetales and the family Treponemataceae (Fig. 16-1). The genus *Treponema* includes a number of species that reside in the gastrointestinal and genital tracts of humans. *T. pallidum, T. pertenue,* and *T. carateum* (see box) are human pathogens responsible for significant worldwide morbidity.

Direct examination of the treponemes is most commonly performed with darkfield microscopy. Microscopically these pathogenic treponemes appear as fine, spiral (8 to 24 coils) organisms approximately 6 to 15 μm long. They have a trilaminar outer membrane similar to that of gram-negative bacteria.

Pathogenic treponemes are not cultivable with any consistency in artificial laboratory media. Outside of the host, the pathogenic treponemes are extremely susceptible to a variety of physical and chemical agents. Treponemes, however, may remain viable for up to 5 days in tissue specimens removed from diseased animals and from frozen, cryoprotected specimens.

EPIDEMIOLOGY

Pathogenic treponemes are transmitted almost uniformly by direct contact. Syphilis is a venereal disease. The three treponematoses—yaws, pinta, and bejel—are rarely seen in the United States but are prevalent in other countries. These diseases are associated with poverty, overcrowding, and poor hygiene.

Yaws, pinta, and bejel are diseases caused by bacteria closely related to *T. pallidum.* Yaws is common in the Caribbean, Latin America, Central Af-

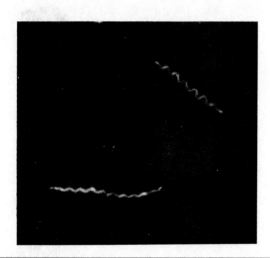

FIGURE 16-1

Treponema pallidum.
(From Bauer JD: Clinical laboratory methods, ed 9, St Louis, 1982, The CV Mosby Co.)

Treponema-Associated Diseases in Humans

Bacteria	*Associated disease*
T. pallidum	Syphilis
T. pallidum (variant)	Bejel
T. pertenue	Yaws
T. carateum	Pinta

rica, and the Far East. Pinta is found only in Latin America, and infection is limited to the skin. Bejel is found in the eastern Mediterranean, the Balkans, and the cooler areas of North Africa.

In these infections, the skin or oral lesions contain many spirochetes that may be transmitted by personal, but not necessarily venereal, contact. These infections are generally acquired during childhood. In each of these diseases, infection elicits antibodies reactive in nontreponemal and treponemal methods.

Syphilis develops in 30% to 50% of the sexual partners of persons with syphilitic lesions. The risk of acquiring syphilis from a single sexual exposure to an infected partner is unknown. A high rate of partners, however, do seek medical treatment within 90 days of contact. Among American civilians, approximately 80,000 cases of syphilis are reported annually. Although the incidence of syphilis declined steadily after World War II, the number of reported cases has been rising over the last several years. The highest incidence of syphilis is among men and women from 20 to 24 years of age. More than one third of infected men are bisexual or exclusively homosexual.

Syphilis can be acquired by kissing a person with active oral lesions. Very few cases of transfusion-acquired syphilis have been reported in recent years in the United States. During the first half of this century, however, syphilis was a major bloodborne infectious disease that was easily transmitted through the prevailing method of direct donor-to-patient blood transfusion. The hazard of transmission of syphilis has not disappeared in some tropical countries, where the organization of blood banks is deficient and where direct blood transfusion prevails in emergency situations. Refrigerated blood storage decreases accidental transmission of the microorganism because *Treponema pallidum* has a short survival period in stored blood. Spirochetes do not appear to survive in units of citrated blood at 4° C for more than 72 hours.

Cases of children who have acquired syphilis by sharing a bed with an infected parent have been reported. In addition, syphilis may be transmitted transplacentally to the fetus. Spirochetes can be transmitted to the fetus during the last trimester of pregnancy, before the mother manifests postpartum evidence of infection.

SIGNS AND SYMPTOMS

Untreated syphilis is a chronic disease with subacute symptomatic periods separated by asymptomatic intervals, during which the diagnosis can be made serologically.

The progression of untreated syphilis is generally divided into stages. Initially, *T. pallidum* penetrates intact mucous membranes or enters the body through tiny defects in the epithelium. Upon entrance, the microorganism is carried by the circulatory system to every organ of the body. Spirochetemia occurs very early in infection, even before the first lesions have appeared or blood tests become reactive. Before clinical or serologic manifestations develop, patients are said to be "incubating syphilis." The incubation period usually last about 3 weeks but can range from 10 to 90 days.

Primary Syphilis

At the end of the incubation period, a patient develops a characteristic primary inflammatory lesion called a *chancre*, at the point of initial inoculation and multiplication of the spirochetes. The chancre begins as a papule and erodes to form a gradually enlarging ulcer with a clean base and indurated edge (Fig. 16-2). Generally, it is relatively painless. In most cases, only a single lesion is present, but multiple chancres are not rare.

Chancres are commonly located around the genitalia, but in about 10% of cases lesions may appear almost anywhere else on the body, e.g., throat, lip, hands. In males, spirochetes are present in the lesion on the penis or discharged from deeper sites with semen. In females, infected lesions are commonly located in the perineal region or on the labia, vaginal wall, or cervix. If the lesion is located inside the urethra, the only symptom may be a scanty serous urethral discharge.

Of patients with primary syphilis of the external genitals, 50% to 70% will subsequently develop in-

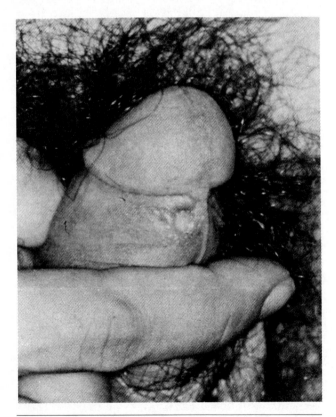

FIGURE 16-2

A primary chancre of syphilis.
(From Kaye D and Rose LF: Fundamentals of internal medicine, St Louis, 1983, The CV Mosby Co.)

guinal adenopathy. Inguinal adenopathy, however, is less common with chancres involving the cervix or proximal portion of the vagina because these sites are drained by the iliac nodes. Regional adenopathy may accompany primary inoculation at other sites; e.g., cervical adenopathy may accompany a syphilitic lesion of the oral cavity. Even without treatment, the primary chancre will persist for 1 to 5 weeks and will heal completely within about 4 to 6 weeks. Regional adenopathy will also resolve itself.

Secondary Syphilis

Within 2 to 8 weeks (but occasionally as long as 6 months) after the appearance of the primary chancre, a patient may develop the signs and symptoms of secondary syphilis. In some cases, primary and secondary syphilis overlap, and the chancre is still obvious. In other situations, some patients never notice the primary chancre and initially have manifestations of secondary syphilis.

The secondary stage is characterized by a generalized illness that usually begins with symptoms suggesting a viral infection: headache, sore throat, low-grade fever, and occasionally a nasal discharge. Blood tests reveal a moderate increase in leukocytes with a relative increase in lymphocytes.

The disease progresses with the development of lymphadenopathy and lesions of the skin and mucous membranes. Approximately 75% of syphilitic patients suffer from generalized adenopathy. Skin lesions are demonstrated by 80% of infected patients. These lesions contain a large number of spirochetes and when located on exposed surfaces are highly contagious. Macular lesions are common and a rash invariably involves the genitalia and often is prominent on the palms and soles. Patients may also develop *condylomata lata*, flat lesions resembling warts in moist areas of the body, for example, around the anus or vagina. These lesions do not reflect areas of inoculation but appear to be caused by hematogenous dissemination of spirochetes. The central nervous system (CNS) is asymptomatically involved in about one third of patients. About 2% of cases manifest themselves as acute syphilitic meningitis. Early involvement of CNS may progress to neurosyphilis if untreated. Hepatitis and immune complex glomerulonephritis occasionally accompany secondary syphilis. Secondary syphilis usually resolves itself within 2 to 6 weeks, even in the absence of therapy.

Latent Syphilis

After resolution of untreated secondary syphilis, the patient enters a latent noninfectious state, in which diagnosis can be made *only* by serologic methods. During the first 2 to 4 years of infection, one fourth of patients will have one or more mucocutaneous relapses in which the manifestation of secondary syphilis reappears. During these relapses, patients are infectious, and the underlying spirochetemia may be passed transplacentally to the fetus. Relapses are extremely rare after 4 years of latency. About one third of patients entering latency are eventually spontaneously cured of the disease; one third will never develop further clinical manifestation of the disease; and the remaining one third will eventually develop late syphilis.

Late (Tertiary) Syphilis

The first manifestations of late syphilis are usually seen from 3 to 10 years after primary infection. About 15% of untreated syphilitic individuals eventually develop late benign syphilis, which is characterized by the presence of destructive granulomas. These granulomas, or gummas, may produce lesions resembling segments of circles that often heal with superficial scarring. The skeletal system is frequently affected, but treponemes are rarely seen.

Of untreated patients 10% develop cardiovascular manifestations. *T. pallidum* may directly affect the aortic endothelium. Weakening of the blood vessels can occur as a syphilitic aneurysm, usually of the aortic arch.

In about 8% of untreated patients, late syphilis involves the CNS. Initially CNS disease is asymptomatic and can be detected only by examination of cerebrospinal fluid (CSF). CSF should be examined in all patients being treated for syphilis of unknown duration or who have had syphilis for more than 1 year. Meningovascular syphilis usually manifests itself as a seizure or cerebrovascular accident (stroke). Spirochetes may also involve the brain tissues and cause general paresis, personality changes, dementia, and delusional states. *Tabes dorsalis* results from involvement of the posterior columns and dorsal roots of the spinal cord and is character-ized by a broad-based gait. Impotence and bladder dysfunction are common in this disorder.

Congenital Syphilis

Congenital syphilis is caused by maternal spirochetemia and transplacental transmission of the microorganism. Congenital syphilis is diagnosed in three fourths of the cases in patients over 10 years of age. Late congenital syphilis may manifest the *hutchinsonian triad:* Hutchinson's teeth (Fig. 16-3), interstitial keratitis, and nerve deafness. Other characteristics include fissuring around the mouth and anus, skeletal lesions, perforation of the palate, and the collapse of nasal bones to produce a saddle-nose deformity.

IMMUNOLOGIC MANIFESTATION

In the treponemes, two classes of antigen have been recognized: those restricted to one or a few species and those shared by many different spirochetes. Specific and nonspecific antibodies are produced in the immunocompetent host. Specific antibodies against *T. pallidum* and nonspecific antibodies against the protein antigen group common to pathogenic spirochetes are formed. Specific antitreponemal antibodies in early or untreated early latent syphilis are predominantly IgM antibodies. The early immune response to infection is rapidly followed by the appearance of IgG antibodies, which soon become predominant. The greatest elevation in IgG concentration is seen in secondary syphilis.

Nontreponemal antibodies, often called *reagin antibodies,* are produced by an infected patient against components of their own or other mammalian cells. Although these antibodies are almost always produced by patients with syphilis, they are

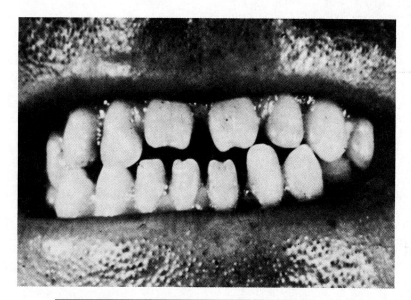

FIGURE 16-3
Congenital syphilis (hutchinsonian triad).
(From Kaye D and Rose LF: Fundamentals of internal medicine, St Louis, 1983, The CV Mosby Co.)

also produced by patients with other infectious diseases. Infectious diseases in which reagin can be demonstrated include measles, chickenpox, hepatitis, infectious mononucleosis, leprosy, tuberculosis, leptospirosis, malaria, rickettsial disease, trypanosomias, and lymphogranuloma venereum (LGV). Reagin can also be exhibited by patients with noninfectious conditions such as autoimmune disorders, drug addiction, old age, pregnancy, and recent immunization.

Delayed hypersensitivity immune mechanisms also contribute to the pathophysiology of syphilis. It is suggested that the granulomatous reactions, or *gummas*, result from delayed hypersensitivity in the immune host. In addition, the manifestations of congenital syphilis apparently result in part from an immune-inflammatory reaction. Antigen-antibody complexes have been detected in the blood of patients with secondary syphilis and are responsible for the syphilis-associated glomerulonephritis. Suppression of the various aspects of cell-mediated immunity have been noted in syphilis and may contribute to prolonged survival of *T. pallidum*.

DIAGNOSTIC EVALUATION

The diagnosis of syphilis depends on clinical skills, demonstration of microorganism in a lesion, and serologic testing. A wide variety of diagnostic procedures for syphilis are available. Classic serologic methods for syphilis measure the presence of two types of antibodies: *treponemal* and *nontreponemal.*

Serologic procedures for syphilis include:
1. *Nontreponemal methods,* e.g., Venereal Disease Research Laboratory (VDRL) and the rapid plasma reagin (RPR) procedures.
2. *Treponemal methods,* e.g., fluorescent *Treponema pallidum*-absorbed (FTA-ABS) and microhemagglutination *Treponema pallidum* (MHA-TP).

Darkfield Microscopy

For symptomatic patients with primary syphilis, darkfield microscopy is the test of choice. A darkfield examination is also suggested for immediate results in cases of secondary syphilis with a VDRL titer follow-up.

Nontreponemal Methods

The VDRL and RPR are the two most widely used nontreponemal serologic procedures. Each is a flocculation (or agglutination) test in which soluble antigen particles coalesce to form larger particles visible as clumps when they are aggregated by antibody.

The VDRL procedure is recommended when a patient who is suspected of having syphilis has a negative darkfield microscopy result or when atypical lesions are present. It is further recommended that a quantitative VDRL assessment be made

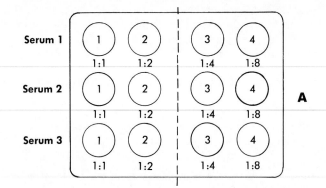

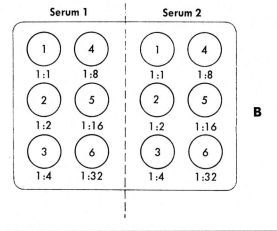

FIGURE 16-4

A, Diagram of slide for quantitative, three-serum, VDRL slide test. *B,* Diagram of slide for quantitative, two-serum VDRL slide test.
(From Bauer JD: Clinical laboratory methods, ed 9, St Louis, 1982, The CV Mosby Co.)

quarterly for 1 year after treatment for syphilis, or to monitor the adequacy of treatment in both latent and early syphilis. The VDRL procedure can be performed on cerebrospinal fluid for the detection of neurosyphilis.

The RPR test can be performed on unheated serum or plasma using a modified VDRL antigen suspension of choline chloride with EDTA. The RPR card test antigen also contains charcoal for macroscopic reading. There are three versions of the RPR test. The original RPR method used unmeasured amounts of plasma and was used as a field procedure for screening large numbers of people. It was about 10% more reactive than the VDRL slide test. The modified RPR uses the unheated serum reagin (USR) test and is performed on measured volumes of unheated serum. This version has a somewhat lower level of reactivity than the VDRL slide test. The RPR (circle) card test uses unheated serum, and less frequently plasma, for testing. It is about as specific as and possibly more sensitive than the VDRL slide test.

Treponemal Methods

The FTA-ABS and MHA represent treponemal methods. The *Treponema pallidum* immobilization test (TPI) method is obsolete. Reactive (positive) reagin tests can be confirmed with these two specific treponemal antigen tests. These procedures, however, should not be used as primary screening methods. Procedures such as the FTA-ABS and MHA can be used to confirm that a positive nontreponemal test result has been caused by syphilis rather than one of the other biologic conditions that can produce a positive VDRL or to determine quantitative titers of antibody, which is useful for following response to therapy. An enzyme-linked immunosorbent assay (ELISA) procedure for syphilis antibody is available, but it is not widely used at present. The ELISA method, however, does offer a sensitive and specific alternative to existing methods.

The FTA-ABS uses as the antigen a killed suspension of *T. pallidum* spirochetes. This procedure is performed by overlaying whole treponemes fixed to a slide with serum from patients suspected of having syphilis because of a previously positive VDRL or RPR test. The patient's serum is first absorbed with non-*T. pallidum* treponemal antigens to reduce nonspecific cross reactivity. Fluorescein-conjugated antihuman antibody (AHG) reagent is then applied as a marker for specific antitreponemal antibodies in the patient's serum.

The microhemagglutination assay for *T. pallidum* is based on agglutination by specific antibodies in the patient's serum with sheep erythrocytes sensitized to *T. pallidum* antigen. The MHA method uses treated red cells coated with treponemal antigens, from a turkey or other animal. The presence of specific antibody produces red cell agglutination that is exhibited by the formation of a flat mat across the bottom of a microdilution well in which the test is performed. If their VDRL is positive, selected asymptomatic persons (including all pregnant women, persons with proven contacts, and persons in demonstrated high-risk groups) should be tested with the microhemagglutination-*Treponema pallidum* method (MHA-TP).

Sensitivity of Commonly Used Serologic Tests for Syphilis

Detection of syphilis by serologic methods is related to both the stage of the disease and the test method (Table 16-1). In the primary stage, about 30% of cases become serologically active after 1 week, and 90% of patients demonstrate reactivity after 3 weeks. Reagin titers increase rapidly during the first 4 weeks of infection and then remain stationary for approximately 6 months. Patients in the secondary stage of syphilis are serologically positive. During latent syphilis there is a gradual return of nonreactive serologic manifestations with nontreponemal method. About one third of patients in the latent stage will remain seroreactive and presumably infectious. In late syphilis, treponemal tests are generally reactive; nontreponemal methods are nonreactive.

TABLE 16-1

Sensitivity of Commonly Used Serologic Tests for Syphilis

Test*	Primary	Stage Secondary	Late
Nontreponemal (reagin tests)			
VDRL	70%	99%	1%†
RPR	80%	99%	
Automated Reagin Test (ART)			0%
Specific treponemal tests			
Fluorescent Treponemal Antibody absorption test (FTA-ABS)	85%	100%	95%
T. pallidum Hemagglutination Assay (TPHA-TP)	65%	100%	95% 95%
Treponemal Immobilization (TPI)	50%	97%	

*Percentage of patients with positive serologic tests in treated or untreated primary or secondary syphilis.
†Treated late syphilis.
From Tramont E: *Treponema pallidum*. In Mandell GL, Douglas RG Jr, and Bennett JE, eds: Principles and practice of infectious diseases, ed 2, New York, 1985, John Wiley & Sons.

PROCEDURE

Serologic Procedures
Venereal Disease Research Laboratory (VDRL) Qualitative Slide Test

PRINCIPLE

During the period of infection with syphilis, *reagin*, a substance with the properties of an antibody, appears in the serum of affected patients. Reagin has the ability to combine with a colloidal suspension extracted from animal tissue and clumps together to form visible masses, a process known as *flocculation*.

In the VDRL procedure, the patient's heat-inactivated serum is mixed with a buffered saline suspension of cardiolipin-lecithin-cholesterol antigen. This serum-antigen mixture is microscopically examined for flocculation. Positive or reactive sera can be serially diluted and titrated. Syphilis and disorders such as pinta, yaws, bejel, and other treponemal diseases can produce positive reactions.

SPECIMEN COLLECTION AND PREPARATION

No special preparation of the patient is required prior to specimen collection. The patient must be positively identified when the specimen is collected. The specimen is to be labeled at the bedside and must include the patient's full name, the date the specimen is collected, and the patient's hospital identification number. The phlebotomist's initials should also appear on the label.

Blood should be drawn by an aseptic technique. The required specimen is a minimum of 2 mL of clotted blood (red top evacuated tube). The specimen should be promptly centrifuged and an aliquot of the serum removed. Severely lipemic or hemolyzed serum is unsuitable for testing. Before testing, the serum must be heat inactivated at 56° C for 30 minutes. Inactivated serum should be reheated at 56° C for 10 minutes, if tested more than 4 hours after the original inactivation.

Cerebrospinal fluid is also an appropriate fluid for testing.

REAGENTS, SUPPLIES, AND EQUIPMENT

1. VDRL antigen—a colorless, alcoholic solution containing 0.03% cardiolipin, 0.9% cholesterol, and sufficient purified lecithin to produce standard reactivity. Each lot must be serologically standardized by comparison with an antigen of known reactivity. Ampules should be stored in the dark at either 6° to 10° C or at room temperature. Antigen that contains precipitate should be discarded.
2. VDRL buffered saline contains 1% sodium chloride, pH 6.0±0.1, available commercially. pH must be checked—discard if out of range, store in screw-capped or glass-stoppered bottles.

WORKING ANTIGEN SUSPENSION

Note: The temperature of the buffered saline and antigen should be in the range of 23° to 29° C (73° to 85° F). The antigen suspension must be used on the day of preparation.

1. Add 0.4 mL of buffered saline to the bottom of the 30 mL, round, glass-stoppered bottle.
2. Rapidly add 0.5 mL of antigen drop by drop (from the lower half of 1.0 mL pipette graduated to the tip) directly to the saline while continuously and gently rotating the bottle in a circular motion on a flat surface. The pipette tip should remain in upper third of the bottle. Take care to avoid splashing saline on the pipette. Blow the last drop of antigen from the pipette without touching the pipette to the saline.
3. Continue to rotate the bottle for 10 seconds.
4. Add 4.1 mL of buffered saline from a 5 mL pipette.
5. Place the top on the bottle and shake up and down approximately 30 times in 10 seconds. The antigen suspension is ready for use but it must be gently mixed at the time of use. Do not force back and forth through the needle and syringe. NOTE: A double volume of antigen may be prepared.
   a. Waterbath, 56° C.
   b. Mechanical rotator (180 rpm) that circumscribes a circle ¾ inch in diameter on a horizontal plane.
   c. 18-gauge hypodermic needle without bevel (this will deliver 60 drops/mL reagent).
   d. Syringe, Luer type, 1 or 2 mL.
   e. Slides with ceramic rings (14 mm diameter).
   f. Flat bottom glass bottle (30 mL) with narrow mouth (35 mm in diameter).

QUALITY CONTROL

1. Include positive control sera of graded reactivity each time serologic testing is performed. The antigen suspension to be used each day is first examined with these control sera. Store control sera frozen at −20° C or liquid form for 7 to 10 days. Thaw, mix thoroughly, and heat inactivate at 56° C before use.
2. Check antigen dispensing needle at the time of use to be sure that it accurately delivers 60 drops/mL reagent. Clean needles and syringes by rinsing with water, alcohol, and acetone. Remove needle from syringe after cleaning.

PROCEDURE

NOTE: The test should be performed at a temperature range of 23° to 29° C (73° to 85° F).

1. Pipette 0.5 mL of inactivated patient serum into one of the rings of the ceramic-ringed slide. Pipette additional specimens and controls into additional rings.
2. Add 1 drop of antigen suspension to each serum with a calibrated 18-gauge needle and syringe held in a vertical position.
3. Rotate the slide on a mechanical rotator for 4 minutes. In extremely dry climates, cover the slides with a lid containing moistened filter paper to prevent evaporation during rotation.
4. Examine each specimen microscopically with the low (10×) objective.

REPORTING RESULTS

Nonreactive: no clumping or very slight roughness
Weakly reactive*: small clumps
Reactive: medium and large clumps

PROCEDURE NOTES

SOURCES OF ERROR. *False-negative reactions* can occur in a variety of situations. These conditions include:

1. Technical error, e.g., unsatisfactory antigen or technique.
2. Low antibody titers. Patients may have syphilis but the reagin concentration is too low to produce a reactive test result. A low concentration of reagin may be caused by several factors: an infection that is too recent to have produced antibodies; the effects of treatment; latent or inac-

---

*When a reactive result is obtained on some dilutions of a serum that produced only a weakly reactive or rough nonreactive result before dilution, the test should be reported as reactive and include a quantitative titer.

tive disease; or patients who have not produced protective antibodies because of immunologic tolerance. These seronegative patients may demonstrate a positive reaction with more sensitive treponemal tests such as the FTA-ABS.

3. The presence of inhibitors in the patient's serum.
4. Reduced ambient temperature (below 23° to 29° C).
5. Prozone reaction.

A *prozone reaction* is encountered occasionally. This type of reaction is demonstrated when complete or partial inhibition of reactivity occurs with undiluted serum, and minimal reactivity is obtained only with diluted serum. The prozone phenomenon may be so pronounced that only a weakly reactive or rough nonreactive result is produced in the qualitative test by a serum that will be strongly reactive when diluted. It is recommended that all sera producing weak reaction or rough nonreactive results in qualitative testing be retested by using a quantitative procedure, before a final report of the VDRL slide test is issued.

Weakly reactive results can be caused by:
1. Very early infection.
2. Lessening of the activity of the disease after treatment.
3. Improper technique or questionable reagents.

False-positive reactions can also be observed. Of all positive serologic tests for syphilis, 10% to 30% may be false biologic positive reactions. Nonsyphilitic positive VDRL reactions have been reported with cardiolipin-type antigen in:
1. Lupus erythematosus
2. Rheumatic fever
3. Vaccinia and virus pneumonia
4. Pneumococcal pneumonia
5. Infectious mononucleosis
6. Infectious hepatitis
7. Leprosy
8. Malaria
9. Rheumatoid arthritis
10. Pregnancy
11. Aging individuals

Contaminated or hemolyzed specimens can also produce false-positive results.

CLINICAL APPLICATIONS. The purpose of the VDRL procedure is to demonstrate reagin in cases of syphilis. The procedure may also be positive in treponemal diseases such as yaws and pinta. Reagin, however, is found in some patients who are not infected with treponemes, which can be partially explained by the necrotizing effect of spirochetes on tissues and in other conditions and disorders. It is important that results of the VDRL procedure be correlated with patient history as well as with signs and symptoms.

LIMITATIONS. The VDRL procedure is not specific for syphilis but may demonstrate positive reactions in other reagin-producing disorders, autoimmune disorders, infectious diseases, and alter-

ations, such as pregnancy or aging, in normal physiology.

REFERENCES

Nicholas L. In Friedman J, Linna TJ, and Prier JE, eds: Immunoserology in the diagnosis of infectious diseases, Baltimore, 1979, University Park Press.

Olansky S. In Samter M and Alexander HL, eds: Immunological diseases, Boston, 1965, Little, Brown, & Co, Inc.

PROCEDURE

VDRL Quantitative Slide Test

PRINCIPLE
Retest quantitatively to an end-point titer all sera that produce reactive, weakly reactive, or questionably nonreactive results in the qualitative VDRL slide test.

SPECIMEN COLLECTION AND PREPARATION (see VDRL qualitative procedure for collection and processing of original undiluted sera.)

PREPARATION OF SERIAL DILUTIONS. Serial dilutions of serum are prepared as follows:
A. Pipette 0.05 mL of 0.9% saline into ring numbers 2, 3, and 4 on ceramic slide (Figs. 16-4 *A* and *B*). Do not spread the saline.
B. Pipette 0.05 mL of serum to ring numbers 1 and 2. Draw the serum and saline mixture up and down in the pipette tip in ring number 2 to mix. Aspirate 0.05 mL of diluted serum and spread the remaining dilution over the entire area of the circle with the pipette tip.
C. Transfer 0.05 mL of the diluted (1:2) serum in ring number 2 to ring number 3. Draw the serum and saline mixture up and down in the pipette tip in ring number 3 to mix. Aspirate 0.05 mL of diluted serum and spread the remaining dilution over the entire area of the circle with the pipette tip.
D. Transfer 0.05 mL of the diluted (1:4) serum in ring number 3 to ring number 4. Draw the serum and saline mixture up and down in the pipette tip in ring number 3 to mix. Aspirate 0.05 mL of diluted serum and spread the remaining dilution over the entire area of the circle with the pipette tip.
E. Discard 0.05 mL of the diluted (1:8) serum from ring number 4, unless greater dilutions are needed for strongly reactive serum, and spread the remaining dilution over the entire area of the circle with the pipette tip.

REAGENTS, SUPPLIES, AND EQUIPMENT
In addition to reagents, supplies, and equipment required for the qualitative VDRL, the following reagent and piece of equipment is needed:
1. 0.9% saline. Prepare by weighing 0.9 g of sodium chloride (chemical grade) to a 1 L volumetric

flask. Dilute to the calibration mark with distilled water.
2. Safety pipette (50 μL or 0.05 mL).

QUALITY CONTROL (see VDRL qualitative procedure)

PROCEDURE

Note: The test should be performed at a temperature range of 23° to 29° C (73° to 85° F)
1. Add 1 drop of antigen suspension to each diluted serum with a calibrated 18-gauge needle and syringe held in a vertical position.
2. Rotate the slide on a mechanical rotator for 4 minutes. In extremely dry climates, the slides may be covered with a lid containing moistened filter paper to prevent evaporation during rotation.
3. Examine each specimen microscopically (low [10×] objective).

REPORTING RESULTS

Report the titer in terms of the highest dilution that produces a reactive (not weakly reactive) result. Example:

Serum Dilutions				Result
1:1 Reactive	1:2 Reactive	1:4 Weakly reactive	1:8 Nonreactive	Reactive, 1:4 dilution or 4 dilutions.

CLINICAL APPLICATIONS. (see VDRL qualitative procedure)

REFERENCES (see VDRL qualitative procedure)

☐ PROCEDURE

VDRL Qualitative Slide Test (Cerebrospinal Fluid)

PRINCIPLE (see VDRL qualitative procedure)

SPECIMEN COLLECTION AND PREPARATION

Centrifuge and decant the specimen. Spinal fluids that are visibly contaminated or that contain gross blood are unsatisfactory for testing. Specimens of spinal fluid do not need to be heat inactivated before testing.

REAGENTS, SUPPLIES, AND EQUIPMENT

See VDRL qualitative procedure for required materials.
PREPARATION OF WORKING ANTIGEN SUSPENSION:
A. Prepare antigen suspension as described for VDRL qualitative slide test.
B. Mix 1 part 10% saline to 1 part VDRL slide test suspension.
C. Mix by gently rotating bottle or inverting tube, and allow to stand for at least 5 minutes but no more than 2 hours before use.
ADDITIONAL SUPPLIES:
1. 22- or 23-gauge hypodermic needle, without bevel. The needle and syringe should dispense 100 ± 2 drops of sensitized antigen suspension per milliliter when the needle and syringe are held vertically.
2. 10% saline. Prepare 10 g sodium chloride/100 mL distilled water.
3. Test slides (2 × 3 inches with concavity measuring 16 mm in diameter and 1.75 mm in depth).

QUALITY CONTROL (see VDRL qualitative procedure)

PROCEDURE

NOTE: The test should be performed at a temperature range of 23° to 29° C (73° to 85° F).
1. Pipette 0.05 mL of spinal fluid into a concavity of the slide.
2. Add 1 drop (0.01 mL) of the working antigen suspension to the specimen from a 21- or 22-gauge needle and syringe held in a vertical position.
3. Rotate the slide for 8 minutes on a mechanical rotator at 180 rpm. In extremely dry climates, the slides may be covered with a slide containing moistened filter paper to prevent evaporation during rotation.
4. Microscopically examine the slide on low (10×) power.

REPORTING RESULTS

Nonreactive: no clumping or very slight roughness
Reactive: definite clumps
A quantitative test should be performed on any reactive specimen.
CLINICAL APPLICATIONS. (see VDRL qualitative procedure)

REFERENCES (see VDRL qualitative procedure)

☐ PROCEDURE

VDRL Quantitative Slide Test (Cerebrospinal Fluid)

PRINCIPLE (see VDRL qualitative slide test)

SPECIMEN COLLECTION AND PREPARATION

Diluted spinal fluid. Prepare the dilutions as follows:
A. Pipette 0.2 mL of 0.9% saline into each of five or more tubes.
B. Add 0.2 mL of unheated spinal fluid to tube 1, mix, transfer to tube 2.
C. Continue mixing and transferring 0.2 mL from one tube to the next until the last tube is reached. Dilutions: 1:2, 1:4, 1:8, 1:16, 1:32.

REAGENTS, SUPPLIES, AND EQUIPMENT (see VDRL qualitative slide test [spinal fluid])

QUALITY CONTROL (see VDRL qualitative slide test [spinal fluid])

PROCEDURE

Treat each dilution as if it were undiluted spinal fluid and see VDRL qualitative slide test (spinal fluid) for the procedural protocol.

REPORTING RESULTS

Report the titer in terms of the highest dilution that produces a reactive (not weakly reactive) result. Example:

Serum dilutions					Result
1:1	1:2	1:4	1:8	1:16	Reactive,
Reactive	Reactive	Reactive	Reactive	Non-reactive	1:8 dilution or 8 dils.

CLINICAL APPLICATIONS. (see VDRL qualitative slide test [spinal fluid])

REFERENCES (see VDRL qualitative slide test [spinal fluid])

◻ PROCEDURE

Rapid Plasma Reagin (RPR) Card Test

PRINCIPLE

The Rapid Plasma Reagin (RPR) test is designed to detect reagin, an antibody-like substance present in serum. In this procedure, serum is mixed with an antigen suspension of a carbon particle cardiolipin antigen. If the specimen contains antibody, flocculation occurs with a coagglutination of the carbon particles of antigen. This flocculation appears as black clumps against the white background of a plastic-coated card. The cards are viewed macroscopically.

This method is a nontreponemal testing procedure for the serologic detection of syphilis; however, pinta, yaws, bejel, and other treponemal diseases may produce positive results. Positive reactions are occasionally observed with other acute or chronic conditions.

SPECIMEN COLLECTION AND PREPARATION

No special preparation of the patient is required before specimen collection. The patient must be positively identified when the specimen is collected. The specimen is to be labeled at the bedside and must include the patient's full name, the date the specimen is collected, and the patient's hospital identification number. The phlebotomist's initials should also appear on the label.

Blood should be drawn by an aseptic technique. The required specimen is a minimum of 2 mL of clotted blood (red top evacuated tube). After allowing the blood to clot, centrifuge the specimen and allow the serum to remain in the original tube. Severely lipemic or hemolyzed serum is unsuitable for testing. NOTE: In special situations when nontreponemal test results are needed rapidly and the specimen is collected in EDTA anticoagulant, plasma can be used for both qualitative and quantitative procedures if the test is performed within 24 hours. Store the specimen at 2° to 8° C and centrifuge before testing.

REAGENTS, SUPPLIES, AND EQUIPMENT

Note: Except for the antigen, all other components should be stored at room temperature in a dry place in the original kit packaging.

1. The following components are provided in Macro-Vue RPR Card Test Kit*
   A. RPR card test antigen. This antigen suspen-sion is similar to VDRL antigen: cardiolipin, lecithin, cholesterol, EDTA, Na_2HPO_4, KH_2PO_4, thimerosal (preservative), charcoal, choline chloride, and distilled water.

   If the ampule of antigen is frozen during shipment, it can be reconstituted once by warming to room temperature. Avoid repeated freezing and thawing.

   Store the antigen suspension in ampules or in the plastic dispensing bottle at 2° to 8° C. Unopened ampules have a shelf life of 12 months from the date of manufacture. Before opening, shake the ampule vigorously for 10 to 15 seconds to resuspend the antigen and dispense any carbon particles that may have become lodged in the neck of the ampule. If any carbon should remain in the neck of the ampule after this shaking, no additional effort should be made to dislodge it as this will only tend to produce a coarse antigen.

   To prepare the antigen, attach the needle to the tapered fitting on the plastic dispensing bottle. Be sure the antigen is below the breakline; snap the ampule neck and withdraw all of the antigen into the dispensing bottle by collapsing the bottle and using it as a suction device. Shake the card antigen dispensing bottle gently before each series of antigen droppings. The needle and dispensing bottle should be discarded when the kit reagents are depleted.

   Once the antigen ampule is opened and placed in the dispensing bottle, it is stable for 3 months or the expiration date on the label (if it occurs sooner) if refrigerated 2° to 8° C. Label dispensing bottle with antigen lot

---

*Hynson, Westcott & Dunning, Division of Becton Dickinson and Co., Baltimore, Md.

number, expiration date, and date antigen is placed in bottle.

Immediate use of refrigerated antigen may result in decreased sensitivity in testing. Allow the antigen to warm to room temperature (23° to 29° C) before use. Do not use beyond expiration date. Avoid bright sunlight.

B. Needle, 18-gauge, without bevel. The needles should deliver 60 ± 2 drops of antigen suspension per milliliter when held in a vertical position. Take care to obtain drops of uniform size. Upon completion of tests, remove needle from dispensing bottle and rinse the needle with distilled or deionized water. Do not wipe needle because this will remove the silicone coating and may affect the accuracy of the drop of antigen being dispensed.

C. Specially prepared, plastic coated cards, each with ten 18 mm circle spots designed for use with RPR card antigen. Take care not to finger-mark the test areas on the card, which may result in an oily deposit and improper test results. Avoid scratching the card when spreading the specimen. If the specimen does not spread to the outer perimeter of the test area, use another test area of the card.

D. Dispenstirs, 0.05 mL/drop.

E. Capillary pipettes, 0.05 mL capacity or the following pipettes: 0.2 mL (graduated in 0.01 mL subdivisions), 0.5 mL (graduated in 0.01 mL subdivisions), or 1.0 mL (graduated in 0.01 mL subdivisions). Dispenstirs are provided with the kit for use with the 18 mm circle qualitative test; however, these stirrers may only be used to transfer a specimen to the card surface. New Dispenstirs or capillary tubes must be used for each specimen. Take care to avoid drawing specimen up into the rubber ball attached to the capillary tube.

F. Rubber bulbs.

G. Stirrers.

2. Rotator (100 rpm) circumscribing a circle 2 cm in diameter on a horizontal plane.

3. Humidifier cover containing a moistened sponge.

4. 0.9% saline (for quantitative test). Prepare by adding 0.9 g of sodium chloride (ACS) to 100 mL of distilled water.

QUALITY CONTROL

A. Controls with established patterns of graded reactivity should be included in each day's testing to confirm optimal reactivity of the antigen suspension. Control sera must be at 23° to 29° C (73° to 85° F) at the time of testing.

Caution: Because the control sera are derived from human sources, they should be handled in the same manner as clinical serum.

Serum that is nonreactive to syphilis in 0.9% saline is required for diluting test specimens producing a reactive result at the 1:16 dilution.

B. A new lot of antigen should be compared with an antigen suspension of known reactivity before being used.

C. The calibration of the delivery needle is an important aspect of quality control. An 18-gauge needle delivers 60 ± 2 drops/mL of reagent. Place the needle on a 2 mL syringe or a 1 mL pipette. Fill the syringe or pipette with the antigen suspension and, holding it in a vertical position, count the number of drops delivered in 0.5 mL. The needle is considered to be satisfactory if 30 ± 1 drop are obtained from 0.5 mL of suspension.

PROCEDURE

Preliminary testing of antigen suspension (see antigen description under *Reagents, supplies, and equipment*).

A. Attach needle hub to tapered fitting on plastic dispensing bottle. Shake antigen ampule to resuspend antigen particles, snap ampule neck at the break line, and withdraw all the RPR card antigen suspension into the dispensing bottle by suction, collapsing the bottle and using it as a bulb. Shake dispenser gently before each series of antigen drops is delivered.

B. Test control sera of graded reactivity each day.

PROCEDURE

1. Place 0.05 mL of unheated serum on an 18 mm circle of the test card with a capillary or serologic pipette. Hold the dispensers in a vertical position directly over the card test area to which the specimen is to be delivered. *Do not touch card surface.*

2. Spread serum in the circle with an inverted Dispenstir (closed end), stirrer (broad end), or serologic pipette to fill the entire circle. Care must be taken not to scratch the card surface.

3. Gently shake antigen dispensing bottle before use. Holding in a vertical position, dispense several drops into the dispensing bottle cap to make sure the needle passage is clear. Add exactly 1 free-falling drop (1/60 mL) of RPR antigen suspension from the 20-gauge (yellow hub) needle to each test area containing serum. Do not stir; mixing is accomplished during rotation.

4. Place card on rotator and cover with humidifier cover. *Note:* The Macro-Vue RPR Card Test (Teardrop Qualitative) Brewer Diagnostic Kit (Hynson, Westcott & Dunning, Div. of Becton Dickinson, Baltimore, Md.) can be hand rocked and used where laboratory equipment is not available.

5. Rotate 8 minutes at 100 rpm (95 to 110 rpm acceptable) on mechanical rotator. If below or above range, there is a tendency for the clumping antigen to be less intense in test with undiluted specimen, so that some minimal reactions may be missed.

6. Observe each specimen *immediately* in the "wet" state under a high-intensity incandescent

lamp or strong daylight. Observation should be without magnification. It is permissible to gently rotate or tilt the card by hand (3 or 4 times) to observe minimally reactive from nonreactive specimens.

7. Specimens producing questionable reactions should be retested by this method and other serologic methods.

8. When testing is completed, the work area should be cleaned. The dispensing needle should be rinsed in distilled water and air-dried. Avoid wiping the needle because this will remove the silicone coating. Recap the antigen solution and store in the refrigerator.

REPORTING RESULTS

Reactive: slight to large agglutination
(black clumps)

Nonreactive: no agglutination, or very slight roughness (even light-gray color)

PROCEDURE NOTES

All reactive tests should be retested using the quantitative procedure to establish a baseline from which changes in titer can be determined, particularly for evaluating treatment. It is desirable to quantitate specimens that are nonreactive-rough so that an infrequent zonal specimen may be revealed.

18 mm Circle Quantitative Card Test

1. For each specimen to be tested, place 0.05 mL of 0.9% saline onto circle numbers 2 to 5 with a capillary or serologic pipette.

2. Pipette 0.05 mL of serum onto circle number 1 and 0.05 ml of serum onto circle number 2.

3. Prepare a serial two-fold dilution by drawing the mixture up and down (avoid formation of bubbles). Transfer 0.05 mL of the dilution to the next circle and repeat procedure to circle number 5. Discard 0.05 mL of the dilution from circle number 5.

4. Beginning with the most dilute specimen (circle number 5), spread the dilution to fill the entire surface of the circle. Use a new stirrer for each circle.

5. Proceed with steps 3 through 8 in the qualitative procedure described above.

REPORTING RESULTS

Report the highest dilution producing a minimal to moderate reaction, i.e., circle 1=1:1 undiluted, circle 2=1:2, circle 3=1:4, circle 4=1:8, and circle 5=1:16. If the 1:16 is reactive, prepare a 1:50 dilution with nonreactive serum in 0.9% saline. This preparation is to be used to prepare subsequent serial dilutions. Pipette 0.05 mL of 1:50 nonreactive serum into each of the circles 2 to 5, pipette 0.05 ml of the 1:16 dilution of test specimen in circle 1, and prepare and test the specimen as described in step 3 above.

SOURCES OF ERROR. Error can be introduced into test results because of factors such as contamination of rubber bulbs or an improperly prepared antigen suspension.

False biologic positive reactions have been reported with cardiolipin-type antigens in the following conditions:

1. Lupus erythematosus
2. Rheumatic fever
3. Vaccinia and viral pneumonia
4. Pneumococcal pneumonia
5. Infectious mononucleosis
6. Infectious hepatitis
7. Leprosy
8. Malaria
9. Rheumatoid arthritis
10. Pregnancy
11. Aging individuals

False-negative reactions can result from poor technique, ineffective reagents, or improper rotation.

If mechanical rotation is below or above the 95 to 110 rpm acceptable range, there is a tendency for the clumping of the antigen to be less intense in procedures with undiluted specimen, so that some minimal reactions may be missed. In quantitative tests, rotation above 110 rpm tends to produce a decrease in titer—approximately one dilution lower.

CLINICAL APPLICATIONS. (see VDRL qualitative procedure)

LIMITATIONS. A diagnosis of syphilis cannot be made based on a single reactive result without clinical signs and symptoms or history. Plasma specimens should not be used to establish a quantitative baseline from which changes in titer can be determined, particularly for evaluating treatment.

RPR cards should not be used for testing cerebrospinal fluid. Little reliance should be place on cord blood serologic testing for syphilis. The RPR procedure has adequate sensitivity and specificity in relation to clinical diagnosis and a reactivity level similar to that of the VDRL slide test.

REFERENCES

Manual of tests for syphilis, Public Health Service Publication, No 411, 1969.

Macro-Vue RPR Card Tests, 18 mm Circle, Brewer Diagnostic Kits Product Insert, BBL Microbiology Systems, Cockeysville, Md.

◻ PROCEDURE

FTA-ABS
(Fluorescent *Treponema pallidum* Antibody Absorption Test)

PRINCIPLE

The Fluorescent *Treponema pallidum* Antibody Absorption test is a direct method of observation. Although not recommended for screening, it is the most sensitive serologic procedure in the detection of primary syphilis.

SPECIMEN COLLECTION AND PREPARATION

No special preparation of the patient is required before specimen collection. The patient must be positively identified when the specimen is collected. The specimen is to be labeled at the bedside and must include the patient's full name, the date the specimen is collected, and the patient's hospital identification number. The phlebotomist's initials should also appear on the label.

Blood should be drawn by an aseptic technique. The required specimen is a minimum of 2 mL of clotted blood (red top evacuated tube). The specimen should be centrifuged and the serum should be removed from the clot. Before testing, the serum should be heated at 56° C for 30 minutes if never inactivated, or for 10 minutes at 56° C if inactivated more than 4 hours before testing. Evidence of hemolysis or bacterial contamination makes the specimen unsuitable for testing.

REAGENTS, SUPPLIES, AND EQUIPMENT

Reagents:

1. *Treponema pallidum antigen.* The antigen for this test is a suspension of *T. pallidum* (Nicols strain) extracted from rabbit testicular tissue, containing a minimum of 30 organisms per high dry field. The antigen may be stored at 6° to 10° C or may be processed by lyophilization. Lyophilized antigen is also stored at 6° to 10° C and is reconstituted for use according to direction when needed. Any antigen that becomes bacterially contaminated or does not give the appropriate reactions with control sera must be discarded.

PREPARATION OF *TREPONEMA PALLIDUM* ANTIGEN SLIDES

A. Mix the antigen suspension with a disposable pipette and rubber bulb, drawing the suspension into and expelling it from the pipette at least 10 times to break the treponemal clumps and to ensure an even distribution of treponemes. Check by darkfield examination for even distribution. Additional mixing may be required.

B. Place one loopful of *T. pallidum* antigen suspension on a glass side with a wire loop. Spread the suspension into a circle about 1 cm in diameter.

C. Allow to air dry for at least 15 minutes.

D. Fix the smears in acetone for 10 minutes, and allow them to air dry. No more than 60 slides should be fixed with each 200 mL of acetone.

E. After the slides are thoroughly dry, the smears should be stored in a freezer at −20° C or lower. Fixed, frozen smears can be used indefinitely, if satisfactory results are achieved with controls. Antigen smears cannot be thawed and refrozen.

2. FTA-ABS test sorbent. This is a standardized product prepared from culture of Reiter treponemes. It may be purchased lyophilized or liquid state, and should be stored according to the manufacturer's directions.

3. Fluorescein-labeled antihuman globulin (conjugate). This should be proven quality for FTA-ABS test. Each new lot of conjugate should be tested to ensure its dependability with respect to working titer, and to verify that it meets the criteria concerning nonspecific staining and standard reactivity. The lyophilized conjugate should be stored at 6° to 10° C. Rehydrated conjugate should be dispensed in not less than 0.3 mL quantities and should be stored at −38° C or lower. For practical purposes, a conjugate with a working titer of 1:400 or higher may be diluted 1:10 with sterile phosphate-buffered saline (containing Merthiolate in a concentration of 1:5000 before storage). When conjugate is thawed for use, it should not be refrozen but should be stored at 6° to 10° C. It may then be used as long as acceptable reactivity is obtained with test controls. If a change in FTA-ABS test reactivity is noted in routine testing, the conjugate should be retitered to determine whether this is the contributing factor.

CONJUGATE

Prepare serial doubling dilutions of the new conjugate in PBS containing 2% Tween-80 to include the titer indicated by the manufacturer. Examples are: (1) 1:2.5, 1:5, 1:10, 1:20, 1:40, 1:80, 1:160; or (2) 1:12.5, 1:25, 1:50, 1:100, 1:200, 1:400, 1:800. Prepare higher dilutions if necessary.

Test each conjugate dilution with the reactive (4+) control serum diluted 1:5 with PBS (follow the procedure below). Include a nonspecific staining control with each conjugate dilution. A standard conjugate, at its titer, is set up at the same time with a reactive (4+) control serum, a minimally reactive (1+) control serum, and a nonspecific staining control with PBS for the purpose of controlling reagents and test conditions. Table 16-2 illustrates the titration of a new conjugate.

Read slides in the following order:

1. Examine the three control slides to ensure that the reagents and testing conditions are satisfactory.

2. Examine the slides with new conjugate, starting with the lowest dilution of conjugate.

3. Record readings as graded reactions from negative to 4+.

The endpoint of the titration is the highest dilution giving maximal (4+) fluorescence. The working titer of the new conjugate is one doubling dilution below the endpoint. In Table 16-2, the dilution selected for the working titer is 1:200. The new conjugate should not stain nonspecifically at three doubling dilutions below the working titer of the conjugate. In Table 16-2 the conjugate would meet this criterion, since there is no nonspecific staining with the 1:25 dilution.

Dispense conjugate in not less than 0.3 mL quan-

TABLE 16-2

New Conjugate Titration

Conjugate	Nonspecific staining control (PRS)	Reactive (4+) control serum (dil. 1:5)	Reactive (1+) control serum
Standard titer			
1:400	Negative	4+	1+
New conjugate titer			
1:12.5	1+	4+	
1:25	Negative	4+	
1:50	Negative	4+	
1:100	Negative	4+	
1:200	Negative	4+	
1:400	Negative	4+	
1:800	Negative	3+	

tities and store at $-20°$ C or lower. For practical purposes, a conjugate with a working titer of 1:400 or higher may be diluted 1:10 with sterile PBS containing thimerosal (Merthiolate in a concentration of 1:5000) before storage in the freezer. Verify the titer of the conjugate after at least 3 days storage in the freezer.

CHECK TESTING

If the criterion of acceptability for the nonspecific staining has been met and a working titer has been determined, the new conjugate should be check-tested in parallel with a standard conjugate before being placed in routine use. Testing should be performed on more than one testing day with control sera, individual sera of graded reactivity, and nonreactive sera. Individual sera tested parallel with a standard and a new conjugate are read against the minimally reactive (1+) controls set up with the respective conjugates. A new conjugate is considered to be satisfactory when comparable test results are obtained with both conjugates.

4. Phosphate-buffered saline (PBS), pH 7.2 ± 0.1. Prepare, per liter of distilled water, 7.65 g NaCl, 0.724 g Na_2HPO_4, 0.21 g KH_2PO_4.
5. 2% Tween-80, pH 7.0 to 7.2. Prepare heat PBS and Tween-80 in 56° C water bath. To 98 mL of PBS, add 2 mL of Tween-80. Refrigerate to store. Discard if precipitate forms or if pH is outside the acceptable range (check pH periodically).
6. Mounting medium, consisting of one PBS, pH 7.2, plus 9 parts glycerin (reagent quality).
7. Acetone (A.C.S.).
8. Pipettes.
9. 12×75 test tubes.
10. 35° to 37° C incubator.
11. Darkfield fluorescent microscope assembly.
12. Bibulous paper.
13. Slide holder.
14. Moist chamber.
15. Loop—bacteriologic, standard 2 mm, 26-gauge platinum wire loop.
16. Oil-immersion, low-fluorescence, nondrying.

TABLE 16-3

Control Pattern Examples

Control	Reaction
Reactive	
1:5 PBS dilution	Reactive (4+)
1:5 Sorbent dilution	Reactive (3+ to 4+)
Minimally reactive (1+)	*Reactive (1+)*
Nonspecific serum	
1:5 PBS dilution	Reactive (2+ to 4+)
1:5 Sorbent dilution	Nonreactive
Nonspecific staining	
Antigen, PBS & conjugate	Nonreactive
Antigen, sorbent & conjugate	Nonreactive

17. Microscope slides—1×3 inch.
18. Cover slips.
19. Dish—stains, glass or plastic with removable slide carriers.
20. Glass stirring rods.

QUALITY CONTROL

Control sera must be run concurrently with each set of patient specimens. Controls should be prepared as follows: Reactive (4+) control. This control should demonstrate 4+ fluorescence when diluted 1:5 in PBS and only slightly reduced fluorescence when diluted 1:5 in sorbent. These controls are prepared as follows:

1. PBS dilution. Pipette 0.2 mL of PBS into a small test tube. Add 0.2 mL of reactive (4+) control serum. Mix.
2. Sorbent dilution. Pipette 0.2 mL of sorbent into a small test tube. Add 0.2 mL of reactive (4+) control serum. Mix.

Minimal (1+) control. Dilutions of reactive serum demonstrating the minimal degree of fluorescence report as reactive for use as a reading standard. The 4+ reactive control may be used for this control when diluted in PBS.

Nonspecific serum control. A nonsyphilis serum known to demonstrate at least 2+ nonspecific reactivity in the FTA test at a dilution of PBS of 1:5 or higher should be used. Prepare as follows:

1. PBS dilution. Pipette 0.2 mL of PBS into a small test tube. Add 0.05 mL of nonspecific control serum. Mix.
2. Sorbent dilution. Pipette 0.2 mL of sorbent into a small test tube. Add 0.05 mL of nonspecific control serum. Mix.

NONSPECIFIC STAINING CONTROLS

A. Antigen smear treated with 0.03 mL of PBS.
B. Antigen smear treated with 0.03 mL of sorbent.

Controls 1, 3, and 4 are included for the purpose of controlling reagents and test conditions. Control 2 (minimally reactive control serum) is included as the reading standard.

Each new lot of reagents should be tested in parallel with reagents giving satisfactory results before being used.

TREPONEMA PALLIDUM ANTIGEN

A new lot of antigen should be compared with a standard antigen before being placed in routine use. Testing should be performed on more than one testing day with control sera, individual sera of graded reactivity, and nonreactive sera.

A sufficient number of organisms should remain on the slide after staining so that tests may be read without difficulty. The antigen should not contain background material that stains so as to interfere with the reading of the tests. The antigen should not stain nonspecifically with a standard conjugate at its working titer. Reportable test results on controls and individual sera should be comparable with those obtained with the standard antigen.

FTA-ABS TEST SORBENT

A new lot of sorbent should be compared with a standard sorbent before being placed in routine use. Testing should be performed on more than one testing day with control sera, including sera of graded reactivity, and nonsyphilitic sera demonstrating nonspecific reactivity. The new sorbent should remove nonspecific reactivity of the nonspecific serum control. The new sorbent should not reduce the intensity of fluorescence of the reactive (4+) control serum to less than 3+. The nonspecific staining control with the new sorbent should be nonreactive. Reportable test results on controls and individual sera should be with those obtained with standard sorbent. The sorbent should be usable when rehydrated to the indicated volume on the label or according to accompanying direction.

FLUORESCEIN-LABELED ANTIHUMAN GLOBULIN (CONJUGATE)

A satisfactory conjugate should not stain a standard antigen nonspecifically at three doubling dilutions below the working titer of the conjugate.

Reportable test results on controls and individual sera should be comparable with those obtained with the standard conjugate. Most manufacturers designate on the label the working titer of the conjugate that was determined under the testing conditions and with the equipment in their laboratories. Since conditions and equipment vary from one laboratory to another, it is necessary to titer and to check-test a new lot of conjugate with a fluorescence microscope.

PROCEDURE

1. Label test tubes for patient and control sera.
2. Pipette 0.2 mL into each tube.
3. Using a 0.2 mL pipette, add 0.05 mL of inactivated sera to the appropriately labeled test tubes. Mix 8 times.
4. Label a previously prepared antigen suspension slide for each of the patient sera and controls being tested.
5. Cover each antigen preparation with 0.03 mL of a serum dilution, i.e., patient or control.
6. Cover an antigen suspension slide with either 0.03 mL of PBS or sorbent. These are the nonspecific staining controls.
7. Place a moist chamber of the slides to prevent evaporation, and incubate at 35° to 37° C for 30 minutes.
8. Fill two staining dishes with PBS.
9. Place slides in a slide carrier and rinse slides with running PBS for approximately 5 seconds.
10. Place the slides in the staining dish containing PBS solution. Process for 5 minutes. After 5 minutes, dip the slides in and out of the solution at least 10 times.
11. Transfer the slide carrier to the fresh PBS solution in the second staining dish. Process for 5 minutes. After 5 minutes, dip the slides in and out of the solution at least 10 times.
12. Rinse the slides in running distilled water for 5 seconds.
13. Gently blot each smear with bibulous paper to remove all water droplets.
14. Dilute conjugate to its working titer in PBS containing 2% Tween-80.
15. Pipette 0.03 mL of diluted conjugate onto each smear. Spread the conjugate uniformly over the slide with a glass rod.
16. Repeat steps 7 through 13.
17. Mount slides immediately by placing a small drop of mounting medium on each smear and apply a coverslip to each.
18. Microscopically examine slides as soon as possible. The microscope should be equipped with an ultraviolet light source and a high-power dry objective. A combination of BG 12 exciting filter, not more than 3 mm in thickness, and OG 1 barrier filter or equivalent has been found to

be satisfactory. If a delay in reading is encountered, place the slides in a darkened room and read within 4 hours.

19. Using the minimally reactive (1+) control slide as the reading standard, record the intensity of fluorescence of the treponemes.

RECORDING OF FLUORESCENCE

Reading	Fluorescence intensity	Report
0	None or vaguely visible	Nonreactive
<1+	Weak reacting	Borderline*
1+	Equivalent to 1+ control	Reactive*
2+ to 4+	Moderate to strong	Reactive

*A new specimen from these patients should be retested. If repeat testing produces a 1+ or greater reaction, the test is considered to be reactive. If the repeat test continues to be weaker than 1+, it is considered to be a borderline reaction.

20. Check nonreactive smears by using illumination from a tungsten light source to verify the presence of treponemes.

REPORTING RESULTS

REPORTING PROTOCOL

Reading	Repeat Test	Report
0		Nonreactive
<1+	Negative, <1+, or 1+	Borderline
1+	Negative, <1+	Borderline
1+	1+ or greater	Reactive
2+ to 4+		Reactive

CLINICAL APPLICATIONS. If a patient has two borderline tests results, it is impossible to definitively conclude that the patient has or does not have serologic evidence of syphilitic infection. The attending physician should review the patient's history and physical findings. Diagnosis will rely on the clinical evidence in conjunction with the borderline serologic findings.

The false-positive rate of this test is very low but it can be associated with autoimmune disorders, such as systemic lupus erythematosus (SLE). False-positive FTA-ABS results occur in patients suffering from other treponematoses, such as pinta, yaws, or bejel, or in those who have high titer of antinuclear antibodies (ANA) or rheumatoid factor. There is evidence that pregnant women occasionally have false-positive FTA-ABS test results.

LIMITATIONS. This test is recommended as a confirmatory procedure for syphilis. Its use is discouraged as a screening test. Screening with a reagin test such as the VDRL and RPR is recommended for screening.

REFERENCES

Hunter EF, Deacon WE, and Meyer PC: An improved test for syphilis—the absorption procedure (FTA-ABS), Public Health Rep 79:5, 1964.

Jaffe HW, et al: Tests for treponemal antibody in CSF, Arch Intern Med 138:252, 1978.

Leclerc G et al: Study of fluorescent treponemal antibody test on cerebrospinal fluid using monospecific anti-immunoglobulin conjugates IgG, IgM, and IgA, Br J Vener Dis 54:303, 1978.

Chapter Review

HIGHLIGHTS

Syphilis is caused by a spirochete, *Treponema pallidum*. In 1906, the first diagnostic blood procedure, the Wasserman test, was developed to detect this disease. The genus *Treponema* contains four principal species: *T. pallidum* (syphilis in humans), *T. pertenue* (yaws), *T. careteum* (pinta), and *T. cuniculi* (syphilis in rabbits). Outside of the host, *T. pallidum* is extremely susceptible to various physical and chemical agents.

Syphilis in humans is ordinarily transmitted by sexual contact. In males, the micro-organism is transmitted from lesions on the penis or discharged from deeper sites with semen. Lesions in females are commonly located in the perineal region or on the labia, vaginal wall, or cervix. In a small percentage of cases, the primary infection is extragenital and is usually in or around the mouth.

Untreated syphilis is a chronic disease with subacute symptomatic periods separated by asymptomatic intervals, during which the diagnosis can be made serologically. The progression of untreated syphilis is generally divided into stages from the time of contact and initial infection. Primary syphilis is characterized by the presence of chancre, which persists for 1 to 5 weeks and heals spontaneously. During this stage, the serum in about one third of cases becomes serologically reactive after 1 week and becomes serologically demonstrable in the majority of cases after 3 weeks. The reagin titer increases rapidly during the first 4 weeks and then remains stationary for approximately 6 months.

Within 2 to 8 weeks after the appearance of the primary chancre, a patient enters the stage of secondary syphilis. This stage is usually characterized by a generalized illness that is suggestive of a viral infection. The majority of patients manifest skin lesions that contain a large number of spirochetes and are highly contagious if located on exposed surfaces. These lesions subside spontaneously after 2 to 6 weeks even if untreated. In this noninfectious latent stage, serologic tests for syphilis are positive. Relapses, however, with manifestations of secondary syphilis occur in about one fourth of patients during the first 2 to 4 years of infection.

The late (tertiary) stage is usually seen from 3 to 10 years after primary infection. Destructive lesions called gummas, can appear in about 15% of untreated syphilitic persons who eventually develop late benign syphilis. Complications of this stage of the disease can include lesions of the nervous system causing tabes dorsalis or cardiovascular complications. Meningovascular syphilis can manifest itself as seizures or as a cerebrovascular accident. In about one fourth of untreated cases, the tertiary stage is asymptomatic and recognized only by serologic testing. Occasionally, the lesions heal so completely that even serologic tests become nonreactive.

Classic serologic tests for syphilis measure the presence of two types of antibodies: treponemal and nontreponemal. Treponemal antibodies are produced against the antigens of the organisms themselves. Nontreponemal antibodies, often called reagin antibodies, are produced by an infected patient against components of their own or other mammalian bodies. Darkfield microscopy is the test of choice for symptomatic patients with primary syphilis. The two most widely used nontreponemal serologic tests are the VDRL and the RPR methods. Both of these procedures are flocculation methods in which soluble antigen particles are coalesced to form larger particles visible as clumps when they are agglutinated by antibody. Specific treponemal serologic tests include the FTA-ABS (fluorescent treponemal antibody absorption) test and the MHA (microhemagglutination) test. The TPI *(Treponema pallidum* immobilization) test, yet another procedure, is obsolete.

REVIEW QUESTIONS

Questions 1-4.
Match the following *Treponema* associated diseases in humans with their respective causative organism:
1. *T. pallidum*
2. *T. pallidum* (variant)
3. *T. pertenue*
4. *T. carateum*
   A. Yaws
   B. Syphilis
   C. Pinta
   D. Bejel
Questions 5-8.
Match the following stages of syphilis with the appropriate signs and symptoms:
5. Primary syphilis
6. Secondary syphilis
7. Latent syphilis
8. Late (tertiary) syphilis
   A. Diagnosis only by serologic methods
   B. Presence of gummas
   C. Development of a chancre
   D. Hutchinsonian triad
   E. Generalized illness followed by macular lesions in most patients
9. A term for nontreponenal antibodies produced by an infected patient against components of their own or other mammalian cells is:
   A. Autoagglutinins
   B. Reagin antibodies
   C. Alloantibodies
   D. Nonsyphilitic antibodies
   E. Either A or D

Questions 10-13.
Match the following.
10. VDRL
11. FTA-ABS
12. MHA-TP
13. RPR
    A. Treponemal method
    B. Nontreponemal method
14. All of the following are possible causes of a false-negative VDRL reaction except:
    A. Inhibitors in patient sera
    B. Hemolyzed serum specimen
    C. Prozone reaction
    D. Low antibody titer
    E. Technical error
15. In the RPR procedure, a false-positive reaction can result from all of the following except:
    A. Infectious mononucleosis
    B. Leprosy
    C. Rheumatoid arthritis
    D. Streptococcal pharyngitis
    E. Pregnancy

Answers

1. B 2. D 3. A 4. C 5. C 6. E 7. A 8. B 9. B 10. B
11. A 12. A 13. B 14. B 15. D

BIBLIOGRAPHY

Baron EJ and Finegold SM: Bailey and Scott's Diagnostic microbiology, ed 8, St Louis, 1990, The CV Mosby Co.
Boyd RF and Hoerl BG: Basic medical microbiology, ed 3, Boston, 1986, Little, Brown & Co Inc.
Brown ST et al: Serologic response to syphilis treatment: a new analysis of old data, JAMA 253:1296-1299, 1985.
Cerny EH: Adenovirus ELISA for the evaluation of cerebrospinal fluid in patients with suspected neurosyphilis, Am J Clin Path 84:505-508, 1985.
Farshy CE: Four-step enzyme-linked immunosorbent assay for the detection of *Treponema pallidum* antibody, J Clin Microbiol 21:387-389, 1985.
Gardner MF and Clark ME: The *Treponema pallidum* hemagglutination (TPHA) test, WHO/VDT/ReS 75:332, 1975.
Hart G: Syphilis testing in diagnostic and therapeutic decision making, Ann Intern Med 104:368-376, 1986.
Hunter EF, Deacon WE and Meyer PC: An improved test for syphilis—the absorption procedure (FTA-ABS), Public Health Rep 79:5, 1964.
Izzat NN et al: Validity of the VDRL test on cerebrospinal fluid contaminated by blood, Br J Vener Dis 47:162-164, 1971.
Larson SA et al: Cerebrospinal fluid serologies in syphilis: treponemal and nontreponemal test, Internation Conjoint S T D Meeting, 1984. Abstract 166:218, Montreal, Canada.
Mandell GL, Douglas RG, and Bennett JE, eds: Principles and practice of infectious diseases, ed 2, New York, 1985, John Wiley & Sons.
Muller F: Specific immunoglobulins M and G antibodies in the rapid diagnosis of human treponemal infections, Diagn Immunol 4:1-9, 1986.
Muller F and Moskophidis J: Estimation of the local production of antibodies to *Treponema pallidum* in the central nervous system of patients with neurosyphilis, Br J Vener Dis 59:80-84, 1983.
Radolf JD et al: Serodiagnosis of syphilis by enzyme-linked immunosorbent assay with purified recombinant *Treponema pallidum* antigen 4D, J Infect Dis 153:1023-1027, 1986.
Rein MF: Infection caused by Treponema (syphilis, yaws, pinta, bejel). In Stein J, editor: Internal medicine, ed 2, Boston, 1987, Little, Brown & Co, Inc.

Cytomegalovirus

ETIOLOGY

Cytomegalovirus (CMV) is a ubiquitous human viral pathogen. The first descriptive report of histologic changes characteristic of the changes now associated with CMV infection was originally published in 1904 when protozoan-like cells in the lungs, kidneys, and liver of a syphilitic fetus were seen. It was not until 1956 and 1957, however, that the CMV was isolated in the laboratory (Fig. 17-1). In 1966, the actual isolation of the virus following transfusion, as well as the observation of elevated antibody titers, was noted.

Human cytomegalovirus is classified as a member of the herpes family of viruses. There are presently five recognized human herpes viruses: herpes simplex I, herpes simplex II, varicella-zoster virus, Epstein-Barr virus, and cytomegalovirus. All of the herpes viruses are relatively large, enveloped DNA viruses that undergo a replicative cycle involving DNA expression and nucleocapsid assembly within the nucleus. The viral structure gains an envelope when the virus buds through the nuclear membrane that is altered to contain specific viral proteins.

Although the herpes family produces diverse clinical diseases, the viruses share the basic characteristics of being cell associated. The requirements for cell association vary, but all five herpes family viruses may spread from cell to cell, presumably via intercellular bridges and in the presence of antibody in the extracellular phase. This common characteristic may play a role in the ability of these viruses to produce subclinical infections that can be reactivated under appropriate stimuli.

EPIDEMIOLOGY

Cytomegalovirus infection is endemic worldwide. Dissemination of the virus may be by oral, respiratory, or venereal routes. It may also be transmitted parenterally by organ transplantation or via the transfusion of fresh blood. Transmission of CMV appears to require intimate contact with secretions or excretions (primarily urine, respiratory, and genital secretions, tears, and feces of infected persons. The most likely mode of acquisition is via a venereal route through contact with infectious virus in body secretions.

The virus can be present in blood, urine, and breast milk. It has been recognized for more than 15 years that transfusion of blood from healthy asymptomatic blood donors is occasionally followed by active CMV infection in the recipient. There is strong evidence to incriminate peripheral blood leukocytes and transplanted tissues as sources of CMV.

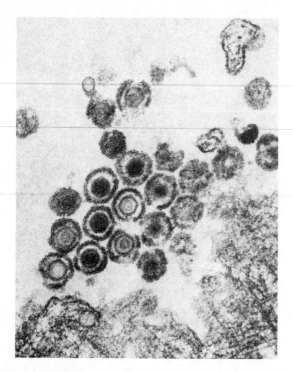

FIGURE 17-1

A group of negatively stained CMV particles propagated in human lung fibroblasts. The typical hexagonal capsid (actually icosahedral in three dimensions) of a herpesvirus can be seen, surrounded by a tegument and double-layered envelope. (× 155.000; Courtesy Janet D. Smith, Ph.D.; from Krugman S, et al: Infectious diseases of children, ed 8, St. Louis, 1985, The CV Mosby Co.)

Acquired Infection

Although fatal infections have been reported in children with leukemia and premature infants of less than 1200 g birth weight, the incidence of primary infections during childhood is low. The rate of exposure to the virus, however, may be accelerated during the first years of life in toddlers and children in daycare centers. During adolescence the infection rate rises significantly. By adulthood, most individuals have experienced asymptomatic contact with CMV. Because CMV can persist latently, active infections may develop under a variety of conditions, such as pregnancy or immunosuppression, or subsequent to organ or bone marrow transplantation. Active CMV infection is a major cause of morbidity and often mortality in patients with acquired immunodeficiency syndrome (AIDS).

Of patients who are immunosuppressed, only seronegative patients appear to be at a significant risk of developing CMV infection. Patients at the highest risk of mortality from cytomegalovirus infections are allograft transplant seronegative patients who receive tissue from a seropositive donor. The great majority of infections in allograft recipients are transmitted by the donor kidney or arise from the reactivation of the recipient's latent virus.

Transmission of CMV by transfusion of blood or blood components containing white cells is assuming increased importance in patients with severely impaired immunity who require supportive therapy. Low birth weight neonates are also at high risk to CMV infection through transfusion of CMV-infected blood products. In these patients, effective donor screening, leukocyte-depleted blood products, and immune globulin containing passively acquired cytomegalovirus antibodies are all methods of prevention.

Healthcare professionals are one of the groups becoming increasingly concerned about the risks associated with exposure to CMV. Nosocomial transmission from patients to health care workers has not been documented, but observance of good personal hygiene and handwashing offer the best measures for preventing transmission.

Latent Infection

Persistent infections characterized by periods of reactivation are frequently termed *latent* infections, although this condition has not been clearly defined for CMV. True viral latency is defined by the presence of the genetic information in an unexpressed state in the host cell. An operational definition of latency can include the conditions of a dynamic relationship between the virus and the host, along with evidence of latency and reactivation of a latent infection.

Evidence that CMV produces latent infections in humans is circumstantial and indirect. The mechanism of latency and identity of the host cells that harbor the latent virus remain undocumented. Leukocytes from the peripheral blood of patients with active CMV infections have been cultured with the subsequent recovery of cytomegalovirus; but attempts to recover the virus from the leukocytes of healthy donors has remained unsuccessful, with the exception of one report. In animal models, the virus is present and recoverable from neutrophilic leukocytes in active infections, but it is also believed that splenic B lymphocytes, and possibly monocytes, may harbor latent infections. Additionally, salivary gland, heart, and prostate tissue may be sites of latent infections. The types of cells and the mechanism of latency remain to be demonstrated in humans. The estimated CMV carrier rate among blood donors, which is defined as the number of seroconversions (patients changing from being negative for antibodies to the virus to demonstrating antibodies) per 100 units of blood transfused, ranges from 1% to 12%.

Congenital Infection

CMV is one of the most important causes of congenital viral infections in the United States. Primary as well as recurrent maternal CMV infection can be transmitted in utero. CMV is recognized as the cause of congenital viral infection in 0.5% to 2.4% of all live births. The majority of CMV-infected newborns are asymptomatic, but 1% manifest damage caused by CMV. Infected infants can

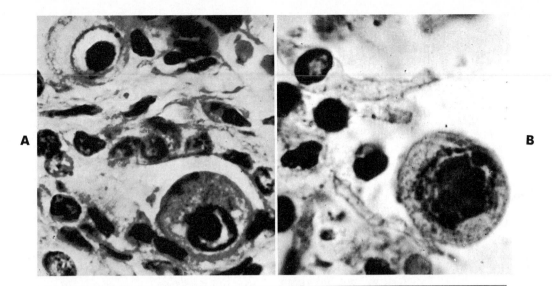

FIGURE 17-2
Cytomegalovirus infection of kidney. **A,** Section showing two huge nuclear inclusions in tubular epithelium. **B,** Diagnostic cell in hematoxylin and eosin-stained urinary sediment (lower right). Compare with normal-appearing tubular epithelial cell (upper left).
(From Kissane JM: Anderson's Pathology, ed 9, St. Louis, 1990, The CV Mosby Co.)

become severely ill, and death may result in premature infants.

SIGNS AND SYMPTOMS
Acquired Infection
Acquired CMV infection is usually asymptomatic and can persist in the host as a chronic or latent infection. In the majority of patients, CMV infection is asymptomatic. Occasionally a self-limited, heterophile-negative, mononucleosis-like syndrome results. The symptoms include a sore throat and fever, chills, profound malaise, and myalgia. Lymphadenopathy and splenomegaly may be observed. Infections occurring in healthy immunocompetent individuals usually result in seroconversion. Virus may be excreted in the urine during both primary and recurrent CMV infection (Fig. 17-2); it can persist sporadically for months or years. Persons experiencing acquired infection, reinfection with the same or different strains of CMV, or reactivation of a latent infection can excrete the virus in titers as high as 10^6 infective units/mL in the urine and/or saliva for weeks or months.

Normal adults and children usually experience CMV infection without serious complications. Infrequent complications of CMV infection in previously healthy individuals, however, include interstitial pneumonitis, hepatitis, Guillian-Barre syndrome, meningoencephalitis, myocarditis, thrombocytopenia, and hemolytic anemia.

CMV infection, however, can be life-threatening in immunosuppressed patients. Infections in these patients may result in disseminated multisystem involvement including pneumonitis, hepatitis, gastrointestinal ulceration, arthralgias, meningoencephalitis, and retinitis. Interstitial pneumonitis, frequently associated with CMV infection, is a major cause of death following allogeneic bone marrow transplantation. In premature infants, acquired CMV infection can result in atypical lymphocytosis, hepatosplenomegaly, pneumonia, or death.

Transfusion-acquired cytomegalovirus infections may cause not only mononucleosis-like syndrome but hepatitis and an increase in rejection of transplanted organs, as well. Three types of CMV infections are possible in blood transfusion recipients:
1. Primary infection occurs when a previously unexposed (seronegative) recipient is transfused with blood from a actively or latently infected donor. This type of infection is accompanied by the presence of virus in the blood and urine, an immediate antibody response, and eventual seroconversion. Primary infections may be symptomatic, but the great majority are not.
2. Reactivated infections can be manifested when a seropositive recipient is transfused with blood from either a CMV antibody-positive or negative donor. Donor leukocytes are thought to trigger an allograft reaction, which in turn reactivates the recipient's latent infection. Such infections may be accompanied by significant increases in CMV-specific antibody. Some reactivated infections exhibit viral shedding as their only manifestation. Reactivated infections are largely asymptomatic.
3. Reinfection by a strain of cytomegalovirus in the donor's blood that is different from the one originally infecting the recipient can occur. A significant antibody response is observed in this situation and viral shedding occurs. Although it is

difficult to differentiate a reactivated infection if both the patient and the donor are CMV antibody positive before transfusion, reinfections can be documented if isolates can be obtained from both donor and recipient.

Congenital Infection

The classic congenital CMV syndrome is manifested by a high incidence of neurologic symptoms as well as neuromuscular disorders, jaundice, hepatomegaly, and splenomegaly. Congenitally infected newborns, especially those who acquire CMV during a maternal primary infection, are more prone to develop severe *cytomegalic inclusion disease* (CID). The severe form of CID may be fatal or can cause permanent neurologic sequelae, such as mental retardation, deafness, vision defects, microcephaly, and motor dysfunction. Psychomotor retardation is seen in 51% to 75% of survivors. Hearing loss is observed in 21% to 50% of cases, and visual impairment in 20% of cases. Infants without symptoms at births may develop hearing impairment and neurologic impairment at a later date.

IMMUNOLOGIC MANIFESTATIONS
Alterations in the Immune System

CMV infection is known to alter the immune system as well as to produce overt manifestations of infection. Infection interferes with immune responsiveness in both normal and immunocompromised individuals. This diminished responsiveness results in a decreased proliferative response to the CMV antigen, which persists for several months. In patients with CMV mononucleosis-like syndrome, alterations of T lymphocyte subsets result, producing an increase in the absolute number of suppressor (OKT8) lymphocytes, and a decrease in helper (OKT4) lymphocytes. These subset abnormalities persist for months.

Questions have been raised regarding CMV as a potentially oncogenic virus because viral antigens and/or nucleic acid have been found in human malignancies, which include adenocarcinoma of the colon, carcinoma of the cervix, cancer of the prostate, and Kaposi's sarcoma. CMV does have transforming properties in vitro. Although considerable circumstantial evidence exists linking cytomegalovirus to human malignancies (especially Kaposi's sarcoma), a direct cause-and-effect relationship has not been established.

Serologic Markers

In cells infected by CMV, several antigens appear at varying times following infection. Before replication of viral DNA takes place, immediate-early antigens and early antigens are present in the nuclei of infected cells. Immediate-early antigens appear within 1 hour of cellular infection, and early antigens are present within 24 hours. At about 72 hours after infection, or the end of the viral replication cycle, late antigens are demonstrable in the nucleus and cytoplasm of infected cells.

The immune antibody response to these various antigens differs in incidence and significance. The presence of antibodies against immediate-early and early antigens is associated with active infection of either a primary or reactivated nature.

Antibody to early antigen undergoes a relatively rapid decline after recovery but can persist for up to 250 days, and it may identify patients with recent as well as active infections. The presence of antibody to early antigen is strongly associated with viral shedding. Antibodies to late antigens persist in high titer long after the recovery from an active infection.

The incidence of viral exposure and subsequent antibody formation (seropositivity) varies greatly depending on the socioeconomic status and living conditions of the population surveyed. The prevalence of CMV antibody varies with age and geographic location but ranges from 40% to 100%.

The incidence of antibodies against CM-induced immediate-early antigens, early antigens, and late antigens was studied in a population of healthy blood donors. Antibodies to immediate-early antigens were found in 9.6%, antibodies to early antigens in 10.2%, and antibodies to late antigens in 76% of the donors. The incidence of antibodies to CMV-induced immediate-early and early antigens increased with age and was higher in females than males. In another study, 51% of donors were seronegative for CMV antibodies. The highest percentage of seronegative findings (60%) was among donors who were 18 to 35 years old. This age group represented 57% of the donors. If viremic donors are a source of transfusion-acquired CMV in high-risk patients, then screening blood for early antigen antibodies is warranted.

The characteristic antibody responses associated with infection are:
1. Primary infection, demonstrated by a transient virus-specific IgM antibody response and eventual seroconversion to produce IgG antibodies to the virus.
2. Reactivation of latent infection in seropositive (IgG) individuals, which may be accompanied by significant increases in IgG antibodies to the virus but which elicit no detectable IgM response.
3. Reinfection by a strain of CMV that is different than the original infecting strain. A significant IgG antibody response is demonstrated. Whether an IgM response occurs is unknown.

DIAGNOSTIC EVALUATION

In cytomegalovirus infection, hematologic examination of the blood usually reveals a characteristic leukocytosis. A slight lymphocytosis with over 20% variant lymphocytes is common. Clinical chemistry assays may demonstrate abnormal liver function tests. Another assessment of the presence of infection is the demonstration of inclusion bodies in leukocytes in urinary sediment.

A definitive diagnosis, however, can only be made by isolating the cytomegalovirus from urine

TABLE 17-1

Methods of Testing for Cytomegalovirus

Method	Constituent Tested
Complement fixation	Antibody
Latex particle agglutination	Antibody
Anticomplement immunofluorescence	IgG antibody
Indirect fluorescent antibody	IgM antibody
Enzyme immunoassay	IgG and IgM antibody
Direct electron microscopy	Antigen
Enzyme immunoassay	Antigen
Nucleic acid probe	Cytomegalovirus mRNA
In situ hybridization	cDNA probe

or blood samples or by the demonstration of CMV-specific IgM or increasing CMV-specific IgG antibody titers (Table 17-1). Methods for measuring CMV IgM antibodies include indirect immunofluorescence, radioimmunoassay, or indirect and reverse ELISA tests. Virus detection in urine by electron microscopy is reliable if positive, but a negative result does not rule out CMV infection. Human CMV is indistinguishable by negative staining electron-microscopy from its close relatives, herpes simplex and varicella, which is the cause of chickenpox. Viral culture is the method of choice for confirming CMV infection. Early detection of CMV in viral cultures is done routinely by direct fluorescent antibody (DFA) examination, and demonstration of CMV in bronchoalveolar lavage specimens by DFA examination is possible. More rapid methods, however, are needed.

Serologic methods to detect the presence of IgM antibodies can aid in the diagnosis of primary infection. Detection of CMV-specific IgM can represent primary infection or rare reactivation of infection. False-positive results, however, can occur because of the presence of other antibodies such as rheumatoid factor. Although tests for heterophil, Epstein-Barr virus and *Toxoplasma* antibodies are generally negative, elevated concentrations (titers) of several antibodies may occur. These include antinuclear antibody (ANA), rheumatoid factor (RA) antibodies, and nonspecific cold agglutinins. The inability to demonstrate IgM in a blood specimen can result from the presence of a large amount of virus-specific IgG. Lack of a CMV-specific IgM response is especially common in congenital infections, of which 50% are CMV−IgM negative by IFA (up to 89% positive by RIA and 69% positive by EIA) even in the presence of virus excretion in the urine.

Detection of significant increases in CMV-specific IgG antibody by methods such as complement fixation (CF), anticomplement immunofluorescence (ACIF), and enzyme immunoassay (EIA)

suggest, but do not prove recent infection or reactivation of latent infection. The EIA method for IgM and IgG antibodies to CMV has replaced CF, ACIF, and immunofluorescent antibody (IFA). Latex particle agglutination and indirect hemagglutination are useful screening methods to obtain seronegative donors.

Newer CMV detection methods are being explored. CMV antigen detection in urine by EIA and cDNA is being developed. RNA transcript of CMV DNA is detectable in peripheral blood mononuclear cells of seropositive individuals by *in situ hybridization* (ISH) with cDNA of CMV. The ISH technique, which is more sensitive than dot-blot hybridization (Northern blot), promises to be a new early detection method for CMV expression.

☐ PROCEDURE

Passive Latex Agglutination for Detection of Antibodies to Cytomegalovirus in Human Serum

PRINCIPLE

In this procedure, latex particles that have been previously sensitized with cytomegalovirus (CMV) viral antigen are mixed with serum. If antibody to CMV is present, the agglutinated particles will be macroscopically visible. In the absence of specific antibody or in the event of low antibody concentration, the latex particles will not agglutinate in the reaction mixture and the particles will appear smooth and evenly dispersed. The absence of CMV antibodies suggests that a person has not been exposed to this virus. The presence of CMV antibodies, however, is indicative of previous exposure to the virus. Although recurrent infection is possible, it may not be as severe as in primary infection. Because CMV is a blood-borne pathogen, infection with this virus is of greatest concern to newborn infants in need of transfusion and to immunosuppressed allograft recipients.

SPECIMEN COLLECTION AND PREPARATION

No special preparation of the patient is required before specimen collection. The patient must be positively identified when the specimen is collected and the specimen is to be labeled at the bedside. Specimen labels must include the patient's full name, the date the specimen is collected, the patient's hospital identification number, and the phlebotomist's initials.

Blood should be drawn by an aseptic technique. A minimum of 2 mL of clotted blood (red top evacuated tube) or anticoagulated blood (lavender top evacuated tube) is required. The specimen should be centrifuged promptly and an aliquot of serum or plasma removed. Plasma specimens containing EDTA or heparin as an anticoagulant can be used for qualitative or quantitative testing using the same technique as for serum samples. Plasma specimens containing CPDA-1 as an anticoagulant can also be used for qualitative or quantitative testing after a 1% dilution is made with the buffer.

Serum or plasma specimens may be stored for up to 1 week at 2° to 8° C or frozen at −18° C or lower, if longer storage is required. Serum specimens with obvious microbial contamination should not be used for testing. The presence of mild lipimea or hemolysis will not affect the test.

Testing of CPDA-1 plasma specimens from platelet units stored at 22° C for 5 days and from red cell units prepared for transfusion stored at 2° to 6° C for 14 days has been successful.

REAGENTS, SUPPLIES, AND EQUIPMENT

The following reagents and equipment are supplied with the CMV Scan Kit (Becton Dickinson):
1. Kit components
   A. Latex antigen. CMV antigen-coated latex particles prepared from disrupted CMV that has been judged to be inactivated by bioassay procedures. This preparation contains 0.02% gentamicin and 0.02% sodium azide. Refrigerate at 2° to 8° C to store and return to refrigerator when not in use. Do not freeze and do not use beyond expiration date on the label.
   B. Dilution buffer. Phosphate buffered saline solution, pH 7.4, containing bovine serum albumin with 0.02% sodium azide. Refrigerate at 2° to 8° C to store and return to refrigerator when not in use. Do not freeze and do not use beyond expiration date on the label.
   C. Test cards. These cards must be flat for proper reactions. If necessary, flatten cards by bowing back in a direction opposite to that of the curl. Care should be taken not to finger-mark the test areas, since this may result in an oily deposit and improper test results. Use each card once and discard. Store the cards in their original packaging in a dry area at room temperature.
   D. Plastic stirrers.
   E. Dispensing needle, 21 gauge, green hub. Upon completion of daily tests, remove the needle from the dispensing bottle and recap the bottle. Rinse the needle with distilled water to maintain a clear passage and accurate drop delivery. Do not wipe the dispensing needle because it is silicone coated and wiping can remove the silicone.

ADDITIONAL REQUIRED EQUIPMENT AND SUPPLIES:
1. Centrifuge.
2. Rotator with humidifying cover. The recommended rotation speed is 100 rpm, but rotation between 95 and 110 rpm does not significantly affect the results obtained. The rotator should circumscribe a circle approximately 2 cm in diameter in the horizontal plane. A moistened humidifier cover must be used to prevent drying of test specimens during rotation.
3. High-intensity incandescent lamp.
4. Micropipettors, 25 μL delivery.
5. Vortex mixer.
6. General equipment necessary for preparation, storage, and handling of serologic specimens.

QUALITY CONTROL

High reactive control serum (human serum) with 0.1% sodium azide. This control should demonstrate agglutination when tested.

Low reactive control serum (human serum) with 0.1% sodium azide. This control should demonstrate agglutination when tested.

Nonreactive control serum (human serum) with 0.1% sodium azide. This control should demonstrate no agglutination when tested.

NOTE: If controls do not produce appropriate reactions, the test results are invalid (see procedure notes).

CAUTION: Because the control serum is derived from human sources, it should be handled in the same manner as clinical serum specimens (see *Universal blood and body fluid precautions* in Chapter 6).

WARNING: The latex reagent, controls, and buffer contain sodium azide as a preservative. Sodium azide may react with lead and copper plumbing to form highly explosive metal azides. Upon disposal, flush with a large volume of water to prevent azide buildup. Sodium azide is toxic if inhaled.

PROCEDURE

PRELIMINARY PREPARATION
1. Allow the reagents to come to room temperature before testing.
   NOTE: Do not mix reagents from different kit lot numbers, and avoid microbial contamination of reagents.
2. The latex reagent should be mixed for 5 to 10 seconds (use the highest speed setting for variable speed mixers). Vortexing is necessary at the beginning of each batch of specimens even if more than one batch is tested per day.
3. Remove the cap from the latex reagent and attach the green hub needle to the tapered fitting.
4. Label each circle of the card with the appropriate identification of patient sera and controls.

PROCEDURE

1. (*Qualitative method*) Using a micropipettor, place 25 μL of each specimen (patient, high reactive control, and negative reactive control) on the appropriately labeled, separate circles, using a new tip each time.

OPTIONAL: QUANTITATIVE METHOD

a. Using a micropipettor, place 25 μL of the negative control onto circle number 1 in the row marked *nonreactive control.* This control requires no dilution.

b. Move to a new row. With a micropipettor, place 25 μL of dilution buffer in circle numbers 2 through 7. Leave circle number 1 empty.

c. Pipette 25 μL of high reactive control onto circle number 1.

d. Using the same micropipettor and tip, add an additional 25 μL of high reactive control directly into the buffer in circle number 2. Mix the serum and buffer by drawing the constituents up and down with the micropipettor 7 times. The serum in this circle (circle number 2) is now a 1:2 dilution.

e. Using the same micropipettor and tip, transfer 25 μL of the 1:2 dilution directly into the buffer in circle number 3. Mix as in step d. Continue this method of preparing serial twofold dilutions to circle number 7.

f. Withdraw 25 μL of serum-buffer dilution from circle number 7 and discard. The dilution in circle number 7 is now 1:64.

   NOTE: If further dilutions are required, continue the process described in steps b through e. To continue the dilutions, 25 μL of the serum-buffer in circle number 7 is transferred to the next row of circles. When the final desired dilution is prepared, discard 25 μL of the serum-buffer dilution from the last circle.

g. Repeat steps a through f for the low reactive control and each patient specimen.

2. Using a new plastic stirrer for each circle, spread the serum to fill the entire circle.

3. Hold the bottle cap over the tip of the needle and gently invert the latex reagent dispensing bottle several times. While holding the bottle in an inverted, vertical position, dispense several drops of the latex reagent into the bottle cap until a drop of uniform size has been formed. This predropped reagent may be recovered *after testing* by aspirating it back into the bottle.

4. Dispense one free-falling drop (approximately 15 μL) of latex reagent onto each circle containing the serum.

   NOTE: To ensure proper drop delivery when dispensing latex antigen, the dispensing bottle *must* be inverted *vertically.*

5. Hand rotate the card (back and forth) 3 or 4 times to distribute the latex antigen throughout each circle. Avoid cross-contamination with adjacent circles.

6. Place the card on a rotator and mix for 8 minutes under a moistened humidifying cover.

7. Immediately after rotation, read the card macroscopically in the wet state. To help differentiate weak agglutination from no agglutination, a brief hand rotation of the card (3 or 4 back-and-forth motions) must be made following mechanical rotation. Results should be read under a high-intensity incandescent lamp. Fluorescent light is generally insufficient to distinguish minimally reactive results.

REPORTING RESULTS

QUALITATIVE METHOD. Positive (reactive): any agglutination of the latex reagent.
Negative (nonreactive): suspension remains evenly dispersed with no agglutination.

QUANTITATIVE METHOD. Report reactivity in terms of the highest dilution showing any agglutination of the latex reagent. Serum showing no agglutination at any dilution is reported as nonreactive.

Reference range The incidence of CMV infection depends on geographic and socioeconomic factors and the age of the patient. Serologic studies indicate that 25% to 50% of the American population demonstrate CMV antibodies present by the age of 15. In adult populations, the incidence of antibodies to CMV has been reported between 15% and 70%.

PROCEDURE NOTES

Procedure can be performed qualitatively on undiluted serum to determine presence of antibodies to CMV. Quantitative procedures using serial twofold dilutions can be performed to determine the titer of CMV antibody.

The control serum must react appropriately. Examples of appropriate reactions are presented in Table 17-2.

SOURCES OF ERROR. Incorrect test results may be caused by a variety of factors. Specimens that are incorrectly collected or stored can produce errors in the test results. The use of components or procedures other than those previously described may also lead to erroneous results.

CLINICAL APPLICATIONS. The absence of CMV antibodies suggests that a patient has not been previously exposed to cytomegalovirus; however, in the early stages of a primary infection, antibodies may not be detectable. The presence of CMV antibodies in qualitative testing on a single acute or convalescent phase specimen is an indication of previous exposure to the virus but does not indicate immunity to subsequent reinfection.

When paired specimens are tested simultaneously, the absence of a four-fold titer rise does not definitively rule out the possibility of exposure and infection. Demonstration of seroconversion in quantitative testing (or a four-fold or greater rise in antibody titer) on paired specimens collected at least 2 weeks apart may suggest recent infection. Conversion from seronegativity to positivity or a change in antibody titer between paired specimens may occasionally be caused by influenza A or *Mycoplasma pneumoniae* infections, suggesting stress reactivation of CMV antibody.

TABLE 17-2

Serum Dilutions

	Undiluted	1:2	1:4	1:8	1:16	1:32	1:64
High reactive control	R	R	R	R	R	R	R
Low reactive control	R	R	R	R	N	N	N
Nonreactive control	N						
Patient #1	R	R	N	N	N	N	N
Patient #2	R	R	R	R	R	R	N

R=reactive
N=nonreactive
Report as:
High reactive control=positive, $\geq$ 1:64 dilution
Low reactive control=positive, 1:8 dilution
Nonreactive control=negative
Patient #1= positive, 1:2 dilution
Patient #2= positive, 1:32 dilution

Clinically, the selection of CMV seronegative blood donors or organs by screening with a serologic test for antibody has been reported to be effective in reducing the occurrence of CMV infection in CMV seronegative recipients. The most suitable candidates for seronegative blood for transfusion are newborn and unborn infants and immunocompromised organ-transplant recipients.

LIMITATIONS. Several limitations are inherent in CMV antibody detection. These limitations include:

1. Patients with acute infection may not have detectable antibody.
2. Seroconversion may indicate recent infection, but an increase in antibody titer by this method does not differentiate between a primary and a secondary antibody response.
3. The timing of antibody response during a primary infection may differ slightly. The pattern of antibody response during a primary CMV infection has not been demonstrated.
4. Test results from neonates should be interpreted with caution because the presence of CMV antibody is usually the result of passive transfer from the mother to the fetus.
5. Although the CMV latex procedure will detect IgM and IgG antibodies, detection of IgA and IgE antibodies, has not yet been demonstrated.
6. A negative CMV test result may be useful in excluding possible infection, but the diagnosis of an actual CMV infection should be documented by demonstrating the presence of the virus directly or by viral culture.

REFERENCES

Package insert CMV Scan, Becton Dickinson Microbiology Systems, Cockeysville, Md.

☐ PROCEDURE

Quantitative Determination of IgM Antibodies to Cytomegalovirus (CMV) in Human Serum

PRINCIPLE

The cytomegalovirus (CMV) IgM assay is an indirect enzyme-labeled immunosorbent assay for determination of IgM antibodies to cytomegalovirus using antigen-coated microwells as a solid phase. CMV antigens are attached to wells of microplates. Test samples are diluted in sample diluent containing an absorbent that removes any CMV-specific IgG and IgM rheumatoid factor, which can interfere with the test. Diluted test samples are added to the coated wells and incubated. During incubation, antibodies to CMV present in the sample will bind to the antigen-coated well. After washing to remove unbound material, antibodies to human IgM labeled with alkaline phosphatase (conjugate) are added. The conjugate binds to any IgM antibodies bound to CMV antigens. The well is washed to remove unbound conjugate and incubated with p-nitrophenyl phosphate. The p-nitrophenyl phosphate is hydrolyzed by alkaline phosphatase to form p-nitrophenol, a yellow end product with absorbance maximum at 405 nm. The intensity of the absorbance at 405 nm is proportional to the amount of IgM antibody to CMV present in the sample. The serologic detection of IgM antibodies to CMV is a clinically useful aid in the diagnosis of primary CMV infection.

SPECIMEN COLLECTION AND PREPARATION

No special preparation of the patient is required before specimen collection. The patient must be positively identified when the specimen is collected and the specimen is to be labeled at the bedside. Specimen labels must include the patient's full name, the date the specimen is collected, the patient's hospital identification number, and the phlebotomist's initials.

Blood should be drawn by an aseptic technique. Serum or plasma can be used. A minimum of 2 mL of clotted blood (red top evacuated tube) or anticoagulated blood (lavender top evacuated tube) is required. The specimen should be centrifuged promptly and an aliquot of serum removed. Lipemia, hemolysis, or contamination with bacteria renders a specimen unsuitable for testing. Although icteric and turbid specimens have given valid results, fresh non-heat inactivated serum is *recommended* for use in the test.

If the test cannot be performed immediately, the specimen should be refrigerated (2° to 8° C). If the specimen must be kept for more than 7 days, it should be frozen at −18° C or below. Frozen serum should be thawed rapidly at 37° C.

Specimens containing visible particulate matter should be clarified by centrifugation before testing. The test specimens should not be heat inactivated since this may cause false-positive results.

REAGENTS, SUPPLIES, AND EQUIPMENT

Kit reagents available commercially in the SIA CMV IgM Procedure (Sigma Chemical Co, St. Louis, Mo.)

NOTE: Store reagents at 2° to 6° C. The reagents are stable until the expiration date on the label.

1. Kit components
   a. Antigen wells. Microplate wells coated with CMV antigen (strain AD 169). Store these antigen wells with desiccant in the reusable plastic bag and carefully reseal the bag after opening.
   b. Holder for wells.
   c. Sample diluent. This is a buffered protein solution containing surfactant and blue dye, pH 7.5. It contains absorbent (heat-aggregated human IgG) and 0.1% sodium azide as a preservative.
   d. Calibrator. This is human serum containing IgM antibodies to CMV at 100 arbitrary units (AU/mL). It contains 0.1% sodium azide as a preservative.
   e. Conjugate. This component contains goat antibodies to human IgM labeled with calf alkaline phosphatase. It contains a pink dye and 0.02% sodium azide as a preservative.
   f. Substrate. The substrate contains p-nitrophenyl phosphate, disodium, hexahydrate 1 mg/mL, pH 9.6. This solution may develop a slight yellow color on storage. Do not use if the absorbance of the undiluted substrate is greater than 0.4 at 405 nm when measured against water using a microplate reader or a spectrophotometer with a 1 cm lightpath.
   g. Wash concentrate. This is a buffer solution concentrate with surfactant. It contains 0.1% sodium azide as a preservative. The wash solution is prepared by adding the contents of the wash concentrate bottle to 1 liter of deionized water. Mix well.
   h. Stop solution. An alkaline solution, pH 12.0. Store at room temperature. This reagent is stable until the expiration date on the label. WARNING: Stop solution causes irritation. Avoid contact with eyes, skin, and clothing. Avoid breathing vapor. Wash thoroughly after handling.

NOTE: Do not interchange reagents from different lots.

WARNING: The reagents and controls contain sodium azide as a preservative. Sodium azide may react with lead and copper plumbing to form highly explosive metal azides. On disposal, flush with a large volume of water to prevent azide buildup. Sodium azide is also toxic. Take care to avoid ingestion.

ADDITIONAL REQUIRED EQUIPMENT AND SUPPLIES

1. Spectrophotometer that accommodates a 1 mL volume, or microplate reader capable of accurately measuring absorbance at 405 nm.
2. Pipettes (10 μL, 100 μL, and 200 μL) and pipettor.
3. Timer.
4. 1-liter measuring cylinder.
5. Squeeze bottle for dispensing wash solution.
6. Dilution plates or tubes.
7. Test tubes or cuvettes, 1.0 mL.

QUALITY CONTROL

POSITIVE CONTROL. This is a human serum containing IgM antibodies to CMV. Content (expected range, expressed as percent of calibrator) indicated on the label. It contains 0.1% sodium azide.

NEGATIVE CONTROL. This is a human serum containing no detectable antibodies to CMV. It contains 0.1% sodium azide. The negative control should be less than 30% of the calibrator.

NOTE: If these requirements are not satisfied, the results may be inaccurate and the assay should be repeated.

CAUTION: Because the antigen wells and control and calibrator sera are derived from human sources, they should be handled in the same manner as clinical serum specimens (see *Universal blood and body fluid precautions* in Chapter 6).

PROCEDURE

1. Dilute calibrator, positive and negative controls, and test specimens by combining 10 μL of each with 200 μL of sample diluent in labeled tubes or dilution plates.
2. Place the desired number of antigen wells in the holder.
3. Using a pipette tip, mix the samples and diluent by drawing up and expelling 2 or 3 times.

Transfer 100 μL of each diluted specimen to the appropriate antigen well.

4. Include one well that contains only 100 μL sample diluent. This serves as the reagent blank and is used to zero the photometer.

5. Allow the plate to stand at room temperature (18° to 26° C) for 30 ± 2 minutes.

6. Shake out or aspirate contents of wells. Wash the wells by filling them with wash solution from a squeeze bottle and shaking out or aspirating. Wash three times. Drain the wells on a paper towel to remove excess fluid.

    NOTE: Thorough washing is necessary to achieve accurate results. Avoid bubbles.

7. Place 2 drops (or 100 μL) conjugate in each well, including the reagent blank well.

8. Allow to stand at room temperature (18° to 26° C) for 30 minutes ± 2 minutes.

9. Wash wells by repeating step 6.

10. Place 2 drops (or 100 μL) substrate into each well, including the reagent blank well.

11. Allow to stand at room temperature (18° to 26° C) for 30 minute ± 2 minutes.

12. Place 2 drops (or 100 μL stop solution into each well.

13. Read and record absorbance of each test at 405 nm within 2 hours after the reaction has been stopped:

    MICROPLATE READER. Set absorbance at 405 nm to 0 with water as reference. Read and record absorbance of reagent blank (A blank). Then set absorbance to 0 with the reagent blank as a reference. Read and record absorbance of samples (A sample) and calibrator (A calibrator).

SPECTROPHOTOMETER

Completely remove contents of each well and transfer to cuvette or test tube. Add 800 μL of deionized water to each sample and mix. Set absorbance at 405 nm to 0 with water as a reference. Read and record the absorbance of each sample including the reagent blank. Subtract the absorbance of the reagent blank for the absorbance of each sample.

CALCULATION

CMV IgM Antibody concentration as percent of

$$\text{calibrator} = \frac{\text{A sample}}{\text{A calibrator}} \times 100$$

Example:

ABSORBANCE MEASURED USING A MICROPLATE READER

$$\text{A sample} = 0.413$$

$$\text{A calibrator} = 0.571$$

Antibody concentration as percent of

$$\text{calibrator} = \frac{0.413}{0.571} \times 100 = 72$$

ABSORBANCE MEASURED USING A SPECTROPHOTOMETER

$$\text{A blank} = 0.009$$

$$\text{A sample} = 0.083$$

$$\text{A calibrator} = 0.115$$

$$\text{A sample} - \text{A blank} = 0.083 - 0.009 = 0.074$$

$$\text{A calibrator} - \text{A blank} = 0.115 - 0.009 = 0.106$$

Antibody concentration as percent of

$$\text{calibrator} = \frac{0.074}{0.106} \times 100 = 70$$

REPORTING RESULTS

± 30% of calibrator: positive for IgM antibody to CMV and indicates the probability of current or recurrent infection <30% of calibrator: negative for IgM antibody to CMV.

PROCEDURE NOTES

Specimens giving absorbance values above that of the calibrator should be diluted appropriately and reassayed. The value obtained should be multiplied by the dilution factor.

If cord blood is tested, contamination with maternal blood should be avoided. A follow-up specimen directly from the newborn should be tested to confirm positive IgM antibody results.

SOURCES OF ERROR. False-negative and false-positive test results may occur in IgM assays for a variety of reasons.

The reasons for false-negative results include:

1. A low level of specific IgM antibodies is known to produce falsely negative reactions. If the specimen is obtained too early in the development of the infection, it may contain no detectable IgM antibody by serum assay. To avoid this situation, a subsequent specimen should be obtained 7 to 14 days later for retesting.

2. In many IgM assays, interference by competitive antigen specific IgG can result in false-negative reactions. High levels of CMV-specific IgG may be present in the serum of congenitally infected newborn infants because of the presence of maternal IgG. In this procedure, however, comparative testing before and after removal of IgG has no significant effect on the CMV IgM assay results.

The reasons for false-positive results include:

1. Interference by IgM rheumatoid factor can produce false-positive results. Thus IgM assays must be designed to eliminate these interfering substances. In the SIA method, the sample diluent contains heat-aggregated IgG sufficient to neutralize the immunologic activity of up to 348 IU/mL of IgM rheumatoid factor.

2. Interference by specific IgG antibody can produce false-positive results. Serum containing very high levels of antibody to DNA (>2000 IU/

mL), e.g., systemic lupus erythematosus (SLE) patients, may yield false-positive results in the CMV IgM SIA test.

Viral infections have also been reported to elicit heterotypic CMV IgM responses. Approximately 30% of sera from patients with heterophil (antibody positive) mononucleosis show heterotypic CMV IgM responses. In addition, varicella-zoster virus has been reported to cause heterotypic CMV IgM response.

CLINICAL APPLICATIONS. The presence of IgM antibodies to CMV is, in general, indicative of primary CMV infection. Specific IgM antibody, however, has been reported in reactivations and reinfections. IgM antibody may persist for as long as 9 months in immunocompetent individuals and for longer periods in immunosuppressed patients.

IgM responses vary between different individuals. Of infants congenitally infected with CMV, 10% to 30% fail to develop IgM antibody responses. Approximately 27% of adults with primary CMV infection may not demonstrate an IgM response. In pregnant women, the presence or absence of CMV IgG or IgM response is of limited value in predicting congenital CMV infection. However, the presence of CMV-specific IgM antibody in the circulation of the newborn is indicative of infection.

LIMITATIONS. The detection of IgM is of limited value in determining the timing of primary infection. In addition, testing results should serve only as an aid to diagnosis and should not be interpreted as diagnostic in themselves.

REFERENCES

SIA CMV IgM Product Brochure, Sigma Chemical Co, St Louis, Mo.

Chapter Review

HIGHLIGHTS

Cytomegalovirus (CMV) is a ubiquitous human viral pathogen. Human cytomegalovirus is classified as a member of the herpes family of viruses. All of the herpes viruses are relatively large, enveloped DNA viruses that undergo a replicative cycle involving DNA expression and nucleocapsid assembly within the nucleus. Although the herpes family produces diverse clinical diseases, the viruses share the basic characteristics of being cell associated. These characteristics may play a role in the ability of the virus to produce subclinical infections that can be reactivated under appropriate stimuli. Dissemination of the virus may occur by oral, respiratory, or venereal routes. It may also be transmitted parenterally by organ transplantation or by transfusion of fresh blood.

The incidence of primary infections during childhood is low. Of patients who are immunosuppressed, only seronegative patients appear to be at a significant risk of developing CMV infection. Patients at the highest risk of mortality from CMV infections are allograft transplant seronegative patients who receive tissue from a seropositive donor. The majority of infections in allograft recipients are transmitted by the donor kidney or arise from the reactivation of the recipient's latent virus.

Transmission of CMV by transfusion of blood or blood components containing white cells is assuming increasing importance in patients with severely impaired immunity who require supportive therapy. Low-birth-weight neonates are also at high risk to CMV infection through transfusion of CMV-infected blood products. Persistent infections characterized by periods of reactivation of CMV are frequently termed latent infections, although this condition has not been clearly defined for CMV.

CMV is considered to be one of the most important causes of congenital viral infections in the United States because primary as well as recurrent maternal CMV infection can be transmitted in utero. Acquired CMV infection is usually asymptomatic and can persist in the host as a chronic or latent infection. In the majority of patients, CMV infection is asymptomatic. Occasionally a self-limited, (heterophil-negative, mononucleosis-like syndrome results. CMV infection is known to alter the immune system as well as produce overt manifestations of infection. Infection interferes with immune responsiveness in both normal and immunocompromised individuals. This diminished responsiveness results in a decreased proliferative response to the CMV antigen, which persists for several months. In patients with CMV mononucleosis-like syndrome, alterations of T lymphocyte subsets result, producing an increase in the absolute number of suppressor (OKT8) lymphocytes, and a decrease in helper (OKT4) lymphocytes. These subset abnormalities persist for months. In addition, questions have been raised regarding CMV as a potentially oncogenic virus because viral antigens and/or nucleic acid have been found in some human malignancies.

In cells infected by CMV, several antigens appear at varying time intervals after infection. Before replication of viral DNA takes place, immediate-early antigens and early antigens are present in the nuclei of infected cells. Immediate-early antigens appear within 1 hour of cellular infection and early antigens are present within 24 hours. At about 72 hours postinfection or at the end of the viral replication cycle, late antigens are demonstrable in the nucleus and cytoplasm of infected cells. The immune antibody response to these various antigens differ in incidence and significance. The presence of antibodies against immediate-early and early antigens is associated with active infection of either a primary or reactivated nature. The characteristic antibody responses associated with infection are primary infection, which is demonstrated by a transient virus-specific IgM antibody response and eventual seroconversion to produce IgG antibodies to the virus; reactivation of latent CMV infection in seropositive (IgG) individuals, which may be accompanied by significant increases in IgG antibodies to the virus but elicits no detectable IgM response; and reinfection by a strain of CMV that is different than the original infecting strain in which a significant IgG antibody response is demonstrated but in which it is unknown whether an IgM response occurs.

Serologic methods to detect the presence of IgM antibodies can aid in the diagnosis of primary infection. Detection of CMV-specific IgM can represent primary infection or rare reactivation of infection. Detection of significant increases in CMV-specific IgG antibody by methods such as complement fixation (CF), anticomplement immunofluorescence (ACIF), and enzyme immunoassay (EIA) suggest, but do not prove, recent infection or reactivation of latent infection. The EIA method for IgM and IgG antibodies to CMV has replaced CF, ACIF, and immunofluorescent antibody (IFA). Latex particle agglutination and indirect hemagglutination are useful screening methods to obtain seronegative blood donors. Newer CMV detection methods are being explored. CMV antigen detection in urine by EIA and cDNA is being developed. RNA transcript of CMV DNA are detectable in peripheral blood mononuclear cells of seropositive individuals by in situ hybridization (ISH) with cDNA of CMV. The ISH technique, which is more sensitive than dot-blot hybridization (Northern blot), promises to be a new early detection method for CMV expression.

REVIEW QUESTIONS

1. All of the following descriptive characteristics are true of cytomegalovirus except:
   A. A herpes family virus
   B. A DNA virus
   C. A cell-associated virus
   D. Is epidemic worldwide
   E. Can be transmitted by organ transplantation or transfusion of fresh blood
2. Because CMV can persist latently, an active infection may develop as a result of all of the following conditions except:
   A. Pregnancy
   B. Immunosuppression therapy
   C. Organ or bone marrow transplantation
   D. AIDS
   E. Transfusion of leukocyte-poor blood

3. CMV is recognized as the cause of congenital viral infection in _____% of all live births:
   A. 0.1 to 0.4
   B. 0.5 to 2.4
   C. 2.5 to 4.9
   D. 5.0 to 9.9
   E. Over 10
4. Transfusion-acquired CMV infection can cause:
   A. Mononucleosis-like syndrome
   B. Hepatitis
   C. Rejection of a transplanted organ
   D. Rejection of transplanted bone marrow
   E. All of the above

Match the three types of CMV infection with their appropriate description:
5. Primary infection
6. Reactivated infection
7. Reinfection
   A. A significant antibody response and viral shedding caused by a different strain of virus
   B. When a seronegative recipient is transfused with blood from an actively or latently infected donor
   C. When a seropositive recipient is transfused with blood from either a CMV antibody-positive or negative donor

Match the following serologic markers of CMV infection:
8. Early antigens
9. Immediate-early antigens
10. Late antigens
    A. Appear at about 72 hours post-infection or at the end of the viral replication cycle
    B. Appear within 1 hour of cellular infection
    C. Present within 24 hours
11. Antibodies to immediate-early and early antigens are associated with:
    A. Primary active infection
    B. Reactivated active infection
    C. Latent infection
    D. Increasing age and sex of the patient

Match the following:
12. Primary infection
13. Reactivation of latent infection in seropositive IgG patient
14. Reinfection with a different strain of CMV than original strain
    A. IgG but IgM response unknown
    B. Specific IgM antibody response
    C. IgG (no detectable IgM)

Match the following:
15. Latex particle agglutination
16. Indirect fluorescent antibody
17. Enzyme immunoassay
    A. Antibody
    B. IgM
    C. IgG and IgM antibody

ANSWERS

1. D 2. E 3. B 4. E 5. B 6. C 7. A 8. C 9. B 10. A 11. D 12. B 13. C 14. A 15. A 16. B 17. C

BIBLIOGRAPHY

Adler SP: Transfusion-associated cytomegalovirus infections, Rev Infect Dis 5:977-993, 1983.

Alpaugh K and Beckwith DG et al: A donor population classified for viral exposure and infection: cytomegalovirus and hepatitis B, with an addendum on HTLV-III test results, Lab Med 16(8):485-488, Aug 1986.

Betts RF: The relationship of epidemiology and treatment factors to infection and allograft survival in renal transplantation. In Platkin SA et al, editors: CMV pathogenesis and prevention of human infection, New York, 1984, Alan R Liss, Inc.

Bowden R et al: Cytomegalovirus immune globulin and seronegative blood products to prevent primary cytomegalovirus infection after marrow transplantation, Engl J Med 314:1006-1010, 1986.

Brady MT: Cytomegalovirus infections: occupational risk for health professionals, Am J Infect Control 14(5):197-203, Oct 1986.

Chernesky MA, Ray CG, and Smith TF: Laboratory diagnosis of viral infections, Cumitech 15:9-11, May 1982.

Demmler GJ et al: Enzyme-linked immunosorbent assay for the detection of IgM-class antibodies to cytomegalovirus, J Infect Dis 153:1152-1155, 1986.

Feng CS et al: A comparison of four commercial test kits for detection of cytomegalovirus antibodies in blood donors, Transfusion 26(2):203, 1986.

Fiesthumel S et al: Cytomegalovirus (CMV) infection in blood donors: correlation of serologic markers with viral shedding, American Red Cross Blood Services, Syracuse, New York. Abstract of paper to be presented at the 39th annual American Association of Blood Banks Meeting, Oct 1986, Transfusion 26(6):554.

Hanshaw JV: Cytomegalovirus. In Remington JS and Klein J, editors: Infectious diseases of the fetus and newborn infant, Philadelphia, 1983, WB Saunders Co.

Hanshaw JV et al: School failure and deafness after "silent" congenital cytomegalovirus infection, N Engl J Med 295:486, 1976.

Ho M: Characteristics of cytomegalovirus. In James HV, editor: Cytomegalovirus—biology and infection, New York, 1982, Plenum Publishing Corp.

Joassin L and Riginster M: Elimination of nonspecific cytomegalovirus immunoglobulin M activities in the enzyme-linked immunosorbent assay by using antihuman immunoglobulin G, J Clin Microbiol 23:576-581, 1986.

Kinney JS et al: Cytomegaloviral infection and disease, J Infect Dis 151:772-774, 1985.

Lamberson HV: Cytomegalovirus (CMV): The agent, its pathogenesis, and its epidemiology. In Daniels JS, editor: Infection, immunity and blood transfusion, New York, 1985, Alan R Liss, Inc.

Martin WJ II and Smith TF: Rapid detection of cytomegalovirus in bronchoalveolar lavage specimens by monoclonal antibody method, J Clin Microbiol 23:1006-1008, 1986.

McHugh TM et al: Comparison of six methods for the detection of antibody to cytomegalovirus, J Clin Microbiol 22:1014-1019, 1985.

McKeating JA et al: Detection of cytomegalovirus in urine samples by enzyme-linked immunosorbent assay, J Med Virol 16:367-373, 1985.

Musianim M et al: Serological screening for the prevention of transfusion-acquired cytomegalovirus infections, J Infect 9:148-152, 1984.

Panjwani AJ et al: Virological and serological diagnosis of cytomegalovirus infection in bone marrow allograft recipient, J Med Virol 16:357-365, 1985.

Prince AM et al: A serologic study of cytomegalovirus infections associated with blood transfusions, N Engl J Med 284:1125, 1971.

Reynolds DW et al: Inapparent congenital cytomegalovirus, N Engl J Med 290:281, 1974.

Schrier RD, Nelson JA, and Nelson MB: Detection of human cytomegalovirus in peripheral blood lymphocytes in a natural infection, Science 230:1048-1051, 1985.

Schuster V et al: Detection of human cytomegalovirus in urine by DNA-DNA and RNA-DNA hybridization, J Infect Dis 154:309-314, 1986.

Shuster EA et al: Monoclonal antibody for rapid laboratory detection of cytomegalovirus infections: characterization and diagnostic application, Mayo Clin Proc 60:577-585, 1985.

Stagno S et al: Immunoglobulin M antibodies detected by enzyme-linked immunosorbent assay and radioimmunoassay in the diagnosis of cytomegalovirus infections in pregnant women and newborn infants, J Clin Microbiol 21:930-935, 1985.

Stagno S and Whitley RJ: Herpes virus infections of pregnancy, part I: cytomegalovirus and Epstein-Barr virus infections, N Engl J Med 313:1270-1274, 1985.

Stagno S et al: Congenital cytomegalovirus infection, N Engl J Med 306:945, 1982.

Stagno S et al: Immunoglobulin M antibodies detected by enzyme-linked immunosorbent assay and radioimmunoassay in the diagnosis of cytomegalovirus infections in pregnant women and newborn infants, J Clin Microbiol 21:930, 1985.

Starr SE, Friedman HJ: Human cytomegalovirus. In Lennette EH, Balows A, Hausler WJ et al, editors: Manual of clinical microbiology, ed 4, Washington, DC, 1985, American Soc Microbiol.

Stern H: Cytomegalovirus vaccine: justification and problems. In Waterson AP, ed: Recent advances in clinical virology, New York, 1977, Churchill-Livingstone, Inc.

Sullivan JL and Hanshaw JV: Cytomegalovirus infections. In Glaser R and Gotlieb-Stematsky T, eds: Human herpes virus infections—clinical aspects, New York, 1982, Marcel Dekker, Inc.

Taswell HF, Reisner RK, et al: Comparison of three methods for detecting antibody to cytomegalovirus, Transfusion 26(3):285-289, 1986.

Tegtmeier GE: Cytomegalovirus and blood transfusion. In Infection, immunity and blood transfusion, New York, 1985, Alan R Liss, Inc.

Turgeon ML: Clinical hematology, Boston, 1988, Little, Brown & Co, Inc.

Turgeon ML: Fundamentals of immunohematology, Philadelphia, 1989, Lea & Febiger.

CHAPTER 18

Infectious Mononucleosis

ETIOLOGY

The Epstein-Barr virus (EBV) was first discovered in 1964 as the cause of infectious mononucleosis (IM). This disorder is usually an acute, benign, and self-limiting lymphoproliferative condition. EBV is also the cause of Burkitt's lymphoma (a malignant tumor of the lymphoid tissue occurring mainly in African children), nasopharyngeal carcinoma, and neoplasms of the thymus, parotid gland, and supraglottic larynx. EBV infections can result in complications involving the cardiac, ocular, respiratory, hematologic, digestive, renal, and neurologic systems. EBV-associated neurologic syndromes include Bell's palsy, Guillain-Barré syndrome, meningoencephalitis, Reye's syndrome, myelitis, cranial nerve neuritis, and psychotic disorders. Respiratory paralysis caused by bulbar involvement can be fatal.

EPIDEMIOLOGY

EBV is widely disseminated. It is estimated that 95% of the world's population is exposed to the virus, which makes it the most ubiquitous virus known to man. EBV is a human herpes DNA virus. In IM the virus infects B lymphocytes, but the variant lymphocytes produced in response to and seen in microscopic examination of the peripheral blood have T-cell characteristics. One of the habitats of the persisting viral genome in hosts with a latent infection is the B lymphocytes of the lymphoreticular system and in epithelial cells of the oropharynx.

Although EBV appears to be transmitted primarily by close contact with infectious oral-pharyngeal secretions, the virus has been reported to be transmitted by blood transfusion and transplacental routes. Under ordinary conditions transmission of the virus through transfusion or transplacental exposure is unlikely.

The frequency of *seronegative* patients is nearly 100% in early infancy and declines with increasing age, more or less rapidly, depending on socioeconomic conditions, to less than 10% in young adults. After primary exposure a person is considered to be immune and generally no longer susceptible to overt reinfection. In Western society primary exposure to EBV occurs in two waves. Approximately half of the population is exposed to the virus before the age of 5 years; a second wave of *seroconversion* occurs during late adolescence (15 to 24 years of age). Approximately 90% of adult patients demonstrate antibodies to the virus.

Individuals at risk include those who lack antibodies to the virus. EBV is only a minor problem for immunocompetent persons, but it can become a major one for immunologically compromised patients. Blood transfusion from an immune donor to a nonimmune recipient may produce a primary infection in the recipient known as IM postperfusion syndrome. IM or IM-like illness following blood transfusion often may be the result of a concomitant cytomegalovirus infection rather than the EBV.

A low percentage of patients experience symptomatic reactivation. Reactivation of latent infection has been implicated in a persistent illness referred to as the EBV-associated fatigue syndrome, but this phenomenon is not universally accepted.

Clinically apparent IM has an estimated frequency of 45:100,000 in adolescents. In immunosuppressed patients the incidence of EBV infection ranges from 35% to 47%. As occurs with other herpes viruses, there is a carrier state after primary infection.

SIGNS AND SYMPTOMS

The majority of individuals seroconvert without any significant clinical signs and symptoms of disease. In children under 5 years of age, infection is either asymptomatic or frequently characterized by mild, poorly defined signs and symptoms. Although anyone can suffer from this viral disorder, it is typically manifested in young adults.

The incubation period of IM is from 10 to 50 days and once fully developed lasts for 1 to 4 weeks. Clinical manifestations include extreme fatigue, malaise, sore throat, fever, and cervical lymphadenopathy. Splenomegaly occurs in about 50% of cases. Jaundice is infrequent, although the most common complication is hepatitis. A smaller percentage of patients develop hepatomegaly or splenomegaly and hepatomegaly. Because abnormal liver function is more marked with EBV-induced IM than in CMV-associated mononucleosis, EBV must be considered in the differential diagnosis of hepatitis. A significant number of cases of IM do not manifest classic signs and symptoms.

IMMUNOLOGIC MANIFESTATION
Heterophil Antibodies

Heterophil antibodies comprise a broad class of antibody. These antibodies are defined as ones that are stimulated by one antigen and react with an entirely unrelated surface antigen present on cells from different mammalian species. Heterophil antibodies may be present in normal individuals in low concentrations (titers), but a titer of 1:56 or greater is clinically significant in suspected cases of IM.

The IgM type of heterophil antibody usually appears during the acute phase of IM, but the antigen that stimulates its production remains unknown. IgM heterophil antibody is characterized by the following features:

1. Reacts with horse, ox, and sheep erythrocytes
2. Absorbed by beef erythrocytes
3. Not absorbed by guinea pig kidney cells
4. Does not react with EBV-specific antigens

Paul and Bunnell first associated IM with sheep cell agglutination and developed a test for the IM heterophil. Davidsohn modified the original Paul-Bunnell test, introducing a differential adsorption aspect to remove the cross-reacting *Forssman* and *serum sickness* heterophil antibodies. Since then, the Davidsohn test has become the classic laboratory reference test (see p. 206) for the diagnosis of IM. The Davidsohn test, however, is time-consuming and cumbersome.

Rapid slide tests (see p. 207), based on the principle of agglutination of horse erythrocytes are now available. The use of horse erythrocytes appears to increase the sensitivity of the test.

EBV Serology

Within the adult population, 10% to 20% of individuals with acute IM do not produce IM heterophil antibody. The pediatric population is of particular concern because more than 50% of children under 4 years of age with IM are heterophil negative. In diagnostically inconclusive cases of IM, a more definitive assessment of immune status may be obtained through an EBV serologic panel. Candidates for EBV serology include those who do not exhibit classic symptoms of IM, who are heterophil negative, or who are immunosuppressed.

EBV-infected B lymphocytes express a variety of "new" antigens encoded by the virus. Infection with EBV results in the expression of viral capsid antigen (VCA), early antigen (EA), and nuclear antigen (NA), with corresponding antibody responses. Assays for IgM and IgG antibodies to these EBV antigens are available. EBV-specific serologic studies (Table 18-1) are beneficial in defining immune status, and their time of appearance may be indicative of the stage of disease. This can provide important information for both the diagnosis and management of EBV-associated disease.

Viral Capsid Antigen

Viral capsid antigen (VCA) is produced by infected B cells and can be found in the cytoplasm. Anti-VCA IgM is usually detectable early in the course of infection, but it is low in concentration and disappears within 2 to 4 months. Anti-VCA

TABLE 18-1

Characteristic Antibody Formation in Infectious Mononucleosis

	VCA IgM	VCA IgG	EA-D	EA-R	EBNA IgG	Heterophil
No previous exposure	−	−	−	−	−	−
Recent (acute) infection	+	+	+/−	−	−	+
Past infection (convalescent) period	−	+	−	−	+	−
Reactivation of latent infection	+/−	+	+/−	+/−	+	+/−

VCA = Viral capsid antigen
EA-D = Early antigen (diffuse)
EA-R = Early antigen (restricted)
EBNA = Epstein-Barr nuclear antigen

IgG is usually detectable within 4 to 7 days after the onset of signs and symptoms and persists for an extended period of time, perhaps lifelong.

Early Antigen

Early antigen (EA) is a complex of two components, *early antigen–diffuse (EA-D)*, which is found in both the nucleus and the cytoplasm of the B cells, and *early antigen–restricted (EA-R)*, which is usually found as a mass only in the cytoplasm.

Anti-EA-D of the IgG type is highly indicative of acute infection, but it is not detectable in 10% to 20% of patients with IM. EA-D disappears in about 3 months; however, a rise in titer is demonstrated during reactivation of a latent EBV infection.

Anti-EA-R IgG is not usually found in young adults during the acute phase, but it is sometimes demonstrated in the serum of very young children during the acute phase. Anti-EA-R IgG appears transiently in the later convalescent phase. In general, anti-EA-D and anti-EA-R IgG are not consistent indicators of the disease stage.

Epstein-Barr Nuclear Antigen

Epstein-Barr nuclear antigen (EBNA) is found in the nucleus of all EBV-infected cells. Although the synthesis of NA precedes EA synthesis during the infection of B cells, EBV-NA does not become available for antibody stimulation until after the incubation period of IM, when activated T lymphocytes destroy the EBV genome-carrying B cells. As a result, antibodies to NA are absent or barely detectable during acute IM.

Anti-EBNA IgG does not appear until a patient has entered the convalescent period. EBV-NA antibodies are almost always present in sera containing IgG antibodies to VCA of EBV unless the patient is in the early acute phase of IM. Patients with severe immunologic defects or immunosuppressive disease may not have EBV-NA antibodies, even if antibodies to VCA are present.

Under normal conditions, antibody titers to NA gradually increase through convalescence and reach a plateau between 3 and 12 months postinfection. The antibody titer remains at a moderate, measurable level indefinitely because of the persistent viral carrier state established following primary EBV infection. Most healthy individuals with previous exposure to EBV have antibody titers to EBV-NA that range from 1:10 to 1:160. In EBV-associated malignancies, the levels of EBNA antibody are usually high in patients with nasopharyngeal carcinoma and can range from barely detectable to very high in patients with Burkitt's lymphoma.

Test results of antibodies to EBV-NA should be evaluated in relationship to patient symptoms, clinical history, and antibody response patterns to EBV-VCA and EA to establish a diagnosis. The antibody profile can be especially useful. For example, a patient with an IM-like illness caused by reactivation of a persistent EBV infection resulting from an immunosuppressive malignancy or nonmalignant disease can demonstrate high titers of both IgM and IgG VCA antibodies. If the antibody to EBV-NA, however, is also elevated, a diagnosis of primary EBV infection can be excluded.

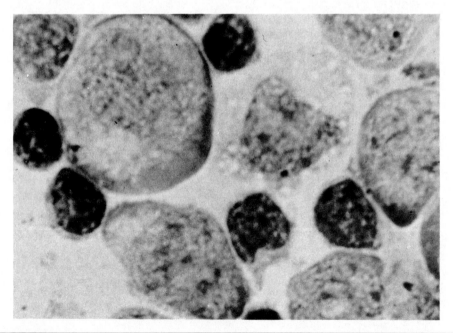

FIGURE 18-1

Lymph node imprint, infectious mononucleosis. (Wright's stain; × 1,200; courtesy Dr. JC Sieracki.)
(From Miale JB: Hematology, ed 6, St Louis, 1982, The CV Mosby Co.)

Additional Testing

A test commonly used in the EBV serology is based on immunofluorescence (IF). Antigen substrate slides containing EBV-infected B cells are incubated with the patient's serum. The presence of specific antibody is detected by the addition of fluorescein-conjugated antihuman IgG or IgM. The disadvantages of this type of testing are that it is time-consuming, difficult to interpret, and prone to interference from other serum components, such as rheumatoid factor.

Diagnostic Evaluation

In addition to clinical signs and symptoms, laboratory testing is necessary to establish or confirm the diagnosis of IM.

Hematologic studies reveal a leukocyte count ranging from 10 to 20 × 10/L in about two thirds of patients; about 10% of the patients with this disorder demonstrate *leukopenia*. A differential leukocyte count may initially disclose a neutrophilia, although mononuclear cells usually predominate as the disorder develops. Typical relative lymphocyte counts range from 60% to 90% with 5% to 30% *variant lymphocytes*. These variant lymphocytes exhibit diverse morphologic features and persist for 1 to 2 months and as long as 4 to 6 months (Fig. 18-1).

If the classic signs and symptoms of IM are absent, a diagnosis of IM is more difficult to make. A definite diagnosis of IM can be established by serologic antibody testing. The antibodies present in IM are heterophil and EBV antibodies.

☐ PROCEDURE

The Paul-Bunnell Screening Test

PRINCIPLE

The Paul-Bunnell test is a hemagglutination test designed to detect heterophil antibodies in patient serum when mixed with antigen-bearing sheep erythrocytes. Dilutions of inactivated patient serum are mixed with sheep erythrocytes, incubated, centrifuged, and macroscopically examined for agglutination. Positive reactions are preliminarily associated with the manifestation of infectious mononucleosis (IM).

SPECIMEN COLLECTION AND PREPARATION

No special preparation of the patient is required prior to specimen collection. The patient must be positively identified when the specimen is collected. The specimen shall be labeled at the bedside and shall include the patient's full name, the date the specimen is collected, and the patient's hospital identification number. The phlebotomist's initials should also appear on the label.

Blood should be drawn by an aseptic technique.

The required specimen is a minimum of 2 mL of clotted blood (red-top evacuated tube). The presence of hemolysis makes the specimen unsuitable for testing.

Centrifuge the tube of blood and remove an aliquot of clear serum. Inactivate the serum at 56° C for 30 minutes before testing.

REAGENTS, SUPPLIES, AND EQUIPMENT

2% suspension of washed sheep cells in normal saline (prepared by pipetting 0.2 mL of packed erythrocytes into 9.8 mL of saline)
0.9% sodium chloride (normal physiologic saline)
12 × 75 mm test tubes
NOTE: The cell should be no more than 1 week old.
Graduated serologic pipettes
Centrifuge
37° C incubator (optional)

QUALITY CONTROL

A known positive control should be run concurrently.

PROCEDURE

1. Label two sets of test tubes. Each set should consist of 10 tubes.
2. Pipette 0.5 mL of saline into tube 1 and 0.25 mL of saline into each of the remaining 9 tubes.
3. To the first set of tubes, add 0.1 mL of patient's inactivated serum to tube 1; mix and transfer 0.25 mL of the dilution to the second tube; mix and transfer 0.25 mL of the dilution to the third tube. Repeat this process to tube 10. Discard 0.25 mL from the final tube, tube 10.
4. To the second set of tubes, add 0.1 mL of the control serum and proceed to dilute it as in step 3.
5. Add 0.1 mL of 2% sheep cells to each tube.
6. Gently shake the tubes until mixed.
7. Incubate the tubes at 37° C for 1 hour or overnight at room temperature.
8. Centrifuge the tubes for 1 minute at 1500 rpm.
9. Gently shake each tube and examine macroscopically for agglutination.
10. Record the results.

REPORTING RESULTS

A titer of greater than 1:56 is considered to be a positive presumptive test.

PROCEDURE NOTES

The antigens on sheep erythrocytes are associated with infectious mononucleosis, serum sickness, and the Forssman antigen.

SOURCES OF ERROR. False positive reactions have been observed in conditions such as hepatitis infection and Hodgkin's disease. An improperly inactivated serum will produce hemolysis.

CLINICAL APPLICATIONS. The Paul-Bunnell test is a useful screening test for the presence of heterophil antibodies because it is simple and inexpensive. Although the specificity of the heterophil assay is rated as good, negative results are demonstrated in individuals who do not produce IM heterophil antibody. If negative results are displayed, however, EBV serology may be indicated.

LIMITATIONS. The test is only indicative of the presence or absence of heterophil antibodies. Demonstrating agglutination by using sheep erythrocytes does not make a distinction between antibodies associated with infectious mononucleosis, serum sickness, or the Forssman antigen.

Heterophil antibody assay lacks sensitivity as a diagnostic criterion for IM. Sheep erythrocytes are less sensitive than erythrocytes from other species, such as the horse. A patient may take as long as 3 months to develop a detectable heterophil titer.

REFERENCES

Paul JR and Bunnell WW: The presence of heterophile antibodies in infectious mononucleosis, Am J Med Sci 183:90-104, 1932.
Sumaya CV: Infectious mononucleosis and other EBV infections: diagnostic factors, Lab Management 24:37-45, 1986.

☐ PROCEDURE

Davidsohn Differential Test

PRINCIPLE

This classic test distinguishes between the heterophil antibodies that agglutinate the antigen-bearing erythrocytes of sheep. The differential nature of the test is predicated on the fact that sheep and beef (ox) erythrocytes bear some common antigens that are not present on the kidney cells of the guinea pig. Exposure of patient serum to both guinea pig cells, which are rich in Forsmann antigen, and beef erythrocytes, which are poor in Forsmann antigen, produces differential absorption. Any absorbed antibodies are removed by centrifugation, and the supernatant fluid is tested with sheep erythrocytes. This test classically differentiates the heterophil types of antibody associated with infectious mononucleosis (IM), serum sickness, or Forssman antigen.

SPECIMEN COLLECTION AND PREPARATION

No special preparation of the patient is required prior to specimen collection. The patient must be positively identified when the specimen is collected. The specimen shall be labeled at the bedside and shall include the patient's full name, the date the specimen is collected, and the patient's hospital identification number. The phlebotomist's initials should also appear on the label.

Blood should be drawn by an aseptic technique. The required specimen is a minimum of 2 mL of clotted blood (red-top evacuated tube). The presence of hemolysis makes the specimen unsuitable for testing.

Centrifuge the tube of blood and remove an aliquot of clear serum. Inactivate the serum at 56° C for 30 minutes before testing.

REAGENTS, SUPPLIES, AND EQUIPMENT

0.9% sodium chloride (normal physiologic saline)
2% suspension of washed sheep cells in normal saline (prepared by pipetting 0.2 mL of packed erythrocytes into 9.8 mL of saline)
12 × 75 mm test tubes
NOTE: The cell should be no more than 1 week old.
20% beef erythrocytes
20% suspension of guinea pig kidney cells
NOTE: Sheep, beef, and guinea pig kidney cells are commercially available from Baltimore Biological Laboratories, Cockeysville, Maryland.
12 × 75 mm test tubes
2 conical centrifuge tubes
Graduated serologic pipettes
Test tube racks

QUALITY CONTROL

A known positive control should be run concurrently.

PROCEDURE

PRELIMINARY SPECIMEN PREPARATION
A. Pipette 1.0 mL of beef cells into an appropriately labeled conical centrifuge tube.
B. Pipette 1.0 mL of guinea pig cells into an appropriately labeled conical centrifuge tube.
C. Pipette 0.25 mL of inactivated patient serum into each tube and shake.
D. Incubate the tubes at room temperature for 5 minutes. Shake the tubes periodically to resuspend the cells.
E. Centrifuge for 10 minutes at 1500 rpm.

PROCEDURE
1. Label two sets of test tubes: beef 1-8 and guinea pig 1-8.
2. Pipette 0.25 mL of saline into each test tube.
3. Carefully pipette 0.25 mL of clear supernatant from the beef erythrocyte conical centrifuge tube to the first tube of the beef set of test tubes.
4. Carefully pipette 0.25 mL of clear supernatant from the guinea pig conical centrifuge tube to the first tube of the guinea pig set of test tubes.
5. Mix the contents of the first beef tube and transfer 0.25 mL of the dilution to the next tube. Continue to mix and transfer 0.25 mL until the last tube, tube 8, is reached. Discard 0.25 mL from the last tube.
6. Mix the contents of the first guinea pig tube and transfer 0.25 mL of the dilution to the next tube. Continue to mix and transfer 0.25 mL until the last tube, tube 8, is reached. Discard 0.25 mL from the last tube.
7. Pipette 0.1 mL of sheep erythrocytes into each tube.
8. Shake gently until the cells are well mixed.
9. Incubate at room temperature for 2 hours.

10. Gently shake each tube and examine macroscopically for agglutination. Record the results.

REPORTING RESULTS

Agglutination patterns are presented below. If the pattern of reactivity demonstrates reduced titers with either beef or guinea pig cells, the antibody source can be attributed to one of the heterophil antibody types.

DIFFERENTIAL ABSORPTION PATTERNS

Type of heterophil antibody	Absorbed by guinea pig kidney cells	Absorbed by beef erythrocytes
Forssman	Yes	No
IM	No	Yes
Serum sickness	Yes (partially)	Yes (completely)

PROCEDURE NOTES

The Davidsohn differential is performed only if the preliminary Paul-Bunnell test is positive in a titer of 1:56 or above. Serum sickness occurs as the result of sensitization to animal serum, usually horse serum.

SOURCES OF ERROR. Incorrect pipetting or the use of noninactivated serum can contribute to errors.

CLINICAL APPLICATIONS. The Davidsohn differential can distinguish between three types of heterophil antibodies.

LIMITATIONS. The test is time-consuming.

REFERENCES

Davidsohn I: Serologic diagnosis of infectious mononucleosis, *JAMA* 108:289, 1937.

◻ PROCEDURE

Monospot*

PRINCIPLE

This procedure is based on agglutination of horse erythrocytes by heterophil antibody present in infectious mononucleosis. Because horse red cells exhibit antigens directed against both Forssman and infectious mononucleosis antibodies, a differential absorption of the patient's serum is necessary to distinguish the specific heterophil antibody from those of the Forssman type. The basic principle of the absorption steps in this procedure is comparable to those originally described by Davidsohn in his sheep agglutinin test. Serum or plasma are absorbed with both guinea pig kidney and beef erythrocyte stroma. Guinea pig kidney contains only the Forssman antigen, and beef erythrocytes contain only the antigen associated with infectious mononucleosis. Guinea pig kidney will absorb only heterophil antibodies of the Forssman type, and beef erythrocytes will absorb only the heterophil antibody of infectious mononucleosis. Agglutination of horse red blood cells by the absorbed patient specimen is indicative of a positive reaction for heterophil antibody.

SPECIMEN COLLECTION AND PREPARATION

No special preparation of the patient is required prior to specimen collection. The patient must be positively identified when the specimen is collected. The specimen shall be labeled at the bedside and shall include the patient's full name, the date the specimen is collected, and the patient's hospital identification number. The phlebotomist's initials should also appear on the label.

Blood should be drawn by an aseptic technique. The required specimen is a minimum of 2 mL of whole blood. Serum or plasma mixed with anticoagulants including EDTA, sodium oxalate, potassium oxalate, sodium citrate, ACD solution, or heparin may be used.

Centrifuge the tube of blood and remove an aliquot of serum. Serum or plasma samples should be clear and particle-free. The presence of hemolysis makes the specimen unsuitable for testing. Inactivation of the serum is not necessary; however, inactivated serum may be used. Serum or plasma may be stored at 2° to 8° C for several days following collection before testing. If prolonged storage is desired, the serum or plasma may be frozen.

CAPILLARY SPECIMENS

1. Using a standard heparinized or nonheparinized capillary pipette (75 mm length, 1.1 mm to 1.2 mm inside diameter, 85 μL volume) obtain a minimum of four full capillary tubes of blood from a finger puncture. The required 0.05 mL of serum or plasma can be recovered by this procedure, if the patient's hematocrit is less than 50%. If the hematocrit is greater than 50% (e.g., newborn infants or patients with polycythemia), additional tubes must be collected.
2. Seal the dry end of each capillary tube and centrifuge for 5 minutes in a microhematocrit centrifuge.
3. Break the capillary tubes at the interface between the serum or plasma and the cells.
4. Use the serum or plasma from two tubes as the patient sample for each side of the slide according to the directions for use.

REAGENTS, SUPPLIES, AND EQUIPMENT

All of the following required materials are provided in the Monospot kit:

1. Guinea pig antigen. A suspension of guinea pig kidney antigen preserved with 1% sodium azide. Store at 2° to 8° C. Do not freeze. If properly stored, the reagent is stable until the expiration date.
2. Beef erythrocyte stroma. A suspension of beef erythrocyte stroma antigen preserved with 1% sodium azide. Store at 2° to 8° C. Do not freeze.

---

*Ortho Diagnostics, Raritan, NJ.

If properly stored, the reagent is stable until the expiration date.

3. Horse erythrocytes. A suspension of stabilized horse red blood cells preserved with 1:3000 chloramphenicol and 1:10,000 neomycin sulfate. Store at 2° to 8° C. Do not freeze. If properly stored, the reagent is stable until the expiration date. Hemolysis will indicate that the cells are deteriorating, but proper reactivity may be verified by use of the positive control serum.
   WARNING: The reagents and controls contain sodium azide as a preservative. Sodium azide may react with lead and copper plumbing to form highly explosive metal azides. Upon disposal, flush with a large volume of water to prevent azide buildup.
4. Glass slide
5. Microcapillary pipettes (20 lambda) for indicator cells
6. Rubber bulbs
7. Plastic pipettes for delivery of serum or plasma samples
8. Wooden applicator sticks
   ADDITIONAL REQUIRED EQUIPMENT
Stopwatch or laboratory timer

QUALITY CONTROL

Positive control serum (human). A human serum containing the heterophil antibody of IM, preserved with 0.1% sodium azide.

Negative control serum (human). A human serum not containing the heterophil antibody of IM, preserved with 0.1% sodium azide. The control sera should be checked when the kit arrives and periodically during the dating period.
   CAUTION: Because the control sera are derived from human sources, they should be handled in the same manner as clinical serum specimens (see *Universal blood and body fluid precautions* in Chapter 6).

PROCEDURE

NOTE: All of the reagent cells should be shaken well to provide a homogeneous suspension before testing. Reagents should be kept at room temperature.
   QUALITATIVE METHOD
1. Place the slide on a flat surface under a direct light source.
2. Invert the vial horse (indicator) erythrocytes to resuspend the cells. Using a clean microcapillary tube, place 10 lambda of cells on one corner of both squares on the slide.
   To use the microcapillary tube, insert the end of the pipette marked with a heavy black line one quarter inch into the neck of the rubber tube. Hold the rubber bulb between the thumb and the third finger. Tilt the vial of cells and insert the pipette. Allow the pipette to fill to the top (20 lambda)

mark by capillary action. *Do not draw the cells into the bulb.*
   To deliver 10 lambda of cells to the slide, place the index finger over the hole in the top of the bulb and squeeze gently until the level of cells in the pipette reaches the first mark. Touch the pipette tip to a corner of square I to release the cells. Repeat the process to deliver the remaining 10 lambda of cells to the corner of square II.
3. Put one drop of thoroughly mixed guinea pig antigen (reagent I) in square I.
4. Put one drop of thoroughly mixed beef erythrocyte stroma (reagent II) in square II.
5. Using a disposable plastic pipette, add one drop of the patient serum or plasma to the center of each square on the slide.
6. Mix the serum/plasma and the guinea pig antigen in square I at least 10 times with a clean wooden applicator stick. *Avoid the horse erythrocytes.*
7. Mix the serum/plasma and the beef erythrocyte stroma in square II at least 10 times with a clean wooden applicator stick. *Avoid the horse erythrocytes.*
8. Blend the horse (indicator) erythrocytes over the entire surface of each square. Use a clean wooden applicator for each side, and use no more than 10 stirring motions to blend.
9. Start a timer upon completion of the final mixing. Do not move or pick up the slide during the reaction period.
10. Observe for agglutination for no longer than 1 minute after the final mixing.

REPORTING RESULTS
   QUALITATIVE METHOD
Positive = If the agglutination pattern is stronger on the left side (square I), the test is positive.

Negative = If the agglutination pattern is stronger on the right side (square II), the test is negative.

If no agglutination appears on either side (I or II) of the slide, or if agglutination is equal on both squares of the slide, the test is negative.

PROCEDURE NOTES

If a positive qualitative result is demonstrated, a titration procedure may be performed to provide a semiquantitative indication of the level of heterophil antibody.
   TITRATION PROCEDURE FOR SEMIQUANTITATIVE METHOD
A. Serial dilutions of serum (see p. 209) can be prepared by pipetting 0.5 mL of 0.85% saline into each of the desired number of tubes. Pipette 0.5 mL of patient serum into the first tube, mix, and transfer 0.5 mL of the diluted serum to the second tube. Repeat this process unit the final tube is reached. Discard 0.5 mL of the diluted serum from the last tube.

Tube	Dilution
1	1:2
2	1:4
3	1:8
4	1:16
5	1:32
6	1:64

B. Place a titration slide on a flat surface under a direct light source. Treat each of the dilutions as if they were individual sera and follow the steps for the qualitative procedure for each of the appropriately labeled squares. *Omit the use of beef stroma, and use only guinea pig antigen.*

C. The highest dilution in which visible agglutination occurs is the end point. If agglutination is present in all of the dilutions, extend the serial dilutions. Record the titration value.

NOTE: the titer with Monospot *cannot* be compared with titration values obtained with other slide or tube test procedures because there are significant variations in sensitivity. Fresh, stabilized horse erythrocytes have been shown to be more sensitive than sheep erythrocytes or formalinized horse erythrocytes.

The relative value of titers performed on specimens with different techniques is proportional to the concentration of heterophil antibody present. Although the titration value is not indicative of the severity of the disease, sequential examinations may provide information of value to the clinician.

SOURCES OF ERROR. To obtain accurate results, only clear, particle-free serum or plasma specimens should be used.

False positive results can be caused by:

1. Observing agglutination after the 1 minute observation time.
2. Misinterpreting agglutination that occurs because the slide is moved or rocked.
3. Simultaneous occurrence of infectious mononucleosis and hepatitis has been reported. A result that may be interpreted as a false positive may be caused by residual heterophil antibody present after clinical symptoms have subsided.

CLINICAL APPLICATIONS. Infectious diseases such as influenza, rubella, and hepatitis may cause clinical symptoms that mimic infectious mononucleosis and present problems in diagnosis. Although the final diagnosis of infectious mononucleosis depends on clinical, hematologic, and serologic findings, a positive test result is indicative of the presence of the heterophil antibody specific for infectious mononucleosis.

LIMITATIONS. Because the clinical symptoms of infectious mononucleosis are similar to those of many other diseases, it is often difficult to disprove the theoretical possibility of a concomitant infection. In addition, seronegative infectious mononu-cleosis has been reported because of a delayed heterophil antibody response, it is possible that clinical and hematologic symptoms of infectious mononucleosis will appear before serologic confirmation is possible.

REFERENCES

Monospot Product Brochures, May 1984, Ortho Diagnostics, Raritan, NJ.

Chapter Review

HIGHLIGHTS

The Epstein-Barr virus (EBV) was first discovered in 1964 as the cause of infectious mononucleosis (IM). This disorder is usually an acute, benign, and self-limiting lymphoproliferative condition. EBV is also the cause of Burkitt's lymphoma (a malignant tumor of the lymphoid tissue occurring mainly in African children), nasopharyngeal carcinoma, and neoplasms of the thymus, parotid gland, and supraglottic larynx.

EBV is widely disseminated. It is estimated that 95% of the world's population is exposed to the virus, which makes it the most ubiquitous virus known to man. EBV is a human herpes DNA virus. In IM the virus infects B lymphocytes. Although EBV appears to be transmitted primarily by close contact with infectious oral-pharyngeal secretions, the virus has been reported to be transmitted by blood transfusion and transplacental routes. Under ordinary conditions transmission of the virus by transfusion or transplacental exposure is unlikely. The frequency of *seronegative* patients is nearly 100% in early infancy and declines with increasing age, more or less rapidly, depending on socioeconomic conditions, to less than 10% in young adults. After primary exposure a person is considered to be immune and generally no longer susceptible to overt reinfection. In Western society primary exposure to EBV occurs in two waves among children and adolescents. EBV is only a minor problem for immunocompetent persons, but it can become a major one for immunologically compromised patients.

The antibodies present in IM are heterophil and EBV antibodies. Heterophil antibodies comprise a broad class of antibodies. They are defined as antibodies that are stimulated by one antigen and react with an entirely unrelated surface antigen present on cells from different mammalian species. The IgM type of heterophil antibody usually appears during the acute phase of IM, but the antigen that stimulates its production remains unknown. EBV-infected B lymphocytes express a variety of "new" antigens encoded by the virus. Infection with EBV results in the expression of viral capsid antigen

(VCA), early antigen (EA), and nuclear antigen (NA), with corresponding antibody responses. Assays for IgM and IgG antibodies to these EBV antigens are available. EBV-specific serologic studies are beneficial in defining immune status, and their time of appearance may be indicative of the stage of disease. This can provide important information for both the diagnosis and management of EBV-associated disease.

REVIEW QUESTIONS

1. The Epstein-Barr virus can cause all the following *except:*
   A. Infectious mononucleosis
   B. Burkitt's lymphoma
   C. Nasopharyngeal carcinoma
   D. Neoplasms of the bone marrow
   E. Neoplasms of the thymus, parotid gland, and supraglottic larynx
2. The *primary* mode of EBV transmission is:
   A. Exposure to blood
   B. Exposure to oral-pharyngeal secretions
   C. Congenital transmission
   D. Fecal contamination of drinking water
   E. Exposure to infected urine
3. IgM heterophil antibody is characterized by all the following features *except:*
   A. Reacts with horse, ox, and sheep RBC
   B. Absorbed by beef erythrocytes
   C. Absorbed by guinea pig kidney cells
   D. Does not react with EBV-specific antigens
   E. Both B and D
4. Characteristics of EBV-infected lymphocytes include all the following *except:*
   A. B type
   B. Express viral capsid antigen
   C. Express early antigen
   D. Express nuclear antigen
   E. Express the EBV genome
5. Which of the following stages of IM infection is characterized by antibody to EBNA?
   A. No previous exposure
   B. Recent (acute) infection
   C. Past infection (convalescent) period
   D. Reactivation of latent infection
   E. Both C and D
6. Heterophil antibody can be found in patients with:
   A. No previous exposure
   B. Recent (acute) infection
   C. Past infection (convalescent) period
   D. Reactivation of latent infection
   E. Both B and D

Answers

1. D 2. B 3. C 4. E 5. E 6. E

BIBLIOGRAPHY

Andiman W: Use of cloned probes to detect Epstein-Barr viral DNA in tissues of patients with neoplastic and lymphoproliferative diseases, J Infect Dis 148:967-977, 1983.

Borysiewicz LK et al: Epstein-Barr virus–specific immune defects in patients with persistent symptoms following infectious mononucleosis, Q J Med 58:111-121, 1986.

Chretien JH et al: Predictors of the duration of infectious mononucleosis, South Med J 70:437-439, 1977.

Evans AS and Niederman JC: Epstein-Barr virus. In Evans AS, editor: Viral infections of human epidemiology and control, ed 2, New York, 1982, Plenum Medical.

Evans AS et al: A prospective evaluation of heterophile and Epstein-Barr virus specific antibodies in clinical and subclinical infectious mononucleosis: specificity and sensitivity of the tests and persistence of antibodies, J Infect Dis 132:546-554, 1975.

Fleisher GR: Epstein-Barr virus. In Belshe M, editor: Textbook of human virology, Littleton, Mass, 1984, PSG Publishing.

Fleisher GR et al: Primary Epstein-Barr virus infection in association with Reye Syndrome, J Pediatr 97:935-937, 1980.

Gallo D, Walen KH, and Riggs JL: Improved immunofluorescence antigens for detection of immunoglobulin M antibodies to Epstein-Barr viral capsid antigen and antibodies to Epstein-Barr virus nuclear antigen, J Clin Microbiol 15:243-248, 1982.

Geltosky JE, Smith RS, Whalley A, and Rhodes G: Use of a synthetic peptide-based ELISA for the diagnosis of infectious mononucleosis and other diseases, J Clin Lab Anal 1:153-162, 1987.

Gotlieb-Stematsky T and Glaser R: Association of Epstein-Barr virus with neurologic diseases. In Glaser R and Gotlieb-Stematsky T, editors: Human herpesvirus infections: clinical aspects, New York, 1982, Marcel Dekker.

Henle W and Henle G: Epstein-Barr virus and infectious mononucleosis, N Engl J Med 288:263-264, 1973.

Henle W and Henle G: Epstein-Barr virus and infectious mononucleosis. In Glaser R and Gotlieb-Stematsky T, editors: Human herpesvirus infections: clinical aspects, New York, 1982, Marcel Dekker.

Henle W and Henle G: Epstein-Barr virus and blood transfusions, Infection, immunity, and blood transfusion, New York, 1985, Alan R. Liss, Inc, pp 201-209.

Henle W et al: Antibodies to early antigens induced by Epstein-Barr virus in infectious mononucleosis, J Infect Dis 124:8-67, 1971.

Horwitz CA et al: Heterophil-negative infectious mononucleosis and mononucleosis-like illnesses: laboratory confirmation in 43 cases, Am J Med 63:947-957, 1977.

Horwitz CA et al: Long-term serological follow-up of patients for Epstein-Barr virus after recovery from infectious mononucleosis, J Infect Dis 151:1150-1153, 1985.

Lennette ET and Henle W: Epstein-Barr virus infections: clinical and serologic features, Lab Management 25:23-28, 1987.

Leyvraz S et al: Association of Epstein-Barr virus with thymic carcinoma, N Engl J Med 312:1296-1299, 1985.

Mandell GE, editor: Principles and practices of infectious disease, ed 2, New York, 1985, John Wiley & Sons.

Paul JR and Bunnell WW: The presence of heterophile antibodies in infectious mononucleosis, Am J Med Sci 183:90-104, 1932.

Ray CG, Hicks MJ, and Minnich LL: Viruses, rickettsia, and chlamydia. In Henry JB, editor: Clinical diagnosis and management by laboratory methods, Philadelphia, 1984, WB Saunders, pp 1290-1291.

Saemundsen AK et al: Epstein-Barr virus in nasopharyngeal and salivary gland carcinomas of Greenland Eskimoes, Br J Cancer 46:721-728, 1982.

Schmitz H: Acute Epstein-Barr virus infections in children, Med Microbiol Immunol 158:58-63, 1972.

Smith RS et al: A synthetic peptide for detecting antibodies to Epstein-Barr virus nuclear antigen in sera from patients with infectious mononucleosis, J Infect Dis 154:885-889, 1986.

Sumaya CV: Serological testing for Epstein-Barr virus—development in interpretation, J Infect Dis 151:984-987, 1985.

Sumaya CV: Epstein-Barr virus serologic testing: diagnostic indications and interpretations, Pediatr Infect Dis 5:337-342, 1986.

Sumaya CV: Infectious mononucleosis and other EBV infections: diagnostic factors, Lab Management 24:37-45, 1986.

Sumaya CV and Ench Y: Epstein-Barr virus infectious mononucleosis in children. I. Clinical and general laboratory findings, Pediatrics 75:1003-1010, 1985.

Sumaya CV and Ench Y: Epstein-Barr virus infectious mononucleosis in children. II. Heterophil antibody and viral-specific responses, Pediatrics 75:1011-1019, 1985.

Turgeon ML: Leukocytes: the lymphocytes and plasma cells. In Clinical hematology, Boston, 1988, Little, Brown & Co, pp 107-108.

Turgeon ML: Fundamentals of immunohematology, Philadelphia, 1989, Lea & Febiger, pp 388-390.

CHAPTER 19

Hepatitis

Viral hepatitis is the most common liver disease worldwide. Approximately one half of the population of Western society has serologic evidence of prior infection with viral hepatitis. The viral agents of acute hepatitis can be divided into two major groups: (1) primary hepatitis viruses: A, B, and non-A, non-B; and (2) secondary hepatitis viruses: Epstein-Barr virus, cytomegalovirus, Herpesvirus, and others.

Primary hepatitis viruses account for approximately 95% of the cases of hepatitis. These viruses are classified as primary hepatitis viruses because they attack primarily the liver and have little direct effect on other organ systems. The secondary viruses involve the liver secondarily in the course of systemic infection of another body system. The viruses for type A, type B, and delta agent as well as secondary viruses such as Epstein-Barr and cytomegalovirus have been isolated and identified. The hepatitis C virus has been recently associated with non-A, non-B hepatitis.

As a clinical disease hepatitis can occur in acute or chronic forms. The signs and symptoms of hepatitis are extremely variable. It can be mild, transient, and completely asymptomatic, or it can be severe, prolonged, and ultimately fatal. The course of viral hepatitis can take one of four forms (Table 19-1).

TABLE 19-1

Forms of Hepatitis

Form	Characteristics
Acute hepatitis	This form of hepatitis is the typical form with associated jaundice. It has four phases: *incubation, pre-icteric, icteric,* and *convalescence.* The incubation period, from the time of exposure and the first day of symptoms, ranges from a few days to many months. The average length of time is 75 days (range of 40-180 days) in hepatitis B.
Fulminant acute hepatitis	This rare form of hepatitis is associated with hepatic failure.
Subclinical hepatitis without jaundice	This form of hepatitis probably accounts for persons with demonstrable antibodies in their serum but no reported history of hepatitis.
Chronic hepatitis	This form of hepatitis is accompanied by hepatic inflammation and necrosis that lasts for at least 6 months. It occurs in about 10% of hepatitis B patients.

HEPATITIS A VIRUS
Etiology

The hepatitis A (HA) virus is a small RNA virus that belongs to the picornavirus class. The structure is a simple nonenveloped virus with a nucleocapsid designated as the hepatitis A antigen (HA Ag). Inside the capsid is a single molecule of single-stranded RNA. It is believed that the RNA has a positive polarity and that proteins are translated directly from the RNA.

Epidemiology

HA, formerly called *infectious hepatitis* or *short-incubation hepatitis*, is the most common form of hepatitis. Seroepidemiologic studies indicate that the prevalence of antibody in a given population increases with age, reaching approximately 40% of the U.S. population by age 50. In other parts of the world, more than 90% of adults have hepatitis A antibody.

Susceptibility to infection is independent of sex and race. Crowded, unsanitary conditions are a definite risk factor. The hepatitis A virus is transmitted by a fecal-oral route during the early phase of acute illness. Large outbreaks are usually traceable to a common source such as an infected food handler or contaminated water supply. It is noted for occurring in isolated outbreaks or as an epidemic, but it also may occur sporadically.

The incidence of HA is not increased among health care workers or in dialysis patients. HA is very rarely a transfusion-acquired hepatitis and only rarely causes fulminant acute hepatitis.

Signs and Symptoms

Nonimmune adult patients infected with HA virus will develop clinical symptoms within 2 to 6 weeks after exposure. Initially elevated serum enzymes are exhibited, with jaundice developing several days later. Many patients will be anicteric. Viremia and fecal shedding of virus disappear at the onset of jaundice. Although protracted illness lasting from 3 to 6 months can occur, protracted cholestasis has been described. A chronic carrier state and chronic hepatitis do not occur.

Immunologic Manifestation

Shortly after the onset of fecal shedding, an IgM antibody is detectable in serum followed within a few days by the appearance of an IgG antibody. IgM anti-HA is almost always detectable in patients with acute HA. IgG anti-HA peaks after the acute illness and remains detectable indefinitely, perhaps lifelong.

The finding of IgM anti-HA in a patient with acute viral hepatitis is highly diagnostic of acute HA. Demonstration of IgG anti-HA indicates previous infection. The presence of IgG anti-HA protects against subsequent infection with HA virus, but it is not protective against HBV or other viruses.

Diagnostic Evaluation

Testing methods for HA include:
1. Total antibody by enzyme immunoassay (EIA)
2. IgM antibody by radioimmunoassay (RIA)
3. HA antigen by radioimmunoassay (RIA)

The short period of viremia makes detection difficult. Specific IgM antibody (measured for total antibodies to HAV) persists for an indefinite time, although the antibody level decreases to undetectable levels in those who are infected when they are very young. Specific IgG antibody apparently protects an individual from symptomatic infection, but specific IgM may increase with reinfection.

Prevention

After close personal contact with a person with hepatitis A or if traveling to an endemic area, individuals should receive immune globulin intramuscularly. If a person remains in an endemic area for more than 3 months, he/she should receive immune globulin injections every 5 months.

HEPATITIS B
Etiology

Hepatitis B virus (HBV), formerly called the Australia or hepatitis-associated antigen, was discovered in 1966. This discovery permitted characterization of the biochemical and epidemiologic characterization of the virus.

HBV is a complex DNA virus that belongs to a new class called the hepadna viruses. The intact virus is a double-shelled particle referred to as the *Dane particle* (Fig. 19-1). It has an outer surface structure, hepatitis B surface antigen (HB$_s$Ag), and an inner core component, the hepatitis B core antigen (HB$_c$Ag). Inside this core is the viral genome, a single molecule of partially double-stranded deoxyribonucleic acid (DNA).

The unique structure of the DNA of HBV is one of the distinguishing characteristics of the hepadna class of viruses. The DNA is circular and double-stranded, but one of the strands is incomplete, leaving a single-stranded or gap region that comprises 10% to 50% of the total length of the molecule. The other DNA strand is nicked (the 3 and 5 ends are not joined). The entire DNA molecule is small, and all the genetic information for producing both

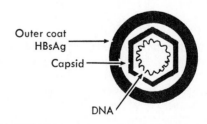

FIGURE 19-1

The hepatitis B virus (Dane particle).
(From Bauer JD: Clinical laboratory methods, ed 9, St Louis, 1982, The CV Mosby Co.)

the surface and core antigens is on the complete strand. In addition to the DNA configuration, the core of the virus also contains an enzyme that is a DNA-dependent DNA polymerase. This polymerase acts to complete the single-stranded region of the DNA.

Epidemiology

HBV infection was previously called *serum hepatitis* or *long incubation hepatitis*. This name was partially derived from the fact that the causative agent is a blood-borne pathogen. Soon after the discovery of HBV, the relationship between the presence of the antigen in donor blood and posttransfusion hepatitis was documented. In the past, HBV infection was one of the most frequent clinical infections transmitted by blood transfusion.

HBV does not seem capable of penetrating the skin or mucous membranes; therefore some break in these barriers is required for disease transmission. HBV is largely a disease spread by the parenteral route through blood transfusion, needlestick accidents, and contaminated needles, although the virus can be transmitted in the absence of obvious parenteral exposure. About half of the patients with acute type B hepatitis have a history of parenteral exposure. Inapparent parenteral exposure involves close intimate or sexual contact with an infectious individual. HBV has been found in saliva, semen, and other biologic fluids of HBV carriers. Urine and stool are not believed to be infectious.

The incidence of transfusion-acquired HBV has been severely reduced since high-risk donor groups, such as paid donors, prison inmates, and military recruits, have been eliminated as a major source of donated blood. This shift to an all-voluntary donor supply probably accounts for a 50% to 60% reduction in transfusion-related hepatitis. The overall incidence of HBV, however, is high among patients who have received multiple transfusions or blood components prepared from multiple donor plasma pools, dialysis patients, drug addicts, and medical personnel.

Signs and Symptoms

A number of factors, for example, the dose of the agent and an individual's immunologic host response ability, influence the clinical course of the infection.

Asymptomatic Infection

The most frequent clinical response to HBV is an asymptomatic or subclinical infection. In patients developing clinical symptoms of transfusion-associated hepatitis B, jaundice and abnormal serum enzymes, transaminase (ALT/SGPT) levels can be manifested from a few weeks to up to 6 months after a single transfusion episode. There is, however, rarely any doubt about the diagnosis in patients with a classic serologic response associated with HBV, even in the absence of significant symptoms. Diagnosis is more difficult to make in asymptomatic patients with negative HBV serology, who develop a mild elevation of serum enzyme, transaminase, levels a few weeks after a transfusion. Elevated enzyme levels may persist for 1 or 2 weeks.

Chronic Infection

HBV leads to chronic infection, and these patients have been shown to have the viral DNA actually incorporated into their liver cells' DNA. This integration may be an important factor in the eventual development of liver cell cancer, hepatocellular carcinoma, a well-known long-term outcome of chronic HBV infection.

Carrier State

Carriers can be divided into two categories based on differing infectivity, depending on the presence in their serum of another antigen, hepatitis Be antigen (HB$_e$Ag), or its antibody, (anti-HBe). The types of carrier states include:
1. The more commonly identified carriers have anti-HBe in their serum and are at a later stage of infection. Anti-HBe carriers are less infectious but may transmit infection through blood transfusion. HB$_s$Ag positive carriers will become anti-HBe positive carriers at a rate of about 5% to 10% per year. All HB$_s$Ag positive individuals must be excluded from giving blood for transfusion.
2. About one in four carriers has HB$_e$Ag in his/her serum. It is likely that these individuals have recently become carriers and their blood is highly infectious.

Immunologic Manifestation

The incidence of serologic markers for HBV exposure is 3.5% to 10% in the general population and 60% to 68% for homosexuals. Several serologic markers for HBV infection have been defined (Table 19-2):
1. Hepatitis B surface antigen (HB$_s$Ag)
2. Hepatitis Be antigen (HB$_e$Ag)
3. Antibody to the hepatitis B core antigen (anti-HBc)
4. Antibody to hepatitis Be antigen (anti-HBe)
5. Antibody to hepatitis B surface antigen (anti-HBs)

Hepatitis B Surface Antigen

The initial detectable marker found in serum during the incubation period of HBV infection is hepatitis B surface antigen (HB$_s$Ag). The titer of HB$_s$Ag rises and generally peaks at or shortly after the onset of elevated serum enzymes, for example, ALT/SGPT. Clinical improvement of the patient's condition and a decrease in serum enzyme concentrations are paralleled by a fall in the titer of HB$_s$Ag, which subsequently disappears. There is, however, variability in the duration of HB$_s$Ag positivity and in the relationship between clinical recovery and the disappearance of HB$_s$Ag (Fig. 19-2).

Among persons infected with HBV with detectable HB$_s$Ag in their serum, not all of the HB$_s$Ag represents complete Dane particles. HB$_s$Ag positive serum also contains two other viruslike structures. These viruslike structures are incomplete spherical and tubular forms, consisting entirely of HB$_s$Ag and devoid of any HB$_c$Ag, DNA, or DNA polymerase. The incomplete HB$_s$Ag particles can be present in serum in extremely high concentrations and form the bulk of the circulating HB$_s$Ag.

Hepatitis Be Antigen

A hepatitis B-related antigen, the hepatitis Be antigen (HB$_e$Ag), is found in the serum of some patients who are HB$_s$Ag positive. It is rarely found in the absence of HB$_s$Ag. HB$_e$Ag appears to be associated with the HBV core; however, the relationship between HB$_e$Ag and the structure of HBV is unclear. HB$_e$Ag appears to be a reliable marker for the presence of high levels of virus and a high degree of infectivity.

TABLE 19-2

Serologic Markers for Hepatitis B Virus (HBV) Infection

	Early (asymptomatic)	Acute or chronic	Low-level carrier	Immediate recovery	Long after infection	Immunized with HB$_s$Ag
HB$_s$Ag	+	+	−	−	−	−
Anti-HBs	−	−/+	−	−	−/+	+
Anti-HBc	−	+	+	+	−/+	−
Anti-HBc (IgM)	−	+	−	+	−	−

Modified from Hoofnagle JH: Type A and type B hepatitis, Lab Med 14(11):713, 1983.

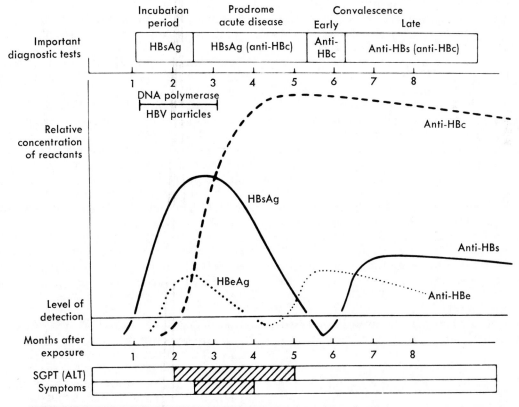

FIGURE 19-2

Serologic and clinical patterns observed during acute hepatitis B viral infection.
(From Hollinger FB and Dreesman GR. In Rose NR and Friedman H, editors: Manual of clinical immunology, ed 2, Washington, DC, 1980, American Society for Microbiology.)

Hepatitis B Core Antibody

During the course of most HBV infections, HB_sAg forms immune complexes with the antibodies produced as part of the recovery process. Because the HB_sAg contained in these complexes is usually undetectable, HB_sAg disappears from the serum of up to 50% of symptomatic patients. During this phase an indicator of a recent hepatitis B infection is anti-HBc, the antibody to the core antigen. The period of time between the disappearance of detectable HB_sAg and the appearance of detectable antibody to HB_sAg (anti-HBs) is called the *anti-core window* or hidden antigen phase of hepatitis B virus infection. This window phase may last for a few weeks, several months, or a year; during this time anti-HBc may be the only serologic marker. Anti-HBc occurs in 3% to 5% of persons. Of 100 anti-HBc positive persons, 97 will have anti-HBs, 2 will have HB_sAg, and 1 may have only anti-HBc.

Antibodies to HB_eAg and HB_sAg

Antibodies to HB_eAg (anti-HBe) and Hb_sAg (anti-HBs) develop during convalescence and recovery from HBV infection. The development of anti-HBe in a case of acute hepatitis is the first serologic evidence of the convalescent phase. Antibody to HB_sAG (anti-HBs), unlike anti-HBc and anti-HBe, does not arise during the acute disease; it is manifested during convalescence. Anti-HBs is a serologic marker of recovery and immunity. Anti-HBs is probably the major protective antibody in this disease. Thus hepatitis B immune globulin is so named because it contain high levels of anti-HBs.

Diagnostic Evaluation

Appropriate diagnostic procedures should be ordered depending on clinical factors, such as patient history, signs and symptoms, being evaluated, or in cases of donated blood. The various components of HBV infection can be measured by laboratory assay (see box).

HB_sAg

The initial laboratory screening procedure for hepatitis was for the detection of HB_sAg. This procedure screens for the presence of the major coatprotein of the virus (HB_sAg) in serum and is considered to be the most reliable method of choice for preventing the transmission of HBV via blood. The presence of HB_sAg indicates active HBV infection, either acute or chronic.

Test protocols for Hb_sAg range from immunodiffusion and its electrophoretic modifications to solid-phase assays including reverse passive hemagglutination (RPHA), radioimmunoassay (RIA), which is more correctly called immunoradiometric assay (IRMA), enzyme-linked immunosorbent assay (ELISA), and immunofluorescent assay (IFA). One of the most popular methods is the Ayszyme II EIA (Enzyme Immuno Assay) procedure.

In the Ayszyme II (Abbott Laboratories) EIA test for hepatitis B surface antigen, 200 µL of the serum sample is added to the assigned well. Beads coated with hepatitis B surface antibody are incubated for 30 minutes at 38° to 41° C, washed, and incubated with goat antibody to HB_sAg conjugated with horseradish peroxidase. The beads are washed again and transferred to assay tubes to which the substrate of o-phenylenediamine-2.HCl is added. The addition of hydrochloric acid stops the enzyme reaction. As in the other tests, the color change is read spectrophotometrically at 492 nm, and the reactivity is calculated against controls included in each test run.

Anti-HBc

Testing for antibody to the core of the virus (anti-HBc) may provide some additional advantage, since it may lead to the identification of a person recently recovered from a hepatitis B virus infection, who may still be infectious.

An anti-HBc test is the Corzyme (Abbott Laboratories) EIA test. In this method 200 µL of antibody to hepatitis B core antigen–horseradish perioxidase conjugate is added to each sample well. Then 100 µL of the serum sample is added to each well. Beads coated with hepatitis B core antigen are incubated for 2 hours at 40° C with the serum sample anti-HBc mixture, washed, and transferred to assay tubes to which an O-phenylenediamine-2.HCl substrate is added. The enzyme reaction is stopped by the addition of sulfuric acid. The color change is then read spectrophotometrically at 492 nm, and the reactivity is calculated against controls included in each test run.

The most recent assay to be developed is the test for IgM antibody to hepatitis B core antigen (anti-HBc IgM). This test is considered to be a reliable marker during the so-called core window period, when most other markers may be absent. The IgM anti-HBc titer rises rapidly in the acute phase and becomes negative in most patients in 3 to 9 months, although it may persist for many years.

Interrelationship of Test Results

If HB_sAg is negative and anti-HBc is positive, the anti-HBs will confirm previous HBV infection or immunity. The presence of anti-HBc IgM in the absence of HB_sAg in the serum indicates a recent HBV infection. An absence of IgM anti-HBc in the presence of HB_sAg and HB_eAg suggests high infectivity in chronic HBV disease; the presence of anti-HBe in this situation indicates low infectivity.

A vaccine-type response includes test results that are negative for anti-HBc and positive for anti-

---

Enzyme Immunoassay Measurement of HBV
Serologic Markers

HB_sAg	IgM anti-HBc
Total anti-HBs	HB_eAg
Total anti-HBc	Anti-HBe

HBs. In evaluation of individuals prior to vaccination, positive results for both anti-HBc and anti-HBs should be required as proof of immunity, especially if the result for anti-HBs displays a low positive reaction. Because there is a positive relationship between the amount of HB_sAg present and a positive reaction for HB_eAg, testing for HB_eAg is usually not necessary except in pregnant women. In these cases a positive HB_sAg during pregnancy results in an 80% to 90% risk of infection in the newborn in the absence of prophylaxis.

Prevention

The use of the vaccine against hepatitis B licensed in 1982 is warranted for high-risk persons. Among those who are at high risk of contracting HBV are medical personnel who handle blood specimens.

Vaccination offers a new approach to preventing transfusion-acquired hepatitis in patients who are likely to need ongoing transfusion therapy, such as nonimmune patients with hemophilia, sickle cell anemia, or aplastic anemia. In cases of accidental needlestick exposure or exposure of mucous membranes or open cuts to HB_sAg positive blood, hepatitis B immune globulin (HBIG) should be administered within 24 hours of exposure and again 25 to 30 days later. Infants born to mothers with acute hepatitis B in the third trimester or with HB_sAg at the time of delivery should be given HBIG as soon as possible and no later than 24 hours after birth. Persons who are either HB_sAg positive or who have anti-HBs need not be given HBIG.

The most important factors in preventing transfusion-acquired HBV are donor interviewing, screening of donor blood, the use of hepatitis-free products when possible, or the appropriate use of blood and blood components. Elimination of high-risk donors has accounted for at least a 50% reduction in the incidence of hepatitis, and routine testing of donated blood for HB_sAg has further reduced the incidence by another 20% to 30%. Testing for anti-HBc will detect almost 100% of Hb_sAg positive persons, the rare asymptomatic donor who is in the core window, and the large number of donors who have had subclinical hepatitis B infections and are now immune. In addition, the avoidance of high-risk blood components, such as untreated factor VIII prepared from multiple donor pools, reduces the incidence of HBV.

DELTA HEPATITIS
Etiology

The *delta agent* was first described in 1977 as a pathogen that "superinfects" some patients who are already infected with HBV. HBV is required as a "helper" to initiate delta infection. Only persons with acute or chronic HBV infection as demonstrated by serum HB_sAg can be infected with delta agent.

The delta agent is a defective or incomplete RNA virus that is unable by itself to cause infection. Delta agent consists of viral RNA coated in HB_sAg produced by HBV, its "helper" virus. This agent is unique because it can replicate only in HBV infected hosts. Therefore the delta virus infects only patients who are HB_sAg positive.

Epidemiology

In Italy and the Middle East, delta infection is common and found in HB_sAg carriers. In the United States, northern Europe, and Asia, infection is uncommon and occurs only in individuals with multiple parenteral exposures, such as hemophiliacs and intravenous drug addicts.

Signs and Symptoms

Delta infection may be benign and brief, but fulminate hepatitis and chronic hepatitis are being attributed with increasing frequency to the delta agent. Chronic delta infection is associated with increased hepatic damage and a more severe clinical course than is expected from chronic HBV infection alone. The occurrence of sequential attacks of HBV in the same patient is probably attributable in most cases to delta infection superimposed on a previous acute HBV infection.

Infection with delta agent can occur in several conditions, and the symptoms would be typical of either acute or chronic hepatitis. These situations are:
1. Acute delta hepatitis with a concurrent acute type B hepatitis
2. Acute delta hepatitis in a chronic HB_sAg carrier
3. Chronic delta hepatitis in a chronic HB_sAg carrier

Immunologic Manifestation

The delta agent probably partially suppresses HBV replication. Delta infection is diagnosed by the appearance of delta antigen in serum or by development of IgM or IgG anti-delta antibodies that appear sequentially in a timeframe similar to that described for hepatitis A or B antibodies.

Diagnostic Evaluation

The delta agent appears in the circulating blood as a particle with a core of delta antigen and a surface component of HB_sAg. A person with delta hepatitis will have detectable delta antigen in the liver and antibody to the delta agent in the serum. Test methodologies for delta agent include:
1. Total antibody by enzyme immunoassay (EIA)
2. IgM assay by radioimmunoassay (RIA)
3. Antigen detection by double immunodiffusion (DIF)

In addition, delta agent antigen can be demonstrated in liver biopsies by direct immunofluorescence (DIF) and immunoperoxidase (IP) and in serum by cloned DNA (cDNA). The importance of detection of antibodies to delta agent is largely prognostic. Detection of IgG anti-delta in the presence of IgM anti-HBc antibody strongly suggests simultaneous infection (coinfection). Detection of IgM anti-delta in a patient with chronic HBV infection is evidence of HDV superinfection.

Screening for total anti-delta antibodies in serum is important in the identification of a subpopulation of apparently healthy HB_sAg carriers whose risk of serious liver damage is fourfold higher than that in anti-delta negative carriers. The combined presence of total anti-delta antibody plus abnormal liver function tests in a symptom-free carrier suggests parenchymal damage and is considered an indication for liver biopsy. Hepatic lesions in anti-delta positive carriers often consists of chronic active hepatitis or advanced cirrhosis. A positive test result for IgM anti-delta increases the likelihood of occult active HBV infection.

NON-A, NON-B HEPATITIS
Etiology

Non-A, non-B (NANB) hepatitis was first recognized in 1974. In the past, NANB hepatitis was diagnosed if the other primary causes, such as hepatitis A (HA) and hepatitis B (HBV) and the secondary causes of hepatitis such as Epstein-Barr virus (EBV) could be excluded.

Recently the genome of a NANB agent, designated the hepatitis C virus (HCV), has been cloned and a recombinant-based assay for HCV antibodies has been developed. The data suggest that HCV is a major cause of chronic NANB hepatitis throughout the world. With a specific and sensitive antibody test and the availability of HCV hybridization probes, it should be possible to address the issue of whether other parenteral NANB hepatitis agents exist.

Epidemiology

Transmission of the virus or viruses is by both parenteral and nonparenteral routes. Blood or blood component transfusions and accidental needlesticks comprise a clearly documented route of transmission. Blood donors as well as patients incubating acute NANB are primary sources in the transmission of this blood-borne pathogen. NANB hepatitis is the principal cause of posttransfusion hepatitis and is the major source of hepatitis among dialysis patients. In cases of posttransfusion hepatitis, NANB is believed to be responsible for 80% to 90% of these cases.

Epidemic water-borne acute NANB hepatitis has an epidemiology similar to that of HA virus. Between 25% to 50% of sporadic hepatitis cases in the United States that are unrelated to parenteral exposure are of the NANB type. A chronic carrier state also exists.

Signs and Symptoms

In the past, the diagnosis of NANB hepatitis was one of exclusion in patients with hepatitis in the absence of evidence of other causes. NANB more closely resembles HBV than HA in regard to transmission and clinical features. NANB, like HBV, can be acute, ranging from mild anicteric illness to ful-

minant disease. Less than 25% of patients develop jaundice.

A number of different patterns of NANB hepatitis exist. Transfusion-associated NANB can be divided into short and long incubation types, with incubation periods of short duration ranging from 1 or 2 to 5 weeks and of longer duration ranging from 7 to 12 weeks to 6 months or longer.

The diagnosis of NANB hepatitis has a guarded prognosis. Between 20% to 40% of patients with this disease will become chronic carriers or develop chronic active hepatitis followed by a progressive disease eventually leading to cirrhosis.

Immunologic Manifestation

In the absence of a specific antibody assay, surrogate testing using serum transaminase and the absence of HA and HBV markers have been used. Elevated serum transaminase levels and the absence of serologic markers, however, are of little value in diagnosing or monitoring individual patients.

In 1989, an assay for circulating antibodies to a major etiologic virus of human NANB hepatitis was reported. In this specific assay for blood-borne NANB hepatitis virus, a polypeptide synthesized in recombinant yeast clones of hepatitis C virus (HCV) is used to capture circulating antibodies. Preliminary studies by Kuo et al[*] demonstrated that 10 cases of transfusion-acquired NANB seroconverted during their illness. In addition, the same study found that 58% of NANB hepatitis patients from the United States with no identifiable source of parenteral exposure to HCV were also positive for HCV antibody.

Diagnostic Evaluation

In the absence of serologic markers, surrogate testing procedures have been instituted. Surrogate procedures consist of transaminase enzyme (alanine aminotransferase ALT/SGPT) and hepatitis B core antibody testing.

Many NANB infections are detected by a mild elevation of the concentration of the serum enzyme, transaminase. An elevation of the ALT/SGPT is usually defined as a value that is 2.5 times the upper limit of normal on two or more separate occasions. In studies of blood donors, one center demonstrated that the chance of NANB occurring in a recipient was eight times greater if the donor's serum ALT was greater than 45 IU/L above normal. In this same study, however, 62% of transfusion-acquired NANB hepatitis cases occurred in recipients of blood that were below the cutoff value. Therefore the predictive effectiveness of ALT screening is difficult to assess. In addition, the test is not specific and is influenced by a large number of physiologic variables. Elevation of ALT can be

---

[*]Kuo G et al: An assay for circulating antibodies to a major etiologic virus of human Non-A, Non-B hepatitis. Science 244:4902, April 1989, pp 362-364.

TABLE 19-3

Characteristics of Viral Hepatitis

	Type A Travelers	Type B Hospital personnel	Delta	Non-A, Non-B Posttransfusion
Agent	Hepatitis A	Hepatitis B	Delta agent	Hepatitis C (one agent recently identified)
Antigens	RNA HA Ag	DNA HB$_s$Ag, HB$_c$Ag, HB$_e$Ag, HB$_c$Ag	RNA Delta	DNA HCV
Antibodies	Anti-HAV	Anti-HBs, Anti-HBc, Anti-HBe	Anti-delta	Anti HCV
Epidemiology	Fecal-oral	Parenteral	Parenteral	Parenteral and nonparenteral
Incubation period (in days)	15-45	40-180	30-50	15-150

Modified from Hoofnagle JH: Type A and type B hepatitis, Lab Med 14(11):715, 1983.

the result of a variety of causes such as medications, alcohol intake, and obesity.

The relationship between the presence of antibody to hepatitis B core antigen (anti-HBc) in donor blood and the development of hepatitis in recipients of that blood has been studied. Of 193 recipients of at least 1 unit of blood positive for anti-HBc, 11.9% developed NANB hepatitis compared with 4.2% of recipients of only anti-HBc negative blood. In addition, donor anti-HBc status was not significantly associated with the development of hepatitis B. The significance of using the anti-HBc assay as a surrogate marker for NANB hepatitis remains unclear.

In the foreseeable future, HCV antibody testing will be implemented in the testing of blood donors. This should significantly reduce the risk of blood-borne transmission of hepatitis C.

Prevention

Preventive practices among health care workers to avoid needlestick injuries should be exercised. Recent investigations have shown that removing blood from donors with anti-HB$_c$Ag from the blood supply may reduce the incidence of posttransfusion NANB. As an alternative there is some evidence that it may be possible to identify donors belonging to "high-risk" populations, but it is questionable if using anti-HBc as a marker for high-risk donors is generally applicable.

Chapter Review

HIGHLIGHTS

Viral hepatitis is the most common liver disease worldwide. Approximately one half of the population of Western society has serologic evidence of prior infection with viral hepatitis. The viral agents of acute hepatitis can be divided into two major groups: (1) primary hepatitis viruses A, B, and non-

A, non-B, and (2) secondary hepatitis viruses, including Epstein-Barr virus, cytomegalovirus, *Herpesvirus*, and others. Primary hepatitis viruses account for approximately 95% of the cases of hepatitis. These viruses are classified as primary hepatitis viruses because they attack primarily the liver and have little direct effect on other organ systems. The secondary viruses involve the liver secondarily in the course of systemic infection of another body system. The viruses for type A, type B and delta agent as well as the secondary viruses have been isolated and identified. One of the agents that cause non-A, non-B hepatitis has been recently identified. As a clinical disease hepatitis can occur in an acute or chronic forms. The signs and symptoms of hepatitis are extremely variable. The disease can be mild, transient, and completely asymptomatic, or it can be severe, prolonged, and ultimately fatal.

Hepatitis A (HA) virus is a small RNA virus. HA, formerly called infectious hepatitis or short-incubation hepatitis, is the most common form of hepatitis. Shortly after the onset of fecal shedding, an IgM antibody is detectable in serum followed within a few days by the appearance of an IgG antibody.

Hepatitis B virus (HBV), previously called the Australian antigen or hepatitis-associated antigen, was discovered in 1966. HBV is a complex DNA virus that belongs to a new class called the hepadna viruses. The intact virus is a double-shelled particle referred to as the Dane particle. HBV infection was previously called *serum hepatitis* or *long incubation*. This name was partially derived from the fact that the causative agent is a blood-borne pathogen. Soon after discovery of HBV, the relationship between the presence of the antigen in donor blood and posttransfusion hepatitis was documented. In the past, HBV infection was one of the most frequent clinical infections transmitted by blood transfusion. HBV does not seem capable of penetrating through intact skin or mucous membranes, and it is mostly a disease spread by the parenteral route through blood transfusion, needlestick accidents, and contaminated needles. The most frequent clinical response to HBV is an asymptomatic or subclinical infection. In patients developing clinical symptoms of transfusion-associated hepatitis B, jaundice and abnormal serum enzymes can be manifested from a few weeks to up to 6 months after a single transfusion episode. There is, however, rarely any doubt about the diagnosis in patients with a classic serologic response associated with HBV, even in the absence of significant symptoms. HBV leads to chronic infection, and these patients have been shown to have the viral DNA actually incorporated into their liver cells' DNA. This integration may be an important factor in the eventual development of liver cell cancer, hepatocellular carcinoma. Carriers of HBV can be divided into two categories based on differing infectivity, depending on the presence of another antigen, hepatitis Be antigen (HB_eAg) or its antibody (anti-HBe) in their serum.

The initial detectable marker found in serum during the incubation period of HBV infection is HB_sAg. A hepatitis B–related antigen, the hepatitis B e antigen (HB_eAg), is found in the serum of some patients who are HB_sAg positive. It is rarely found in the absence of HB_sAg. HB_sAg appears to be associated with the HBV core; however, the relationship between HB_eAg and the structure of HBV is unclear. HB_eAg appears to be a reliable marker for the presence of high levels of virus and a high degree of infectivity. During the course of most HBV infections, Hb_sAg forms immune complexes with the antibodies produced as part of the recovery process. Because the HB_sAg contained in these complexes is usually undetectable, HB_sAg disappears from the serum of up to 50% of symptomatic patient. During this phase, an indicator of a recent hepatitis B infection is anti-HBc, the antibody to the core antigen. The period of time between the disappearance of detectable HB_sAg and the appearance of detectable antibody to HB_sAg (anti-HBs) is called the anti–core window or hidden antigen phase of hepatitis B virus infection. Antibodies to HB_eAg (anti-HBe) and Hb_sAg (anti-HBs) develop during convalescence and recovery from HBV infection. The development of anti-HBe in a case of acute hepatitis is the first serologic evidence of the convalescent phase. Antibody to HB_sAG (anti-HBs), unlike anti-HBc and anti-HBe, does not arise during the acute disease; it is manifested during convalescence. Anti-HBs is a serologic marker of recovery and immunity. Anti-HBs is probably the major protective antibody in this disease. Thus hepatitis B immune globulin is so named because it contains high levels of anti-HBs.

The delta agent was first described in 1977 as a pathogen that "superinfects" some patients who are already infected with HBV. HBV is required as a "helper" to initiate delta infection. Only persons with acute or chronic HBV infection as demonstrated by serum HB_sAg can be infected with delta agent. The delta agent is a defective or incomplete RNA virus that is unable by itself to cause infection. The delta agent appears in the circulating blood as a particle with a core of delta antigen and a surface component of HB_sAg. A person with delta hepatitis will have detectable delta antigen in the liver and antibody to the delta agent in the serum. Test methodologies for delta agent include total antibody by enzyme immunoassay (EIA), IgM assay by radioimmunoassay (RIA), and antigen detection by double immunodiffusion (DIF). In addition, delta agent antigen can be demonstrated in liver biopsies by direct immunofluorescence (DIF) and immunoperoxidase (IP) and in serum by cloned DNA (cDNA). The importance of detection of antibodies to delta agent is largely prognostic. Detection of IgG anti-delta in the presence of IgM anti-HBc antibody strongly suggests simultaneous infection (coinfection). Detection of IgM anti-delta in a patient with chronic HBV infection is evidence of HBV superinfection.

Non-A, non-B (NANB) hepatitis was first recognized in 1974. In the past other primary and secondary causes of hepatitis were excluded before non-A, non-B hepatitis was considered. One of the agents responsible for NANB hepatitis has been recently identified. Epidemiologic studies, however, suggest that at least two forms of non-A, non-B hepatitis exist, which may indicate that more than one viral agent is responsible for NANB hepatitis. Transmission of the virus or viruses is by both parenteral and nonparenteral routes. Blood or blood component transfusions and accidental needlesticks comprise a clearly documented route of transmission. In the absence of serologic markers, surrogate testing procedures were instituted. Surrogate procedures consist of transaminase enzyme (alanine aminotransferase ALT/SGPT) and hepatitis B core antibody testing. An assay for HCV antibody has been recently developed.

REVIEW QUESTIONS

Questions 1-4
Match each of the following forms of hepatitis with its representative description.
1. Acute hepatitis
2. Fulminant acute hepatitis
3. Subclinical hepatitis without jaundice
4. Chronic hepatitis
   A. This rare form is associated with hepatic failure
   B. Typical form of hepatitis with associated jaundice
   C. Probably accounts for persons with serum antibodies but no history of hepatitis
   D. Accompanied by hepatic inflammation and necrosis

Match (use an answer only once)

5. Hepatitis A
6. Hepatitis B

7. Delta hepatitis
8. Non-A, non-B hepatitis

A. Intact virus is the Dane particle
B. Transmission by both parenteral and nonparenteral routes
C. Requires HBV as a helper
D. Most common form of hepatitis

Match (use an answer only once)

9. Hepatitis A

10. Hepatitis B
11. Delta agent
12. Non-A, non-B hepatitis

A. Should receive immunoglobin intramuscularly after exposure
B. A defective or incomplete RNA virus
C. Has an epidemiology similar to HA virus
D. Previously called Australian antigen

Match
13. HBs Ag
14. HBe Ag
15. Anti-HBc
16. Anti-HBe
17. Anti-HBs

A. Indicator of recent HBV infection may be only serologic marker during the window phase
B. Found in the serum of some patients who are HBs Ag positive; marker for level of virus, infectivity
C. A serologic marker of recovery and immunity
D. Initial detectable marker found in serum during incubator period of HBV infection
E. Antibody to HBs Ag; does not arise during acute disease

Answers

1. B 2. A 3. C 4. D 5. D 6. A 7. C 8. B 9. A 10. D
11. B 12. C 13. D 14. B 15. A 16. E 17. C

BIBLIOGRAPHY

Ahtone J and Maynard JE: Laboratory diagnosis of hepatitis B, JAMA 249:2067-2069, 1983.

Alter HJ and Holland PV: Indirect test to detect the non-A, non-B hepatitis carrier state, Ann Intern Med 101:859-861, 1984.

An assay for circulating antibodies to a major etiologic virus of human non-A, non-B hepatitis, JAMA 262:13, 1989.

Arico S et al: Clinical significance of antibody to the hepatitis delta virus in symptomless HB$_s$Ag carriers, Lancet 2:356-358, 1985.

Baker CH and Brennan JM: Keeping health-care workers healthy: legal aspects of hepatitis B immunization programs, N Engl J Med 311:684-688, 1984.

Chaudhary RK: Detection of hepatitis A virus by a modified commercial radioimmunoassay, Am J Clin Pathol 81:337-338, 1984.

De Cock KM et al: Delta hepatitis in the Los Angeles area: a report of 126 cases, Ann Intern Med 105:108-114, 1986.

Farci P et al: Diagnostic and prognostic significance of the IgM antibody to the hepatitis delta virus, JAMA 255:1443-1446, 1986.

Feinstone SM and Hoofnagle JJ: Non-A, maybe-B hepatitis, N Engl J Med 311:185-189, 1984.

Hegarty J and Williams R: Chronic hepatitis in the 1980s, Br Med J 290:877-878, 1985.

Khan NC and Hollinger FB: Non-A, non-B hepatitis agent, Lancet 1:41, 1986.

Koziol DE et al: Antibody to hepatitis B core antigen as a paradoxical marker for non-A, non-B hepatitis agents in donated blood, Ann Intern Med 104:488-495, 1986.

Kuo G et al: An assay for circulating antibodies to a major etiologic virus of human non-A, non-B hepatitis, Science 244:4902, 1989.

Lemon SM: Type A viral hepatitis: new developments in an old disease, N Engl J Med 313:1059-1067, 1985.

Nicholson KG: Hepatitis delta infections, Br Med J 290:1370-1371, 1985.

Rizzetto M and Verme G: Delta hepatitis—present status, J Hepatology 1:187-193, 1985.

Seto B et al: Detection of reverse transcriptase activity in association with the non-A, non-B hepatitis agents(s), Lancet 2:941-943, 1982.

Smedile A et al: Radioimmunoassay detection of IgM antibodies to the HBV-associated delta antigen: clinical significance in delta infection, J Med Virol 9:131-138, 1982.

Soloway HB: Hepatitis panels revised, Diagn Med 5(4):23-26, 1985.

Stevenson EE et al: Hepatitis B virus antibody in blood donors and the occurrence of non-A, non-B hepatitis in transfusion recipient, Ann Intern Med 101:733-738, 1984.

Turgeon ML: Clinical hematology, Boston, 1988, Little, Brown & Co.

Turgeon ML: Fundamentals of immunohematology, Philadelphia, 1989, Lea & Febiger.

Rubella Infection

ETIOLOGY

The rubella virus was first isolated in 1962. Acquired rubella, also known as German or 3-day measles, is caused by an enveloped, single–stranded RNA virus of the togavirus family. Because the virus is endemic to humans, the disease is highly contagious and transmitted through respiratory secretions. Before widespread rubella immunization, this viral infection occurred most commonly in childhood, although it affected adults as well.

EPIDEMIOLOGY

Three strains of live attenuated rubella vaccine virus were developed and first licensed for use in the United States in 1969. Before widespread rubella immunization in the United States and Canada, rubella infections occurred in epidemic proportion at 6- to 9-year intervals. In 1964, more than 20,000 cases of *congenital rubella syndrome* and an unknown number of stillbirths occurred in the United States as the result of epidemic that year. As of August 23, 1989, 1123 confirmed cases of measles were reported by the Chicago Department of Health in a measles outbreak in that city. Of these cases, 78% occurred in preschool-aged children with blacks and Hispanics accounting for 94% of the cases. In countries where vaccination is uncommon, the incidence of rubella infection is high and epidemics are frequent.

Because vaccination programs have prevented the rubella epidemics that once gave people naturally acquired immunity, individuals who have not been vaccinated have a higher level of susceptibility to rubella infection. Since 1983, the number of reported measles cases increased annually until 1986, then decreased in 1987 and 1988 (a provisional total of 3411 cases in 1988.) In 1988, the age distribution of cases was similar to that in previous years. Primarily two types of outbreaks have occurred in the United States in the recent past: those among highly vaccinated school-aged children and those among unvaccinated preschool-aged children. The epidemiology of measles points to two major impediments to measles elimination—unvaccinated preschool-aged children, a factor that allows large outbreaks, like the Chicago epidemic, in inner-city areas and vaccine failures, which account for outbreaks in highly vaccinated school-aged populations. On American college and university campuses, the susceptibility to rubella infection among students is estimated to be as high as 20%. There have been six documented rubella outbreaks on college campuses since 1983; however, the actual number of outbreaks among college students is suspected to be much higher. Many incidences have been either unrecognized or unreported because many cases of rubella infection are mild or subclinical.

Contracting the infection or vaccination against rubella are the only routes to developing immunity. Individuals should be immune to rubella, if they have a dated record of rubella vaccination on or after their first birthday or if they have demonstrable rubella antibody. Even when antibody titers fall to relatively low levels, previous infection or successful vaccination appear to confer permanent immunity to rubella, except in cases of congenital rubella. The only proof of immunity is a positive serologic screening test for rubella antibody. History of rubella infection, even if verified by a physician, is not acceptable evidence of immunity.

It is critical to continue to determine the rubella immune status of women of childbearing age and to vaccinate those who are not immune. Individuals requiring rubella immune status determination include those belonging to the following groups:
1. Preschool and school-age children.
2. All females at or just prior to childbearing age.
3. Women who are about to be married.
4. Married women. If the woman is not rubella-immune, she should be vaccinated and advised not to become pregnant for 3 months because there is a remote possibility that the vaccination could lead to an infected fetus.
5. Pregnant women. A positive test confirms immunity, but to rule out any possibility of unsuspected current infection, an IgM screening procedure may also be ordered. If the patient is not rubella immune, she should be cautioned to avoid exposure to rubella infection. Vaccination is contraindicated in pregnant women; however, a woman should be vaccinated immediately after termination of the pregnancy.
6. Health care personnel. Both men and women should be vaccinated to prevent possible spread of nosocomial infection to pregnant patients.

SIGNS AND SYMPTOMS

A diagnosis of acquired rubella is not based solely on clinical manifestation. The signs and symptoms of rubella vary widely from person to person and may not be recognized in some cases, especially if the characteristic rash is light or absent, as it may be in a substantial number of cases. Rubella infection may resemble other disorders, such as infectious mononucleosis and drug-induced rashes.

Acquired Infection

The incubation period of acquired rubella infection varies from 10 to 21 days, and 12 to 14 days is typical. Infected persons are usually contagious for 12 to 15 days, beginning 5 to 7 days before the appearance (if present) of a rash. Acute rubella infection lasts from 3 to 5 days and generally requires little treatment. Permanent effects are extremely rare in acquired infections.

The clinical presentation of acquired rubella is usually mild. The clinical manifestation of infection usually begins with a prodromal period of catarrhal symptoms, followed by involvement of the retroauricular, posterior cervical, and postoccipital lymph nodes, and finally by the emergence of a maculopapular rash on the face and then on the neck and trunk (Figs. 20-1 and 20-2). A fever of less than 101° F is usually present. In older children and adults, self-limiting arthralgia and arthritis are common.

Congenital Infection

Although rubella infection is usually a mild self-limiting disease with only rare complications in children and adults, rubella infections in pregnant women, especially those infected in their first trimester of pregnancy, can have devastating effects on the fetus (Fig. 20-3). In utero infection can result in fetal death or manifestation of *rubella syndrome*. This syndrome represents a spectrum of congenital defects. Ten to 20% of newborn infants infected in utero fail to survive past the first 18 months of life.

The point in the gestation cycle at which maternal rubella infection occurs greatly influences the severity of congenital rubella syndrome (Table 20-1), and the extent of congenital anomalies varies from one infant to another. Some infants manifest nearly all the defects associated with rubella, while others exhibit few, if any, consequences of infection. Clinical evidence of congenital rubella infection may not be recognized for months or even years after birth.

Rubella syndrome encompasses a number of congenital anomalies. In addition to stillbirth, fetal abnormalities associated with maternal rubella infection include encephalitis, hepatomegaly, bone defects, mental retardation, cataracts, thrombocytopenic purpura, cardiovascular defects, splenomegaly, and microcephaly. Severely afflicted children are likely to have multiple defects in different organ systems. In neonates with congenital rubella syndrome, low birthweight and failure to thrive are common.

Rubella immunity develops in almost all children who have had congenital rubella. In late childhood, however, about one third of these patients lose antibody and become susceptible to acquired rubella. If acquired rubella occurs, it follows a typically benign course. Children who are afflicted with congenital rubella should be screened for rubella immunity in late childhood and vaccinated if necessary.

IMMUNOLOGIC MANIFESTATION
Acquired Infection

In a patient suffering from a primary rubella infection, the appearance of both IgG and IgM antibodies is associated with the appearance of clinical signs and symptoms when present.

IgM antibodies become detectable a few days after the onset of signs and symptoms and reach peak levels at 7 to 10 days. These antibodies persist but rapidly diminish in concentration over the next 4 to 5 weeks until antibody is no longer clinically detectable. The presence of IgM antibody in a single specimen suggests that the patient has recently experienced a rubella infection. In most cases the infection probably occurred within the preceding month.

Production of IgG is also associated with the appearance of clinical signs and symptoms. Antibody levels increase rapidly for the next 7 to 21 days, then level off or even decrease in strength. IgG antibodies, however, remain present and protective indefinitely. The detection of IgG antibody is a useful indicator of rubella infection *only* in cases where the acute and convalescent blood specimens

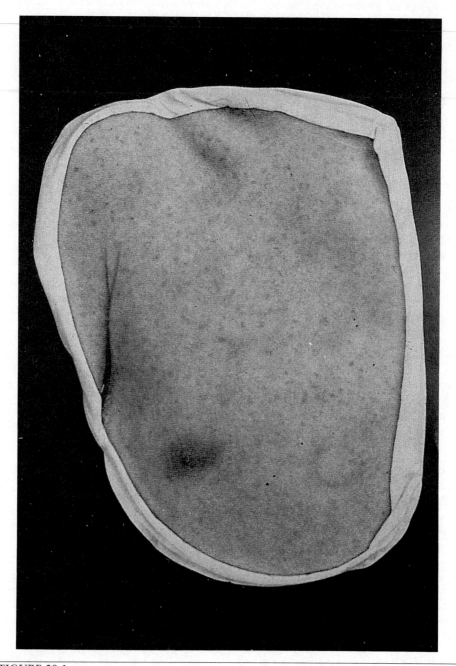

FIGURE 20-1
Rubella.
(From Habif TP: Clinical dermatology, St Louis, 1985, The CV Mosby Co.)

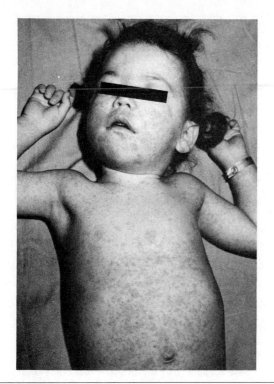

FIGURE 20-2

Rubella rash.

(From Krugman S et al: Infectious diseases of children, ed 8, St Louis, 1985, The CV Mosby Co.)

TABLE 20-1

Manifestation of Anomalies in Maternal Rubella

Period of gestation	Risk of anomaly
First month	50%
First trimester	25%
Third month	>10%
Fourth or fifth month	6%
After fifth month	No risk

Rubella: a clinical update, ACOG Technical Bulletin, No 62, p 4, Chicago, 1981, American College of Obstetricians and Gynecologists.

are drawn several weeks apart. Optimum timing for paired testing for the diagnosis of a recent infection is 2 or more weeks apart, with the first (acute) specimen taken before or at the time signs and symptoms appear, or within 2 weeks of exposure.

Paired specimen testing may demonstrate that the antibody levels are the same. In these cases the patient was either previously immunized or the acute sample was taken after the antibody had already reached maximum levels. Demonstration of an unequivocal increase in IgG antibody concentration between the acute and convalescent specimens is suggestive of either a recent primary infection or

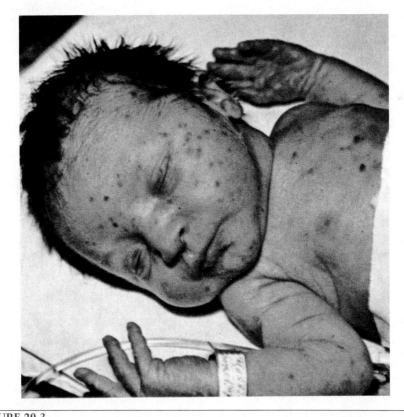

FIGURE 20-3

Congenital malformations of Rubella.

(From Krugman S et al: Infectious diseases of children, ed 8, St Louis, 1985, The CV Mosby Co.)

a secondary (anamnestic) antibody response to rubella in an immune individual. In cases of an anamnestic response, IgM antibodies are not demonstrable, but IgG production begins quickly. No other
signs or symptoms of disease are exhibited.

If both IgM and IgG test results are negative, the
patient has never suffered from rubella infection or
been vaccinated. Such patients are susceptible to
infection. If no IgM is demonstrable but IgG is
present in paired specimens, the patient is immune. In evaluation of the immune status of patients, IgG antibodies present in a dilution of 1:8 or
greater indicate past infection with rubella virus
and clinical protection against future rubella infection. The clinical significance of lower levels is not
currently known. Titers of 1:16, 1:64, 1:512 or
greater may be found in both acute and past infections; however, to diagnose acute infections would
require an IgM antibody titer on the same specimen
or a paired specimen comparison. It should be
noted that IgM also appears after vaccination for a
transient period.

Congenital Rubella Syndrome

Because IgG antibody is capable of crossing the placental barrier, there is no way of distinguishing between IgG antibody of fetal origin and IgG antibody
of maternal origin in a neonatal blood specimen.

Testing for IgM antibody is invaluable in the diagnosis of congenital rubella syndrome in the neonate. IgM does not cross an intact placental barrier;
therefore demonstration of IgM in a single neonatal
specimen is diagnostic of congenital rubella syndrome. In the newborn, serologic confirmation of
rubella infection can be made by testing for IgM antibody for at least the first 6 months of life. This is
especially useful in instances where clinical evidence of congenital rubella is slow in emerging or
is of uncertain origin.

DIAGNOSTIC EVALUATION

Physicians apply the results of rubella testing independently, frequently without the benefit of clinical signs and symptoms. Historically, hemagglutination inhibition (HAI) antibody testing has been
the most frequently used method of screening for
the presence of rubella antibodies. Within the past
few years, the HAI test has been challenged by a
number of assays that are more convenient as the
screening method of choice for the determination
of rubella immune (IgG) status. In some cases, such
as pregnant women, it also may be necessary to determine if a recent infection has been experienced.
The assays for determination of immune status and
evidence of recent infection are presented in Table
20-2.

Hemagglutination Inhibition

Despite wide acceptance and use of these other assays, HAI testing continues to be the reference
method for detection and quantitation of rubella

TABLE 20-2

Diagnostic Tests for Immune Status/Serodiagnosis

Method	Immunity	Serodiagnosis
Hemagglutination inhibition (HAI)	Yes	Yes*
Passive hemagglutination (PHA)	Yes	No
Fluorescent immunoassay (FIA)	Yes	Yes*
Latex agglutination	Yes	No
Radioimmunoassay	Yes	No
Enzyme immunoassay (EIA-IgM)	No	Yes
Enzyme immunoassay (EIA-IgG)	Yes	Yes*

*Serodiagnosis may not differentiate between primary infection
and reinfection. An IgM specific procedure must be used.

antibody. Rubella methods vary in sensitivity and
specificity when samples with antibody levels near
the breakpoint of *immune* versus *nonimmune* are
analyzed. A gray area exists around the cutoff point
of any test, but marginal results may be encountered with some methods. False negatives with
some methodologies are most frequently seen
when HAI titers are at or near the cutoff antibody
level of 1:8. It is important that the method used
for screening demonstrates sensitivity, specificity,
and reproducibility of >/ 95% based on an assay of
200 or more serum samples compared with HAI. A
disadvantage of HAI, however, is that although the
procedure detects a combination of IgM and IgG antibodies, it does not distinguish between them. If
IgG is separated from IgM, this procedure can be
used as a differential method. Separation of IgM can
be by sucrose density gradient fractions, protein A-
Sepharose or an affinity column.

Other Methods

Latex procedures provide more rapid and convenient alternatives to HAI. If more quantitative results are desired, enzyme immunoassay (EIA) and
fluorescent immunoassay (FIA) appear to be as reliable as HAI. Widespread use of EIA for assessment
of immune status (IgG) and recent infection (IgM)
should result in the near future in simplification of
rubella serology.

EIA can be used to measure total antibody, IgG,
or IgM. IgM antibodies can be detected by EIA in
100% of patients between days 11 and 25 after onset of signs and symptoms of acquired infection, in
60% to 80% of persons at days 15 to 25 after vaccination, and in 90% to 97% of infants with congenital rubella between 2 weeks and 3 months after
birth. The rubella-specific IgM often persists for 20
to 30 days after acute infection or vaccination and
also in infants with congenital rubella. Persons
with infectious mononucleosis sometimes have ru-

bella-specific IgM in low concentrations. Cross-reactions of rubella IgM-positive sera can result from Parvovirus IgM. Occasionally, pregnant women will demonstrate IgM antibodies not only to rubella but also to cytomegalovirus, varicella-zoster virus and measles virus. In these cases diagnosis of rubella can be made only by assessment of rubella-specific IgG antibodies by HAI and/or EIA procedures supported by a detailed clinical history. Rubella-specific IgG is regularly detected by EIA only at more than 15 to 25 days after infection and at more than 25 to 50 days after vaccination.

Passive hemagglutination (PHA) methods are not licensed for serodiagnosis of recent rubella infection. PHA is faster and less complex than HAI. In PHA, erythrocytes are coated with rubella antigen. In the presence of rubella antibody, agglutination occurs.

PROCEDURE

Passive Latex Agglutination Test (Rubrascan)

PRINCIPLE
Latex particles are sensitized with solubilized rubella virus antigens from disrupted virions that have been judged to be inactivated. When the latex reagent is mixed with serum containing rubella antibodies on a dark surface, the antigen-antibody complex will form visible clumps. In the absence of antibody or if the concentration is insufficient to react, the latex particles will remain smooth and evenly dispersed. If a qualitative procedure is performed, the presence of rubella antibodies is an indication of previous infection, and presumptive immunity can be used to evaluate the immune status of that individual with regard to resistance or susceptibility to primary rubella infection.

SPECIMEN COLLECTION AND PREPARATION
The protocol for specimen collection will vary depending on the testing objectives. Single specimens are required for qualitative antibody level determinations. In suspected clinical infections or exposure, two specimens for quantitative testing should be obtained. The first should be collected within 3 days of the onset of rash or at the time of exposure and tested upon arrival in the laboratory. This specimen should be frozen and stored until the second specimen is collected 7 to 21 days after the onset of the rash or at least 30 days after exposure, if no clinical symptoms occur. Both specimens should be tested simultaneously.

No special preparation of the patient is required prior to specimen collection. The patient must be positively identified when the specimen is collected and the specimen is to be labeled at the bedside. Specimen labels must include the patient's full name, the date the specimen is collected, the patient's hospital identification number, and the phlebotomist's initials.

Blood should be drawn by an aseptic technique. A minimum of 2 mL of clotted blood (red-top evacuated tube) is required. The specimen should be centrifuged promptly and an aliquot of serum removed. Specimens may be stored up to 48 hours at 2° to 8° C. Specimens should be frozen if longer storage is required. Do not heat-inactivate the serum. The presence of particulate matter, lipemia, or hemolysis does not affect the test.

REAGENTS, SUPPLIES, AND EQUIPMENT
WARNING: The latex reagent, buffer, and controls contain sodium azide as a preservative. Sodium azide may react with lead and copper plumbing to form highly explosive metal azides. Upon disposal, flush with a large volume of water to prevent azide buildup.
1. Reagents and supplies provided in the Rubrascan kit (Becton Dickinson Microbiology Systems, Cockeysville, Md.):
   A. Latex antigen. This reagent contains 0.02% gentamicin and 0.2% sodium azide. Store at 2° to 8° C and return to refrigeration when not in use. DO NOT FREEZE.
   B. Card dilution buffer. Phosphate buffered saline solution containing bovine serum albumin with 0.02% sodium azide. Store at 2° to 8° C and return to refrigeration when not in use. DO NOT FREEZE.
   C. Test cards. Cards must be flat for proper reactions. If necessary, flatten cards by bowing back in a direction opposite to that of the curl. Care should be taken not to finger-mark the test areas, since this may result in an oily deposit and improper test results. Use each card once and discard. Store cards in the original package in a dry area at room temperature.
   D. Plastic stirrers
   E. Dispensing needle (21 G, green hub). Upon completion of daily tests, remove the needle from the dispensing bottle and recap the bottle. Rinse the needle with distilled water to maintain clear passage and accurate drop delivery. Do not wipe the dispensing needle since it is silicone-coated.
2. Centrifuge
3. Rotator. The recommended rotation speed is 100 rpm, but rotation between 95 and 110 rpm does not significantly affect the results obtained. The rotator should circumscribe a circle approximately 2 cm in diameter in the horizontal plane. A moistened humidifying cover should be used to prevent drying of test specimens during rotation.
4. Humidifying cover
5. High-intensity incandescent lamp
6. Micropipettors, 25 μL and 100 μL

7. Other equipment and glassware for preparation, storage, and handling of serologic specimens

QUALITY CONTROL

The following controls are provided in the Rubrascan kit (Becton Dickinson Microbiology Systems, Cockeysville, Md.):

1. Low reactive control with 0.1% sodium azide. This control is used for both the qualitative and the quantitative assay.
2. Nonreactive control with 0.1% sodium azide. This control is used for both the qualitative and the quantitative assay.
3. High reactive control with 0.1% sodium azide. This control is used in the quantitative assay only.

Each of these controls must be tested with each series of unknown patient specimens.

CAUTION: Because the control sera are derived from human sources, they should be handled in the same manner as clinical serum specimens (see *Universal blood and body fluid precautions* in Chapter 6).

PROCEDURE

NOTE: The test area, reagents, specimens, and test components must be at 23° to 29° C before testing. Do NOT mix reagents from different lot numbers. The dispensing bottle must be held vertically.

QUALITATIVE TESTING

1. Remove the cap from the bottle of latex agglutination and attach the green hub needle to the tapered fitting.
2. Mark the card to identify the low reactive and nonreactive controls and all samples.

WITH UNDILUTED SPECIMENS

A. With a micropipettor, place 25 uL of low reactive control on the appropriately marked circle.

B. With the same micropipettor and a clean tip each time, repeat the procedure in step a, using the nonreactive control and each specimen to be tested.

ALTERNATE PROCEDURE: 1:10 SPECIMEN DILUTION*

A. Using the micropipettor, add 100 uL of buffer to the appropriate squares for each control and specimen to be tested. These squares will be used to prepare the 1:5 dilution in step c below.

B. Using the micropipettor, add 25 uL of buffer to the appropriate squares for each control and specimen to be tested. These squares will be used to prepare the 1:10 dilution in step d below.

C. With the micropipettor and a clean tip, pipette 25 uL of low reactive control directly into the buffer in the appropriately labeled circle and mix the serum and buffer by drawing up-and-down with the micropipettor 12 times. Caution should be exercised to avoid the formation of bubbles. The serum in this circle is now a 1:5 dilution.

D. Using the same micropipettor and tip, transfer 25 uL of the 1:5 dilution from the circle and place directly into the buffer in the corresponding numbered circle and mix by drawing up-and-down with the micropipettor six times. Withdraw 25 uL from the circle and discard. The serum in this circle is now a 1:10 dilution.

E. Repeat the procedure in step C for the nonreactive control and for each specimen to be tested.

3. Using a new plastic stirrer for each circle, spread each of the specimens to be tested (either 25 uL of serum or 25 uL of 1:10 diluted serum) to fill the entire circle.

4. Place the bottle cap over the tip of the needle and gently invert the bottle of latex reagent several times to mix.

5. While holding the latex reagent bottle in a *vertical position,* dispense several drops of antigen into the bottle cap until a drop of uniform size has been formed. Dispense one free-falling drop of antigen (approximately 15 uL) on each circle containing diluted serum. Care must be taken to avoid contamination of the bottle tip. The predropped antigen can be recovered from the bottle cap and reused.

6. Place the card on a rotator and rotate for 8 minutes under a moistened humidifying cover.

7. Immediately following mechanical rotation, read the card macroscopically in the wet state with the aid of a high-intensity incandescent lamp. A brief hand rotation of the card (three or four back-and-forth motions) must be made following mechanical rotation to help differentiate weak agglutination from no agglutination. Fluorescent lighting is generally insufficient to distinguish minimally reactive results. The use of magnification in reading test results is not recommended.

8. The reactive control should exhibit agglutination; the nonreactive control should demonstrate no agglutination.

REPORTING RESULTS

A positive reaction = demonstrates agglutination
A negative reaction = demonstrates no agglutination

PROCEDURE NOTES

A single specimen can be used to estimate the immune status of the individual because any detectable antibody is indicative of immunity and protection against subsequent viremic infection. The alternate procedure using specimens diluted 1:10 should be used when data at a sensitivity level approximating that expected with hemagglutination inhibition methods is needed. Optimal sensitivity can be ensured by screening all serum samples un-

---

*The alternate (1:10 dilution) is equivalent in sensitivity and specificity to results obtained with HAI methods.

diluted and repeating negative specimens at a 1:10 dilution.

NOTE: The National Committee for Clinical Laboratory Standards (NCCLS) advises that the specimen should not be frozen in a frost-free freezer because the freeze-thaw cycle may be detrimental to serum proteins. The guidelines of this agency further suggest that frozen specimens be retained for *at least 1 year* for later follow-up, especially for women of childbearing age who are inadvertently exposed to the virus.

The acute-phase specimen should be collected as nearly as possible to the time of exposure, and no later than 3 days after the onset of rash. The convalescent phase specimen should be taken 7 to 21 days after the onset of the rash or at least 30 days after exposure, if no clinical symptoms appear because of a possible inapparent infection. BOTH SPECIMENS SHOULD BE TESTED SIMULTANEOUSLY.

SOURCES OF ERROR. False negative results may occur in the following conditions:

1. Reduction in the degree of agglutination has been reported with rare high-titered specimens when the test is performed undiluted.
2. In undiluted specimens, strong reactivity may cause the center of the test circle to appear clear, because agglutinated latex has migrated to the periphery.
3. If only a 1:10 dilution is used, the procedure may fail to detect a low-level antibody that might have otherwise been detected with an undiluted specimen.
4. The absence of a fourfold titer rise does not necessarily rule out the possibility of exposure and infection. If the first (acute phase) sample is taken too late or the second (convalescent phase) sample is taken too soon, seroconversion or a fourfold rise in titer characteristic of recent infection may not be seen.

CLINICAL APPLICATIONS. The presence of antibodies in a single patient specimen is an indication of previous exposure and immunity to rubella virus. Demonstration of any detectable antibody is indicative of immunity and protection against subsequent viremic infection; however, a test configuration using an undiluted specimen may be preferred.

Demonstration of seroconversion, or a fourfold or greater rise in antibody titer with properly collected paired specimens, is diagnostic of a recent or current infection with rubella virus. Seroconversion means a positive test result of 1:5 or greater after an initial nonreactive result of less than 1:5.

LIMITATIONS. A single specimen determines immunity; it is not a serodiagnosis of infection/reinfection.

The qualitative card test is designed to detect the presence of rubella antibody. At a single dilution the qualitative protocol will perform satisfactorily with both acute-phase and convalescent-phase antibodies; however, in cases where the presence or absence of a fourfold titer rise in paired specimens must be demonstrated, the quantitative protocol is required.

REFERENCES

Rubrascan Product Brochure, Becton Dickinson Microbiology Systems, Cockeysville, Md, 1988.

Skendzel LP: New guidelines and standards for rubella antibody testing from NCCLS and CAP, Lab Med 18(7):461, 1987.

PROCEDURE

Semi-Quantitative Immunoassay for Determination of IgG Antibodies to Rubella Virus*

PRINCIPLE

The following procedure is an indirect enzyme-labeled immunoabsorbent assay using microwells as a solid phase. Rubella antigen is attached to wells of microplates. Diluted test samples are added to the coated wells and incubated. During incubation, antibodies to rubella present in the specimen will bind to the antigen-coated well. After washing to remove unbound material, antibodies to human IgG labeled with alkaline phosphatase (conjugate) are added. The conjugate binds to any rubella antibody bound to rubella antigen. The well is washed to remove unbound conjugate and incubated with *p*-nitrophenyl phosphate. The *p*-nitrophenyl phosphate is hydrolyzed by alkaline phosphatase to form *p*-nitrophenol, a yellow-colored end product with absorbance maximum at 405 nm. The intensity of absorbance at 405 nm is proportional to the amount of IgG antibodies to rubella present in the specimen. The clinical application of this procedure is to determine the rubella immune-status and susceptibility to rubella infection in individuals.

SPECIMEN COLLECTION AND PREPARATION

No special preparation of the patient is required prior to specimen collection. The patient must be positively identified when the specimen is collected and the specimen is to be labeled at the bedside. Specimen labels must include the patient's full name, the date the specimen is collected, the patient's hospital identification number, and the phlebotomist's initials.

Blood should be drawn by an aseptic technique. A minimum of 2 mL of clotted blood (red-top evacuated tube) is required. The specimen should be centrifuged promptly and an aliquot of serum removed.

If the test cannot be performed immediately, the specimen should be refrigerated (2° to 8° C) for no longer than 72 hours. If additional delay occurs, the serum should be frozen at −20° C or below. Frozen

---

*Sigma Chemical Company, St. Louis, MO.

serum should be thawed rapidly at 37° C. Specimens containing visible particulate matter should be clarified by centrifugation prior to testing. The serum sample should not be heat-inactivated prior to testing.

The NCCLS advises that the specimen should not be frozen in a frost-free freezer because the freeze-thaw cycle may be detrimental to serum proteins. The guidelines of this agency further suggest that frozen specimens be retained for *at least 1 year* for later follow-up, especially for women of childbearing age who are inadvertently exposed to the virus.

REAGENTS, SUPPLIES, AND EQUIPMENT*

NOTE: Store reagents at 2° to 6° C. The reagents are stable until the expiration date on the label.

1. Antigen wells. Microplate wells coated with rubella antigen (Gilchrist strain). Store antigen wells with dessicant in the reusable plastic bag. Reseal the bag after opening.
2. Holder for wells.
3. Sample diluent. Buffered protein solution containing surfactant and blue dye, pH 7.5. Contains 0.1% sodium azide as a preservative.
4. Calibrator. Human serum containing antibodies to rubella at 100 arbitrary units/mL (AU/mL). This constituent contains 0.1% sodium azide as a preservative.
5. Conjugate. Goat antibodies to human IgG labeled with calf alkaline phosphatase. This solution contains a pink dye and 0.02% sodium azide as a preservative.
6. Substrate. Contains *p*-nitrophenyl phosphate, disodium, hexahydrate 1 mg/mL, pH 9.6. The substrate may develop a slight yellow color upon storage. Do not use if absorbance of the undiluted substrate is greater than 0.4 at 405 nm when measured against water using a microplate reader or a spectrophotometer with a 1-cm lightpath.
7. Wash concentrate. Buffer solution concentrate with surfactant. This solution contains 0.1% sodium azide as a preservative. The wash solution is prepared by adding the contents of wash concentrate bottle to 1 liter of deionized water. Mix well. Wash solution may be stored at room temperature (18° to 26° C).
8. Stop solution. This is an alkaline solution pH 12.0. Store at room temperature. Reagent is stable until expiration date on the label.
   WARNING: Stop solution causes irritation. Avoid contact with eyes, skin, and clothing. Avoid breathing vapor. Wash thoroughly after handling.
   NOTE: Do not interchange reagents from different lots.
   WARNING: Sample diluent, calibrator, controls, and

buffer contain 0.1% sodium azide as a preservative. Sodium azide may react with lead and copper plumbing to form highly explosive metal azides. Upon disposal, flush with a large volume of water to prevent azide buildup. Sodium azide is also toxic. Care should be taken to avoid ingestion.

Wells contain rubella antigen (Gilchrist strain) and have been tested for noninfectivity. No method, however, can assure that all infectious agents are absent. Employ universal precautions when handling this material.

Additional required supplies and equipment:

1. Spectrophotometer or microplate reader capable of accurately measuring absorbance at 405 nm
2. Pipetting device for the accurate delivery of volumes required for the assay
3. Timer
4. 1-Liter measuring cylinder
5. Squeeze bottle for dispensing wash solution
6. Dilution plates or tubes
7. Test tubes or cuvettes, 1.0 mL

QUALITY CONTROL

Positive control: Human serum containing antibodies to rubella. Content (expected range, expressed as % of calibrator) indicated on the label. This serum contains 0.1% sodium azide. The assay value of the positive control should be within the range shown on the label.

Negative control: Human serum containing no detectable rubella antibodies. This serum contains 0.1% sodium azide. The negative control should be less than 15% of the calibrator. If this requirement is not satisfied, test results may be inaccurate and the assay should be repeated.

CAUTION: Because the antigen wells and control and calibrator sera are derived from human sources, the specimen should be handled in the same manner as clinical serum specimens (see *Universal blood and body fluid precautions* in Chapter 6).

PROCEDURE

1. Dilute calibrator, positive and negative controls, and test samples by combining 5 uL of each of with 200 uL sample diluent in labeled tubes or dilution plates.
2. Place the desired number of antigen wells in holder.
3. Using a pipette tip, mix the samples and diluent by drawing up and expelling 2 or 3 times. Transfer 100 uL of each diluted sample to the appropriate antigen well.
4. Include one well that contains only 100 uL sample diluent. This serves as the reagent blank and is used to zero the photometer.
5. Allow the plate to stand at room temperature (18° to 26° C) for 30 +/− 2 minutes.
6. Shake out or aspirate contents of wells. Wash wells by filling them with wash solution from a squeeze bottle and shaking out or aspirating. Wash 3 times. Drain wells on paper towels to remove excess fluid.

---

*SIA Rubella Kit Reagents available commercially from Sigma Chemical Co., St. Louis, Mo.

NOTE: Thorough washing is necessary to achieve accurate results. Avoid bubbles.

7. Place 2 drops (or 100 uL) conjugate into each well, including the reagent blank well.
8. Allow to stand at room temperature (18° to 26° C) for 30 minutes +/− 2 minutes.
9. Wash wells by repeating step 6.
10. Place 2 drops (or 100 uL) substrate into each well, including the reagent blank well.
11. Allow to stand at room temperature (18° to 26° C) for 30 minutes +/− 2 minutes.
12. Place 2 drops (or 100 uL) stop solution into each well.
13. Read and record absorbance of each test at 405 nm within 2 hours after reaction has been stopped:

    Microplate reader. Set absorbance at 405 nm to zero with water as reference. Read and record absorbance of reagent blank (A blank). Then set absorbance to zero with a reagent blank as a reference. Read and record absorbance of samples (A sample) and calibrator (A calibrator).

    SPECTROPHOTOMETER. Completely remove contents of each well and transfer to cuvette or test tube. Add 800 uL of deionized water to each sample and mix. Set absorbance at 405 nm to zero with water as a reference. Read and record the absorbance of each sample including the reagent blank. Subtract the absorbance of the reagent blank for absorbance of each sample.

CALCULATION

Concentration of IgG antibodies to rubella in sample is calculated as follows:

Antibody concentration as percent of calibrator =

$$\frac{\text{A sample}}{\text{A calibrator}} \times 100$$

EXAMPLE:
Absorbance measured using a microplate reader
A sample = 0.840
A calibrator = 1.543

Antibody concentration as percent of calibrator =

$$\frac{0.8402}{1.5430} \times 100 = 54$$

Absorbance measured using a spectrophotometer
A blank = 0.006
A sample = 0.357
A calibrator = 0.659
A sample = A blank = 0.357 = 0.006 = 0.351
A calibrator = A blank = 0.659 = 0.006 = 0.653

Antibody concentration as percent of calibrator =

$$\frac{0.3510}{0.653} \times 100 = 54$$

REPORTING RESULTS

It is recommended that each laboratory establish an expected reference range that is characteristic of the local population.

Positive (immune) = >/ 15% of calibrator
Negative (nonimmune) = <15% of calibrator

PROCEDURE NOTES

Absorbance values will vary with temperature of room and incubation time. The absorbance value of the reagent blank when read against water at 405 nm should be less than 0.4 using a microplate reader or less than 0.09 using a spectrophotometer with a 1-cm lightpath. The absorbance value of the calibrator should be greater than or equal to 0.5 using a microplate reader when the assay is performed at 22° C.

Specimens giving absorbance values above that of the calibrator should be diluted appropriately with sample diluent and reassayed. The obtained value should be multiplied by the dilution factor.

SOURCES OF ERROR. Inappropriately collected specimens can fail to detect IgG antibodies.

CLINICAL APPLICATIONS. Determination of the presence of IgG antibodies establishes the immune status of a patient.

LIMITATIONS. The results obtained with the assay should serve only as an aid to diagnosis and should not be interpreted as diagnostic in itself.

REFERENCES

Horvath LM and LeBar WD: A comparison of methods for the determination of rubella antibody, ACPR, pp 18-19, April 1987.

Skendzel LP: New guidelines and standards for rubella antibody testing from NCCLS and CAP, Lab Med, 18(7):461, 1987.

SIA Rubella Product Brochure, Sigma Chemical Co, 1988.

Chapter Review

HIGHLIGHTS

Acquired rubella, also known as German or 3-day measles, is caused by an enveloped, single-stranded RNA virus of the togavirus family. Because the virus is endemic to humans, the disease is highly contagious and transmitted through respiratory secretions. Contracting the infection, or vaccination against rubella, are the only routes to developing immunity. It is critical, however, to continue to determine the rubella immune status of women of childbearing age and to vaccinate those who are not immune. A diagnosis of acquired rubella is not based solely on clinical manifestation. The signs and symptoms of rubella vary widely from person to person and may not be recognized in some cases. Although rubella infection is usually a mild self-limiting disease with only rare complications in children and adults, rubella infections in pregnant women, especially those infected in their first trimester of pregnancy, can have devastating effects on the fetus. In utero infection can result in fetal death or manifestation of rubella syndrome. This syndrome represents a spectrum of congenital defects.

In a patient suffering from a primary rubella infection, the appearance of both IgG and IgM antibodies is associated with the appearance of clinical signs and symptoms when present. IgM antibodies become detectable a few days after the onset of signs and symptoms and reach peak levels at 7 to 10 days. These antibodies persist but rapidly diminish in concentration over the next 4 to 5 weeks until antibody is no longer clinically detectable. The presence of IgM antibody in a single specimen suggests that the patient has recently experienced a rubella infection. Demonstration of an unequivocal increase in IgG antibody concentration between the acute and convalescent specimens is suggestive of either a recent primary infection or an anamnestic antibody response to rubella in an immune individual. If both IgM and IgG test results are negative, the patient has never suffered from rubella infection or been vaccinated. Such patients are susceptible to infection. If no IgM is demonstrable but IgG is present in paired specimens, the patient is immune.

Testing for IgM antibody is invaluable in the diagnosis of congenital rubella syndrome in the neonate. IgM does not cross an intact placental barrier; therefore demonstration of IgM in a single neonatal specimen is diagnostic of congenital rubella syndrome. In the newborn, serologic confirmation of rubella infection can be made by testing for IgM antibody for at least the first 6 months of life. This is especially useful in instances where clinical evidence of congenital rubella is slow in emerging or is of uncertain origin.

Historically, hemagglutination inhibition (HAI) antibody testing has been the most frequently used method of screening for the presence of rubella antibodies. Within the past few years, the HAI test has been challenged by a number of assays that are more convenient as the screening method of choice for the determination of rubella immune (IgG) status. In some cases, such as in pregnant women, it also may be necessary to determine if a recent infection has been experienced.

Despite wide acceptance and use of these other assays, HAI testing continues to be the reference method for detection and quantitation of rubella antibody. Latex procedures provide more rapid and convenient alternative to HAI. If more quantitative results are desired, enzyme immunoassay (EIA) and fluorescent immunoassay (FIA) appear to be as reliable as HAI. Widespread use of EIA for assessment of immune status (IgG) and recent infection (IgM) should soon result in simplification of rubella serology. EIA can be used to measure total antibody, IgG, or IgM. Passive hemagglutination (PHA) methods are not licensed for serodiagnosis of recent rubella infection. PHA is faster and less complex than HAI. In PHA, erthrocytes are coated with rubella antigen. In the presence of rubella antibody, agglutination occurs.

REVIEW QUESTIONS

1. All of the following groups of individuals should receive rubella vaccinations *except:*
   A. School-age children
   B. Women of childbearing age
   C. Pregnant women
   D. Health care personnel
   E. Preschool children
2. The greatest risk of the manifestation of anomalies in maternal rubella is _____ of gestation.
   A. During the first month
   B. During the first trimester
   C. During the third month
   D. During the fourth or fifth month
   E. After the fifth month
3. In a patient suffering from a primary rubella infection, the appearance of _____ antibodies is associated with the clinical signs and symptoms when present.
   A. IgG
   B. IgM
   C. IgD
   D. IgA
   E. both A and B
4. Testing for _____ antibody is invaluable in the diagnosis of congenital rubella syndrome.
   A. IgM
   B. IgG
   C. IgD
   D. IgE
   E. IgA
5. The reference method for detection and quantitation of rubella antibody is:
   A. Latex agglutination
   B. Hemagglutination inhibition
   C. Passive hemagglutination
   D. Enzyme immunoassay
   E. Fluorescent immunoassay

Answers

1. C 2. A 3. E 4. A 5. B

BIBLIOGRAPHY

Bellamy K et al: IgM antibody capture enzyme linked immunosorbent assay for detecting rubella specific IgM, J Clin Path 38:1150-1154, 1985.

Chernesky MA and Mahoney JB: Rubella virus. In Rose NR, Friedman H, and Fahey HJL, editors: Manual of clinical laboratory immunology, ed 3, Washington, DC, 1986, American Society of Microbiology, pp 536-539.

Enders G, Knotek F, and Pacher U: Comparison of various serological methods and diagnostic kits for the detection of acute, recent, and previous rubella infection, vaccination, and congenital infections, J Med Virol 16:219-232, 1985.

Fennes FJ and White DO: Medical virology, ed 2, New York, 1976, Academic Press, p 440.

Herrmann KL: Rubella virus. In Lennette EH et al, editors: Manual of clinical microbiology, ed 4, Washington, DC, 1985, American Society of Microbiology, pp 779-784.

Horvath LM and LeBar WD: A comparison of methods for the determination of rubella antibody, ACPR, April 1987, pp 18-19.

Kurtz JB and Anderson MJ: Cross-reactions in rubella and parvovirus specific IgM tests, Lancet 2:1356, 1985.

MMWR: Measles—United States, 1988, JAMA 262:13, 1989.

MMWR: Measles outbreak—Chicago, 1989, JAMA 262:12, 1989.

Morgan-Capner P, Tedder RS, and Mace JE: Reactivity for rubella-specific IgM in sera from patients with infectious mononucleosis, Lancet 1:589, 1983.

Mushahwar II: Rubella on college campuses, Infectious Disease and Immunology Forum, July 1985, Abbott Laboratories.

Sever JL: Laboratory advances in rubella diagnosis, North Chicago, Ill, 1983, Abbott Laboratories.

Skendzel LP: New guidelines and standards for rubella antibody testing from NCCLS and CAP, Lab Med 18(7):461-462, 1987.

Toxoplasmosis

ETIOLOGY

Toxoplasmosis is a widespread disease that occurs in man and animals. The microorganism *Toxoplasma gondii* causes this infection. Recently the *Toxoplasma* organism was recognized as a tissue coccidia.

EPIDEMIOLOGY

Toxoplasma gondii was first discovered in a North African rodent and has been observed in numerous birds and mammals around the world, including humans. It is a parasite of cosmopolitan distribution that is able to develop in a wide variety of vertebrate hosts. Human infections are common in many parts of the world. For unknown reasons, the incidence rates vary from place to place. The highest recorded rate (93%) occurs in Parisian women who prefer undercooked or raw meat; a 50% rate of occurrence exists in their children.

The definitive host is the house cat and certain other Felidae. Domestic cats are a source of the disease because oocysts are often present in their feces. Accidental ingestion of oocysts by humans and animals, including the cat, produces a proliferative infection in the body tissues. Fecal contamination of food or water, soiled hands, inadequately cooked or infected meat, and raw milk can be major sources of human infection. The hazard of transfusion-transmitted toxoplasmosis has been recently recognized in connection with the use of leukocyte concentrates. Patients at risk are those who are receiving immunosuppressive agents or corticosteroids.

All mammals, including humans, can transmit the infection transplacentally. Transplacental transmission usually takes place in the course of an acute but inapparent or undiagnosed maternal infection. New evidence indicates that the number of infants born in the United States each year with congenital *T. gondii* infection is considerably higher than the 3000 previously estimated. It is estimated that 6 out of every 1000 pregnant women in the United States will acquire primary infection with *Toxoplasma* during a 9-month gestation. Approximately 45% of the women who acquire the infection for the first time and who are not treated will give birth to congenitally infected infants. Consequently, the expected incidence of congenital toxoplasmosis is 2.7 per 1000 live births.

It is recommended that all pregnant women be tested for toxoplasmosis immunity. If a patient is susceptible, screening should be repeated during pregnancy and at delivery. Prevention of infection (see box) in pregnant women should be practiced in order to avert congenital toxoplasmosis. In order to further prevent infection of the fetus, women who are at risk should be identified by serologic testing and drug therapy should be provided to pregnant women suffering from primary infections. Treatment consists of a combination of drugs (pyrimethamine and sulphadiazine). These drugs, with

---

Methods for Prevention of Congenital Toxoplasmosis

Avoid touching mucous membranes of the mouth and eye while handling raw meat.
Wash hands thoroughly after handling raw meat.
Wash kitchen surfaces that come in contact with raw meat.
Cook meat to >66°; smoke it or cure it in brine.
Wash fruits and vegetables before consumption.
Prevent the access of flies, cockroaches, and other insects to fruits and vegetables.
Avoid contact with or wear gloves when handling materials that are potentially contaminated with cat feces, e.g., cat litter boxes, or when gardening.

leucovorin to counter the side effects, can be administered orally from midpregnancy to delivery. The newborn is treated with the same drugs for the first 2 weeks postpartum.

SIGNS AND SYMPTOMS
In adults and children other than newborn babies, the disease is usually asymptomatic. A generalized infection probably occurs. Although spontaneous recovery follows acute febrile disease, the organism can localize and multiply in any organ of the body or the circulatory systems.

Acquired Infection
When symptoms are seen, they are frequently mild. The disease can simulate infectious mononucleosis, with chills, fever, headache, lymphadenopathy, and extreme fatigue. A chronic form of toxoplasmic lymphadenopathy exists. *T. gondii* presents a special problem in immunosuppressed or otherwise compromised hosts. In such patients some have developed reactivation of a latent toxoplasmosis. The types of cases in which this has been observed include Hodgkin's and non-Hodgkin's type of lymphoma, as well as in recipients of organ transplants. Reactivation of cerebral toxoplasmosis is not uncommon in patients with acquired immunodeficiency syndrome (AIDS). Primary infection may be promoted by immunosuppression.

Congenital Infection
Congenital toxoplasmosis can result in central nervous system malformation or prenatal mortality. In infants who are serologically positive at birth,

many fail to display neurologic, opthalmic, or generalized illness at birth. In as many as 75% of the cases of congenitally infected newborns who are not serologically diagnosed at birth, the disease remains dormant, only to be discovered when other symptoms such as choriorentinitis, unilateral blindness, or severe neurologic sequelae become apparent.

IMMUNOLOGIC MANIFESTATIONS
Because *T. gondii* is difficult to culture, diagnosis must be supported by serologic methods. Both clinical and laboratory findings in this disease resemble infectious mononucleosis. An increased number of variant lymphocytes can be seen on a peripheral blood smear. The diagnosis is established by serologically demonstrating marked elevations of toxoplasma antibodies. Antibodies are demonstrable within the first 2 weeks after infection, rising to high levels early in the infection, and falling slightly but persisting at an elevated level for many months before declining to low levels after many years.

Levels of IgM and IgG specific antibodies to *T. gondii* can be determined serologically. The presence of IgM to *T. gondii* in an adult is indicative of an active infection. In the newborn, detection of IgM also suggests an active infection because IgM antibodies are able to cross the placenta; therefore they are of fetal origin.

DIAGNOSTIC EVALUATION
The enzyme-linked immunosorbent assay (EIA) is considered by many to be the method of choice for

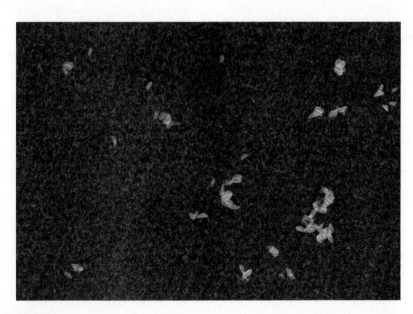

FIGURE 21-1
Indirect fluorescent antibody test for *Toxoplasma gondii* antibodies. *Toxoplasma* organisms affixed to the slide bind specific antibodies in the patient's serum. Antihuman antibody conjugated with fluorescein binds in turn to the bound patient's antibodies, causing the organisms to fluoresce.
(From Finegold SM and Baron EJ: Bailey and Scott's diagnostic microbiology, ed 8, St Louis, 1990, The CV Mosby Co.)

detection of IgM antibodies in toxoplasmosis. Serologic testing methods for *T. gondii* antibody can include:
1. Indirect fluorescent antibody (IFA)
2. Indirect hemagglutination (IHA)
3. Enzyme-linked immunoassay (EIA)
4. Complement fixation
5. Sabin-Feldman dye test

For the detection of IgM antibodies to *T. gondii*, indirect immunofluorescence (Fig. 21-1) and enzyme-linked immunoassays have been developed. A major problem associated with EIA in the measurement of IgM is interference with rheumatoid factor and specific IgG antibodies. These problems, however, have been generally overcome in enzyme-linked assays with new methodology. Serial samples for detection of specific IgG and IgM by EIA offer the best chance of early diagnosis and recognition of remote infection. Specific IgM levels demonstrated by the EIA method usually are elevated for 4 to 8 months, compared to IFA titers, which have usually fallen by the second to fourth month. IgM measured by EIA for *Toxoplasma*-specific IgM is positive in about 75% of infants with proven congenital infection, compared to 25% positivity with IgM evaluation by IFA methodology.

Complement fixation commonly shows a four-fold rise in titer with sera taken during each of the first 3 months following symptomatic onset, and is particularly useful when early sera are not available for specific IgM tests. Indirect hemagglutination (IHA) is least useful for diagnosis because an increase in titer or seroconversion usually requires 4 to 10 weeks.

The Sabin-Feldman dye test (DT) titers peak is useful because it peaks very early—usually in less than 4 weeks—and is persistent. The DT procedure has high sensitivity and specificity and has been found to be useful in problem cases. Detection of circulating antigen, e.g., in immune complexes, is being researched.

☐ PROCEDURE

Quantitative Determination of IgM Antibodies to *Toxoplasma gondii**

PRINCIPLE

Soluble antigens from *Toxoplasma gondii* (RH strain) are attached to wells of microplates. Test specimens are diluted in a diluent containing an absorbent that removes any interfering rheumatoid factor. Diluted test specimens are added to the coated wells and incubated. If antibodies to *T. gondii* are present in the specimen, they will bind to the antigen-coated well during incubation. After washing to remove unbound material, antibodies to

*Sigma Diagnostics, Sigma Chemical Company, St. Louis, Mo.

human IgM labeled with alkaline phosphatase (conjugate) are added. The conjugate binds to any IgM antibodies bound to *Toxoplasma* antigens. The well is washed to remove unbound conjugate and incubated with *p*-nitrophenyl phosphate. The *p*-nitrophenyl phosphate is hydrolyzed by alkaline phosphatase to form *p*-nitrophenol, a yellow-colored end product. The intensity of the absorbance is proportional to the amount of *Toxoplasma* IgM specific antibody present in the specimen.

SPECIMEN COLLECTION AND PREPARATION

No special preparation of the patient is required prior to specimen collection. The patient must be positively identified when the specimen is collected and the specimen is to be labeled at the bedside. Specimen labels must include the patient's full name, the date the specimen is collected, the patient's hospital identification number, and the phlebotomist's initials.

Blood should be drawn by an aseptic technique. A minimum of 2 mL of clotted blood (red-top evacuated tube) or anticoagulated blood (lavender-top evacuated tube) is required. The specimen should be centrifuged promptly and an aliquot of serum or plasma removed.

Specimens should be stored in a refrigerator (2° to 6° C) or frozen (−20° C) if kept for more than 7 days. Specimens containing visible particulate matter should be clarified by centrifugation prior to testing. Serum sample should not be heat-inactivated as this may cause false positive results.

REAGENTS, SUPPLIES, AND EQUIPMENT

Kit reagents are available commercially from Sigma Chemical Company, St. Louis, Mo.
NOTE: Store reagents at 2° to 6° C. The reagents are stable until the expiration date on the label.
1. Kit components:
   A. Antigen wells. Microplate wells coated with *T. gondii*. Store antigen wells with dessicant in the reusable plastic bag and reseal the bag after opening.
   B. Holder for wells.
   C. Sample diluent. This is a buffered protein solution containing surfactant and blue dye, pH 7.5. It contains absorbent (heat aggregated human IgG) and 0.1% sodium azide as a preservative.
   D. Calibrator. This human serum contains IgM antibodies to *T. gondii*. It also contains 0.1% sodium azide as a preservative.
   E. Conjugate. The conjugate contains goat antibodies to human IgM labeled with calf alkaline phosphatase. It contains a pink dye and 0.02% sodium azide as a preservative.
   F. Substrate. The substrate contains *p*-nitrophenyl phosphate, disodium, hexahydrate 1mg/mL, pH 9.6. The substrate may develop a slight yellow color upon storage. Do not use if absorbance of the undiluted substrate is greater than 0.4 at 405 nm when

measured against water using a microplate reader or a spectrophotometer with a 1-cm lightpath.

G. Wash concentrate. This is a buffer solution concentrate with surfactant. It contains 0.1% sodium azide as a preservative. The wash solution is prepared by adding the contents of the wash concentrate bottle to 1 liter of deionized water. Mix well.

H. Stop solution. This is an alkaline solution, pH 12.0. Store at room temperature. Reagent is stable until expiration date on the label. *Warning*: Stop solution causes irritation. Avoid contact with eyes, skin and clothing. Avoid breathing vapor. Wash thoroughly after handling.

NOTE: Do not interchange reagents from different lots.

Additional required supplies and equipment:

2. Spectrophotometer that accommodates a 1-mL volume or microplate reader capable of accurately measing absorbance at 405 nm
3. Pipetting device for the accurate delivery of 5 uL, 100 uL, and 200 uL volumes
4. Timer
5. 1-liter measuring cylinder
6. Squeeze bottle for dispensing wash solution
7. Dilution plates or tubes
8. Test tubes or cuvettes, 1.0 mL

QUALITY CONTROL

Positive control: Human serum containing IgM antibodies to *T. gondii*. Content (expected range, expressed as % of calibrator) indicated on the label. It also contains 0.1% sodium azide.

Negative control: Human serum containing no detectable antibodies to *T. gondii*. It also contains 0.1% sodium azide.

CAUTION: Because the antigen wells, and control and calibrator sera, are derived from human sources, it should be handled in the same manner as clinical serum specimens (see *Universal blood and body fluid precautions* in Chapter 6).

WARNING: The reagents and controls contain sodium azide as a preservative. Sodium azide may react with lead and copper plumbing to form highly explosive metal azides. Upon disposal, flush with a large volume of water to prevent azide buildup. Sodium azide is also toxic. Care should be taken to avoid ingestion.

PROCEDURE

1. Dilute the calibrator, positive and negative controls and test samples by combining 5 uL of the respective sera with 200 uL of sample diluent in labeled tubes or dilution plates.
2. Place the desired number of antigen wells in the holder.
3. Using a clean pipette tip for each specimen, mix the samples and diluent by drawing up and expelling 2 or 3 times. Transfer 100 uL of each diluted specimen to the appropriate antigen well.

4. Include one well that contains only 100 uL sample diluent. This serves as the reagent blank and is used to zero the photometer.
5. Allow the plate to stand at room temperature (18° to 26° C) for 30 +/− 2 minutes.
6. Shake out or aspirate contents of wells. Wash wells by filling them with wash solution from a squeeze bottle and shaking out or aspirating. Wash 3 times. Drain wells on paper towel to remove excess fluid.

NOTE: Thorough washing is necessary to achieve accurate results. Avoid bubbles.

7. Place 2 drops (or 100 uL) conjugate into each well, including the reagent blank well.
8. Allow to stand at room temperature (18° to 26° C) for 30 minutes +/− 2 minutes.
9. Wash wells by repeating step 6.
10. Place 2 drops (or 100 uL) of substrate into each well, including the reagent blank well.
11. Allow to stand at room temperature (18° to 26° C) for 30 minutes +/− 2 minutes.
12. Place 2 drops (or 100 uL stop solution into each well.
13. Read and record absorbance of each test at 405 nm within 2 hours after the reaction has been stopped.

Microplate reader. Set absorbance at 405 nm to zero with water as reference. Read and record absorbance of reagent blank (A blank). Then set absorbance to zero with the reagent blank as a reference. Read and record the absorbance of samples (A sample) and calibrator (A calibrator).

SPECTROPHOTOMETER. Completely remove contents of each well and transfer to cuvette or test tube. Add 800 uL of deionized water to each sample and mix. Set absorbance at 405 nm to zero with water as a reference. Read and record the absorbance of each sample including the reagent blank. Subtract the absorbance of the reagent blank from the absorbance of each specimen.

CALCULATION

Antibody concentration as percent of calibrator =

$$\frac{\text{A sample}}{\text{A calibrator}} \times 100$$

EXAMPLE:
Absorbance measured using a microplate reader
A sample =0.597
A calibrator = 0.842

Antibody concentration as percent of calibrator =

$$\frac{0.597}{0.842} \times 100 = 71$$

Absorbance measured using a spectrophotometer
A blank = 0.006
A sample = 0.242
A calibrator = 0.332
A sample - A blank = 0.242 - 0.006 = 0.236
A calibrator - A blank = 0.332 - 0.006 = 0.326

Antibody concentration as percent of calibrator =

$$\frac{0.236}{0.326} \times 100 = 72$$

REPORTING RESULTS

Reference ranges should be established by each laboratory to reflect the characteristics of the populations of the area in which it is located.

>40% = Positive for IgM antibodies to *T. gondii*

and indicates the probability of current or recent infection.

<40% = Negative for IgM antibodies to *T. gondii*.

PROCEDURE NOTES

Specimens giving absorbance values above that of the calibrator should be diluted appropriately and reassayed. The value obtained should be multiplied by the dilution factor.

SOURCES OF ERROR. **False positive** results can be caused by the presence of rheumatoid factor in the specimen. In this procedure, the sample diluent contains heat-aggregated IgG sufficient to neutralize the immunoglobulin activity of up to 348 IU/mL of IgM rheumatoid factor.

False negative results have been reported in assays detecting IgM antibodies due to the competition between specific IgG antibodies and low levels of specific IgM antibodies. In addition, specimens taken from patients very early in the course of infection may contain no detectable level of IgM specific antibody to *T. gondii*.

CLINICAL APPLICATIONS. Demonstration of *Toxoplasma* IgM antibody is indicative of a recent or current acute infection in adults or children and a congenital infection in the newborn. *Toxoplasma* IgM antibodies should be absent in noninfected individuals.

LIMITATIONS. Detection of Toxoplasma-specific IgM is reliable except when the specimen is collected too early (an increase is sometimes apparent within 1 month) or too late (more than 4 to 8 months after infection).

An additional limitation is that the detection of IgM antibodies to *T. gondii* is designed to serve as an aid to definitive diagnosis. Clinical considerations should be integrated with serologic findings.

Chapter Review

HIGHLIGHTS

Toxoplasmosis is a widespread disease that occurs in man and animals. The microorganism *Toxoplasma gondii* causes this infection. It is a parasite of cosmopolitan distribution with the definitive host being the house cat and certain other Felidae. Domestic cats may be a source of the disease because oocysts are often present in their feces. Accidental ingestion of oocysts by humans and animals, including the cat, produces a proliferative infection in the body tissues. Fecal contamination of food or water, soiled hands, inadequately cooked or infected meat, and raw milk can be important sources of human infection. All mammals, including humans, can transmit the infection transplacentally. Transplacental transmission usually occurs in the course of an acute but inapparent or undiagnosed maternal infection.

In adults and children other than newborns, the disease is usually asymptomatic. A generalized infection probably occurs. Although spontaneous recovery follows acute febrile disease, the organism can localize and multiply in any organ of the body or the circulatory systems. In acquired infection, when symptoms are seen, they are frequently mild. The disease conditions may simulate infectious mononucleosis. In contrast, congenital toxoplasmosis can result in central nervous system malformation or prenatal mortality. Because *T. gondii* is difficult to culture, diagnosis must be supported by serologic methods. Levels of IgM and IgG specific antibodies to *T. gondii* can be determined serologically. The presence of IgM to *T. gondii* in an adult is indicative of an active infection. In the newborn, detection of IgM also suggests an active infection because IgM antibodies are able to cross the placenta; therefore they are of fetal origin. The enzyme-linked immunosorbent assay is considered by many to be the method of choice for detection of IgM antibodies in toxoplasmosis. Serologic testing methods for *T. gondii* antibody can include indirect fluorescent antibody (IFA), indirect hemagglutination (IHA), enzyme-linked immunoassay (EIA), complement fixation, and the Sabin-Feldman dye test.

REVIEW QUESTIONS

1. Toxoplasmosis is a _____ infection.
   A. Bacterial
   B. Mycotic
   C. Parasitic
   D. Viral
   E. Fungal
2. The definitive host of *T. gondii* is the _____.
   A. Horse
   B. Pig
   C. Dog
   D. House cat
   E. Goat
3. All of the following are specific methods for preventing congenital toxoplasmosis *except:*
   A. Avoid touching mucous membranes while handling raw meat
   B. Wash hands thoroughly after handling raw meat
   C. Eliminate food contamination by flies, cockroaches, and other insects
   D. Disposal of fecally contaminated cat litter into plastic garbage bags
   E. Cooking meat to temperature higher than 66° F
4. The presence of IgM to *T. gondii* in an adult is indicative of:
   A. Carrier state
   B. Active infection
   C. Chronic infection
   D. Latent disease
   E. Relapse

Answers

1. C 2. D 3. D 4. B

BIBLIOGRAPHY

Bruce-Chwatt LJ: Transfusion associated parasitic infections. In Infection, immunity, and blood transfusion, New York, 1985, Alan R Liss, Inc, pp 101-125.

Franco EL, Walls KW, and Sulzer AJ: Reverse enzyme immunoassay for detection of specified anti-toxoplasma immunoglobulin M antibodies, J Clin Microbiol 13:859, 1981.

Hall SM: The diagnosis of toxoplasmosis, Br Med J 289:570-571, 1984.

Krogstasd DJ et al: Blood and tissue protozoa. In Lennette EH et al, editors: Manual of clinical microbiology, ed 4, Washington, DC, 1985, American Society of Microbiology, pp 612-630.

Markell EK et al: Medical parasitology, ed 6, Philadelphia, 1986, WB Saunders Co, pp 112-117, 131-138.

SIA Toxoplasma IgM Product Literature, Sigma Chemical Co, St Louis, Mo, 1988.

Turgeon ML: Clinical hematology, Boston, 1988, Little, Brown & Co, pp113-114.

Turgeon ML: Fundamentals of immunohematology, Philadelphia, 1989, Lea & Febiger.

Walls KW: Serodiagnostic tests for parasitic diseases. In Lennette EH et al, editors: Manual of clinical microbiology, ed 4, Washington, DC, 1985, American Society of Microbiology, pp 945-948.

Walls KW and Wilson M: Immunoserology in parasitic infections. In Immunodiagnostics, New York, 1983, Alan R Liss, Inc, pp 191-214.

Wilson CB and Remington JJ: What can be done to prevent toxoplasmosis? Am J Obstet Gynecol 138:357-363, 1980.

CHAPTER 22

Acquired Immunodeficiency Syndrome (AIDS)

T he *human T-lymphotropic virus type III* is also referred to as HTLV-III, LAV, or most recently, the *human immunodeficiency virus* (HIV). HIV-1 is the predominant virus responsible for acquired immunodeficiency syndrome (AIDS). Although HIV has been only recently recognized, it has been tentatively concluded that HIV-1 has infected human beings for more than 20 but less than 100 years.

ETIOLOGY

At the beginning of the 1980s no infectious retroviruses had been found in human beings, and many believed that no human retroviruses would be found. In spite of this skepticism, however, the first human retrovirus, human T-lymphotropic virus type I (HTLV-I), was isolated in 1980; HTLV-II was isolated in 1982.

Introduction

In 1983 researchers at the Pasteur Institute in Paris isolated a retrovirus from a homosexual man with lymphadenopathy. The virus was named the *lymphadenopathy-associated virus* (LAV), but the researchers were unable to prove that this agent caused acquired immunodeficiency syndrome (AIDS). The American research team headed by Dr. Robert Gallo isolated the same class of virus, which they labeled *human T-lymphotropic retrovirus* (HTLV) type III. In 1984 the Gallo team was able to demonstrate conclusively through virologic and epidemiologic evidence that HTLV-III was the cause of AIDS. When it was demonstrated that LAV and HTLV-III were the same virus, an interna-

tional commission changed the name of the virus to HIV to eliminate confusion caused by two names for the same entity and to acknowledge that the virus does cause AIDS. The intent of the designation of the HIV nomenclature is that HIV would refer to the generic virus class of HTLV-III/LAV, including the AIDS-related virus. Individual viral strains as well as specific viral reagents developed from isolates and analyses based on those reagents are to continue to be referenced by the names as originally assigned.

In addition to the original HIV type 1 (HIV-1), a second AIDS-causing virus, HIV type 2 (HIV-2), was identified in 1985. In evolutionary terms, the two viruses are related and have a similar overall structure. The pathogenic potential of HIV-2, however, is not as well established as that of HIV-1.

Viral Characteristics
Viral Structure

The HIV virus is a type D retrovirus that belongs to the *lentivirus* subfamily. Examination of HIV-infected cells can be done with an electron microscope. The virus may appear as buds of the cell membrane particles. The virion has a double membrane envelope and electron-dense laminar crescent or semicircular cores. An intermediate less electron-dense layer lies in between the envelope and core. In a free extracellular mature virion, the core appears as a bar-shaped nucleoid structure in cross section. This structure appears circular and is frequently located eccentrically. It is composed of structural proteins and glycoproteins that occupy the core and envelope regions of the particle. The

TABLE 22-1

HIV Proteins of Serodiagnostic Importance

Virus	Protein	Location	Gene
HIV-1	gp41	Envelope (transmembrane protein)	env
	gp160/120	Envelope (external protein)	env
	p24	Core (major structural protein)	gag
HIV-2	gp34	Envelope (transmembrane protein)	env
	gp140	Envelope (external protein)	env
	p26	Core (major structural protein)	gag

TABLE 22-2

Encoding Genes and Antigens of AIDS Virus

Encoding gene	Antigen
gag	p55
gag	p24
gag	p17
pol	p66
pol	p51
sor	p24
env	gp160
env	gp120
env	gp41
3'orf	p27

Summary of HIV-1 Life Cycle

1. The virus attaches to the CD4 membrane receptor and sheds its protein coat, exposing its RNA core.
2. Reverse transcriptase converts viral RNA into proviral DNA.
3. The proviral DNA is integated into the genome (genetic complement of the host cell).
4. New virus particles are produced as the result of normal cellular activities of transcription and translation. Once the viral genome is integrated into host cell DNA, the potential for viral production always exists and the viral infection of new cells can continue.
5. New particles bud from the cell membrane.

virion structure consists of knoblike structures composed of a protein called gp 120, which is anchored to another protein called gp41. Each knob includes three sets of these protein molecules. The core of the virus includes a protein called p25 or p24. Following human exposure, these viral components as well as others may induce an antibody response that is important in serodiagnosis (Table 22-1). Retroviruses contain a single positive-stranded RNA with the virus's genetic information and a special enzyme called *reverse transcriptase* in their core. Reverse transcriptase enables the virus to convert viral RNA into DNA. This reverses the normal process of transcription where DNA is converted to RNA; hence the term *retrovirus.*

The *genomes* of all known retroviruses are organized in a similar way. In the provirus, which is formed when complementary DNA synthesis is completed from the retroviral RNA template, viral core and envelope proteins and the enzyme reverse transcriptase are encoded by the **gag, env,** and **pol** genes, respectively, while viral gene expression is regulated by **tat, trs, sor,** and **3'orf** gene products. The gag gene encodes a polyprotein found at high levels in infected cells and is subsequently cleaved to form p17 and p24, both of which are viral particle-associated. The pol gene encodes for reverse transcriptase, endonuclease, and protease activities. The sor gene stands for small open-reading frame. The sor gene product is a protein that induces antibody production in the natural course of infection. The tat gene represents a small open-reading frame; the protein product has not been identified to date.

The env gene encodes for a polyprotein that contains numerous glycosylation sites. The glycoprotein form, gp160, is found on infected cells but is deficient on viral particles. Gp160, however, gives rise to two glycoproteins, gp120 and gp41, which are associated with the viral envelope. The encoding genes and gene products, or antigens, of the AIDS virus that may induce an antibody response following human exposure are presented in Table 22-2. *Long terminal redundancies,* or **LTRs,** which

exist at each end of the proviral genome, play an important role in the control of viral gene expression and the integration of the provirus into the DNA of the hosts. Although a structural similarity exists between the genomes of HIV-1 and HIV-2 (HTLV-IV), the nucleotide sequence homology is limited. There is a nucleotide sequence homology of only 60% between the gag genes and 30% to 40% between the remainder of the genes of HIV-1 and HIV-2.

Viral Replication

The replication of HIV is complicated and involves several steps (see box). The HIV life cycle is that of a retrovirus. Retroviruses are so named because they reverse the normal flow of genetic information. In body cells the genetic material is DNA. When genes are expressed, DNA is first transcribed into messenger RNA (mRNA), which then serves as the template for the production of proteins. The genes of a retrovirus are encoded in RNA; before they can be expressed, the RNA must be converted into DNA. Only then are the viral genes transcribed and translated into proteins in the usual sequence.

Target cells. The infectious process begins when the gp120 protein on the viral envelope binds to the protein receptor, called CD4, located on the surface of a target cell. Fusion of the virus to the membrane of this host cell enables the viral RNA and reverse transcriptase to invade the cell's cytoplasm.

HIV has a marked preference for the helper-inducer subset of T lymphocytes. These cells, however, are not the only cells that have CD4 antigen embedded in their membrane. Macrophages, as many as 40% of the peripheral blood monocytes, and cells in the lymph nodes, skin, and other organs, also express measurable amounts of CD4 and can be infected by HIV. In addition, about 5% of the B lymphocytes may express CD4 and be susceptible to HIV infection.

Although some cells do not produce detectable amounts of CD4, they do contain low levels of messenger RNA encoding the CD4 protein, which indicates that they do produce some CD4. Because these cells can be infected by HIV in culture, the expression of only a very small amount of CD4 or an alternate receptor molecule may be necessary for HIV infection to take place. These cell types include certain cells of the brain, **glial cells,** a variety of malignant brain-tumor cells, and some cells derived from cancers of the bowel. In addition, cells of the gastrointestinal system do not produce appreciable amounts of CD4, but gut cells called *chromaffin cells* do sometimes appear to be infected by HIV in vivo. This suggests that gastrointestinal infection may be what leads to the AIDS-associated weight loss and emaciation known in Africa as *slim disease.*

Replication. The viral replication cycle begins when HIV binds CD4 receptor on the outer cell membrane and injects its core into the cell. The core includes two identical strands of RNA. The enzyme, DNA polymerase, is responsible for converting the viral genetic information into DNA. Initially, this enzyme makes a single-stranded DNA copy of the viral RNA. An associated enzyme, *ribonuclease,* destroys the original RNA, and the polymerase makes a second complimentary copy of DNA using the first DNA strand as a template. The DNA polymerase and ribonuclease together are often called *reverse transcriptase.*

After the viral genetic information is in the form of double-stranded DNA (the same form in which the cell carries its own genetic makeup), it migrates to the cell nucleus. A third viral enzyme, called an *integrase,* may then splice the HIV genome (the full complement of genetic information) into the host cell's DNA. After the viral genome is integrated into the host DNA, the provirus will be duplicated together with the cell's own genes every time the cell divides. At this stage the HIV is permanent.

The second half of the HIV life cycle (the production of new virus particles) takes place only sporadically and only in some infected cells. This phase begins when nucleotide sequences in the LTRs at the ends of the viral genome direct enzyme belonging to the host cell to copy the DNA of the integrated virus into RNA. Some of the RNA will provide the genetic material for a new generation of virus; other RNA strands serve as the mRNAs that guide the synthesis of structural proteins and enzymes of the new virus. When formed, the viral proteins are reassembled into a complete virus particle. The HIV particles bud from the cell membrane; once released into the circulation, they have the ability to infect new target cells.

An elaborate set of genetic controls determines if the cycle of replication will occur and at what speed it will proceed. In addition to the genes for expression of core and envelope proteins, the HIV genome includes at least six other genes. Some—perhaps all—of these genes act to regulate the production of viral proteins.

EPIDEMIOLOGY
Incidence

The AIDS pandemic is still in its early stages, and its ultimate dimensions are difficult to assess accurately. The thousands of AIDS cases now being reported every year are due to HIV infection that began spreading silently and extensively in the 1970s, before the disease was recognized. Based on current knowledge of the disease, it is estimated that over 250,000 cases of AIDS have already occurred and that between 5 and 10 million people worldwide are infected with HIV. By 1993, about 1 million new AIDS cases are expected to develop globally. Africa has been the continent hardest hit by the AIDS pandemic.

AIDS has become a major cause of morbidity and mortality in the United States. The number of reported cases of AIDS has increased each year since the disease was first recognized. Geographically, the northeastern area of the United States has been most severely affected. The highest number of cases (more than 5 per 10,000 of population) has occurred in the state of New York and the District of Columbia. Other states with a high incidence (2 to 5 reported cases of AIDS per 10,000 population) are Massachusetts, Connecticut, Maryland, Georgia, Florida, Texas, California, and Nevada.

As of March 31, 1989, the number of American adults and children reported as suffering from AIDS was 89,501. More than 80% of the patients diagnosed before 1985 have died. The incidence of AIDS will increase in the next few years as some of the estimated 1 to 1.5 million Americans who are already infected with HIV develop the signs and symptoms of AIDS. The majority of adult cases of AIDS will be among homosexual or bisexual men and IV drug abusers. A significant proportion of these cases will be in the black and Hispanic population. Other identifiable groups that have demonstrated the signs and symptoms of AIDS include sexual partners of IV drug users; children below the age of 13 (pediatric AIDS), primarily infants, toddlers; and recipients of unscreened blood or blood products, e.g., hemophiliacs. Of these cases of pediatric AIDS, 91% were in children under 3 years of age, and the majority of these children were born to parents who either had AIDS or who practiced high-risk behaviors.

Transfusion-acquired AIDS in patients with no other risk factors accounts for only 1% to 2% of the total number of AIDS cases. Transfusion-associated AIDS is defined as the occurrence of AIDS in persons with no other known risk factor for AIDS and who received a transfusion with blood or blood components within 5 years of the onset of illness. In addition, a small number health care workers— 4 of 1035—who had accidentally punctured or cut their skin with HIV-contaminated needles or sharps demonstrated seroconversion. None of the 136 workers whose intact mucous membranes or skin had been exposed to HIV-positive blood have seroconverted to date.

Infectious Patterns

HIV-1 and HIV-2 are distinct but related viruses. The two viruses are similar in their overall structure, and both can cause AIDS. HIV-1 is responsible for the main AIDS epidemic, but the pathogenic potential of HIV-2 is not as well established. The discovery of HIV-2 suggests that other HIVs may also exist.

Three infection patterns of HIV virus have been traced worldwide. Pattern 1 is found in North and South America, Western Europe, Scandinavia, Australia, and New Zealand. In these countries it is primarily a disease of homosexuals and IV drug abusers. The male to female ratio of reported AIDS cases in pattern 1 areas ranges from 10:1 to 15:1. Pattern 2 is found in Africa, the Caribbean, and some areas of South America. In the pattern 2 areas AIDS is primarily a heterosexual disease; the number of infected females and males is approximately equal. Pattern 3 is typically demonstrated in Eastern Europe, North Africa, the Middle East, Asia, and the Pacific, excluding Australia and New Zealand. In the pattern 3 areas relatively few cases of AIDS have been identified; most of the affected individuals have had contact with pattern 1 or pattern 2 countries.

Modes of Transmission

Transmission of HIV is believed to be restricted to intimate contact with body fluids from an infected person (Table 22-3); casual contact with infected persons has not be documented as a mode of transmission. Although the mode of transmission is considered to be predominantly sexual, the virus can be transmitted through contact with infected blood through blood transfusion (if the blood has not been screened for HIV) or by HIV-contaminated needles. Post-transfusion AIDS is now well documented both from cellular blood components and cell-free preparations, such as unheated factor VIII concentrate and plasma.

Although HIV has been isolated from blood, semen, vaginal secretions, saliva, tears, breast milk,

TABLE 22-3

Classification of infected male	% Female sex partner with no other risk— HIV positive
Intravenous drug abuser	48
Bisexual	26
Transfusion	20
Hemophilia	9

Human immunodeficiency virus infection in the United States: A review of current knowledge, MMWR 36:S-6, 1-48, 1987.

cerebrospinal fluid (CSF), amniotic fluid, and urine, only blood, semen, vaginal secretions, and possibly breast milk have been implicated in transmission of HIV to date. Evidence of the role of saliva in the transmission of virus is unclear; however, universal precautions (see Chapter 6) do not apply to saliva uncontaminated with blood. HIV may be *indirectly* transmitted. Viral transmission can result from contact with inanimate objects such as work surfaces or equipment recently contaminated with infected blood or certain body fluids, if the virus is transferred to broken skin or mucous membranes by hand contact.

Prevention

A variety of practices have been advocated for the prevention of HIV transmission. Sexual abstinence or the practice of safe sex is essential to curtailing HIV transmission. The screening of blood donors and donors of organs, tissues, and semen as well as blood products for HIV has reduced the risk of HIV transmission to minimal levels. In addition, heat treatment and techniques such as monoclonal absorption have eliminated the risk of blood-borne HIV transmission to hemophiliacs. Guidelines from the Centers for Disease Control for clinical and laboratory personnel who work with AIDS patients and blood specimens suggest that the same precautions should be used as when the risk of hepatitis B infection is present.

SIGNS AND SYMPTOMS
Early Stages

The early phase of HIV infection may last from many months to many years after the initiation of infection. Typically, patients in the early stages of HIV infection are either completely asymptomatic or may show mild, chronic lymphadenopathy. When HIV first enters the body, the virus often replicates abundantly and free virus appears in CSF surrounding the brain and spinal cord and in circulating blood. Within a few weeks the viral concentration in the bloodstream and CSF drops precipitously and the initial symptoms disappear.

An unknown number of infected patients experience a brief, infectious, mononucleosis-like or flu-like illness with fever, malaise, and possibly a skin rash. Neurologic complaints may also be reported. These symptoms parallel the first wave of HIV replications and develop at about the time antibodies produced by the body against HIV can first be detected. This is usually between 2 weeks and 3 months after infection, rarely later. Following HIV infection and any clinically manifested signs and symptoms, a person may remain symptom-free for years.

Late Phase

HIV causes a predictable progressive derangement of immune function, and AIDS is just one late manifestation of that process. From 2 to 10 years after HIV infection, replication of the virus flares again and the infection enters its final stage. An average of 8 or 9 years may pass before AIDS is fully developed. The virus behaves differently depending on the kind of host cell and the cell's own level of mitotic activity. In T cells, however, the virus can

Opportunistic Infections in Immunosuppressed and Immunodeficient Patients

Oral/esophageal candidiasis
Cytomegalovirus
Pneumocystis carinii
Herpes simplex
Entamoeba histolytica
Giardia lamblia
Herpes zoster
Atypical acid fast bacilli
Shigella
Campylobacter
Cryptococcosis
Adenovirus
Hepatitis
Chlamydia
Salmonella
Syphilis
Anal candidiasis
Dientamoeba fragilis
Blastocystic hominis
Toxoplasmosis

lie dormant indefinitely, but it can destroy the host cell in a burst of replication. HIV grows continuously but slowly in macrophages-monocytes. This slow growth of the virus saves the cell from destruction but probably alters its function.

Clinical symptoms of the later phase of HIV infection include extreme weight loss, fever, and multiple secondary infections. The end stage of AIDS is characterized by the occurrence of neoplasms and/or opportunistic infections. Lethal *Pneumocystis carinii* pneumonia has been a hallmark of AIDS (Fig. 22-1). Other opportunistic infections, however, are frequent and may exist concurrently (see box). *Cryptosporidiosis* and *Histoplasmosis capsulatum* are being recognized with increasing frequency.

The most frequent malignancy observed is an aggressive, invasive varient of *Kaposi's sarcoma* discovered in many cases through autopsy (Fig. 22-2). Kaposi's sarcoma produces tumors in the skin and linings of internal organs, lymphomas, and cancers of the rectum and tongue. Malignant B cell lymphomas are also being more commonly recognized in patients with AIDS or those at high risk for AIDS. Because certain lymphomas can develop quite early, it is hypothesized that B cell hyperactivity plays a role in their development. Lymphomas and other cancers that appear late in HIV disease could also stem from the failure of the compromised immune system to recognize and destroy cancer cells.

Classification of Patients with HIV Infection

A system for grouping patients has been developed at the Walter Reed Army Medical Center. In this system of classification (Table 22-4) as the disease progresses, the patient moves through six stages, the last of which is AIDS. The system is based on several indicators of the immune impairment that underlies HIV infection, e.g., OKT4 cell count. The presence of opportunistic infection is a criterion for the diagnosis of AIDS, but the presence of Kaposi's sarcoma is omitted as a criterion because this form of cancer is not caused by immune suppression and can appear early in the course of HIV infection.

TABLE 22-4

Walter Reed Classification System

Stage	HIV antibody and/or virus	Chronic lymph-adenopathy	T4 cell mm³	Delayed hypersensitivity	Opportunistic infection
0	−	−	>400	Normal	−
1	+	−	>400	Normal	−
2	+	+	>400	Normal	−
3	+	+/−	<400	Normal	−
4	+	+/−	<400	Partial	−
5	+	+/−	<400	Abnormal	−
6	+	+/−	<400	Abnormal	+

Modified from Redfield RR and Burke DS: HIV infection: the clinical picture, Sci Am 259(4):93, 1988.

In addition to the OKT4 cell count as an indicator of the disease stage, other indicators include the onset of chronic lymphadenopathy or swollen lymph nodes, the patient's response to a set of skin tests that reflect the overall function of cell-mediated immunity, and the presence of opportunistic infection.

Initially, the patient's OKT4 lymphocyte concentration is often close to the normal level of about 800×10^9L, and the patient feels well. Usually within 6 months to a year chronic lymphaden-opathy develops. Within a few years evidence of more severe, subclinical immune defects, e.g., a declining OKT4 count and an abnormal skin test, begin to be manifested. As the OKT4 cell count drops, chronic infections of the skin and mucous membranes initially develop followed by disseminated systemic infections. In addition, HIV infection may result in replication in brain cells or the induction of the secretion of neurotoxic cytokines. Psychologic disorders such as dementia can result.

Initially the immune system limits viral replica-

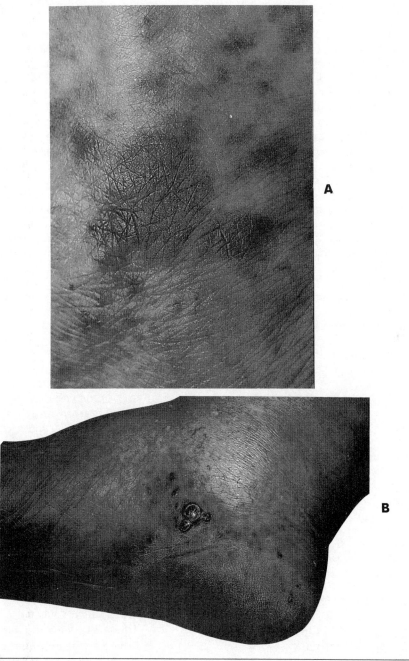

FIGURE 22-1

Kaposi's sarcoma. **A,** Early lesion consisting of violaceous macules and plaques. **B,** Purple nodules are most commonly seen on the lower legs.
(From Habif TP: Clinical dermatology, St Louis, 1985, The CV Mosby Co.)

tion, but the HIV virus slowly gains ground. Eventually, a threshold is reached, probably between stages 3 and 5. At this time the decline in OKT4 cells is so significant that the immune system can no longer function efficiently enough to hold HIV in abeyance and the disease progresses.

Disease Progression

Although a large enough dose of the right strain of HIV can cause AIDS on its own, co-factors can influence the progression of disease development. Debilitated patients, weakened by a pre-existing medical condition before HIV infection, may progress toward AIDS more quickly than others. Stimulation of the immune system in response to later infections can also hasten disease progression. Other pathogenic microorganisms, such as a herpes virus called *human B-cell lymphotropic virus* (HBLV) or *human herpes virus 6* (HHV-6), can interact with HIV in a way that may increase the severity of HIV infection. HHV-6 is usually easily controlled by the immune system. If HIV compromises the immune system, however, HHV-6 may replicate more freely and become a health threat. The main host of HHV-6 is the B cell, but this virus can also infect T4 cells. If T cells are simultaneously infected by HIV, HHV-6 can stimulate the virus, which further impairs the immune system and promotes disease progression.

The progressive decline of OKT4 cells leads to a general decline in immune function and is the primary factor in determining the clinical progression of AIDS.

Infection with HIV is presently considered to lead to death. Several experimental treatments, however, are being tested. At the present time the interval between diagnosis of AIDS and death varies greatly. In developed countries, 50% of patients die within 18 months of diagnosis and 80% die within 36 months.

IMMUNOLOGIC MANIFESTATIONS
Cellular Abnormalities

HIV has a marked preference for the helper/inducer subset of lymphocytes. It displays an affinity for these cells because the CD4 surface marker protein on these cells serves as a receptor site for the virus. Recent studies have demonstrated that immunologic activation, such as participation in an immune response to HIV or to viruses in other cells, of T-helper cells latently infected with HIV induces the production of multiple viral particles leading to cell death. The extensive destruction of T cells leads to the gradual depletion of the helper–inducer type of lymphocytes. The major phenotypic cell populations affected by AIDS are helper/inducer (OKT4, Leu 3) and suppressor/cytotoxic (OKT8, Leu 2) subsets of T lymphocytes. Normally, this ratio is 2:1 in heterosexuals and 1.5:1 in homosexuals. A reversal of these subsets is evident in but not diagnostic of AIDS. In patients with AIDS

it is less than 0.5:1. It is important to note that this results from a marked decrease in the absolute number of circulating helper or OKT4 cells, rather than from an absolute increase in suppressor or OKT8 cells. This abnormality exists in the lymph nodes as well as in circulating T cells. A diminished OKT4 to OKT8 ratio (altered lymphocyte subpopulation) can also be seen in individuals with other disorders, such as cutaneous T cell lymphoma, systemic lupus erythematosus (SLE) and acute viral infections. The ratio, however, reverts back to normal after recovery from a viral infection in non-AIDS patients.

A decreased lymphocyte proliferative response to soluble antigens and mitogens exists in AIDS; functional testing reveals a diminished response to pokeweed mitogen (PWM). This disease also demonstrates defective natural killer (NK) cell activity.

Alterations in Immune System

HIV is fragile, and as the virus particle leaves its host cell, a molecule called gp120 frequently breaks off the virus's outer coat. Gp120 can bind to the CD4 molecules of uninfected cells, and when that complex is recognized by the immune system, these cells can be destroyed. The lysis of infected cells and gp120-bound uninfected cells leads to the gradual depletion of the helper–inducer type of lymphocytes. Defects in immunity are related to this T cell depletion. Progressive defects in the immune system also include a severe B cell failure, defects in monocyte function, and defects in granulocyte function.

Although HIV destroys OKT4 cells directly and hampers the immune system, this process does not cause the severe immune deficiency seen in AIDS. The severe deficiency can only be explained if the cells are also destroyed by other means. Several indirect mechanisms have been suggested. Infection by HIV can cause infected and uninfected cells to fuse into giant cells called **syncytia**, which are not functional. Autoimmune responses, in which the immune system attacks the body's own tissues, may also be at work. In addition, HIV-infected cells may send out protein signals that weaken or destroy other cells of the immune system. It is possible that the binding of HIV to a target cell triggers the release of the enzyme protease. Proteases digest proteins; if released in abnormal quantities, they might weaken lymphocytes and other cells and decrease cell survival. The decline in T cells and subsequent alteration of the immune mechanism is the underlying factor in progression of HIV infection.

Serologic Markers
Detection of Core Antigen

Following initial infection, the body mounts a vigorous immune response against the *viremia*. Immunologic activities include the production of different types of antibodies against HIV. Some anti-

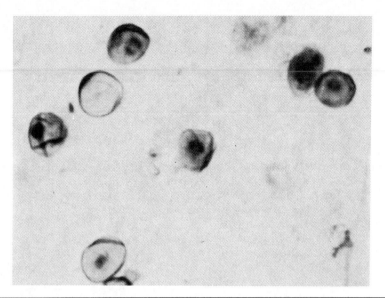

FIGURE 22-2

Pneumocystis carinii from tracheobronchial aspirate; stained with methenamine silver.

(From Markell EK and Voge M: Medical parasitology, ed 5, Philadelphia, 1981, WB Saunders Co.)

bodies neutralize it, others prevent it from binding to cells, and others stimulate cytotoxic cells to attack HIV-infected cells.

The time and sequence of appearance and disappearance of antibodies specific for the serologically important antigens of HIV-1 during the course of infection varies. A "window" period of seronegativity exists from the time of initial infection to 6 or 12 weeks or longer thereafter. Through enzyme immunoassay methods based on defined HIV-1 proteins produced by recombinant DNA methods, antibodies specific for gp41 are detectable for weeks or months before assays specific for p24. The appearance of antibodies specific for p24, however, has been shown in several studies to precede that of anti-gp41 when serum specimens were tested by Western Blot (WB) analysis. This discrepancy in the sequence of antibody appearance is believed to be due to the greater sensitivity of the WB technique compared to viral lysate-based EIAs used for the detection of anti-p24. Gp41 antibodies persist throughout the course of infection. Antibody specific for p24 not only rise to detectable levels after gp41 but can also disappear unpredictably and abruptly.

Increased production of core antigen is believed to be associated with a burst of viral replication and host cell lysis. The disappearance of antibody directed against p24 has been demonstrated to occur concomitantly with an increase in the concentration of core antigen in the serum. This parallel activity may be due to the sequestration of antibody in immune complexes, and the sudden decrease in

anti-p24 is considered to be a grave prognostic sign in HIV-1 infected patients.

Antibodies to HIV-1

Antibodies to HIV-1 appear after a lag period of about 6 weeks between the time of infection and a detectable antibody response. Because of this, some virus-positive, antibody-negative individuals would escape initial screening assays.

In addition to a positive HIV antibody test in 85% to 90% of patients, increased antibody titers to viruses—such as *cytomegalovirus*, *Epstein-Barr* virus, hepatitis A and B, *T. gondii*—and circulating immune (antigen-antibody) complexes can be found. A variety of other ancillary findings including polyclonal hypergammaglobulinemia, elevated levels of alpha interferon, alpha $(\alpha)_1$ thymosin, and beta microglobulin, and reduced levels of interleukin-1 or interleukin-2 have been noted.

Specific intrathecal synthesis of HIV antibody should be assessed simultaneously with an assay for total CSF IgM and for intrathecal synthesis of total IgG, as well as for intrathecal synthesis of IgG specific for an appropriate control organism such as adenovirus. In progressive encephalopathy related to AIDS, an increase in HIV antibody may suggest intrathecal synthesis compared to extrathecal synthesis.

DIAGNOSTIC EVALUATION

Laboratory evaluation of HIV-infected patients consists of assessment of cellular and humoral components. Screening of blood donors and patients at risk is usually done by serologic methods. In patients who have developed the signs and symptoms of AIDS, assessment of cellular concentrations and function become important, along with the diagnosis and treatment of opportunistic infections. Both leukopenia and lymphocytopenia exist in the AIDS patient. Total leukocyte and absolute lymphocyte concentrations need to be periodically assessed. The common denominator of the disease is a deficiency of a specific subset of thymus-derived (T4) lymphocytes. Enumeration of lymphocyte subsets is usually performed by flow cell cytometry. Decreased lymphocyte proliferative response to soluble antigens and mitogens, such as a diminished response to pokeweed mitogen (PWM), exists in this disorder. A variety of other ancillary findings, including polyclonal hypergammaglobulinemia, elevated levels of alpha interferon, alpha $(\alpha)_1$ thymosin, and beta microglobulin, and reduced levels of T cell growth factor or interleukin-2, have been noted.

TESTING METHODS
HIV Antibody

Antibodies to HIV are usually detected by enzyme immunoassay (EIA) and confirmed by the Western Blot technique. The vast majority of, and probably all, seropositive patients are also infectious, as manifested by isolation of HIV from peripheral blood.

EIA Procedures

The development of first-generation serologic procedures was rapid and has had a significant effect on reducing the transmission of HIV in donor blood. Serologic tests detect antibodies to HIV. Because HIV is located inside T cells, it does not produce a protein in excess as does HB_sAg; therefore the quantity of viral protein in the blood of infected persons is very low. HIV antibody, however, is present in much greater quantity, and with present techniques the antibody is much easier to detect.

The EIA screening tests for HIV-1 antibody currently licensed in the United States use microwells or beads coated with antigenic preparations of inactivated and lysed whole virus. In the EIA assay, diluted patient serum is added to a microwell, and HIV-1 specific antibody, if present, is allowed to react with the immunosorbent. After incubation and a thorough washing to remove extraneous serum proteins and unbound antibody, an enzyme-conjugated second antibody specific for human immunoglobulin is added and allowed to react with antibody bound to the absorbed viral lysate. After washing, an appropriate substate is then added to the microwell and the color change resulting from hydrolysis of the substrate by the enzyme is measured spectrophotometrically. When compared to a reference standard of known concentration, this color change is directly proportional to the amount of HIV-1 specific antibody present in the patient specimen.

TABLE 22-5

Problems Encountered in HIV Antibody Testing

False negative results	
HIV-infected patient	Insufficient p24 antigen in the viral reaction mixture
	Lack of detectable antibody for approximately 6 weeks following initial infection "window period"
AIDS patients	Diminished antibody titer associated with late-stage disease
	Loss of viral envelope accompanying the purification of viral lysate
False positive results	
Autoimmune disorders Malignancy	Contamination of immunosorbent with HTLV and related antigens from the human cells in which the virus was cultivated in the preparation of immunosorbent
	Circulating antibodies to nuclear or other cellular antigens
Autoimmune disorders Multiparous women	Circulating HLA antibodies
Alcoholism	Immune dysfunction associated with liver disease
Lymphoproliferative disease	Possible hypergammaglobulinemia
Normal donors	Heat treatment or prolonged storage of serum or plasma; possibly cellular antibodies

The manufacturer's claimed specificity and sensitivity in this method range is from 98% to 100%. Specificity is defined as the proportion of negative EIA test results obtained in the population of individuals who actually lack the antibody in question, e.g., anti-HIV. Sensitivity is defined as the frequency of positive EIA results obtained in the testing of a population of individuals who are truly positive for antibody, e.g., anti-HIV. Difficulties with assay sensitivity are based on the use of crude viral lysate. In clinical use, however, the sensitivity of the procedure ranges from 76% to 96%.

Problems can be encountered in detecting HIV antibodies (Table 22-5). Inherent difficulties in the preparation of viral lysate can cause lot-to-lot variability of results. For example, loss of envelope glycoprotein, e.g., gp41, can result from overstringent purification schemes, which causes insufficient antigen in the reaction mixture result and decreased test sensitivity with potential false negative results. The lack of detectable antibody for approximately 6 weeks following infection can also result in virus-positive, antibody-negative individuals going undetected in an initial screening assay. In addition, because HIV represents an enveloped particle, its membrane shares many antigenic similarities with the cell line used as virus producer. These include T cell antigens, HLA antigens, and other potential targets of the humoral response, which can produce false positive results. In a healthy person, a positive test result may indicate a subclinical infection, immunity, an active carrier state, or a biologic false positive.

At the present time, donor blood samples that are initially reactive in HIV antibody testing are rechecked in duplicate in order to rule out technical errors. With repeat testing, if one or more of the duplicate tests is positive, the specimen is considered "repeatably reactive." If the specimen is from a unit of blood, it is not used for transfusion. In order to rule out false positive results, it is necessary to confirm repeatably reactive test results by an alternate protocol.

Western Blot Test

Before an HIV result is considered to be positive, the results should be both reproducible and confirmable by at least one additional test. The Western Blot (WB) analysis is currently the standard method for confirming HIV-1 seropositivity. If the test is positive for bands gp41 and/or p24 in conjunction with a positive ELISA test, it is regarded as a confirmatory test. The WB test appears to work best with samples that contain high levels of antibody.

In the Western Blot procedure, purified HIV-1 viral antigens are electrophoresed on SDS gels and the separated polypeptides are then transferred onto sheets of nitrocellulose paper that are incubated with the serum specimen. Any antibody that binds to the separated peptides present on the nitrocellulose paper is detected by a secondary antihuman antibody and is conjugated to a suitable enzyme marker and incubated with the appropriate enzyme substrate. Antibody specificities against known viral components (generally the core component p24 and envelope component gp41) are considered true positive results, whereas antibodies specific against nonviral cellular contaminants are nonspecific, false positive results. The Western Blot technique, however, is time-consuming and expensive. It is also open to considerable interpretation and has many sources of error. Variables in the test include:
1. The technical skill and experience of the technologist performing the procedure.
2. Characteristics of the technical methodology.
3. General sensitivity of the WB technique in detecting antibodies specific for various HIV-1 antigens (especially during the window period of seronegativity).
4. Frequent lack of specificity due to contamination of the viral reference preparation by histocompatibility and other antigens that electrophoretically migrate with p24 and gp41.
5. Variation in band reactivity patterns in sera

from an individual over the course of HIV-1 infection.

Alternate Antibody Testing Methods

Alternate testing procedures are currently being used as research tools. These procedures are similar to the original first-generation tests in format and principle, with the exception that the antigen sources are recombinant DNA-derived products rather than crude or purified viral antigens. Sensitivities of gene-derived assays may not be significantly improved, but the specificity of newer tests may be superior because the problems associated with antibody reactivities against cell-substrate components will be nonexistent.

The **synthetic peptide approach** (solid phase EIA) for HIV-1 antibodies is an example of one technique that has been developed. This technique uses microwells to which have been adsorbed defined peptide homologs (produced by chemical synthesis or recombinant DNA technology) of serologically relevant proportions of immunodominant viral proteins. The advantages of synthetic p24/gp41 peptide-based assay over existing viral lysate-based antibody screening methods include increased specificity, increased sensitivity, and earlier detection of specific HIV-1 antibodies. Seroconversion in several patients has been detected from 1 to 5 weeks before it was detected by means of viral lysate-based tests and from 2 to 5 weeks before it was detected by the WB technique with high lot-to-lot reproducibility. In addition, the method demonstrates an absolute correlation with seropositivity exhibited by WB analysis. Future applications of synthetic peptides adsorbed to plastic dipsticks or to latex particles might include the ability to screen for the presence of HIV antibody in small laboratories and rural locations, such as underdeveloped nations in which retrovirus-related diseases are endemic.

To confirm antibody reactivities in a more objective manner than the Western Blot methodology, an immunofluorescent test has been developed that can accurately and rapidly confirm initially reactive serum specimens. In this procedure an HIV-1 induced cell line and an uninfected control cell line are separately deposited onto a microscope slide. The serum specimen to be tested is incubated on each cell spot, followed by an incubation with a goat antihuman antibody conjugated to fluorescein isothiocyanate (FITC). The microscope slides are examined using an ultraviolet microscope. With this technique it is possible to distinguish true positive from false positive test results. A dipstick version has also been developed for clinical laboratories, physicians' offices, and field testing conditions.

HIV Antigen and Genome Testing

In the United States current HIV screening programs identify individuals with anti-HIV-1. Screening of blood for antibodies, however, does not confirm the absence of virus. There are a small number of individuals who for a short period after HIV infection are virus positive by culturing technique but are antibody negative. In these cases detection of HIV antigen is of value. Because of the potential transmissibility of HIV-1 from asymptomatic seronegative individuals to others and the need to monitor patients on therapeutic agents, sensitive assays for the detection of virus are needed. Immunologic assays for antigens, however, may not detect any virus particles at some stages of infectivity. Different procedures have been described that can be used for the detection of HIV-1 antigen.

Cell Culturing and Reverse Transcriptase Methods

Cell culture methods provide valuable information regarding the presence of infectious viral particles. Lymphocytes are incubated in the presence of phytohemagglutinin (PHA) and interleukin-2 (IL-2) to promote growth of the virus-infected helper T cell population. The culture is maintained with IL-2 over a period of several weeks and continuously monitored for the presence of the viral enzyme, reverse transcriptase (RT)—a particle associated RNA-dependent DNA polymerase enzyme. Although this technique is cumbersome, it is capable of detecting viral growth within a 2- to 3-week period. The presence of reverse transcriptase, however, is only indicative of the presence of retrovirus, not necessarily HIV. Virus capture assay detects HIV in cell culture specimens and is more sensitive than classic RT assays.

Immunofluorescence Assay

Immunofluorescence assay (IFA) is commonly used to locate HIV-1 antigen in infected cells. Infected cells are treated with polyclonal or monoclonal antibody against p17 or p24. After washing, the cells are incubated with fluorescein isothiocyanate (FITC) or rhodamine conjugate as a secondary antibody, washed, mounted, and examined using a fluorescent microscope. The limitations of this technique include the need for expensive equipment and the fact that fluorescence fades quickly.

Immunohistochemical Staining

In this technique infected cells are incubated with HIV-1 antibody. After incubation the cells are treated with an enzyme-labeled secondary antibody (usually alkaline phosphatase or horseradish peroxidase), and an appropriate substrate is added. The cells are washed and examined using simple light microscopy. This method has the advantages of IFA but is simple, inexpensive, and does not require extensive expertise. Morphologic changes can also be observed.

ELISA Method

The ELISA method has been developed for antigen detection in culture medium, serum, plasma, or other tissue fluids. HIV antigen ELISA may de-

tect special HIV core antigens. With this technique microwells are coated with monoclonal antibody to the p24 core protein. The specimen is added to the well, incubated, and washed. A probe antibody (biotin conjugate) is then added to the wells. The well is incubated again, washed, and streptavidin-conjugated horseradish peroxidase is added and incubated. After washing, a substrate solution, such as tetramethylbenzidine solution, is added. If a color formation has taken place, it can be measured spectrophotometrically. This research procedure provides a quantitative estimation of the presence of HIV antigen. The method is considered to be more sensitive than reverse transcriptase assay, which is routinely used in many laboratories to detect retrovirus growth in culture medium. The ELISA technique is very specific for HIV-1. Commercial kits presently licensed for research use for the detection of p24 antigen by enzyme immunoassay are manufactured by Abbott Laboratories, Coulter Immunologic Division of Coulter Electronics, DuPont Biotechnology Systems, and Cellular Product, Inc.

Radioimmunoassay

Both solid-phase and liquid-phase RIA techniques have been developed for antigen testing. In the solid phase, microtiter wells are coated with monoclonal or polyclonal antibody to HIV-1 proteins. The test sample is added and incubated. After washing, an appropriate ^{125}I-labeled IgG (anti-HIV-1) solution is added and incubated. After washing, the wells are cut, and radioactivity is measured with a gamma counter. In liquid phase RIA, test specimens, such as serum or culture medium containing HIV-1, are mixed with ^{125}I-labeled IgG (anti-HIV-1) in a small volume of liquid. Following incubation, the mixture is centrifuged, the pellet is washed, and radioactivity is measured. A liquid competition RIA for the detection and quantitation of HIV-1 p24 using monoclonal antibody has also been developed.

Genetic Technologies

Advanced technologies are being developed to directly detect the presence of the viral gene rather than their products. These technologies are appropriate for use when the production of virus is low or when the virus may exist in a latent condition. Genetically based technologies include in situ hybridization, filter hybridation, Southern Blot analysis, and DNA amplification.

In situ hybridization. In this technique, the presence of HIV-1 in lymphocytes in primary lymph node and peripheral blood from AIDS- and HIV-infected patients is demonstrated. The method uses ^{35}S-labeled RNA probe, which binds with viral nucleic acids and is very specific for viral RNA. The procedure involves fixation of infected cells on a slide, acetylation and application of hybridization mixture containing radioactive probe on the slide, and autoradiograph. After processing, the slides are dipped in photographic emulsion, dried, and kept in the dark for 2 days at 4° C, during which time the probe emits radioactive particles and creates a latent image. After 2 days the slides are developed, dried, stained with Wright stain, and analyzed by light microscopy. The location of HIV-1 is represented by microscopic black dots. Twenty to 100 grains (dots) are observed per infected cell. One to three copies are represented by each grain and the grains are located over the nucleus and cytoplasm. Modifications of this technique use nonradioactive probes.

Filter hybridization. Filter hybridization has been successfully used to HIV-1 RNA in infected cells. It is able to detect one infected cell in 1000 peripheral blood leukocytes. The technique involves isolation and denaturation of cytoplasmic RNA from infected cells, transfer of the denatured material to a nylon filter, incubation of the filter with a radioactive probe, and, finally, autoradiography. Prehybridization and hybridization are performed using ^{32}P-labeled DNA. The cloned fragment represents the entire HIV-1 genome, excluding the leftmost 224 nucleotides.

RNA filter hybridization is more sensitive than the RT assay. The procedure is relatively rapid, simple, and inexpensive for detection of nucleic acids in infected cells and can be conveniently used to monitor viral growth in cell culture.

Southern Blot analysis. Southern Blot hybridization technique can be used to detect HIV-1 sequence in peripheral blood cells and tissues such as lymph nodes, liver, and kidney. The procedure involves the digestion of DNA isolated from HIV-1 infected cells or primary tissues with a panel of restriction enzymes and the separation of DNA fragments according to size using agarose gel electrophoresis. The DNA fragments are then transferred (or blotted) onto a membrane from the gel. The membrane is incubated with a cloned HIV-1 probe. With this technique hybridization of 18 viral DNA isolates to the full length of the cloned probe has been achieved. The method avoids complications due to the presence of unintegrated linear and circular DNA, as well as integrated proviral DNA within the infected cells. The enzymes, whose site in the viral LTR are well converted. It is an excellent technique for detecting a specific sequence that may be present in integrated or unintegrated form in infected cells.

DNA amplification. This technique allows for the direct detection of HIV-1 by DNA amplification. This ultrasensitive polymerase chain reaction technique is beginning to revolutionize HIV-1 detection. In addition to confirmatory testing, DNA amplification can be used to monitor the inactivation of HIV-1 by drugs. As this technique matures, it will provide more accurate and predictive HIV-1 testing and better testing for other latent viruses.

The goal of direct detection of active virus in patient specimens by an ultrasensitive method is to detect less than 100 molecules of viral nucleic acid in the peripheral blood cells isolated from 1 mL of blood. This number is the assay target because as few as 1 in 10,000 lymphocytes express viral RNA in HIV-1 infected individuals. Therefore, out of approximately 10^6 lymphocytes per mL of blood, about 100 contain viral nuclei acid, corresponding to 100 to 150 copies of HIV-1 DNA. The presence of HIV-1 DNA in lymphocytes of antibody-positive, asymptomatic persons can be used to confirm exposure to the virus; the presence of viral RNA might be a sensitive indication of viral replication and possibly an indication of further disease progression.

The basis of this technology lies in amplification of minute amounts of viral nucleic acid in lymphocyte DNA. In HIV-1 infected cells the DNA template is a provirus, which exists either as integrated or episomal DNA. After amplification, isotope or nonisotope methods can detect the amplified product. The most effective means of target amplification is the polymerase chain reaction. A pair of specific oligomer primers initiate DNA synthesis in combination with heat-stable Taq I DNA polymerase. Following this first round of primer extension, the material is heated to denature the product from its template and cooled to 37° C to permit annealing of the primer molecules to the original template DNA, as well as to the newly synthesized DNA fragments. Primer extension is then resumed. By repeating these cycles of denaturation, annealing and extension, the original DNA can be increased exponentially.

Viral RNA can also be specifically amplified with some additional steps. The gag region is probably the best choice of a sequence for amplification. Detection of viral RNA as well as DNA in clinical specimens might prove to be a better indicator of biologically active virus than DNA detection alone. The presence both of provirus and viral RNA transcriptase would be a strong indication of viral replication.

Sandwich hybridization is an alternative technique. Sandwich hybridization requires two adjacent, nonoverlapping probes: an immobilized capture probe and a labeled detection probe. A sandwich structure can form only if the specimen contains nucleic acid, which resembles the original junction between the two fragments in genomic nucleic acid. Sandwich hybridization is an ideal system for incorporating nonisotopic probes and nonfilter-based hybridization formats.

Chapter Review

HIGHLIGHTS

Human immunodeficiency virus (HIV-1) is the predominant virus responsible for acquired immunodeficiency syndrome (AIDS). In addition to the original HIV type 1 (HIV-1), a second AIDS-causing virus, HIV type 2 (HIV-2), was identified in 1985. In evolutionary terms, the two viruses are related and have a similar overall structure. The pathogenic potential of HIV-2, however, is not as well established as is HIV-1.

The HIV virus is a type D retrovirus. It is composed of structural proteins and glycoproteins that occupy the core and envelope regions of the particle. Retroviruses contain a single positive-stranded RNA with the virus's genetic information and a special enzyme, called reverse transcriptase, in their core. Reverse transcriptase enables the virus to convert viral RNA into DNA. This reverses the normal process of transcription in which DNA is converted to RNA—hence the term *retrovirus*. The genomes of all known retroviruses are organized in a similar way. In the provirus, which is formed when complementary DNA synthesis is completed from the retroviral RNA template, viral core and envelope proteins and the enzyme reverse transcriptase are encoded by the gag, env, and pol genes, respectively, whereas viral gene expression is regulated by tat, trs, sor, and 3° orf gene products. The HIV life cycle is that of a retrovirus. The genes of a retrovirus are encoded in RNA; before they can be expressed, the RNA must be converted into DNA. Only then are the viral genes transcribed and translated into proteins in the usual sequence.

The infectious process with HIV begins when the gp120 protein on the viral envelope binds to the protein receptor, called CD4, located on the surface of a target cell. Fusion of the virus to the membrane of this host cell enables the viral RNA and reverse transcriptase to invade the cell's cytoplasm. HIV has a marked preference for the helper/inducer subset of T lymphocytes. These cells, however, are not the only cells that have CD4 antigen embedded in their membrane. Macrophages, as many as 40% of the peripheral blood monocytes, and cells in the lymph nodes, skin, and other organs also express measurable amounts of CD4 and can be infected by HIV. In addition, about 5% of the B lymphocytes may express CD4 and be susceptible to HIV infection. Although some cells do not produce detectable amounts of CD4, they do contain low levels of messenger RNA encoding the CD4 protein, which indicates that they do produce some CD4. Because these cells can be infected by HIV in culture, the expression of only a very small amount of CD4 or an alternate receptor molecule may be necessary for HIV infection to take place. These cell types include certain cells of the brain, glial cells, a variety of malignant brain tumor cells, and some cells derived from cancers of the bowel. In addition, cells of the gastrointestinal system do not produce appreciable amounts of CD4, but gut cells called *chromaffin cells* do sometimes appear to be infected by HIV in vivo. This suggests that gastrointestinal infection may be what leads to the AIDS-associated weight loss and emaciation known in Africa as *slim disease.*

The viral replication cycle begins after HIV binds to the CD4 receptor and injects its core into the target cell. The core includes two identical strands of RNA. The enzyme, DNA polymerase, is responsible for converting the viral genetic information into DNA. Initially, this enzyme makes a single-stranded DNA copy of the viral RNA. An associated enzyme, ribonuclease, destroys the original RNA, and the polymerase makes a second complimentary copy of DNA using the first DNA strand as a template. The DNA polymerase and ribonuclease together are often called *reverse transcriptase.* After the viral genetic information is in the form of double-stranded DNA (the same form in which the cell carries its own genetic makeup), it migrates to the cell nucleus. A third viral enzyme, called an *integrase,* may then splice the HIV genome into the host cell's DNA. After the viral genome is integrated into the host DNA, the provirus will be duplicated together with the cell's own genes every time the cell divides. At this stage the HIV is permanent. The second half of the HIV life cycle (the production of new virus particles) takes place only sporadically and only in some infected cells.

AIDS has become a major cause of morbidity and mortality in the United States. The number of reported cases of AIDS has increased each year since the disease was first recognized. Three infection patterns of HIV virus have been traced world wide. Pattern 1 is found in North and South America, Western Europe, Scandinavia, Australia, and New Zealand, where it is primarily a disease of homosexuals and IV drug abusers. The male to female ratio in pattern 1 areas ranges from 10:1 to 15:1. Pattern 2 is found in Africa, the Caribbean, and some areas of South America, where it is primarily a heterosexual disease and the number of infected females and males is approximately equal. Pattern 3 is typically demonstrated in Eastern Europe, North Africa, the Middle East, Asia, and the Pacific, excluding Australia and New Zealand. In pattern 3 areas, relatively few cases of AIDS have been identified, and most of the affected individuals have had contact with pattern 1 or pattern 2 countries. Transmission of HIV is believed to be restricted to intimate contact with body fluids from an infected person; casual contact with infected persons has not been documented as a mode of transmission. Although the mode of transmission is considered to be predominantly sexual, the virus can be transmitted through contact with infected blood. Although HIV has been isolated from blood, semen, vaginal secretions, saliva, tears, breast milk, cerebrospinal fluid (CSF), amniotic fluid, and urine, only blood, semen, vaginal secretions, and possibly breast milk have been implicated in transmission of HIV to date. Evidence for the role of saliva in the transmission of the virus is unclear. A variety of practices have been advocated for the prevention of HIV transmission. Sexual abstinence or the practice of safe sex is essential to curtailing HIV transmission. The screening of blood donors and donors of organs, tissues, and semen, as well as blood products for HIV, has reduced the risk of HIV transmission to minimal levels. In addition, heat treatment and techniques such as monoclonal absorption have eliminated the risk of blood-borne HIV transmission to hemophiliacs. Guidelines from the Centers for Disease Control for clinical and laboratory personnel who work with AIDS patients and blood specimens suggest that the same precautions should be used as when the risk of hepatitis B infection is present.

The early phase of HIV infection may last from many months to many years after initial infection. Typically, patients in the early stages of HIV infection are either completely asymptomatic or may show mild, chronic lymphadenopathy. HIV causes a predictable, progressive derangement of immune function, and AIDS is just one late manifestation of that process. From 2 to 10 years after HIV infection, replication of the virus flares again and the infection enters its final stage. An average of 8 or 9 years may pass before AIDS is fully developed. The virus behaves differently depending on the kind of host cell and the cell's own level of mitotic activity. In T cells, however, the virus can lie dormant indefinitely, but it can destroy the host cell in a burst of replication. HIV grows continuously but slowly in macrophages-monocytes. This saves the cell from destruction but probably alters its function. The end stage of AIDS is characterized by the occurrence of neoplasms and/or opportunistic infections.

Lethal *Pneumocystis carinii* pneumonia has been a hallmark of AIDS. Other opportunistic infections, however, are frequent and may exist concurrently. Infection with HIV is presently considered to lead to death. Several experimental treatments, however, are being tested. At the present time the interval between diagnosis of AIDS to death varies greatly. In developed countries 50% of patients die within 18 months of diagnosis and 80% die within 36 months. A system for grouping patients has been developed at the Walter Reed Army Medical Center. In this system of classification the patient moves through six stages, the last of which is AIDS. The system is based on several indicators of the immune impairment that underlies HIV infection. The presence of opportunistic infection is a criterion for the diagnosis of AIDS. In patients with AIDS the helper/suppressor ratio is less than 0.5:1. It is important to note that this results from a marked decrease in the absolute number of circulating helper or OKT4 cells rather than from an absolute increase in suppressor or OKT8 cells. This abnormality exists in the lymph nodes as well as in circulating T cells. A diminished OKT4 to OKT8 ratio can also be seen in individuals with other disorders. The lysis of infected cells and gp120 bound uninfected cells leads to the gradual depletion of the helper/inducer type of lymphocytes. Defects in immunity are related to this T cell depletion. Progressive defects in the immune system also include a severe B cell failure, defects in monocyte function, and defects in granulocyte function.

Immunologic activities associated with HIV infection include the production of different types of antibodies against HIV. Some antibodies neutralize it, others prevent it from binding to cells, and others stimulate cytotoxic cells to attack HIV-infected cells. A "window" period of seronegativity exists from the time of initial infection to 6 or 12 weeks or longer. Using enzyme immunoassay methods based on defined HIV-1 proteins produced by recombinant DNA methods, antibodies specific for gp41 are detectable for weeks or months before assays specific for p24. The appearance of antibodies specific for p24, however, has been shown in several studies to precede that of anti-gp41 when serum specimens were tested by Western Blot (WB) analysis. This discrepancy in the sequence of antibody appearance is believed to be due to the greater sensitivity of the WB technique compared to viral lysate-based EIAs used for the detection of anti-p24. Gp41 antibodies persist throughout the course of infection. Antibody specific for p24 not only rises to detectable levels after gp41 but can also disappear unpredictably and abruptly in a short period of time. Increased production of core antigen is believed to be associated with a burst of viral replication and host cell lysis. The disappearance of antibody directed against p24 has been demonstrated to occur concomitantly with an increase in the concentration of core antigen in the serum. This parallel activity may be due to the sequestration of antibody in immune complexes; the sudden decrease in anti-p24 is considered to be a grave prognostic sign in HIV-1 infected patients.

Laboratory evaluation of HIV-infected patients consists of assessment of cellular and humoral components. Screening of blood donors and patients at risk is usually by serologic methods. In patients who have developed the signs and symptoms of AIDS, both assessment of cellular concentrations and function and the diagnosis and treatment of opportunistic infections, become important. Both leukopenia and lymphocytopenia exist in the AIDS patient. Total leukocyte and absolute lymphocyte concentrations need to be periodically assessed. The common denominator of the disease is a deficiency of a specific subset of thymus-derived (OKT4) lymphocytes. Enumeration of lymphocyte subsets is usually performed by flow cell cytometry. Decreased lymphocyte proliferative response to soluble antigens and mitogens, such as a diminished response to pokeweed mitogen (PWM), exists in this disorder.

A variety of other ancillary findings has also been noted. Antibodies to HIV are usually detected by enzyme immunoassay (EIA) and confirmed by the Western Blot technique. The Western Blot (WB) analysis is currently the standard method for confirming HIV-1 seropositivity. If the test is positive for bands p41 and/or p24 in conjunction with a positive ELISA test, it is regarded as a confirmatory test. Alternate testing procedures are currently being used as research tools. These procedures are similar to the original first-generation tests in format and principle, with the exception that the antigen sources are recombinant DNA-derived products rather than crude or purified viral antigens. Sensitivities of gene-derived assays may not be significantly improved, but the specificity of newer tests may be superior because the problems associated with antibody reactivities against cell-substrate components will be nonexistent.

The synthetic peptide approach (solid-phase EIA) for HIV-1 antibodies is an example of one technique that has been developed. Different procedures have been described that can be used for the detection of HIV-1 antigen. These procedures include cell culturing and reverse transcriptase methods, immunofluorescence assay (IFA), immunohistochemical staining, the ELISA technique, and radioimmunoassay. Advanced genetic technologies are being developed to directly detect the presence of the viral gene rather than their products. These technologies are appropriate for use when the production of virus is low or when the virus may exist in a latent condition. Genetically-based technologies include: in situ hybridization, filter hybridization, Southern Blot analysis, and DNA amplification.

REVIEW QUESTIONS

1. The major structural protein (core) of the HIV-1 virus is:
   A. gp41
   B. p24
   C. gp34
   D. gp140
   E. p26
2. The infectious process of AIDS begins when the gp 120 protein on the viral envelope bends to the protein receptor, _____, on the surface of a target cell.
   A. CD 8
   B. CD 4
   C. p24
   D. p26
   E. gp140
3. HIV can infect all of the following cells except:
   A. Helper-inducer subset of T lymphocytes
   B. Macrophages
   C. Monocytes
   D. Polymorphonuclear leukocytes
   E. Glial cells
4. The most rapidly growing segment of the HIV-infected population is:
   A. Homosexual males
   B. Lesbians
   C. Health care workers
   D. IV drug users and their sexual partners
   E. Pediatric recipients of blood products
5. In HIV infections, a window period of seronegativity exists from the time of initial infection to_____.
   A. 2 weeks
   B. 2 to 6 weeks or longer
   C. 6 to 12 weeks or longer
   D. 4 to 8 months or longer
   E. 6 to 12 months or longer

6. HIV antibodies are usually detected by ____(6)____ and confirmed by ____(7)____.
   A. Latex agglutination
   B. Enzyme immunoassay
   C. Enzyme inhibition
   D. Radioimmunoassay
   E. Immunofluorescent assay
7.
   A. Southern Blot
   B. Northern Blot
   C. Western Blot
   D. DNA hybridization
   E. Enzyme inhibition

Answers

1. B 2. B 3. D 4. D 5. C 6. B 7. C

BIBLIOGRAPHY

Coulis PA et al: Peptide-based immunodiagnosis of retrovirus infections, ACPR, Nov 1987, pp 34-47.
Epstein LB et al: Progressive encephalopathy in children with acquired immune deficiency syndrome, Ann Neurol 17:488-496, 1985.
Faloona GR: Current pharmacological agents used in experimental antiviral and immune modulating treatment for AIDS, ACPR, Nov 1987, pp 20-27.
Gallo RC and Montagnier L: AIDS in 1988, Sci Am 259(4):40-51, 1988.
Gallo D et al: Comparison of detection of antibody to the acquired immune deficiency syndrome virus by enzyme immunoassay, immunofluorescence, and Western Blot methods, J Clin Microbiol 23:1049-1051, 1986.
Goudsmit J et al: Expression of human immunodeficiency virus antigen (HIV-Ag) in serum and cerebrospinal fluid during acute and chronic infection, Lancet 2:177-180, 1986.
Goudsmit J et al: Intrathecal synthesis of antibodies to LAV/TLV-III specific IgG in individuals without AIDS or AIDS-related complex, N Engl J Med 292:1231-1234, 1986.
Goudsmit J et al: Intrathecal synthesis of antibodies to HTLV-III in patients without AIDS or AIDS related complex, Br Med J 192:1231-1234, 1986.
Haseltine WA and Wong-Stall F: The molecular biology of the AIDS virus, Sci Am 259(4):52-63, 1988.
Heyward WL and Curran JW: The epidemiology of AIDS in the US, Sci Am 259(4):72-81, 1988.
Ho DD et al: Isolation of HTLV-III from cerebrospinal fluid and neural tissues of patients with neurologic symptoms related to the acquired immunodeficiency syndrome, N Engl J Med 313:1493-1497, 1985.
Keller GH and Khan NC: Identification of HIV sequences using nucleic acid probes, ACPR, Nov 1988, pp 10-15.
Khan NC, Chatlynne LG, and Hunter E: Isolation of human immunodeficiency virus Type 1 from clinical samples obtained from AIDS patients, ACPR, May 1988, pp 12-17.
Khan NC and Hunter E: Detection of human immunodeficiency virus Type 1, ACPR, May 1988, pp 20-25.
Mann JM et al: The international epidemiology of AIDS, Sci Am 259(4):40-51, 1988.
Mayer KH et al: Human T-lymphotropic virus type III in high-risk, antibody-negative homosexual men, Ann Intern Med 104:194-196, 1986.
MMWR: 38:24, 1989.
Papsidero L et al: Acquired immune deficiency syndrome: detection of viral exposure and infection, Am Clin Prod Rev, 1986, pp 17-23.
Redfield RR et al: The Walter Reed staging classification for HTLV-III/LAV infection, N Engl J Med 314:131-132, 1986.
Redfield RR and Burke DS: HIV infection: the clinical picture, Sci Am 259(4):90-98, 1988.

Resnick L: Intra-blood-brain barrier synthesis of HIV specific IgG in patients with neurologic symptoms associated with AIDS or AIDS-related complex, N Engl J Med 313:1498-1502, 1985.

Sadovsky R: HIV-infected patients: a primary care challenge, Am Fam Phy 40:3, 1989.

Salahuddin SZ: HTLV-III in symptom-free seronegative persons, Lancet 2:1418-1420, 1984.

Shaw GM et al: HTLV-III infections in brains of children and adults with AIDS encephalopathy, Science 227:177-182, 1985.

Turgeon ML: Clinical hematology, Boston, 1988, Little, Brown & Co.

Turgeon ML: Fundamentals of immunohematology, Philadelphia, 1989, Lea & Febiger.

US Department of Health and Human Services: Testing donors of organs, tissues, and semen for antibody to human T-lymphotropic virus type III/lymphadenopathy-associated virus, MMWR 34(20):294, 1985.

US Department of Health and Human Services: Human immunodeficiency virus infection in the United States: a review of current knowledge, MMWR 36:Suppl-6, 1-48, Dec 18, 1987.

US Department of Health and Human Services: Universal precautions for prevention of transmission of HIV, hepatitis B virus, and other blood borne pathogens in health care settings, MMWR 37:377, June 24, 1988.

US Department of Health and Human Services: Update: acquired immunodeficiency syndrome and HIV infection among health care workers, MMWR 37:229, April 22, 1988.

Weber JN and Weiss RA: HIV infection: the cellular picture, Sci Am 259(4):100-109, 1988.

Weiss SH et al: Screening test for HTLV-III (AIDS agent) antibodies: specificity, sensitivity, and applications, JAMA 253:221-225, 1985.

Wong-Stall F and Gallo RC: Human T-lymphotropic retroviruses, Nature 317:395-403, 1985.

PART
IV

Immunologically and Serologically Related Disorders

Hypersensitivity Reactions

The term *immunization,* or *sensitization,* describes an immunologic reaction dependent on the host's response to a subsequent exposure of antigen and not to any significant difference in the cellular and chemical events that follow the injection of the antigen. Small quantities of antigen, however, may favor sensitization by restricting the quantity of antibody formed. An unusual reaction, i.e., an allergic or hypersensitive reaction, that follows a second exposure to antigen reveals the existence of the sensitization. Hypersensitivity has traditionally been separated on the basis of time after exposure to an offending antigen. When this criteria is used, the terms *immediate* and *delayed* are appropriate. As described in Chapter 1, immediate hypersensitivity is antibody-mediated, and delayed hypersensitivity is cell-mediated.

ANAPHYLACTIC AND TYPE I REACTIONS

Type I hypersensitivity reactions can range from life-threatening anaphylactic reactions to milder manifestations associated with food allergies. Atopic allergies include hay fever, asthma, and food allergies.

Etiology

Atopic allergies are mostly naturally occurring, and the source of antigenic exposure is not always known. Atopic illnesses were among the first antibody-associated diseases demonstrating a strong familial or genetic tendency.

Several groups of agents cause anaphylactic reactions. The two most common agents are drugs, e.g., systemic penicillin, and insect stings. Insects of the order *Hymenoptera*, e.g., common hornet, yellow jacket, yellow hornet, and paper wasp, are representative examples of insects causing the most serious reactions.

Immunologic activity

Mast cells (tissue basophils) are the cellular receptors for IgE, which attaches to their outer surface. These cells are common in connective tissues, the lungs and uterus, and around blood vessels. They are also abundant in the liver, kidney, spleen, heart, and other organs. The granules contain a complex of heparin, histamine, and zinc ions, with the heparin existing in an approximate ratio of 6:1 with histamine. The actual heparin content is about 70 to 90 $\mu g/10^6$ cells; the histamine content is about 10 to 15 $\mu g/10^6$ cells. The release of histamine and heparin from mast cell granules occurs when the cells are exposed to specific immunologic or chemical agents. The cellular events during mast cell degranulation and the molecular events that follow degranulation occur within a few seconds.

Anaphylaxis is the clinical response to immunologic formation and fixation between a specific antigen and a tissue-fixing antibody. This reaction is usually mediated by IgE antibody and occurs in three stages:

1. The offending antigen attaches to the IgE antibody fixed to the surface membrane of mast cells and basophils. Cross-linking of two IgE molecules is necessary to initiate mediator release from mast cells.
2. Activated mast cells and basophils release various mediators.
3. The effects of mediator release produce vascular changes, activation of platelets, eosinophils, and neutrophils, and activation of the coagulation cascade.

It is believed that physical allergies such as heat, cold, and ultraviolet light cause a physiochemical derangement of protein or polysaccharides of the skin and transform them into autoantigens responsible for the allergic reaction. Most, if not all of these reactions, are caused by the action of a self-directed IgE.

Anaphylactoid (anaphlaxis-like) reactions are clinically similar to anaphylaxis. They can be caused by immunologically inert materials that activate serum and tissue proteases and the alternate pathway of the complement system. They are not mediated by antigen-antibody interaction but offending substances act directly either on the mast cells, causing the release of mediators, or on the tissues, e.g., anaphylotoxins of the complement cascade—C3a, C5a, etc. Direct chemical degranulation of mast cells may be the cause of anaphylactoid reactions resulting from the infusion of macromolecules, such as proteins.

Signs and symptoms

Local reactions consist of urticaria and angioedema at the site of antigen exposure of angioedema of the bowel after ingestion of certain foods. These reactions are severe but rarely fatal. Physical allergies to heat, cold, sunlight, and pressure are not as life-threatening as those related to injectables.

Anaphylactic reactions are dramatic and rapid in their onset. The signs and symptoms of anaphylaxis are defined by the physiologic effects of the primary and secondary mediator on the target organs such as the cardiovascular or respiratory system, gastrointestinal tract, or the skin. Several important pharmacologically active compounds are discharged from mast cells and basophils during anaphylaxis (Table 23-1).

Histamine release leads to constriction of bronchial smooth muscle, edema of the trachea and larynx, and stimulation of smooth muscle in the gastrointestinal tract, which causes vomiting and diarrhea. The resulting breakdown of cutaneous vascular integrity results in urticaria and angioedema; vasodilation causes a reduction of circulating blood volume and a progressive fall in blood pressure leading to shock. Kinins also alter vascular permeability and blood pressure.

The body's natural moderators of anaphylaxis are the enzymes that decompose the mediators of anaphylaxis. Antihistamines have no effect on histamine release from mast cells or basophils. In humans, antihistamines are effective antagonists of edema and pruritus, which is probably related to their blockage of a histamine-induced increase in capillary permeability. Antihistamines, however, are relatively less effective in humans in preventing bronchoconstriction.

Laboratory evaluation

In vitro evaluation of type I hypersensitivity reactions can be by RIST (RadioImmunoSorbent Test) and RAST (RadioAllergoSorbent Test), and enzyme immunoassays. A nephelometric cryoprecipitation testing may also be used. The RIST procedure depends on the availability of an ^{125}I-labeled IgE myeloma protein and its specific antibody; the latter is used in the solid phase of this RIA procedure. Competition of IgE in any unknown serum sample with the radiolabeled myeloma protein is measured. It is a direct measure of total serum IgE and a typical competitive inhibition RIA test. RAST uses a specific allergen bound to a solid phase carrier, which is then incubated with a serum sample containing an unknown amount of IgE specific for the allergen. The amount of label bound is only a measure of the allergen-specific IgE in the serum. Both the RIST and RAST tests have been adapted to the enzyme immunoassay method.

The advantages of in vitro testing include the lack of risk of a systemic hypersensitivity reaction and the lack of dependence on skin reactivity that can be influenced by drugs, disease, or the patient's age. Disadvantages of the RAST include limited allergen selection, reduced sensitivity compared with intradermal skin testing, and increased expense.

Healthy adults usually have 61 to 100 ng of IgE per mL of serum. IgE in cord serum is about 35% of the adult average. There is no correlation between maternal and newborn serum IgE levels, which indicates that fetal IgE synthesis can occur. In various atopic allergic diseases, especially hay fever and asthma, IgE levels may rise to nearly 6,000 ng/mL. Values over 1,000 are considered to be pathologic.

CYTOTOXIC REACTIONS (TYPE II HYPERSENSITIVITY REACTIONS)

Cytotoxic reactions are characterized by the interaction of IgG or IgM antibody to cell-bound antigen. This binding of an antigen and antibody can result in the activation of complement and destruction of the cell (cytolysis) to which the antigen is bound. Erythrocytes, leukocytes, and platelets can be lysed by this process. Examples of cytotoxic re-

TABLE 23-1

Mediators of Anaphylaxis

Mediator	Primary action
Histamine	Increases vascular permeability
	Promotes contraction of smooth muscle
Leukotrienes	Alters bronchial smooth muscle and enhances the effects of histamine on target organs
Basophil kallikrein	Generates kinins
Serotonin	Contracts smooth muscle
Platelet-activating factor	Enhances the release of histamine and serotonin from platelets that affect smooth muscle tone and vascular permeability
ECF-A Eosinophil chemotactic factors of anaphylaxis	Attracts eosinophils to area of activity; these cells release secondary mediators that may limit the effects of primary mediators
Prostaglandins	Affect smooth muscle tone and vascular permeability

actions include immediate (acute) transfusion reactions and immune hemolytic anemias, such as hemolytic disease of the newborn.

Transfusion reactions

The term *transfusion reaction* generally refers to the adverse consequences of incompatibility between patient and donor erythrocytes. Transfusion reactions can include hemolytic (red cell lysing) reactions occurring during or shortly after a transfusion, shortened post-transfusion survival of red blood cells, an allergic response, or disease transmission.

Transfusion reactions can be divided into hemolytic and non-hemolytic types. Hemolytic reactions are associated with the infusion of incompatible erythrocytes. These reactions can be further classified into acute (immediate) or delayed in their manifestations (see box). Several factors influence whether a transfusion reaction will be acute or delayed. These factors include:

1. The number of incompatible erythrocytes infused
2. The antibody class or subclass
3. The achievement of the optimal temperature for antibody binding

Immediate and Delayed Hemolytic Reactions
Immediate (Acute) Hemolytic Reaction

The most common cause of an acute hemolytic transfusion reaction is the transfusion of ABO-group incompatible blood. In patients with pre-existing antibodies caused by prior transfusion or pregnancy, other blood groups may be responsible.

Epidemiology. Acute hemolytic reactions are

Types of Transfusion Reactions

Immediate hemolytic

Intravascular hemolysis of erythrocytes

Delayed hemolytic

Extravascular hemolysis of erythrocytes

Immediate non-hemolytic

Febrile reactions
Anaphylaxis
Urticaria
Noncardiac pulmonary edema
Fever and shock
Congestive heart failure
Myocardial failure

Delayed non-hemolytic

Graft-*vs*-host disease
Posttransfusion purpura
Iron overload
Alloimmunization to erythrocytes, leukocytes, and/or platelet antigens or plasma proteins
Infectious diseases

---

the most serious and potentially lethal. Most fatalities resulting from acute hemolytic transfusion reactions occur in anesthetized or unconscious patients with the immediate cause of death being uncontrollable hypotension.

Signs and symptoms. Reactions can occur with the infusion of as little as 10 to 15 mL of incompatible blood. The most common initial symptoms are fever and chills, which mimic a febrile, non-hemolytic reaction caused by leukocyte incompatibility. Back pain, shortness of breath, pain at the infusion site, and hypotension are additional symptoms. In addition to shock, the release of thromboplastic substances into the circulation can induce disseminated intravascular coagulation (DIC) and acute renal failure.

Immunologic manifestations. Acute hemolytic reactions occur during or immediately after blood has been infused. Infusion of incompatible erythrocytes in the presence of pre-existing antibodies initiates an antigen-antibody reaction with the activation of the complement, plasminogen, kinin, and coagulation systems. Other initiators of acute hemolytic reactions include bacterial contamination of blood or the infusion of hemolyzed erythrocytes. Many reactions demonstrate both extravascular and intravascular hemolysis. If an antibody is capable of activating complement and is sufficiently active in vivo, intravascular hemolysis occurs producing a rapid increase of free hemoglobin in the circulation. The cause of the immediate clinical symptoms is uncertain, but they may be due to products released by the action of complement on the erythrocytes, which triggers multiple shock mechanisms.

Delayed Hemolytic Reactions

A delayed reaction may not express itself until 7 to 10 days post-transfusion. In contrast to an immediate reaction, a delayed reaction occurs in the extravascular spaces. These reactions are associated with decreased red cell survival because of the coating of the red cells (a positive DAT) that promotes phagocytosis and premature removal of the red cells by the mononuclear phagocytic system. If an antibody does not activate complement or does so very slowly, extravascular hemolysis occurs. Most IgG antibody-coated erythrocytes are destroyed extravascularly, mainly in the spleen.

A delayed hemolytic transfusion reaction may be of two types. It may represent an anamnestic antibody response in a previously immunized recipient upon secondary exposure to transfused erythrocyte antigens or it may result from primary allo-immunization. In an anamnestic response, the antibodies are directed against antigens to which the recipient has been previously immunized by transfusion or pregnancy.

Non-hemolytic Reactions

Non-hemolytic reactions like hemolytic reactions may be of an immediate or delayed nature.

Immediate non-hemolytic reactions include febrile and platelet reactions as well as reactions to plasma constituents. Delayed non-hemolytic reactions include graft versus host disease.

Immediate non-hemolytic reactions—febrile reactions. The most common type of febrile transfusion reaction results from cytotoxic or leukoagglutinins (leukocyte antibodies). If these antibodies are present in the recipient's plasma, a reaction occurs between the antibodies and the antigens present on the cell membrane of transfused leukocytes (lymphocytes or granulocytes) or platelets. Nonspecific leukoagglutinins, as well as those of HLA origin, have been implicated in febrile reactions. Leukoagglutinins have also been implicated in a specific type of delayed reaction referred to as the *noncardiac pulmonary edema syndrome*.

Febrile reactions may be mild to severe and may begin early in the transfusion to an hour or two after the transfusion has been completed. The most common symptom of a febrile reaction is fever, often accompanied by chills, that begins during or soon after transfusion. Although a nonhemolytic febrile reaction is rarely harmful, fever may also be part of the clinical symptoms of a hemolytic transfusion reaction.

Platelet reactions. Two types of immediate reactions to transfused platelets have been documented: febrile reactions and hemolytic reactions. Febrile reactions to platelet transfusions are probably related to the presence of large numbers of leukocytes in the platelet concentrate component.

Reaction to plasma constituents. Immediate reactions to plasma constituents may be classified as *allergic* and *anaphylactoid* or *anaphylactic* in nature.

Allergic and anaphylactoid reactions. Most authorities agree that of allergic and anaphylactoid reactions are caused by a reaction to soluble constituents in donor plasma. There is more discomfort than danger. The second most common transfusion reaction is referred to as an *allergic reaction*. When the reaction is extensive or produces edema, it is referred to as *anaphylactoid*. Anaphylactoid reactions are not uncommon following an intramuscular injection of serum immune globulins that have detectable amounts of IgA.

Allergic and anaphylactoid reactions develop during or shortly after transfusion. Allergic reactions are manifested by urticaria and itching, local erythema but usually no fever. If the cutaneous reaction is extensive or produces oral, pharyngeal, or laryngeal edema, it is an anaphylactoid reaction. Reactions can be controlled with antihistamines.

Anaphylactic reactions. Anaphylactic reactions (discussed in detail in the preceding section) occur in IgA-deficient plasma recipients who have developed anti-IgA antibodies. IgA deficiency is the most frequent of all of the selective deficiencies of serum immunoglobulins occurring in about 1 per 700 persons. 10% of these patients develop antibodies to IgA protein as the result of previous transfusions, pregnancy, or without a known source of stimulation and can suffer acute anaphylactic reactions when infused with blood products containing the protein. Fortunately, anaphylactic reactions due to anti-IgA are very rare. Other potential causes of anaphylactic reaction are the presence of antibodies to soluble plasma antigens or to drugs, such as penicillen, contained in transfused blood.

Clinical signs are seen very suddenly after exposure to the IgA protein, often before 10 mL of plasma has been infused. Symptoms include nausea, abdominal cramps, emesis, and diarrhea. Transient hypertension is followed by hypotension. Shock and loss of consciousness follow.

Delayed Non-Hemolytic Reactions

Graft versus host disease. When immunocompetent lymphocytes are transfused from a donor to a recipient who is not capable of rejecting them, the transfused or grafted lymphocytes recognize the antigens of host as foreign and react immunologically against them. Instead of the usual transplantation reaction of host against graft, the reverse graft-versus-host disease (see Chapter 28) occurs. This reaction produces an inflammatory response.

In a normal lymphocyte-transfer reaction, the results of a graft-versus-host reaction are usually not serious, since the recipient is capable of destroying the foreign lymphocytes. If the recipient, however, cannot reject the transfused lymphocytes, the grafted lymphocytes may cause uncontrolled destruction of the host's tissues and eventually death. Graft-versus-host reactions occur in immunodeficient or immunosuppressed patients. It is now accepted that graft versus host disease may occur whenever immunologically competent allogeneic lymphocytes are transfused into a severely immunocompromised host.

Hemolytic disease of the newborn (HDN). Hemolytic disease of the newborn (HDN), previously called erythroblastosis fetalis, results from excessive destruction of fetal red cells by maternal antibodies. This condition in the fetus or newborn infant is clinically characterized by anemia and jaundice. If the hemoglobin breakdown product that visibly produces jaundice (bilirubin), reaches excessive levels in the newborn infant's circulation, it will accumulate in lipid-rich nervous tissue and can result in mental retardation or death.

Etiology. Antigens possessed by the fetus that are foreign to the mother can provoke an antibody response in the mother. Any blood group antigen that occurs as an IgG antibody is capable of causing HDN.

Although anti-A and anti-B are present in the absence of their corresponding antigens as environmentally stimulated (IgM) antibodies, infrequent IgG forms may be responsible for HDN because of ABO incompatibility. High titers of anti-A,B of the IgG type in group O mothers commonly cause mild HDN. Anti-A and anti-B antibodies are usually 19S (IgM) in character and as such are unable to pass through the placental barrier. In addition, the A and B antigens are not fully expressed on the erythrocytes of the fetus and newborn. In a survey of antibodies that have caused HDN, over 70 different antibodies were identified.

Epidemiology. The incidence of HDN resulting from ABO incompatibility ranges from 1 in 70 to 1 in 180 with an estimated average of 1 in 150 births. The most frequent form of ABO incompatibility occurs when the mother is type O and the baby is type A or type B, usually type A.

Until the early 1970s, the Rh antibody, anti-D, was the most frequent cause of moderate or severe forms of HDN and anti-D either alone or in combination with another Rh antibody; anti-C accounted for approximately 93% of the cases of non-ABO HDN. Since the development of modern treatment to prevent primary immunization to the D antigen, however, the frequency of HDN because of anti-D has significantly decreased.

Signs and symptoms. HDN resulting from ABO incompatibility is usually mild in manifestations because of several factors: fewer A and B antigen sites on the fetal/newborn erythrocytes, weaker antigen strength of fetal/newborn A and B antigens, and competition for anti-A and anti-B between tissues as well as erythrocytes. The number and strength of A and B antigen sites on fetal erythrocytes are less than on adult red blood cell membranes. In addition, A and B substances are not confined to the red cells so that only a small fraction of IgG anti-A and anti-B that crosses the placenta combines with the infant's erythrocytes.

Manifestations of HDN caused by other antibodies can range from mild to severe. In addition to possible death in utero, newborn infants may demonstrate severe anemia and an increase in red blood cell breakdown products, such as bilirubin. Accumulation of bilirubin causes jaundice and may result in mental retardation if methods are not applied to clear bilirubin from the infant's body.

Immunologic mechanism. For antibody formation to take place, the mother must lack the antigen and the fetus must express the antigen (gene product). The fetus would inherit the gene for antigen expression from the father. HDN results from the production of antibodies in the mother that have been stimulated by the presence of these foreign fetal antigens. The actual production of antibodies depends on a variety of factors: the genetic makeup of the mother, the antigenicity of a specific antigen, and the actual amount of antigen introduced into the maternal circulation.

Transplacental hemorrhage (TPH) can occur at any stage of pregnancy. Immunization resulting from TPH can result from negligible doses during the first 6 months in utero; however, significant immunizing hemorrhage usually occurs during the third trimester or at delivery. Fetal erythrocytes can also enter the maternal circulation as the result of physical trauma from an injury, abortion, ectopic pregnancy, amniocentesis or normal delivery.

Abruptio placentae, cesarean section, and manual removal of the placenta are often associated with a considerable increase in TPH.

An example of the normal pattern of immunization is demonstrated by the case of an Rh (D) negative mother whose primary immunization (sensitization) was due to either a previously incompatible Rh (D) positive pregnancy or blood transfusion, which stimulates the production of low titered anti-D, predominantly of the IgM class. Subsequent antigenic stimulation, such as fetal-maternal hemorrhage while pregnant with an Rh (D) positive fetus, can elicit a secondary (anamnestic) response, which is characterized by the predominance of increasing titers of anti-D of the IgG class.

Immune antibodies subsequently react with fetal antigens. Erythrocytic antigens as well as leukocyte and platelet antigens can all induce maternal immunization by the formation of IgG antibodies. In HDN the erythrocytes of the fetus become coated with maternal antibodies that correspond to specific fetal antigens. IgG antibodies, the only immunoglobulin selectively transported to the fetus, are transferred from the maternal circulation to the fetal circulation through the placenta. The mechanism by which IgG passes through the placenta has not been definitely established. Most research on the subject of transplacental passage, however, supports the hypothesis that all IgG subclasses are capable of crossing the placental barrier between mother and fetus.

When the antigen and its corresponding antibody combine in vivo, increased lysis of red cells results. Because of this hemolytic process, the normal 45 to 70 day life-span of the fetal erythrocytes is reduced. To compensate for red cell loss, the fetal liver, spleen, and bone marrow respond by increasing production of erythrocytes. Increased erythrocyte production outside of the bone marrow, *extramedullary hematopoiesis,* can result in enlargement of the liver and spleen and premature release of nucleated erythrocytes from the bone marrow into the fetal circulation. If increased production of erythrocytes cannot compensate for the cell being destroyed, a progressively severe anemia develops that can cause the fetus to develop cardiac failure with generalized edema and death in utero. Less severely affected infants continue to experience erythrocyte destruction after birth, which generates large quantities of unconjugated bilirubin. Bilirubin resulting from excessive hemolysis, can produce the threat of accumulation of free bilirubin in lipid-rich tissue of the central nervous system.

Diagnostic evaluation. The following procedures are generally employed in either the prenatal or postnatal diagnostic evaluation of HDN:
1. ABO blood grouping
2. Rh testing
3. Screening for alloantibodies; identification and titering of any alloantibodies
4. Amniocentesis (prenatal)
5. Serum bilirubin of cord or infant blood

6. Direct antiglobulin test of cord or infant blood
7. Peripheral blood smear
8. The D$^\mu$ Rosette or Kleihauer-Betke test

A complete discussion and the method of performance of these procedures can be found in *Fundamentals of Immunohematology.*

Prevention. Three independent research teams demonstrated that a passive antibody, Rh IgG, could protect most Rh negative mothers from becoming immunized following the delivery of Rh (D) positive infant or similar obstetric conditions. In 1968, Rh IgG was licensed for administration in the United States. Since that time a dramatic decrease in the incidence of HDN caused by anti-D has taken place, although complete elimination may never occur because of the cases in which anti-D is formed before delivery. All pregnant Rh negative women should receive Rh IgG even if the Rh status of the fetus is unknown because fetal D antigen is present on fetal erythrocytes as early as 38 days from conception.

IMMUNE COMPLEX (TYPE III) REACTIONS

The formation of immune complexes under normal conditions protects the host because these complexes facilitate the clearance of various antigens and invading micro-organisms by the phagocytic system. In immune complex reactions, however, antigen-antibody complexes form in the soluble or fluid phase of tissues or in the blood and assume unique biologic functions such as interaction with complement and with cellular receptors. Examples of type III reactions include the Arthus reaction, (Fig. 23-1) serum sickness, and certain aspects of autoimmune disease such as glomerulonephritis in systemic lupus erythematosus. Circulating soluble immune complexes are responsible for or associated with a variety of human diseases, in which both exogenous and endogenous antigens can trigger a pathogenic immune response and result in immune complex disease (Table 23-2).

These reactions are caused by IgG, IgM, or possibly other antibody types. Immune complexes can exhibit a spectrum of biologic activities, including suppression or augmentation of the immune response by interacting with B and T cells; inhibition of tumor cell destruction; and deposition in blood vessel walls, glomerular membranes, and in other sites. These deposits interrupt normal physiologic processes because of tissue damage secondary to the activation of complement and resulting activities such as mediating immune adherence and at-

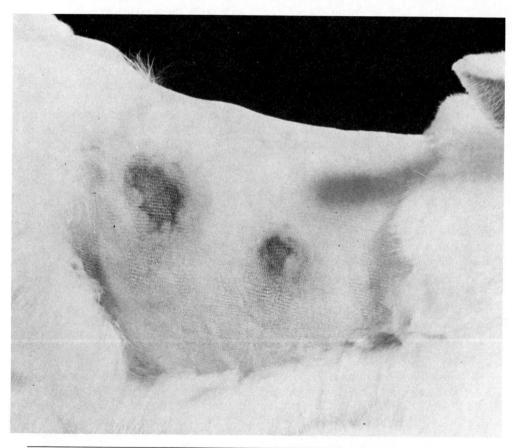

FIGURE 23-1

The arthus reaction. In these two reactions of the skin of a rabbit, the larger reaction has an extensive zone of erythema and edema surrounding its necrotic center.
(From Markell EK and Voge M: Medical parasitology, ed 5, Philadelphia, 1981, WB Saunders Co.)

tracting leukocytes and macrophages to the sites of immune complex deposition. The release of enzymes and possibly other agents damages the tissues. The three general anatomic sites of antigen-antibody interactions are as follows:

1. Antibody can react with soluble antigens in the circulation and form immune complexes that may disseminate and lodge in any tissue with a large filtration area and cause lesions of immune complex disease
2. Antibody can react with antigen secreted or injected locally into the interstitial fluids. The classic example of this is the experimental Arthus reaction, which is the basic model of local immune complex disease
3. Antibody can also react with structural antigens that form part of the cell surface membranes or with fixed intercellular structures such as the basement membranes. The systemic immune complex disease, serum sickness, is an example of soluble and tissue-fixed antigen involvement.

Acute serum sickness develops within 1 to 2 weeks after initial exposure or repeated exposure by injection of heterologous serum protein. There is no pre-existing antibody, and the disease appears as antibody formation begins. The hallmark of serum sickness is the protracted interaction between antigen and antibody in the circulation with the formation of antigen-antibody complexes in an environment of antigen excess. Chronic serum sickness can be experimentally induced if small amounts of antigen are given daily and represent just enough antigen to balance antibody production.

TYPE IV CELL-MEDIATED REACTIONS

Cell-mediated immunity consists of immune activities that differ from antibody-mediated immunity. Cell-mediated immunity is moderated by the link between T lymphocytes and phagocytic cells, i.e., monocytes-macrophages. Lymphocytes (T cells) do not recognize the antigens of micro-organisms or other living cells but are immunologically active through various types of direct cell-to-cell contact and by the production of soluble factors. The delayed type reaction is cell-mediated and involves antigen-sensitized T cells, which respond directly or by the release of lymphokines to exhibit contact dermatitis and allergies of infection (Fig. 23-2).

Cell-mediated immunity is responsible for the following immunologic events:

1. Contact sensitivity
2. Delayed hypersensitivity
3. Immunity to viral and fungal antigens
4. Immunity to intracellular organisms
5. Rejection of foreign-tissue grafts

TABLE 23-2

Diseases associated with immune complexes

Type	Examples
Autoimmune diseases	Rheumatoid arthritis, systemic lupus erythematosus, Sjogren's syndrome, mixed connective tissue disease (MCTD), systemic sclerosis
Glomerulone-phritis	
Neoplastic disease	Solid and lymphoid tumors
Infectious disease	Bacterial infective endocarditis, streptococcal infection, viral hepatitis, infectious mononucleosis

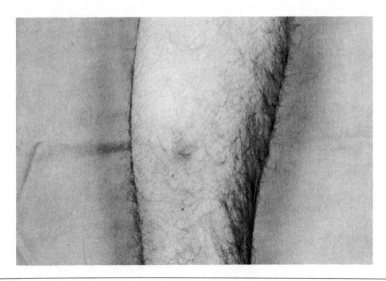

FIGURE 23-2

A delayed skin reaction exhibiting an erythematous but nonedematous zone 15 mm in diameter at 48 hours. A control site, inoculated higher on the forearm, shows no reaction at this time.

(From Barrett JT: Textbook of immunology, ed 5, St Louis, 1988, The CV Mosby Co.)

6. Elimination of tumor cells bearing neoantigens
7. Formation of chronic granulomas
Under some conditions, the activities of cell-mediated immunity may not be beneficial. Suppression of the normal adaptive immune response (immunosuppression) by drugs or other means is necessary in conditions such as organ transplantation, hypersensitivity, and autoimmune disorders.

Chapter Review

HIGHLIGHTS

The term *immunization*, or *sensitization*, is used to describe an immunologic reaction dependent on the response of the host to a subsequent exposure of antigen and not any significant difference in the cellular and chemical events that follow the injection of the antigen. Hypersensitivity has traditionally been separated on the basis of time after exposure to an offending antigen. When this criteria is used, the terms *immediate* and *delayed* are appropriate.

Type I hypersensitivity reactions can range from life-threatening anaphylactic reactions to milder manifestations associated with food allergies. Atopic allergies include hay fever, asthma, and food allergies. Several groups of agents cause anaphylactic reactions. The two most common agents are drugs and insect stings. Mast cells (tissue basophils) are the cellular receptors for IgE, which attaches to their outer surface. The granules consist of a complex of heparin, histamine, and zinc ions. The release of histamine and heparin from mast cell granules occurs when the cells are exposed to specific immunologic or chemical agents. Anaphylaxis is the clinical response to immunologic formation and fixation between a specific antigen and a tissue-fixing antibody. This reaction is usually mediated by IgE antibody and occurs in three stages. In cases of physical allergies such as heat, cold, and ultraviolet light, they are believed to cause a physiochemical derangement of protein or polysaccharides of the skin and transform them into autoantigens that are responsible for the allergic reaction. Anaphylactoid (anaphlaxis-like) reactions are clinically similar to anaphylaxis. They can be caused by immunologically inert materials that activate serum and tissue proteases and the alternate pathway of the complement system.

Local reactions consist of urticaria and angioedema at the site of antigen exposure or angioedema of the bowel after ingestion of certain foods. Physical allergies to heat, cold, sunlight, and pressure are not as life threatening as those related to injectables. By comparison, anaphylactic reactions are dramatic and rapid in their onset. The signs and symptoms of anaphylaxis are defined by the physiologic effects of the primary and secondary mediator on the target organs. Antihistamines have no effect on histamine release from mast cells or basophils.

In vitro evaluation of type I hypersensitivity reactions can be by RIST (RadioImmunoSorbent Test), RAST (RadioAllergoSorbent Test), and enzyme immunoassays. The advantages of in vitro testing include the lack of risk of a systemic hypersensitivity reaction, the lack of dependence on skin reactivity that can be influenced by drugs, disease, or the age of the patient. Disadvantages of the RAST include limited allergen selection, reduced sensitivity compared with intradermal skin testing, and increased expense.

Cytotoxic reactions are characterized by the interaction of IgG or IgM antibody to cell-bound antigen. This binding of an antigen and antibody can result in the activation of complement and cytolysis to which the antigen is bound. Erythrocytes, leukocytes, and platelets can be lysed by this process. Examples of cytotoxic reactions include immediate (acute) transfusion reactions, and immune hemolytic anemias, such as hemolytic disease of the newborn.

Transfusion reactions can be divided into hemolytic and non-hemolytic types. Hemolytic reactions are associated with the infusion of incompatible erythrocytes. These reactions can be further classified into acute or delayed in their manifestations.

The most common cause of an acute hemolytic transfusion reaction is the transfusion of ABO-incompatible blood. In patients with pre-existing antibodies caused by prior transfusion or pregnancy, other blood groups may be responsible. Acute hemolytic reactions are the most serious and potentially lethal. Reactions can occur with the infusion of as little as 10 to 15 mL of incompatible blood. Acute hemolytic reactions occur during or immediately after blood has been infused. Infusion of incompatible erythrocytes in the presence of pre-existing antibodies initiates an antigen-antibody reaction with the activation of the complement, plasminogen, kinin, and coagulation systems. Other initiators of acute hemolytic reactions include bacterial contamination of blood or the infusion of hemolyzed erythrocytes. A delayed reaction may not express itself until 7 to 10 days posttransfusion. Non-hemolytic reactions, like hemolytic reactions, may be of an immediate or delayed nature. Immediate non-hemolytic reactions include febrile and platelet reactions, as well as reactions to plasma constituents. Delayed non-hemolytic reactions include graft-versus-host disease. When immunocompetent lymphocytes are transfused from a donor to a recipient who is not capable of rejecting them, the transfused or grafted lymphocytes recognize the antigens of host as foreign and react immunologically against them. Instead of the usual transplantation reaction of host against graft, the reverse graft-versus-host disease develops. In a normal lymphocyte-transfer reaction, the results of a graft-versus-host reaction are usually not serious because the recipient is capable of destroying the foreign lymphocytes. Graft-versus-host reactions can occur whenever immunologically competent allogeneic lymphocytes are transfused into a severely immunocompromised host.

Hemolytic disease of the newborn (HDN) is another example of a cytotoxic (type II) reaction. This condition in the fetus or newborn infant is clinically characterized by anemia and jaundice and is caused by antibodies in the mother that are stimulated by fetal antigens. The most frequent form of ABO incompatibility occurs when the mother is type O and the baby is type A or type B, usually type A. When the antigen and its corresponding antibody combine in vivo, increased lysis of red cells results. HDN caused by ABO incompatibility, however, is usually mild as compared to HDN caused by other blood groups antigens, such as the D (RH) antigen. In the 1960s, it was demonstrated that passive antibody, Rh IgG, could protect most Rh negative mothers from becoming immunized following the delivery of Rh (D) positive infants or similar obstetric conditions. Since that time a dramatic decrease in the incidence of HDN caused by anti-D has taken place, although complete elimination may never occur because of the cases in which anti-D is formed before delivery. All pregnant Rh-negative women should receive Rh IgG even if the Rh status of the fetus is unknown because fetal D antigen is present in fetal erythrocytes as early as 38 days from conception.

In immune complex reactions, however, antigen-antibody complexes form in the soluble or fluid phase of tissues or in the blood and assume unique biologic functions such as interaction with complement and with cellular receptors. Examples of type III reactions include the Arthus reaction, serum sickness, and certain aspects of autoimmune disease. Immune complexes can exhibit a spectrum of biologic activities, including suppression or augmentation of the immune response by interacting with B and T cells; inhibition of tumor cell destruction; and deposition in blood vessel walls, glomerular membranes, and other sites.

Cell-mediated immunity consists of immune activities that differ from antibody-mediated immunity. Cell-mediated immunity is moderated by the link between T lymphocytes and phagocytic cells. Cell-mediated immunity is responsible for contact sensitivity, delayed hypersensitivity, immunity to viral and fungal antigens, immunity to intracellular organisms, rejection of foreign-tissue grafts, elimination of tumor cells bearing neoantigens, and formation of chronic granulomas.

REVIEW QUESTIONS

Match the following types of hypersensitivity reactions with their respective type of reaction:

1. Type I   A. Cytotoxic
2. Type II   B. Cell-mediated
3. Type III   C. Immune complex
4. Type IV   D. Anaphylactic

5. With which cell type are anaphylactic reactions associated?
   A. T lymphocyte
   B. B lymphocyte
   C. Monocyte
   D. Mast
   E. Polymorphonuclear (PMN)
6. Which one of the following is an example of a delayed non-hemolytic transfusion reaction?
   A. Febrile reactions
   B. Graft versus host disease
   C. Anaphylaxis
   D. Urticaria
   E. Fever and shock
7. Type III reactions are exemplified by all of the following *except:*
   A. Arthus reaction
   B. Serum sickness
   C. Glomerulonephritis
   D. Rheumatoid arthritis
   E. Shingles
8. Type IV reactions are responsible for all of the following *except:*
   A. Contact sensitivity
   B. Delayed hypersensitivity
   C. Immunity to viral and fungal antigens
   D. Immunity to bacteria
   E. Immunity to intracellular organisms

Answers

1. D 2. A 3. C 4. B 5. D 6. B 7. E 8. D

BIBLIOGRAPHY

Ali M and others: Allergy testing from in vivo to in vitro, Diag Med, pp 37-56, June 1982.

Altman LC editor: Clinical allergy and immunology, Boston, 1984, GK Hall & Co.

Barrett JT: Textbook of immunology, St Louis, 1988, The CV Mosby Co.

Endo L, Corman LC, and Panusk RS: Clinical utility of assays for circulating immune complexes, Med Clin No Amer 69(4):623-635, July 1985.

Henriques JF and Phillips TM: Immune complex assays, ACPR, pp 28-31, Oct 1987.

Kaplan AP, editor: Allergy, New York, 1985, Churchill Livingstone Inc.

Lawlor GJ and Rosenblatt HM: Anaphylaxis. In Manual of allergy and immunology, ed 2, Boston, 1988, Little, Brown & Co.

Lockey RF and Bukantz SC, editors: Principles of immunolgy and allergy, Philadelphia, 1987, WB Saunders Co.

Mann R and Neilson EG: Pathogenesis and treatment of immune-mediated renal disease, Med Clin No Amer 69(4):715-719, July 1985.

McDougal JS and McDuffie FC: Immune complexes in man: detection and clinical significance, Adv Clin Chem 24:1-59, 1985.

Sly MR: Textbook of pediatric allergy, New Hyde Park, NY, 1985, Medical Examination Pub Co.

Turgeon ML: Fundamentals of immunohematology, Philadelphia, 1989, Lea & Febiger.

CHAPTER 24

Immunoproliferative Disorders

Hypergammaglobuline-mias are either monoclonal or polyclonal in nature. A monoclonal gammopathy, which can be either a benign or malignant condition, results from a single clone of lymphoid-plasma cells producing elevated levels of a single class and type of immunoglobulin. The elevated immunoglobulin is referred to as a *monoclonal protein, M protein,* or *paraprotein.* In comparison, a polyclonal gammopathy is classified as a secondary disease and characterized by the elevation of two or more immunoglobulins by several clones of plasma cells.

GENERAL CHARACTERISTICS OF MONOCLONAL GAMMOPATHIES

Monoclonal gammopathies are characterized by an uncontrolled proliferation of a single clone of plasma cells at the expense of other clones. The stimulus for proliferation is unknown but it is not believed to be antigenic. This dysfunction, however, leads to the synthesis of elevated quantities of one homogeneous immunoglobulin or immunoglobulin subunits and an associated immunodeficiency because of decreased levels of normal immunoglobulins.

Serum and urine electrophoresis patterns and other immunoglobulin assays can demonstrate strikingly abnormal results in disorders such as multiple myeloma and Waldenstrom's macroglobulinemia. The gamma region of the electrophoresis pattern can show a dense, highly restricted band from uncontrolled proliferation of one cell clone while the other normal immunoglobulins are deficient. Clinical interpretation of some patterns, however, can be difficult. In contrast, some symp-

tomatic patients do not exhibit the characteristic monoclonal band or spike in their serum protein patterns. This is often the case with light-chain disease where only κ (kappa) or λ (lambda) monoclonal light chains are synthesized by the clone. These low-molecular-weight immunoglobulin fragments are filtered through the glomerulus and into the urine, which produces a serum electrophoresis pattern that suggests hypogammaglobulinemia with either a very faint monoclonal band or no band at all. These also suggest the possibility of the presence of a non-secretory clone, which produces no monoclonal immunoglobulins and frequently demonstrates hypogammaglobulinemia because of the inhibition of normal clones.

GENERAL CHARACTERISTICS OF POLYCLONAL GAMMOPATHIES

A polyclonal gammopathy is a common protein abnormality. It is defined as an increase in more than one immunoglobulin and involves several clones of plasma cells. In contrast to a monoclonal protein, a polyclonal protein consists of one or more heavy-chain classes and both light-chain types. Polyclonal increases are exhibited as secondary manifestations of infection or inflammation. They are commonly seen in chronic infections; chronic liver disease, especially chronic active hepatitis; rheumatoid connective tissue (autoimmune) diseases; and lymphoproliferative diseases.

A polyclonal protein is characterized by a broad peak or band, usually of gamma mobility, on electrophoresis, by a thickening and elongation of all heavy- and light-chain arcs on immunoelectrophoresis, and by the absence of a localized band on immunofixation. A polyclonal gammopathy, therefore, resembles a normal pattern with the serum staining more intensely. A selective polyclonal increase is of special interest because only one class of immunoglobulin is significantly elevated but the increase is polyclonal because immunoglobulin is produced by several clones of plasma cells and both κ and λ types are produced. Quantitation by specific assay procedures of the immunoglobulins demonstrates which immunoglobulin is increased. Immunofixation is not recommended in cases of polyclonal gammopathy because it presents no additional information.

MULTIPLE MYELOMA

Multiple myeloma (also referred to as *plasma cell myeloma, myelomatosis,* or *Kahler's disease*) is characterized by a neoplastic or potentially neoplastic proliferation of a single clone of plasma cells that produce a specific type of immunoglobulin. The synthesized immunoglobulin, often referred to as *M protein, myeloma protein,* or *paraprotein,* is monoclonal. It consists of one heavy-chain and one light-chain class.

Etiology

The cause of multiple myeloma is unknown. Radiation may be a factor in some cases; the possibility of a viral cause has been suggested. Other possible factors may be environmental stimulants such as exposure to asbestos, benzene, or industrial toxins. The likelihood of a genetic factor in some cases is supported by well-documented reports of familial clusters with multiple myeloma.

Epidemiology

Multiple myeloma is the most common form of *dysproteinemia.* It accounts for 1% of all types of malignant diseases and slightly more than 10% of hematologic malignancies. The general incidence is estimated to be 3 cases per 100,000 per year in the United States.

Onset of this disorder is between the ages of 40 and 70 years with a peak incidence in the seventh decade. It is uncommon (less than 2% of cases) in patients under 40 years of age. In general, patients with light chain disease and with IgD myeloma are younger than those with IgG or IgA myeloma and have a poorer prognosis because of their high incidence of nephropathy. Males are afflicted with the disease in approximately 62% of cases. The male-to-female ratio is 1.6:1. In addition, blacks are afflicted twice as often as whites.

IgG myeloma is the most common form of multiple myeloma (Table 24-1). Four subtypes of IgG heavy chains are known to exist among patients with IgG myeloma. Cases of IgG myeloma are distributed as follows: 65% are gamma G1, 23% are gamma G2, 8% are gamma G3, and 4% fall into the gamma G4 subclass. The only subclass-dependent difference is the greater propensity for patients with IgG3 myeloma to experience *hyperviscosity syndrome* similar to the manifesta-

TABLE 24-1

Distribution of Immunoglobin Types Produced in Patients Having Multiple Myeloma

Type of protein	Multiple myeloma(%)
IgM	12
IgG	52
IgA	22
IgD	2
IgE	rare
Light chains (κ or λ)	11
Heavy chains	rare
Two or more Monoclonal proteins	<1
Nonsecretory myeloma	1

tion in Waldenstrom's macroglobulinemia.

Multiple myeloma runs a progressive course with most patients dying within 1 to 3 years. The major causes of death are overwhelming infection (sepsis) and renal insufficiency. In cases of sepsis, the death rate exceeds 50% despite antibiotic therapy.

Signs and Symptoms

The signs and symptoms of multiple myeloma include bone pain, typically in the back or chest, and weakness, fatigue, and pallor, associated with anemia or abnormal bleeding. Twenty percent of patients exhibit hepatomegaly and 5% demonstrate splenomegaly. In some cases, the major manifestations of disease result from acute infection, renal insufficiency, hypercalcemia or amyloidosis. Weight loss and night sweats are not prominent until the disease is advanced. Bone pain, anemia, and renal insufficiency constitute a triad of signs and symptoms strongly suggestive of multiple myeloma.

Skeletal Abnormalities

About 90% of patients having multiple myeloma suffer from broadly disseminated destruction of the skeleton, which is responsible for the predominance of bone pain. These abnormalities consist of punched-out lytic areas (Fig. 24-1 *A* and *B*), osteoporosis, and fractures in about 80% of patients. The vertebrae, skull, thoracic cage, pelvis, and proximal humeri and femurs are the most frequent sites of involvement.

Hematologic Features

Diagnosis of multiple myeloma depends on the demonstration of an increased number of plasma cells in a bone marrow aspirate and/or biopsy and supporting laboratory results (discussed later under *Diagnostic evaluation*). Although the bone marrow is typically involved, the disorder may involve other tissues. For example, a positive correlation exists between the production of osteoclast-

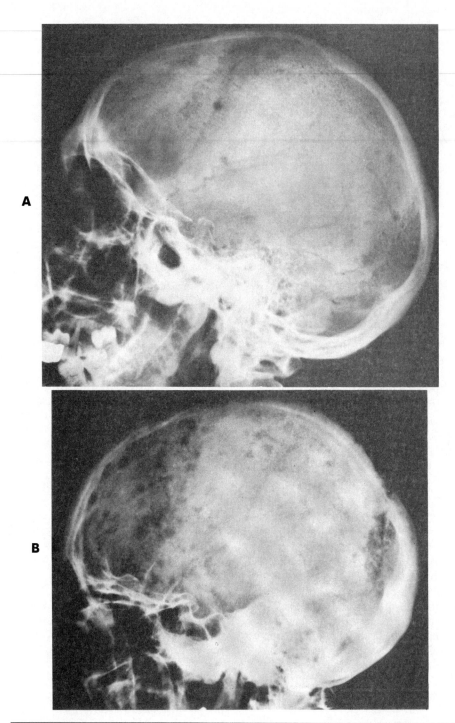

<u>FIGURE 24-1</u>

A, Multiple myeloma. A few scattered small well-marginated lytic lesions appear in calvarium. These are located in normally mineralized bone. Multiple lytic lesions can be seen also in the mandible. **B,** Multiple myeloma. Multiple circumscribed lytic lesions crowd bones throughout. Lesions are still discrete, and margins of most are fairly sharp.

(From Newton TH and Potts DG: Radiology of the skull and brain, vol 1, book 2, St Louis, 1971, The CV Mosby Co.)

activating factor by bone marrow cells and the extent of skeletal destruction. Other hematologic factors contributing to the signs and symptoms of pallor and anemia include bleeding, qualitative platelet abnormalities, inhibition of coagulation factors by M protein, and thrombocytopenia. Intravascular coagulation may be manifested.

Renal Disorders

Acute renal failure occurs in about 5% to 10% of patients. Although acute renal failure may occur at any time in the course of myeloma, it is not uncommon for it to be the initial manifestation of disease. Acute renal failure has been observed following infection, hypercalcemia, dehydration, and intravenous urography. Serum creatinine levels are elevated in about half of these patients, and approximately one third suffer from hypercalcemia.

Chronic renal failure is a common development in patients with multiple myeloma. As many as two thirds of patients display serum creatinine levels of greater than 1.5 mg/dL, and 10% to 20% may develop end-stage renal disease. Patients with IgD or light-chain myeloma are much more likely to develop renal failure than those with IgG or IgA myeloma. Proteinuria is a common finding with over half of all multiple myeloma patients excreting abnormal amounts of *Bence-Jones (BJ) protein* (light chains). Patients with BJ proteinuria are much more likely to have renal tubular defects than those without BJ proteinuria. It has been suggested that BJ proteins may have a deleterious effect on renal function via at least two mechanisms. In one mechanism, renal failure may occur as a result of intratubular precipitation of BJ protein and subsequent intrarenal obstruction. When the distal end collecting tubules become obstructed by large casts consisting mainly of BJ protein, it may be referred to as *myeloma kidney.* The second mechanism of renal failure may be a function of direct tubular cell injury. As a result of these tubular defects, abnormalities in urinary concentrating ability and renal acidification are observed. Although the presence of a large concentration of BJ proteinuria is usually associated with some degree of renal dysfunction, some patients excrete large amounts of BJ protein for years and maintain renal function. Lambda light chains have been implicated in nephrotoxicity, but their role has not been firmly established.

Neurologic Features

Pain is a common characteristic of multiple myeloma, often caused by compression of the spinal cord or nerves. Compression produces back pain with weakness or paralysis of the lower extremities and bowel or bladder incontinence.

Infectious Diseases

The most frequent cause of death is infection. Patients with multiple myeloma have increased susceptibility to infectious micro-organisms because of an inability to cope with bacterial infec-

tions and certain viral diseases. Increased susceptibility principally results from defective antibody synthesis caused by the crowding out and suppression of normal plasma cell precursors.

Repeated bouts of sepsis, often resulting from recurrent infection by micro-organisms such as pneumococci or gram-negative bacteria, are common. Pneumonia, pyelonephritis, meningitis, and arthritis are the leading forms of sepsis; when bacteremia ensues, the death rate is high.

Immunologic Manifestations

Patients with multiple myeloma have defects in humoral but not cellular immunity. Humoral immunity is disrupted because plasma cell tumors induce suppression of antibody synthesis by normal immunoglobulin-secreting cells, and the production of anti-idiotype antibodies suffers proportionately. In addition, selective impairment occurs in the formation of normal antibodies because of increased immunoglobulin catabolism and the release of a protein that incites macrophages to suppress synthesis of normal immunoglobulins by myeloma cells. Depression of normal humoral immunity accounts for the high susceptibility of patients with multiple myeloma to bacterial infection. The normal functioning of cellular immunity, however, is demonstrated by normal resistance to fungal and most viral infections and normal delayed-type hypersensitivity to skin testing antigens.

Initially, in vivo myeloma clones are subject to control by the immune network through specific idiotype-anti-idiotype mechanisms. Each of the million or more potential immunoglobulin variants in every individual carries singular determinants designated *idiotypes.* Anti-idiotypic antibodies directed against autologous immunoglobulin are elicited during a normal immune response. The presumed mission of anti-idiotypic antibodies is to help terminate the immune response by binding complementary idiotypes to form endogenous immune complexes that are removed from the circulation. The anti-idiotype (anti-Id) antibodies in turn stimulate production of antibodies to anti-Id, and so on, to create a modulating network that includes T cells, which recognize idiotype antigens by means of their unique antigen receptors. Anti-Id and Id-sensitized T cells collaborate most efficiently during highly restricted responses during which both antibodies and lymphocytes that specifically recognize the dominant idiotype are activated. These can either inhibit or enhance the response of lymphocytes to receptors expressing the idiotype. The overall net direction of the response is determined by the functional influence of T cells linked by anti-Id receptor interactions to their molecular targets on B cells. In multiple myeloma, idiotype expression is carried to an extreme. Monoclonal paraprotein secreted by plasma cell tumors induces a multitude of immunologic responses capable of acting in concert to contain or modulate tumor growth.

The earliest detectable monoclonal B cell, as identified by idiotypic structures of the myeloma protein, is the transitional form-bearing surface IgM, IgD, and IgG. This and the finding that precursor (early) B cells destined to become myeloma cells possess surface immunoglobulin G (sIgG) indicate that the myeloma tumor clone includes memory B cells that can mature into plasma cells. Use of anti-idiotypic antibodies in identifying IgA myeloma clones has revealed clonal expression at the pre-B state, a finding supported by the observation that B cells in the circulation of myeloma patients are clonally frozen at the pre-B stage. As maturing B cell members of the malignant clone differentiate in the marrow, they lose IgD and IgM in that order, accumulate cIgG and finally shed sIg to become IgG-producing mature plasma cells as programmed by the mutant stem cell. Thus the mature myeloma cell contains abundant cytoplasmic (secretory) IgG but no sIg. IgA myeloma cells proceed along the same normal differentiation scheme of B cell maturation. Although multiple myeloma-associated tumors disseminate widely, the disease is spread through release into the blood circulation of clonal precursors that show lymphoid rather than plasma cell morphology.

The most consistent immunologic feature of multiple myeloma is the incessant synthesis of a dysfunctional single monoclonal protein or of immunoglobulin chains of fragments, with concurrent suppression of the synthesis of normal functional antibody. In 99% of myeloma patients, an M component is usually found in serum, urine, or both. Different types of M components are associated with various clinical syndromes.

Diagnostic Evaluation
Hematologic Assessment

A normochromic normocytic anemia is present in about two thirds of patients at the time of diagnosis. In part, anemia is related to the hypervolemia caused by the increase in plasma volume because of monoclonal protein production. Rouleaux formation is a common finding on peripheral blood smears. The leukocyte count can be normal, although about one third of patients suffer from leukopenia. Relative lymphocytosis is usually present. If lymphocyte subsets are examined, a reduction in OKT4 (helper) and an increase in OKT8 (suppressor) blood lymphocytes can be noted. Defects in the proliferative responses of lymphocytes to mitogens or antigens are explained by the fact that a large portion of B cells in multiple myeloma originates from the malignant stem cell clone. Few mature plasma cells are seen in the circulation except at the terminal phase of the disease, but the covert presence of the malignant B cell clone can be unmasked by the laboratory use of monoclonal antibodies or by transforming agents such as phorbol esters. In rare cases in the terminal stages, plasmablasts and proplasmacytes may amount to 50% of the leukocytes in the peripheral blood. Diagnosis of multiple myeloma, however, depends on the demonstration of an increased number of plasma cells in a bone marrow aspirate (Fig. 24-2) and/or biopsy and supporting laboratory results.

Bleeding is commonly seen. Platelet abnormalities, impaired aggregation of platelets, and interference with platelet function by the abnormal monoclonal protein contribute to bleeding. Inhibitors of coagulation factors and thrombocytopenia from

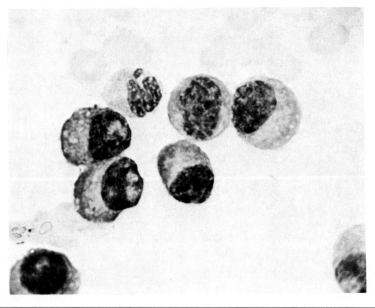

FIGURE 24-2

Myeloma cells in a bone marrow aspirate.
(From Bauer JD: Clinical laboratory methods, ed 9, St Louis, 1982, The CV Mosby Co.)

marrow infiltration of plasma cells or chemotherapy may also contribute to bleeding. Some patients have a tendency toward thrombosis, which may be manifested by a shortened coagulation time, and increased fibrinogen and factor VIII.

Bence-Jones Proteins

Bence-Jones (BJ) proteins may be demonstrated in the urine. In about 10% of multiple myeloma patients only BJ proteins are produced, with no complete IgM, IgG, or IgA. BJ proteins are single-peptide chains with a molecular weight of 20,000 or 22,000, but dimerization occurs spontaneously to form molecules with a molecular weight of 40,000 or 44,000.

Bence-Jones proteins (BJP) are monoclonal κ or λ immunoglobulin light chains that are not attached to the heavy-chain portion of the immunoglobulin molecule. BJPs are seen in two types of syndromes:
1. In conjunction with a typical monoclonal gammopathy or
2. In free light chain disease

Very small amounts of BJP in serum can be associated with significant clinical problems, especially pathologic renal changes. Free light chains filter through the glomerules almost without obstruction because of their small molecular size, and accumulate in the tubules. Renal impairment can result from the toxicity of the light chains. Pathologic changes can range from relatively benign tubular proteinuria to acute renal failure or amyloidosis.

BJP can be detected in serum, urine, or both. The level of monoclonal light chains in serum or urine, however, is related to filtration, reabsorption, or catabolism of the protein by the kidneys. During the early stages of renal disease when the kidneys are only mildly affected, excretion and reabsorption continue normally, but only partial catabolism occurs. At this point, BJP may be detected in the serum but not in the urine. Progressive renal involvement impairs reabsorption so that diminished reabsorption with decreased catabolism results in free light chains in both serum and urine. Later, as reabsorption is totally blocked, light chains are present in urine only. In terminal stages of renal disease, uremia occurs, renal clearance is affected, and BJP again appears in the serum.

BJ proteins are unusual in their response to heating. They are soluble at room temperature, become insoluble near 60° or 70° C, and then resolubilize at 80° C. This pattern reverses when the temperature is lowered, which is a characteristic unique to BJ protein.

Serologically, all BJ proteins (L chains) are not identical. Two types kappa (κ) and lambda (λ) exist. BJ proteins, however, will react with antisera to the L chains of IgG, and L chains react with antisera to BJ protein.

Immunologic Testing

Each monoclonal protein (M protein or paraprotein) consists of two heavy-chain polypeptides of

---

Monoclonal Gammopathies

I. Malignant monoclonal gammopathies
  A. Multiple myeloma (IgG, IgA, IgD, IgE, and free light chains)
  B. Plasmacytoma
  C. Malignant lymphoproliferative diseases
  D. Heavy-chain diseases
  E. Amyloidosis
II. Monoclonal gammopathies of undetermined significance
  A. Benign (IgG, IgA, IgD, IgM, and rarely, free light chains)
  B. Associated with neoplasms of cell types not known to produce monoclonal proteins
  C. Biclonal gammopathies

---

the same class and subclass and two-light chain polypeptides of the same type. The different monoclonal proteins are designated by capital letters corresponding to the class of their heavy chains, which are designated by Greek letters: (γ) in IgG, (α) in IgA, (μ) (mu) in IgM, (δ) in IgD, and (ε) in IgE. The subclasses are IgG1, IgG2, IgG, and IgG4, or IgA1 and IgA2, and their light-chain types are κ and λ. A monoclonal protein is characterized by a narrow peak or a localized band on electrophoresis; by a thickened, bowed arc on immunoelectrophoresis; and by a localized band on immunofixation. Many different entities are associated with M proteins (monoclonal gammopathies); see box above.

Electrophoresis (Fig. 24-3) of the serum or urine reveals a tall, sharp peak on the densitometer tracing or dense localized band in a majority of cases of multiple myeloma. A monoclonal protein is demonstrable in the serum and urine in 90% of patients. Sixty percent of patients exhibit IgG, 20% IgA, 10% light chain only (Bence-Jones proteinemia), and 1% IgD. Electrophoresis of urine shows a globulin peak in 75% of cases, mainly albumin in 10% of patients, and a normal pattern in 15%. When an M spike is observed on serum protein electrophoresis, the suggested sequence of testing (Table 24-2) includes testing by immunoelectrophoresis and immunofixation. Screening for cryoglobulins and viscosity may also be warranted.

DNA hybridization or blotting technology is the newest technology available and can be used to detect abnormal genes in B cells. Although the gene product of monoclonal antibodies is the method of detection, DNA probes that can detect the abnormal gene are now available. Blotting techniques may someday fully or partially replace the current approach to the laboratory evaluation of monoclonal gammopathies.

WALDENSTROM'S PRIMARY MACROGLOBULINEMIA
Etiology

Waldenstrom's macroglobulinemia (WM), or simply macroglobulinemia, is a malignant lymphocyte-plasma cell proliferative disorder that exhibits ab-

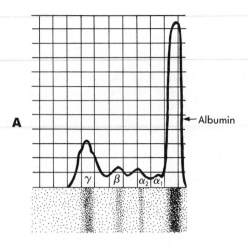

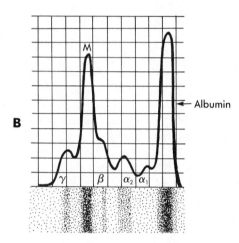

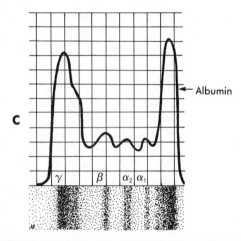

FIGURE 24-3

Serum electrophoretic patterns. **A,** Normal patient. **B,** A patient with multiple myeloma. **C,** A patient with Waldenström macroglobulinemia.

TABLE 24-2

Suggested Sequence of Immunologic Testing for Monoclonal Proteins

M spike on serum protein electrophoresis	
Serum	**Urine**
Immunoelectrophoresis	Screening of urine for increased protein, e.g., sulfosalicylic acid
Immunofixation	Total protein assay of a 24-hour urine specimen
Quantitation of immunoglobulins by radial immunodiffusion or nephelometry	Urinary protein electrophoresis
Screening for cryoglobulins	Urinary immunoelectrophoresis
Determination of serum viscosity, if IgM, IgA or IgG, or signs and symptoms suggestive of hyperviscosity	Immunofixation

normally large amounts of immunoglobulin of the 19S-IgM type. The cause of this disorder is unknown, but a possible genetic predisposition may exist. A greater frequency of IgM monoclonal proteins, as well as quantitative abnormalities, have been observed in some relatives of patients with WM.

WM is a malignant offshoot of B cell development before the myelomas; therefore, the sole gene product is IgM. Patients with WM have chromosomal rearrangements characteristic of B cell neoplasia, including t(8:14) and trisomy 12.

Epidemiology

WM is about one tenth as frequent as multiple myeloma. This disorder has an age-specific incidence; it is most commonly found in older individuals with the mean age of onset at 60 to 64 years. No significant differences in the incidence of WM occur between males and females. Disease onset is usually insidious, and the median survival is approximately 3 years after diagnosis.

Signs and Symptoms

The signs and symptoms of WM have an indolent progression over a period of many years. Initially the onset of the disease is slow and insidious, with the pace of manifestations determined by the rate of proliferation of the IgM-secreting clone. Most of the clinical signs and symptoms of disease stem from intravascular accumulation of high levels of IgM macroglobulin. When the IgM is precipitable at cold temperatures, as it is in 37% of cases, clinical manifestations of cold sensitivity such as Raynaud's phenomenon, arthralgias, purpura of the extremities, renal insufficiency, and peripheral vascular occlusions may develop. Cold hypersensitivity can occur when serum IgM levels exceed 2 to 3 g/dL and the protein precipitates at temperatures exceeding 20° C.

Although the patient experiences weakness and fatigue, it is usually the onset of bleeding from the gums or nose that arouses concern. Patients suffer from weight loss, and the incidence of infection is twice the normal rate. As the disease progresses about 40% of patients develop hepatomegaly, splenomegaly, and lymphadenopathy. Occasionally, the clinical manifestations may simulate diffuse lymphoma. Specific dysfunctions and abnormalities occur in a variety of body systems.

Skeletal Features

In contrast to multiple myeloma, bone pain is virtually nonexistent in WM. Diffuse osteoporosis may be seen, but bone lesions are extremely rare.

Hematologic Abnormalities

Patients with WM usually suffer from chronic anemia and bleeding episodes. Bleeding problems in the form of bruising, purpura, and bleeding from the mouth, gums, nose, and gastrointestinal tract are common. The quantities of circulating platelets may be normal or decreased, but the most notable alteration is a disturbance in platelet function. Therefore, thrombocytopenia or hyperviscosity may contribute to the bleeding disorder.

In addition to anemia caused by chronic or recurrent bleeding, the decrease in red blood cells becomes more severe as the disease progresses because of a dilutional effect caused by increased immunoglobulin production. In addition, the presence of macroglobulin also produces an increased erythrocyte sedimentation rate. Microscopic examination of a peripheral blood smear usually reveals normocytic and frequently hypochromic red cells with striking rouleaux formation. The total blood leukocyte count is either normal or slightly depressed because of moderate neutropenia. In a terminal patient, the blood may be inundated with malignant lymphoplasmacytic cells.

Renal Dysfunction

Renal function becomes mildly or moderately impaired in about 15% of WM patients. Nephrosis is uncommon. Bence-Jones proteinuria, however, is present in about 70% of WM patients but the quantity of light chains excreted is much less than in multiple myeloma.

Glomerular lesions are the predominant form of renal injury. IgM collects on the endothelial side of the basement membrane of the kidney, and sometimes these macroglobulin accumulations obstruct glomerular capillaries.

Ocular Manifestations

Blurred vision is a frequent abnormality of WM. Rouleaux induced by elevations of IgM causes distention of veins and capillaries; retinal oxygenation diminishes as rouleaux-inducing IgM rises. As a result of increased IgM levels, retinal hemorrhage, exudate formation, and varicosities develop, which can lead to more permanent retinal damage unless IgM levels are lowered by therapy.

Neuropsychiatric Problems

The most common serious neurologic consequence of the slowed cerebral perfusion caused by macroglobulinemia is acute cerebral malfunction beginning with headache, fluctuating confusion, forgetfulness, and slowed mentation. This can progress to somnolence, stupor, and coma-diffuse brain syndrome sometimes called *coman paraproteinaemicum*. Neurologic abnormalities can be improved by reduction of plasma viscosity.

Polyneuropathy affects 5% to 10% of patients with WM. This condition is associated with an increase in spinal fluid protein and deposits of monoclonal IgM on myelin sheaths. Monoclonal IgM found in the plasma and attached to damaged nerves has been shown in some instances to share idiotypic determinants. This suggests that polyneuropathy of WM may be an autoimmune process caused by monoclonal IgM possessing antibody activity for a component of nerve tissue.

Cardiopulmonary Abnormalities

Congestive heart failure becomes a serious problem in patients with chronic uncontrolled WM. About 90% of IgM remains trapped in the circulating plasma and exerts an unbalanced transendothelial osmotic effect sufficient to cause marked expansion of the plasma volume. This in turn creates a dilutional anemia and augments cardiac filling and cardiac output. As a result, increased cardiac output and blood viscosity overworks the myocardium.

About 10% of patients develop pulmonary lesions. Pulmonary tumors, diffuse infiltrates, and pleural involvement are all about equally represented. The signs and symptoms of pulmonary dysfunction include coughing and dyspnea.

Cutaneous Manifestations

Cold sensitivity is one of frequent manifestations of WM. Skin lesions, however, are uncommon. A small number of patients develop flat, violaceous, macular skin lesions caused by dense infiltration by lymphoplasmacytoid cells. Pink, pearly looking papules caused by dense deposits of IgM may be exhibited.

Immunologic Manifestations

The basic abnormality in this macroglobulinemia is uncontrolled proliferation of B lymphocyte-plasma cells. As a result there is a heavy accumulation of monoclonal IgM in the circulating plasma and plasmacytoid lymphocytes in the bone marrow.

In many cases, WM is associated with mixed cryoglobulinemia, which reflects the binding of IgG or IgA anti-idiotypic antibody to the mutant IgM. In a small number of patients, dysplastic tumor cells secrete 7S IgM monomers, μ chains, or other monoclonal immunoglobulins or fragments. Therefore, the major IgM production indicates that the immunoglobulin (Ig gene) lesion sometimes degenerates and codes for more than one M component.

Diagnostic Evaluation
Hematologic Assessment

Microscopic examination of a bone marrow aspirate reveals that the lymphocyte-plasma cells vary morphologically from small lymphocytes to obvious plasma cells. Frequently the cellular cytoplasm is ragged and may contain PAS-positive material that is probably identical to the circulating macroglobulin.

The total peripheral blood leukocyte count is usually normal with an absolute lymphocytosis. Moderate-to-severe degrees of anemia are frequently observed on peripheral blood smears as well as rouleaux formation. The patient's plasma volume may be greatly increased and the erythrocyte sedimentation rate (ESR) is increased.

Platelet counts are usually normal. Faulty platelet aggregation and release of platelet factor 3 are caused by nonspecific coating of platelets by IgM. The most common coagulation defect is a prolonged thrombin time as the result of the binding of M component to fibrin monomers and resultant gel clots of IgM-coated fibrin. Bleeding abnormalities, however, can be demonstrated by a variety of procedures. These procedures include:
1. Faulty platelet adhesiveness
2. Defective platelet aggregation
3. Abnormal release of platelet factor 3
4. Impaired clot retraction
5. Prolonged bleeding time
6. Positive tourniquet test
7. Prolonged thrombin/prothrombin time test
8. Decreased levels of factor VIII

Immunologic Assessment

Electrophoresis of serum usually demonstrates the overproduction of IgM (19S) antibodies. Diagnosis is made by demonstration of a homogenous M component composed of monoclonal IgM. Quantitation of immunoglobulins reveals IgM levels ranging from 1 to 12 g/dL (usually more than 3 g/dL), and it accounts for 20% to 70% of the total proteins. Characteristically, blood samples are described as having *hyperviscosity.*

Additionally, *cryoglobulins* can be detected in the patient's serum. Cryoglobulins are proteins that precipitate or gel when cooled to 0° C and dissolve when heated. In most cases, monoclonal cryoglobulins are IgM or IgG. Occasionally, the macroglobulin is both cryoprecipitable and capable of cold-induced anti-i-mediated agglutination of red cells. IgM may also occasionally be a pyroglobulin, which precipitates on heating to 50° to 60° C but does not

redissolve on cooling or intensified heating as do typical BJ pyroglobulins.

OTHER MONOCLONAL DISORDERS
Light-Chain Disease

Light-chain disease (LCD) represents about 10% to 15% of monoclonal gammopathies ranking behind IgG and IgA myelomas, which represent about 60% and 15%, respectively. The incidence of LCD is about as frequent as Waldenstrom's macroglobulinemia. In light-chain disease only κ or λ monoclonal light chains or Bence-Jones proteins are produced.

Diagnostic evaluation of suspected light-chain disease is similar to the protocol for any lymphoproliferative disorder, but certain changes in approach are necessary because of the low levels of paraprotein that can be involved. Agarose high resolution protein electrophoresis of serum and urine should be done to determine the total protein concentration. A 24-hour urine specimen should be examined electrophoretically because almost all of the protein may be Bence-Jones protein. Visual examination of the electrophoresis pattern is essential because a small light-chain band frequently does not exhibit a significant peak on densitometric scanning. Serum protein electrophoresis patterns from patients with monoclonal gammopathies may demonstrate:
1. A typical well-defined monoclonal band
2. A somewhat broad diffuse band caused by polymerization of monoclonal protein
3. A normal gamma region
4. Hypogammaglobulinemia

Heavy-Chain Disease

As the name heavy-chain disease implies, this abnormality is characterized by the presence of monoclonal proteins comprised of the heavy-chain portion of the immunoglobulin molecule. The name *Franklin's disease* is synonymous with gamma heavy-chain disease. Alpha heavy-chain disease is the most frequent of the heavy-chain gammopathies and is frequently seen in men of Mediterranean descent. Mu heavy-chain disease is rare.

Heavy chains may be detected in serum or urine or both (depending on the class of heavy chain involved). When heavy-chain disease is suspected, nonspecific anti-FAB antisera should be used for definitive testing. The serum sample should also be diluted and retested with κ and λ light-chain antisera to rule out prozoning caused by antigen excess.

Gammopathies With More Than One Band

In some cases, more than one monoclonal band is produced. Although gammopathies with two bands may represent a true biclonal condition, routine laboratory techniques cannot distinguish between the various mechanisms that could produce two or more monoclonal bands. Therefore, a serum specimen with an IgG kappa (κ) and an IgA lambda (λ) band should be appropriately reported as a gammopathy with IgG κ and IgA λ monoclonal bands. The appearance of more than one band on electrophoresis is often associated with advanced gammopathies where the asynchronous production of the components of the immunoglobulin molecule occurs. In such cases synthesis of an intact monoclonal immunoglobulin and an excess of monoclonal light chains may be observed. An example of the demonstration of more than one band on electrophoresis can include cases where the pentameric IgM breaks down into 7S subunits, which show up on electrophoresis as one or more "extra" monoclonal bands. In addition, monoclonal IgA molecules have a tendency to dimerize, and the resulting dimer often has a different mobility than the monomer parent molecule.

Chapter Review

HIGHLIGHTS

Hypergammaglobulinemias are either monoclonal or polyclonal in nature. A monoclonal gammopathy can be either a benign or malignant condition that results from a single clone of lymphoid-plasma cells producing elevated levels of a single class and type of immunoglobulin. The elevated immunoglobulin is referred to as a *monoclonal protein, M protein*, or *paraprotein*. A polyclonal gammopathy, however, is classified as a secondary disease and is characterized by the elevation of two or more immunoglobulins by several clones of plasma cells. In monoclonal gammopathies, such as multiple myeloma and Waldenstrom's macroglobulinemia, serum and urine electrophoresis patterns and other immunoglobulin assays can demonstrate strikingly abnormal results. In contrast to a monoclonal protein, a polyclonal protein consists of one or more heavy-chain classes and both light-chain types. Polyclonal increases are exhibited as secondary manifestations of infection or inflammation.

Multiple myeloma, a neoplastic or potentially neoplastic proliferation of a single clone of plasma cells, produces a specific type of immunoglobulin. The cause of this disorder is unknown. Radiation may be a factor; the possibility of a viral cause has also been suggested. Other possible factors in the etiology may be environmental stimuli; the likelihood of a genetic factor in some cases is supported by reports of familial clusters with multiple myeloma. Multiple myeloma is the most common form of dysproteinemia. IgG myeloma is the most common form of multiple myeloma with four subtypes of IgG heavy chains known to exist among patients with IgG myeloma. The signs and symptoms of multiple myeloma include bone pain, typically in the back or chest; weakness; fatigue; and pallor associated with anemia or abnormal bleeding. Bone pain, anemia, and renal insufficiency con-

stitute a triad of signs and symptoms strongly suggestive of multiple myeloma. Proteinuria is a common finding in more than half of all patients excreting abnormal amounts of Bence-Jones (BJ) protein (light-chains). Patients have defects in humoral but not cellular immunity. Humoral immunity is disrupted because plasma cell tumors induce suppression of antibody synthesis by normal immunoglobulin-secreting cells; the production of anti-idiotype antibodies suffers proportionately. Selective impairment occurs in the formation of normal antibodies because of increased immunoglobulin catabolism and the release of a protein that incites macrophages to suppress synthesis of normal immunoglobulins by myeloma cells. Depression of normal humoral immunity accounts for the high susceptibility of multiple myeloma patients to bacterial infection. The normal functioning of cellular immunity, however, is demonstrated by normal resistance to fungal and most viral infections and normal delayed-type hypersensitivity to skin-testing antigens. Laboratory diagnosis includes electrophoresis of the serum or urine, which can reveal a tall, sharp peak on the densitometer tracing or dense localized band in a majority of cases. A monoclonal protein is demonstrable in the serum and urine in 90% of patients. DNA hybridization or blotting technology is the newest technology available and can be used to detect abnormal genes in B-cells. Although the gene product of monoclonal antibodies is the method of detection, DNA probes, which can detect the abnormal gene, are now available. Blotting techniques may someday fully or partially replace the current approach to the laboratory evaluation of monoclonal gammopathies.

Waldenstrom's macroglobulinemia (WM), or simply macroglobulinemia, is a malignant lymphocyte-plasma cell proliferative disorder that exhibits abnormally large amounts of immunoglobulin of the 19S-IgM type. The cause of this disorder is unknown, but a possible genetic predisposition may exist. The signs and symptoms of WM have an indolent progression over a period of many years. Initially the onset of the disease is slow and insidious with the pace of manifestations being determined by the rate of proliferation of the IgM-secreting clone. Most of the clinical signs and symptoms of disease stem from intravascular accumulation of high levels of IgM macroglobulin. The basic abnormality in this macroglobulinemia is uncontrolled proliferation of B lymphocyte-plasma cells. As a result there is a heavy accumulation of monoclonal IgM in the circulating plasma and plasmacytoid lymphocytes in the bone marrow. In many cases, WM is associated with mixed cryoglobulinemia, which reflects the binding of IgG or IgA anti-idiotypic antibody to the mutant IgM. In a small number of patients, dysplastic tumor cells secrete 7S IgM monomers, μ chains, or other monoclonal immunoglobulins or fragments. Therefore, in addition to the major IgM production indicating that the immunoglobulin (Ig gene) lesion sometimes degenerates and codes for more than one M component. Laboratory diagnosis includes electrophoresis of serum, which usually demonstrates the overproduction of IgM (19S) antibodies. Diagnosis is made by demonstration of a homogenous M component composed of monoclonal IgM. Blood samples characteristically display hyperviscosity. In addition, cryoglobulins can be detected in the patient's serum.

Other monoclonal disorders include light-chain disease and heavy-chain disease. Light-chain disease (LCD) represents about 10% to 15% of monoclonal gammopathies. The incidence of LCD is about as frequent as WM. In light-chain disease only kappa (κ) or lambda (λ) monoclonal light chains, or Bence-Jones proteins are produced. Diagnostic evaluation of suspected light-chain disease is similar to the protocol for any lymphoproliferative disorder, but there are certain changes in approach because of the low levels of paraprotein that can be involved. Agarose high-resolution protein electrophoresis of serum and urine should be done to determine the total protein concentration. A 24-hour urine specimen should be examined electrophoretically because almost all of the protein may be Bence-Jones. Visual examination of the electrophoresis pattern is an essential part of the interpretation because a small light-chain band frequently does not exhibit a significant peak on densitometric scanning.

As the name heavy-chain disease implies, this abnormality is characterized by the presence of monoclonal proteins comprised of the heavy chain portion of the immunoglobulin molecule. Alpha heavy chain disease is the most frequent of the heavy chain gammopathies; mu heavy chain disease is rare. Heavy chains may be detected in serum or urine or both (depending on the class of heavy chain involved). When heavy-chain disease is suspected, nonspecific anti-FAB antisera should be used for definitive testing. The serum sample should also be diluted and retested with κ and λ light-chain antisera to rule out prozoning caused by antigen excess.

In some cases, gammopathies with more than one monoclonal band exist. Although gammopathies with two bands may represent a true biclonal condition, routine laboratory techniques cannot distinguish between the various mechanisms able to produce two (or more) monoclonal bands. A serum specimen with an IgG κ and an IgA λ band should be appropriately reported as a gammopathy with IgG κ and IgA λ monoclonal bands. The appearance of more than one band on electrophoresis is often associated with advanced gammopathies, where the asynchronous production of the components of the immunoglobulin molecule occurs. In such cases synthesis of an intact monoclonal immunoglobulin and an excess of monoclonal light-chains may be observed.

REVIEW QUESTIONS

1. Polyclonal gammopathies can be exhibited as a secondary manifestation of all of the following *except:*
   A. Chronic infection
   B. Chronic liver disease
   C. Multiple myeloma
   D. Rheumatoid connective disease
   E. Lymphoproliferative diseases
2. What is the most frequent cause of death in a patient with multiple myeloma?
   A. Skeletal destruction
   B. Chronic renal failure
   C. Neurological disorders
   D. Infectious disease
   E. Hypercalcemia
3. Patients with multiple myeloma have defects in:
   A. Cellular immunity
   B. Humoral immunity
   C. Antigen recognition
   D. Synthesis of normal immunoglobulins
   E. Both B and D
4. What is (are) the most consistent immunologic feature(s) of multiple myeloma?
   A. Synthesis of dysfunctional single, monoclonal proteins
   B. Synthesis of immunoglobulin chains or fragments
   C. Suppression of normal functioning antibody
   D. The presence of M protein in serum and/or urine
   E. All of the above

Bence-Jones protein are soluble at room temperature, become insoluble near_____ and then resolubilize at_____

5. A. 37° C
   B. 50° C
   C. 65° C
   D. 80° C
   E. 100° C

6. A. 37° C
   B. 50° C
   C. 65° C
   D. 80° C
   E. 100° C

7. M proteins are associated with all of the following malignant conditions *except:*
   A. Multiple myeloma
   B. Plasma cytoma
   C. Malignant lymphoproliferative diseases
   D. Lymphoma
   E. Amyloidosis

8. Cryoglobulins are proteins that precipitate at
   A. −18° C
   B. −4° C
   C. 0° C
   D. 4° C
   E. 10° C

Answers

1. C 2. D 3. E 4. E 5. C 6. D 7. D 8. C

BIBLIOGRAPHY

Hoffman EG: Laboratory evaluation of monoclonal gammopathies, Can J Med Tech 49(2):99-115, May 1987.

Jandl JA: Multiple myeloma and other differentiated B cell malignancies. In Blood, Boston, 1988, Little, Brown & Co.

Killingsworth LM and Warren BM: Immunofixation for the identification of monoclonal gammopathies, Beaumont, Texas, 1986, Helena Laboratories.

Kyle A: Multiple myeloma and the dysproteinemias. In Stein J, editor: Internal medicine, ed 2, Boston, 1987, Little, Brown and Co.

Kyle A: Evaluation of monoclonal proteins in serum and urine. In Stein J, editor: Internal medicine, ed 2, Boston, 1987, Little, Brown & Co.

Ritzmann EE: Immunoglobulin abnormalities. In Ritzmann S, editor: Serum protein abnormalities, diagnostic and clinical aspects, Boston, 1976, Little, Brown & Co.

Smolens P and Stein JH: Renal manifestations of dysproteinemias. In Stein J, editor: Internal medicine, ed 2, Boston, 1987, Little, Brown and Co.

Turgeon ML: Clinical hematology, Boston, 1988, Little, Brown & Co.

THE NATURE OF AUTOIMMUNITY

Autoimmunity represents a breakdown of the immune system's ability to discriminate between self and non-self. The term *autoimmune disease* is used in those cases where demonstrable immunoglobulins (autoantibodies) or cytotoxic (T) cells display a specificity for self-antigens or auto-antigens and contribute to the pathogenesis of the disease. The variety of signs and symptoms seen in patients with autoimmune diseases reflects the various forms of the immune response. The sites of organ or tissue damage depend on the location of the immune reaction.

It is also important to note that autoantibodies may be formed in patients secondary to tissue damage or when no evidence of clinical disease exists. Unlike autoimmune disease, autoantibodies can occur as immune correlates of conditions such as blood transfusion reactions. In addition, autoantibodies can be demonstrated in hemolytic disease of the newborn, and graft rejection, or result from disorders such as serum sickness, anaphylaxis, or hay fever where the immune response is clearly the cause of the disease.

THE SPECTRUM OF AUTOIMMUNE DISEASE

Many disorders are believed to be related to immunologic abnormalities and the identification of additional diseases grows continually. Autoimmune diseases exhibit a full spectrum of tissue reactivity. At one extreme are organ-specific diseases, such as Hashimoto's disease of the thyroid; at the other end of the spectrum are diseases that manifest themselves as non-organ–specific diseases such as systemic lupus erythematosus (SLE) and rheumatoid arthritis (RA) (see box below). In organ-specific diseases both the lesions produced by tissue damage and the autoantibodies are directed at a single

Examples of Autoimmune Diseases

Active chronic hepatitis
Addison's disease
Autoimmune atrophic gastritis
Autoimmune hemolytic anemia
Dermatomyositis
Discoid lupus erythematosus
Goodpasture's syndrome
Hashimoto's thyroiditis
Idiopathic thrombocytopenic purpura
Juvenile diabetes
Multiple sclerosis
Myasthenia gravis
Pemphigus vulgaris
Pernicious anemia
Primary biliary cirrhosis
Primary myxedema
Rheumatoid arthritis
Scleroderma
Sjögren's syndrome
Systemic lupus erythematosus
Thyrotoxicosis

target organ, e.g., the thyroid. Midspectrum disorders are characterized by localized lesions in a single organ and autoantibodies that are non-organ specific. An example of a midspectrum disorder is primary biliary cirrhosis. In this disorder the small bile duct is the main target of inflammatory cell infiltration, but the serum autoantibodies are mainly mitochondrial antibodies and are not liver specific. Non-organ–specific disorders are characterized by the presence of both lesions and autoantibodies not confined to any one organ. A summary of the features of organ-specific and non-organ–specific disorder is presented in Table 25-1. Characteristics of some of the organ-specific and midspectrum disorders are discussed later in this chapter. The non-organ–specific disorders of systemic lupus erythematosus and rheumatoid arthritis are discussed in detail in Chapters 26 and 27.

FACTORS INFLUENCING THE DEVELOPMENT OF AUTOIMMUNITY

The potential for autoimmunity, if given appropriate circumstances, is constantly present in every immunocompetent individual because lymphocytes that are potentially reactive with self-antigens exist in the body. Antibody expression appears to be regulated by a complex set of interacting factors. These influences include:

1. Genetic factors
2. Age
3. Exogenous factors

Genetic Factors

Although a direct genetic etiology has not been established in autoimmune disease, there is a tendency for familial aggregates to occur. In addition, a tendency for more than one autoimmune disorder to occur exists in the same individual. For example, patients with Hashimoto's disease have a higher incidence of pernicious anemia than would be expected in a random population matched for age and sex.

The presence of certain HLA antigens is also associated with an increased risk of certain autoimmune states. Another factor related to genetic inheritance is the fact that autoimmune disorders and autoantibodies are found more frequently in women than in men.

Age

Autoantibodies are manifested infrequently in the general population. The incidence of autoantibodies, however, increases steadily with age, reaching a peak at around 60 to 70 years.

Exogenous Factors

Ultraviolet radiation, drugs, viruses, and the presence of chronic infectious disease may all play a role in the development of autoimmune disorders. These factors may alter antigens, which the body then perceives as non-self.

TABLE 25-1

Summary of Organ-Specific and Non-Organ Specific Disorders

Similarities
1. Circulating autoantibodies react with normal body constituents
2. Increased immunoglobulin concentration in serum often found
3. Antibodies may appear in each of the main immunoglobulin classes
4. Disease process not always progressive; exacerbations and remissions occur
5. Autoantibody tests of diagnostic value

Differences	
Organ-specific	*Organ non-specific*
Antibodies and lesions are organ specific	Antibodies and lesions are non-organ specific
Clinical and serologic overlap, e.g., thyroid, stomach, adrenal glands, kidney	Overlap of SLE, RA, and other connective tissue disorders
Antigens only available to lymphoid system in low concentrations	Antigens accessible at higher concentrations
Antigens evoke organ-specific antibodies in normal animals with complete Freund's adjuvant	No antibodies produced in animals with comparable stimulation
Familial tendency to develop organ-specific autoimmunity	Familial tendency to develop connective tissue disease
	Questionable abnormalities in immunoglobulin synthesis in relatives
Lymphoid invasion, parenchymal destruction by questionable cell-mediated hypersensitivity or antibodies	Lesions caused by deposition of antigen-antibody (immune) complexes
Tendency to develop cancer in the organ	Tendency to develop lymphoreticular neoplasia

IMMUNOPATHOGENIC MECHANISMS
An Overview of Immunopathogenicity

Autoimmune disease is usually prevented by the normal functioning of immunologic regulatory mechanisms. When these controls dysfunction, antibodies to self-antigens may be produced and bind to antigens in the circulation to form *circulating immune complexes* or to antigens deposited in specific tissue sites.

The mechanisms governing the deposition in one organ or another are unknown; however, several mechanisms may be operative in a single disease. Wherever antigen-antibody complexes accumulate, *complement* can be activated with the subsequent release of mediators of inflammation. These mediators increase vascular permeability, attract phagocytic cells to the reaction site, and cause local tissue damage. Alternatively, cytotoxic T cells can directly attack body cells bearing the target antigen, which releases mediators that amplify the inflammatory reaction. Autoantibody and complement fragments coat cells bearing the target antigen, which leads to destruction by phagocytes or by antibody-seeking K type lymphocytes.

An individual may develop an autoimmune response in a variety of immunogenic stimuli. These responses may be caused by:
1. Antigens that do not normally circulate in the blood. The *hidden,* or *sequestered, antigen theory* is one of the earliest views with respect to organ-specific antibodies. According to this theory, antigens are sequestered within the organ, and because of the lack of contact with the mononuclear phagocytic system, they fail to establish *immunologic tolerance.* Any conditions producing a release of antigen would then provide an opportunity for autoantibody formation. This situation is true when sperm cells or lens and heart tissues are released directly into the circulation and autoantibodies are formed. Unmodified extracts of tissues involved in organ-specific autoimmune disorders, however, do not readily elicit antibody formation.
2. Altered antigens that arise because of chemical, physical, or biologic processes, such as hapten complexing, physical denaturation, or mutation
3. A foreign antigen that is shared or cross-reactive with self-antigens or tissue components
4. Mutation of immunocompetent cells to acquire a responsive to self-antigens
5. Loss of the immunoregulatory function by T cell subsets

Comprehension of the mechanism of autoimmunity requires an understanding of the regulation of the immune response. The immune response involves interaction of cellular elements, such as lymphocytes and macrophages, antigen, antibody, immune complexes, and complement.

T Cells

Helper and suppressor T cells act together to establish an immunoregulatory balance, which determines the level of immunologic response to a particular antigen. A disequilibrium resulting from either an expansion of helper T cells or a deficiency of suppressor T cells could trigger potentially autoreactive B cell clones to produce autoantibodies.

Auto-reactive T cells can also be demonstrated. Self-reactive effector T cells have been generated when lymphocytes have been cultured with a variety of autologous tissues in the presence of an agent such as mitogenicin lectin. Under normal conditions, it is believed that the body has a homeostatic mechanism to prevent them from being triggered. Presumably these cells are unresponsive because of clonal deletion, T cell suppression, or failure of autoantigen presentation.

B Cells

Intrinsic abnormalities in the B cells themselves can contribute to autoimmunity. According to the theory of B cell abnormality, inappropriate or outlaw B cells are triggered by unknown stimuli. They escape T cell control and may even interact or destroy T cells by producing anti-T cell antibodies.

Macrophages

Abnormalities of macrophages, particularly those expressing Ia antigens, also may contribute to autoimmunity. A major aspect of immunologic control resides with this important cell population.

SELF-RECOGNITION (TOLERANCE)

Self-recognition of membrane idiotypic receptors and the major histocompatibility complex (MHC) antigens appear to be fundamental to facilitating the regulatory interactions between cells. Many of these interactions are mediated through the production of highly specific soluble fraction that contains Ia and idiotypic determinants and transmits signs from one cell to another.

Whether the immunologic response to any given antigen will be expressed as immunity or tolerance is probably determined by a regulatory equilibrium, primarily established by the balance between helper and suppressor T cells. This equilibrium appears to be controlled by immune response (Ir) genes linked to the MHC and expressed on the surface of lymphocytes and macrophages as the Ia antigens. In addition, a new theory suggests that aberrant Ia expression on inflamed cells, such as thyroid cells in autoimmune thyroiditis, could lead to inappropriate antigen presentation by these cells, immune cell activation, and ultimately, to organ-specific autoimmune disease.

Self-tolerance is induced by at least two mechanisms involving contact between antigen and immunocompetent cells:
1. Elimination of the small clone of immunocompetent cells programmed to react with the antigen (Burnet's clonal selection theory).
2. Induction of unresponsiveness in the immunocompetent cells through excessive antigen binding to them and/or through triggering of a sup-

pressor mechanism. The normal immune response is modulated by both antigen-specific and non-specific suppressor cell activity.

The major mechanism in antigen-specific suppression of antibody response appears related to an antiidiotypic immune response induced by the antigen binding site (idiotype) unique for a particular antibody. In the opposite situation, prolonged antigen stimulation, such as in certain chronic infections, leads to polyclonal activation of the B cell response with a resultant *polyclonal hypergammaglobulinemia* (see Chapter 24 for a complete discussion of polyclonal and monoclonal hypergammaglobulinemias).

Receptors for antigens on B cells have the same antigen-binding configurations as the antibody molecules secreted by these cells. In addition, components of the antibody molecule itself elicit the formation of antiidiotype antibody, which can react with antigen receptors on the cell surface and therefore control the immune response. Antibody molecules with the same configuration are known as *idiotypes* and will be represented on the antigen receptor on B cells.

Both T and B cells appear to be targets of suppression by antiidiotypic reactivities represented by antibody and possibly also by specifically reactive T cells. In autoimmunity, T and B cells with antiidiotypic specificity could have the normal function of limiting the immune response to extrinsic antigens. Some types of suppressor T cells may also operate this way. The likelihood that antiidiotype antibodies occur naturally as molecules that are reactive with antigen receptor on T and B cells forms the basis of Jerne's network theory of self-regulation.

MAJOR AUTOANTIBODIES

Major autoantibodies can be detected in different diseases. Many diagnostic laboratory tests are based on detecting these autoimmune responses (see Appendixes B and C). Commonly encountered autoantibodies include thyroid, gastric, adrenocortical, striated muscle, acetylcholine receptor, smooth muscle, salivary gland, mitochondrial, reticulin, myelin, islet cell, and skin antibodies. Antibodies to antinuclear antibodies, which are discussed in detail in Chapter 2, include DNA, histone, and nonhistone protein antibodies. The action of specific autoantibodies and their use in medical diagnosis is as follows.

Acetylcholine receptor (AchR) binding antibody: Measure antibody to acetylcholine receptors at neuromuscular junctions of skeletal muscle. Useful in the diagnosis of myasthenia gravis.

Acetylcholine receptor (AcHR) blocking antibody: Measures antibodies to acetylcholine receptors, which block binding of 125_I-(α)-bungarotoxin. Found in about one third of patients with myasthenia gravis.

Antiadrenal antibody: Measures antibodies to adrenal cortex cells. High antibody titers are char-

acteristic of autoimmune hypoadrenalism in about three fourths of cases but are not found in tuberculous Addison's disease.

Anticardiolipin antibody: Antibodies directed to cardiolipin is present in patients with SLE associated with arterial and venous thromboses and in those with placental infarcts in early pregnancy with or without SLE. Elevation may be predictive of risk of thrombosis or recurrent spontaneous abortions of early pregnancy.

Anticentriole antibody: Measure antibodies to the cellular ultrastructures, centrioles. The appearance of these antibodies is unusual but can be demonstrated in systemic sclerosis.

Anticentromere antibody: Measure anticentromere (antikinetochore) to chromosomal centromeres. The majority of patients with CREST syndrome demonstrate these antibodies. They can also be exhibited by about one third of patients with Raynaud's disease and approximately 10% of patients with systemic sclerosis.

Anti-DNA antibody: Measures antibody to double-stranded deoxyribonucleic acid (DNA). Increased amounts (>25% by membrane assay) and decreased quantities of the C4 complement component confirms the diagnosis of SLE. These tests are also useful in monitoring the activity and exacerbations of SLE. The absence of anti-DNA is demonstrated in about one fourth of SLE patients; therefore, a negative test does not rule out SLE.

Antiglomerular basement membrane antibody: Measure the amount of antibody to glomerular basement membrane (anti-GBM). High titers are suggestive of Goodpasture's disease or anti-GBM nephritis. The test is also useful for monitoring anti-GBM nephritis. Negative results, however, do not rule out Goodpasture's disease.

Antiintrinsic factor antibody: Measures antibody to intrinsic factor (IF). The presence of IF-blocking antibodies is diagnostic of pernicious anemia and found in approximately 60% of cases.

Antiislet-cell antibody: Measures antibody to the islet cells of the pancreas. This test is useful as an early marker of beta pancreatic cell destruction.

Anti-LKM antibody: Measures antibody to components of renal and hepatic microsomes. The presence of a high titer is diagnostic of hepatic disease and suggests aggressive disease.

Antimitochondrial antibody: Measures antibody to the cellular ultrastructures, mitochondria. A high titer strongly suggests primary biliary cirrhosis (PBC); the absence of mitochondrial antibodies is strong evidence against PBC. Other forms of liver disease frequently exhibit low mitochondrial antibody titers.

Antimyelin antibody: Measures antibody tocomponents of the myelin sheath of nerves or myelin basic protein. Antibodies to myelin are associated with multiple sclerosis or other neurologic diseases. Myelin antibodies are not detectable in the cerebrospinal fluid of multiple sclerosis patients.

Antimyocardial antibody: Measures antibody to

components of the myocardium. The presence of myocardial antibodies is diagnostic of Dressler's (cardiac injury) syndrome or rheumatic fever.

Antinuclear antibody (ANA): Measures antibody to nuclear antigens. Antinuclear antibodies are found in most (99%) patients with untreated SLE.

Antiparietal cell antibody: Measures antibody to parietal cells (large cells on the margin of the peptic glands of the stomach). The majority (80%) of patients with pernicious anemia have parietal cell antibodies. In the presence of parietal cell antibodies, gastric biopsy almost always demonstrates gastritis. Low antibody titers to parietal cells are often found with no clinical evidence of pernicious anemia or atrophic gastritis and are sometimes seen in elderly patients.

Antiplatelet antibody: Measures immunologically-attached IgG on platelets. The presence of platelet antibodies, measured indirectly, is associated with immune thrombocytopenia (ITP) SLE.

Antireticulin antibody: Measures antibody to reticulin, an albuminoid or scleroprotein substance present in the connective framework of reticular tissue. The majority (80%) of cases of childhood gluten-sensitive enteropathy demonstrate reticulin antibodies. These antibodies can also be found in dermatitis herpetiformis, adult gluten-sensitive enteropathy, and in about one fifth of patients suffering from chronic heroin addiction.

Anti-rheumatoid arthritis nuclear antigen (Anti-RANA) (also called rheumatoid arthritis precipitin-RAP): Measures an antibody to a component of the Epstein-Barr virus. The antibody is found in the majority of patient with rheumatoid arthritis and in about 15% of patient with SLE. Anti-RANA is not useful in diagnosis or differential diagnosis of arthritis.

Antiribosome antibody: Measures the presence of antibody to the cellular organelles, ribosomes. Ribosomal antibodies are found in about 10% of patients with SLE.

Antinuclear ribonucleoprotein (anti-nRNP) antibody: Measures an antinuclear antibody (ANA), nuclear ribonucleoprotein. A high titer of this antibody is characteristic of *Mixed Connective Tissue Disease* (MCTD) or *Undifferentiated Connective Tissue Disease.* In MCTD, anti-nRNP is found in the absence of various other ANAs. Low titers of anti-nRNP are seen in about one third of patients with SLE and typically found in association with other ANAs, such as anti-DNA or anti-Sm.

Anti-Scl or Anti-Scl-70 antibody: Measures an antibody to a basic nonhistone nuclear protein. The presence of anti-Scl is diagnostic of systemic sclerosis; however, it is demonstrable in only about one fifth of the patients suffering from systemic sclerosis.

Anti-skin antibody (dermal-epidermal): Measures antibody to the basement membrane area of the skin. Antibodies are present in more than 80% of patients with bullous pemphigoid, but the absence of antibodies does not rule out the disorder.

Anti-skin (inter-epithelial) antibody: Measures antibody to intercellular substance of the skin. Antibodies can be detected in most (90%) of patients with pemphigus; the absence of demonstrable antibody usually excludes the diagnosis. The presence of antibodies is also useful in evaluating blistering disease. A rising antibody titer may indicate an impending relapse of pemphigus and a falling titer is suggestive of effective control of the disease.

Anti-Sm antibody: Measures Sm (Smith) antibody to acidic nuclear protein. Sm antibody is demonstrated by about one third of patients with SLE. Presence of the antibody confirms the diagnosis of SLE, but the absence of antibody does not exclude the diagnosis.

Antismooth muscle antibody: Measures antibody to components of smooth muscle. A high and persistent titer is suggestive of the autoimmune form of chronic active hepatitis. Antismooth muscle antibodies are also seen in viral disorders such as infectious mononucleosis.

Antisperm: Evaluates the presence of reproductive cell, sperm, antibodies. Half of vasectomized males demonstrate the antibody as well as 40% of males and females who have fertility problems.

Anti-SS-A (SS-A precipitin; Anti-Ro) antibody: Detects the presence of antibody to acidic nucleoprotein of human spleen extract. SS-A precipitins are demonstrable in more than 70% of patients with Sjögren's syndrome-Sicca complex and are often found in a subset of these patients who are at risk for vasculitis. The antibody is also found in one third of patients with SLE and in those with Sjögren's-rheumatoid arthritis or the annular variety of subacute cutaneous lupus erythematosus (LE). In neonatal LE autoantibodies to SS-A, discoid skin lesions, and congenital heart blocks are common.

Anti-SS-B (SS-B precipitin, anti-La) antibody: Detects antibody to acidic nucleoprotein of rubbati thymus. Anti-SS-B is demonstrated by the majority of patients with Sjörgren's syndrome-systemic lupus erythematosus. One half to three fourths of patients with Sjögren's syndrome-Sicca complex have the antibody; it is frequently found in a subset of these patients at risk for vasculitis.

Antistriational antibody: Measures antibody to components of striated muscle. Antibodies to striated muscles may be detected in patients with myasthenia gravis, thymoma, or with penicillamine treatment. Absence of the antibody in patients with myasthenia gravis generally rules out the presence of thymoma.

Antithyroglobulin and antithyroid microsome antibody: Evaluates the presence of antibodies to the thyroid components: thyroglobulin, an iodine-containing protein secreted by the thyroid gland and stored within its colloid substance; and thyroid microsomes, particles derived from the endoplasmic reticulum. The presence of microsome antibodies is considered to be predictive of an elevated thyroid-stimulating hormone (TSH) level. A positive thyroid antibody test and an elevated TSH titer are associated with a risk of hypothyroidism. Absence of both antibodies is strong evidence against autoimmune thyroiditis.

Histone reactive antinuclear antibody (HRANA): Measures the presence of HRANA. A high titer of HRANA is highly suggestive of drug-induced, e.g., hydralazine, lupus erythematosus. HRANA may occasionally be demonstrated in patients with SLE.

Jo-1 antibody: Detects precipitins to an acidic nuclear protein from calf thymus. Approximately one third of patients with uncomplicated polymyositis and some patients with dermatomyositis demonstrate this antibody.

Ku antibody: Detects precipitins to an acidic nuclear protein from calf thymus. About one-half of patients with overlapping signs and symptoms of scleroderma and polymyositis demonstrate Ku precipitins.

Mi-1-antibody: Detects antibodies to an acidic nuclear protein from calf thymus. Some patients with dermatomyositis and polymyositis demonstrate Mi-1-antibodies.

PM-1 antibody: Detects antibodies to an acidic nuclear protein from calf thymus. These precipitins are found in the majority (87%) of patients with polymyositis-scleroderma. More than half of the patients suffering from polymyositis demonstrate the antibody, but it is detected in less than one fifth of patients with dermatomyositis.

ORGAN SPECIFIC AND MIDSPECTRUM DISORDERS
Endocrine Disorders
Thyroid

Lymphoid (Hashimoto's) thyroiditis is a classic example of an organ-specific autoimmune disorder.

Etiology. The exact mechanism of the disorder is unknown but it is believed to be related an autoimmune process in which the development of circulating cytotoxic antibodies eventually destroys the thryoid gland, producing hypothyroidism.

Epidemiology. This disorder can occur at any age but it is most commonly first diagnosed in the third to fifth decade of life and is much more common in women than in men. The fibrous variant of the disease is more often present in middle-aged and elderly patients. A strong possibility of a genetic tendency to inherit the trait for the development of antibodies against the thyroid gland exists because it is common to have a history of Graves' disease and lymphoid thyroiditis in the same family.

Signs and Symptoms. Lymphoid thyroiditis is believed to be the most common cause of sporadic goiter. Characteristically, there is a firm, diffusely enlarged, nontender thyroid gland that may be lobulated. Hypothyroidism, however, is a common late sequela of lymphoid thyroiditis and patients are usually euthyroid when first seen by a physician. Some individuals have clinical and pathologic

evidence of the coexistence of both (Graves' disease) and lymphoid (Hashimoto's) thyroiditis. Histologically, Hashimoto's thyroiditis is characterized by diffuse lymphocytic infiltration (Fig. 25-1).

Immunologic Manifestations

Patients with lymphocytic thyroiditis as well as other autoimmune thyroid disorders can demonstrate histologic and immunological manifestations of the disease. Antibodies to thyroid constituents may be observed in these patients. Antibodies to the following list of constituents may be demonstrated serologically:
1. Thyroglobulin
2. Thyroid microsome
3. Second colloid antigen (CA2 antigen)
4. Thyroid membrane receptors
5. Thyronine (T_4) and triiodothyronine (T_3)

Thyroglobulin. Thyroglobulin, the major soluble protein in the thyroid gland, was the first antibody discovered against a thyroid component. Immunofluorescent laboratory methods using fluorescein-labeled antihuman immunoglobulin can demonstrate the binding of antithyroglobulin antibody to thin sections of thyroid tissue in abnormal conditions or in approximately 4% of the normal population. It has also been noted that a gradual increase in the frequency of positive titers occurs in the female population with aging. The absence of antithyroglobulin antibodies, however, does not exclude the diagnosis of lymphocytic (Hashimoto's thyroiditis) and, conversely, the presence of antibodies does not establish the diagnosis because it can be positive in Graves' disease and is occasionally positive in thyroid cancer and subacute thyroditis. Testing for antibody may also be used to monitor patients with thyroid cancers.

Thyroid microsomes. Antibodies directed against thyroid microsomes can be detected in about 7% of the population, with titers ranging from 1:100 to 1:1,600. Even a low titer of antithyroid antibodies correlates with a degree of thyroid involvement by an autoimmune process. The absence of antibodies has been documented in diagnosed cases of autoimmune thyoiditis, which may be explained by special characteristics of the antibody or by the fact that it forms complexes with thyroglobulins in the circulation and escapes detection. The presence of such circulating complexes has been documented in patients with thyroid autoimmune disorders.

Second colloid (CA2) antigen. Second colloid antigen (CA2 antigen) is directed against a colloid protein and can be detected by immunofluorescent examination. Antibody to CA2 is present in about 50% of patients who have subacute thyroiditis and is detectable in some patients who have Hashimoto's thyroiditis whose sera shows no other evidence of abnormal antibodies.

Thyroid membrane receptors. The thyroid membrane receptors are a group of IgG antibodies that interact with receptors on thyroid membranes.

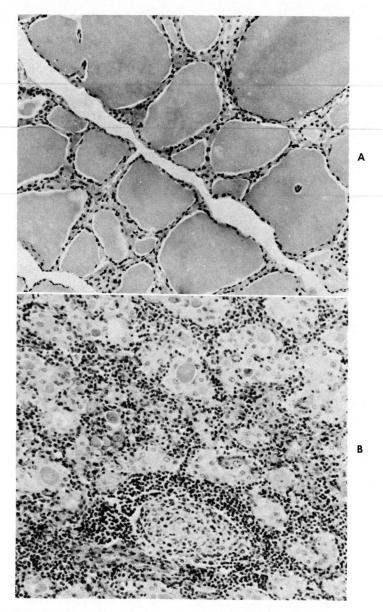

FIGURE 25-1

A comparison of the histologic architecture of the thyroid gland of a normal patient, **A,** and a patient with Hashimoto's disease, **B.** In the normal thyroid, colloid fills the vesicles but in a diseased gland only isolated deposits of colloid are seen. The cell infiltrate is lymphoid in nature. In the lower center is a germinal center.
(From Anderson JR, Buchanan WW, and Goudie RB: Autoimmunity, Springfield, Ill, 1967, Charles C Thomas, Publisher.)

They often produce hyperthyroidism that manifests itself clinically, chemically, and histologically. At present, the classification of these IgG antibodies is operational, based on their method of detection. LATS (long-acting thyroid stimulation) and LATS-P assays are of importance.

Thyronine (T_4) and Triiodothyronine (T_3). Antibodies to T_4 and T_3 have been found in several patients, most of whom had evidence of a thyroid autoimmune process such as goiter and hypothyroidism. In these cases, the underlying autoimmune process is most likely responsible for the hy-

pothyroidism rather than hormone binding by the circulating antithyronine antibodies.

Diagnostic Evaluation

Fine-needle aspiration biopsy of the thyroid in useful in conjunction with clinical evaluation and serologic studies in the diagnosis of lymphocytic (Hashimoto's) thyroiditis.

Histologic examination of thyroid tissue demonstrates variable infiltration of the entire gland with lymphocytes. Germinal lymphoid centers are characteristic, and destruction and distortion of normal

TABLE 25-2

Antithyroid Antibody Tests

Antigen	Test to identify antibody
Thyroglobulin	Precipitin test (Ouchterlony technique)
	Indirect immunofluorescence on fixed thyroid tissues
	Tanned RBC hemagglutination (TRC or TGHA)
	Radioimmunoassay (RIA)
Microsomal antigen	Complement fixation
	Indirect immunofluorescence
	Cytoxicity
	Tanned red cell hemagglutination technique (MCHA)
	Solid phase RIA
Second colloid antigen (CA-2)	Indirect immunofluorescence
Thyroid membrane receptors	LATS (long-acting thyroid stimulator)
	LATS-P (LATS protector)
	In vitro assays for TSI (thyroid-stimulating immunoglobulin) or TBI (TSH-binding inhibition)
Thyronines (T_3 and T_4)	Radioimmunoassay using different separation methods
	Electrophoresis with radioactive-labeled thyronines

thyroid follicles is apparent. The thyroid cells remain intact but are hypertrophied, although the usual heterogenity of small enlarged thyroid follicles, some containing flat epithelium, also can be seen. In advanced cases of disease, there is almost complete destruction of normal thyroid tissue and replacement by lymphocytes or fibrous tissue.

When the disease produces hypothyroidism, a slight increase in the plasma TSH concentration can usually be demonstrated in the early phase, followed by a fall in serum thyroxine and eventually by a fall in serum triiodothyronine. Antithyroglobulin and/or antithyroid microsomal antibodies are found in moderate-to-high titers in more than 50% of patients, but the presence of antimicrosomal antibodies is considered to be more diagnostic.

Antibodies directed against thyroid microsomes can be detected by various techniques (Table 25-2). Hemagglutination tests for microsomal antibody (MCHA) are the most commonly performed. The thyroglobulin precipitin method was originally useful but has been replaced by newer, more sensitive techniques such as indirect hemagglutination. The thyroglobulin precipitin test is frequently negative in the juvenile form of lymphocytic thyroiditis and in the oxyphil variant, but it is frequently positive (96%) in the fibrous variant of Hashimoto's thy-

roiditis. Indirect hemagglutination procedure, which is also referred to as the TGHA test or the tanned red (TRC) test, is the most widely used assay to detect antithyroglobulin antibodies. It uses thyroglobulin-sensitized red cells as detectors when mixed with various dilutions of patient sera. The modification of using turkey cells instead of sheep cells in the procedure has improved the test by reducing nonspecific agglutination and making the method easier and faster to perform. Positive TRC results are usually manifested by 70% of patients with the fibrous and oxyphil variants of Hashimoto's thyroiditis and is frequently absent or present only in low titers in juvenile lymphocytic thyroiditis.

Pancreas

Antibodies reacting with the cells of the pancreatic islets have been found in patients with diabetes accompanying autoimmune endocrine disorders. A higher incidence of these antiislet cell antibodies, however, has been demonstrated in patients with insulin-dependent diabetes.

An immunoglobulin in the sera of patients with insulin-resistant diabetes appears to bind to a tissue receptor for insulin, which prevents some of the biologic effects of insulin. In addition, antibodies that bind to and possibly kill pancreatic islet cells have been found in the majority of young patients with insulin-dependent diabetes.

A small subgroup of patients with insulin-resistant diabetes mellitus has demonstrated antireceptor antibody (InR), an IgG class of antibodies directed against the insulin receptor. Antibodies to InR may be directed to the binding site or to determinants away from the binding site for insulin. This condition is predominant in non-white females of all ages.

Adrenal Glands

More than two thirds of the cases of *Addison's disease* are idiopathic in nature. It is believed that many of these cases are autoimmune in etiology. Approximately 40% to 70% of patients manifest serum antibodies against cortical elements, probably microsomal. Some cases demonstrate antibodies against adrenal cell surfaces. These antibodies generally bind to components in the adrenal cortex but affect only individual zones.

Antibodies are generally low in titer and are not a direct reflection of adrenal cell damage because they are present in only 7% to 18% of patients with adrenal damage, primarily cases involving tuberculosis, and in only 1% of normal individuals.

Ovaries and Testes

Antibodies against cytoplasmic components of different cells of the ovary have been demonstrated in Addison's disease and in premature ovarian failure. In addition, antisperm antibodies have also been detected. Elevated levels of antibodies to sperm have been found in more than 40% of males following vasectomy but only occasionally in males with primary testicular agenesis. Seminal fluid may also contain sperm antibodies of the IgA class.

Autoimmune Hematologic Disorders

Autoimmune Hemolytic Anemia

Autoimmune hemolytic anemia can be classified into four groups:

1. Warm-reactive autoantibodies—the most common
2. Cold-reactive autoantibodies—less than 20% of cases
3. Paroxysmal cold hemoglobinuria (PCH)—rare.
4. Drug-induced hemolysis—less than 20% of cases

Warm autoimmune hemolytic anemia. Warm autoimmune hemolytic anemia (WAIHA) is associated with antibodies reactive at warm temperatures, i.e., 37° C. In more than three fourths of cases the erythrocytes are coated with both IgG and complement, although some may demonstrate coating with IgG alone or, more infrequently, with complement coating. In WAIHA very little serum autoantibody exists because the antibody reacts optimally at 37° C and is being continuously adsorbed by red cells in vivo. Elution of the antibody from the cells (mechanical removal of antibodies) can demonstrate an autoantibody, but testing for specificity is not routinely necessary.

Cold autoimmune hemolytic anemia. Cold hemagglutinin disease (CHAD), either in the acute or chronic form, is the most common type of hemolytic anemia associated with cold-reactive autoantibodies. The acute form is often secondary to *Mycoplasma pneumoniae* infection or lymphoproliferative disorders such as lymphoma. The chronic form is seen in older patients and produces a mild-to-moderate degree of hemolysis with Raynaud's phenomena and hemoglobinuria occurring in cold weather.

In CHAD, a cold-reactive IgM autoantibody reacts with erythrocytes in the peripheral circulation when the body temperature falls to 32° C or below and binds complement to the cells. Hence, comple-

ment is the only globulin detected on the erythrocytes. Elutions prepared from red cells collected at 37° C will not demonstrate antibody reactivity in the eluate.

Paroxysmal cold hemoglobinuria (PCH). Paroxysmal cold hemoglobinuria (PCH) was previously associated with syphilis, but it is now more commonly seen as an acute transient condition secondary to viral infections, particularly in young children. PCH may also occur as an idiopathic chronic disease in older people.

The autoantibody is an IgG protein that reacts with red cells in colder parts of the body, which produce complement components C3 and C4 to bind irreversibly to the cells. At warmer temperatures, red cells are hemolyzed and the antibody elutes from the cells. Eluates are also nonreactive. This IgG autoantibody, a biphasic hemolysin, can be demonstrated by performing the Donath-Landsteiner test. The autoantibody has anti-P specificity and reacts with all except the rare p or p^k phenotypes. Exceptions that include examples with anti-IH specificity have been described.

Drug-induced hemolysis. Coating of red cells demonstrated by a positive direct antihuman globulin test (DAT) may be drug induced (Table 25-3) and may be accompanied by hemolysis. The mechanisms of reactivity have been described as being caused by four basic mechanisms:

1. Drug adsorption
2. Immune complex
3. Membrane modification
4. Autoantibody formation

Drug adsorption. Penicillin is a representative example of a drug that displays drug adsorption. In this type of mechanism, the drug strongly binds to any protein, including red cell membrane proteins. This binding produces a drug red cell hapten complex that can stimulate antibody formation. The antibody is specific for this complex, and no reactions will take place unless the drug is adsorbed on erythrocytes. Massive doses of intravenous (IV) penicillin are needed to coat sufficiently the erythrocytes in order for antibody attachment to occur.

Approximately 3% of affected patients will dem-

TABLE 25-3

Drug-Induced Positive Direct Antiglobulin Test (DAT)

	Drug adsorption	Immune complex	Membrane modification	Autoantibody formation
Common cause	IgG	Complement	Nonserologic	IgG
Antibody screening	Negative*	Positive†	Negative	Variable‡
Eluate reactivity with reagent RBCs	Nonreactive	Nonreactive	Nonreactive	Reactive§
Penicillin-treated RBCs	Reactive with patient's serum and eluate	Nonreactive	Nonreactive	Nonreactive

*Unless alloantibodies are present in the sample.
†If the drug and complement are present in the test system.
‡If the autoantibody is high enough in titer, screening tests may be positive with all cells tested.
§Will react with all normal cells tested, occasionally showing Rh-like specificity.

onstrate a positive DAT and less than 5% will develop hemolytic anemia because of the drug. The hemolysis of red cells is usually extravascular and occurs slowly. It is not life-threatening and will abate when penicillin is discontinued. There appears to be no connection between this type of antibody production and allergic penicillin sensitivity caused by IgE production.

Other drugs that display drug adsorption are cephalothin derivatives, e.g., cephalothin (Keflin) and quinidine.

Immune complex. The mechanism of immune complexing is displayed by a variety of drugs, including phenacetin, quinine, rifampin, and stibophen. In this interaction the drug and antibody form a complex in the serum and attach nonspecifically to the red cells. Once attached, this complex initiates the complement cascade, which culminates in intravascular hemolysis. The immune complex may dissociate from the red cell membrane after complement activation and attach to another red cell. This action allows a small amount of drug to produce a severe anemia. When the offending drug is discontinued, the hemolytic process disappears quickly.

Membrane modification mechanism. Drugs of the cephalosporin type, e.g., cephalothin, occasionally cause a positive DAT with polyspecific and monospecific AHG antisera by membrane modification. In this type of mechanism, the drug alters the membrane so that there is nonspecific adsorption of globulins, including IgG, IgM, IgA, and complement. Hemolysis is not a frequent complication in this type of membrane augmentation.

Autoantibody formation. Drugs such as methyldopa (Aldomet), levodopa, and mefenamic acid (Ponstel) have been implicated in positive DATs caused by autoantibody formation. The autoantibody formed recognizes a part of the red cell and therefore reacts with most normal red cells. Some drug-induced autoantibodies have been shown to have specificities that appear to be of the Rh type but most have no apparent specificity. Antibody production ceases with withdrawal of the drug.

Idiopathic Thrombocytopenia Purpura

Idiopathic thrombocytopenic purpura is now also known as *immunologic thrombocytopenic purpura* (ITP). Patients with ITP usually demonstrate petechiae, bruising, menorrhagia, and bleeding after minor trauma. ITP may be either acute or chronic. Children are most often afflicted with the acute type, while adults predominantly experience the chronic type. This common disorder may complicate other antibody-associated disorders such as SLE.

Although thrombocytopenia (a condition of absent or severely decreased platelets [below 10 to 20×10^9/L]) may result from a wide variety of conditions, such as following the use of extracorporeal circulation in cardiac bypass surgery or in alcoholic liver disease, most thrombocytopenic conditions can be classified into three major categories:
1. Decreased production of platelets
2. Disorders of platelet distribution
3. Increased destruction or use of platelets

Decreased production may result from invasion of the bone marrow by neoplastic cells and is usually not associated with an immunologic cause. Disorders of platelet distribution are associated with a sequestering of platelets in the spleen for a variety of nonimmunologic reasons. Increased destruction or use of platelets, however, is associated with immunologic mechanisms. These mechanisms of destruction are caused by antigens, antibodies, or complement.

Drugs or foreign substances including quinidine, sulfonamide derivatives, heroin, morphine, and snake venom, can produce platelet destruction. Sulfonamide derivative reactions involve the interaction of platelet antigens with drug antibodies. Morphine reactions involve the activation of complement.

Bacterial sepsis causes increased destruction of platelets caused by the attachment of platelets to bacterial antigen-antibody immune complexes. Certain microbial antigens may initially attach to platelets followed by specific antibodies to the micro-organism. This mechanism has been reported to cause the thrombocytopenia that frequently complicates the *Plasmodium falciparum* type of malaria.

Antibodies of either autoimmune or isoimmune origin may produce increased destruction of platelets. Examples of thrombocytopenias of isoimmune origin include posttransfusion purpura and isoimmune neonatal thrombocytopenia. Neonatal autoimmune thrombocytopenia is a condition caused by immunization of a pregnant female by a fetal platelet antigen and transplacental passage of maternal IgG platelet antibodies. The antigen is inherited by the fetus from the father and is absent on maternal platelets. Posttransfusion purpura is a rare form of isoimmune thrombocytopenia.

Pernicious Anemia

Pernicious anemia (PA) is a megaloblastic anemia characterized by a variety of hematologic and chemical manifestations (Table 25-4). PA is caused by a deficiency of vitamin B_{12} caused by the patient's inability to secrete *intrinsic factor* (IF). In the majority of cases of PA, antiintrinsic factors or antiparietal antibodies have been reported. Most authorities consider the demonstration of these antibodies to support the theory that pernicious anemia is an autoimmune disorder.

Assays for anti-intrinsic factor measure antibodies to IF. The presence of IF blocking antibodies is diagnostic of PA. Antibodies can be demonstrated in about 60% of cases. Antiparietal cell assays measure antibodies to parietal cells (large cells on the margin of the peptic glands of the stomach). The majority (80%) of patients with PA have parietal cell antibodies. In the presence of parietal cell anti-

TABLE 25-4

Hematologic and Chemical Findings in Pernicious Anemia

Hematologic manifestations	Hemoglobin	Severely decreased
	Hematocrit (PVC)	Severely decreased
	Erythrocyte count	Decreased
	Leukocyte count	Slightly decreased
	Platelet count	Slightly decreased or normal
	Mean corpuscular volume (MCV)	Increased
Chemical findings	Serum iron	Increased
	Total iron-binding capacity (TIBC)	Normal or decreased
	Percentage of Fe saturation	Increased
	Serum ferritin	Increased

TABLE 25-5

Vitamin B_{12} (Cobalamin) Binding Proteins

	Intrinsic factor	Transcobalamin II	R proteins
Source	Stomach	Liver, other tissues	Leukocytes, ? other tissues
Function	Intestinal absorption	Delivery to cells	Excretion Storage
Membrane receptors	Ileal enterocytes	Many cells	Liver cells

bodies, gastric biopsy almost always demonstrates gastritis. Low-antibody titers to parietal cells are often found with no clinical evidence of PA or atrophic gastritis, and are sometimes seen in elderly patients.

Gastrointestinal Disorders
Atrophic Gastritis and Pernicious Anemia

Immunologic findings. Antibodies against a lipoprotein cytoplasmic component of gastric parietal cells can be detected by immunofluorescence in up to 90% of patients with PA and in about 60% of patients with atrophic gastritis without hematologic abnormalities. These antibodies may also be demonstrated in patients with other autoimmune diseases such as thyroiditis. In addition, antibodies can be found in asymptomatic patients and in persons over 60.

Histologic findings. The histologic findings in atrophic gastritis, which almost always accompanies PA, is characterized by lymphocytic infiltration and the absence of parietal and chief cells. The lesions are associated with decreased synthesis of gastric acid and intrinsic factor. IF normally binds ingested vitamin B_{12} at one site and binds to receptors in the distal ileum at another site. In this manner, vitamin B_1 transport across the ileum is affected.

Vitamin B_{12} (Cobalamin) transport. Cobalamin transport is mediated by three different binding proteins (Table 25-5) that are capable of binding the vitamin at its required physiologic concentrations: *intrinsic factor, transcobalamin II,* and *the R proteins.*

Intrinsic factor (IF), a glycoprotein, is synthesized and secreted by the parietal cells of the mucosa in the fundus region of the stomach in several mammalian species including humans. In health, the amounts of IF secreted by the stomach greatly exceed the quantities required to bind ingested cobalamin in its coenzyme forms. At a very acidic pH, cobalamin splits from dietary protein and combines with IF to form a vitamin-IF complex. Binding by IF is extraordinarily specific and is lost with even slight changes in the cobalamin molecule. This complex is stable and remains unabsorbed until it reaches the ileum. In the ileum, the vitamin-IF complex attaches to specific receptor sites present only on the outer surface of microvillus membranes of ileal enterocytes.

The release of this complex from the mucosal cells with subsequent transport to the tissues depends on transcobalamin II (TC II). TC II is a plasma polypeptide synthesized by the liver and probably several other tissues. Like IF, TC II, which turns over very rapidly in the plasma, acts as the acceptor and principal carrier of the vitamin to the liver and other tissues. Receptors for TC II are observed on the plasma membranes of a wide variety of cells. TC II is also capable of binding a few unusual cobalamin analogues. TC II also stimulates cobalamin uptake by reticulocytes.

The R proteins comprise an antigenically cross-reactive group of cobalamin-binding glycoproteins. The R proteins bind cobalamin and various cobalamin analogs. Their function is unknown, but they appear to serve as storage sites and as a means of eliminating excess cobalamin and unwanted analogs from the blood circulation through receptor sites on liver cells. R proteins are produced by leukocytes and perhaps other tissues. They are present in plasma as transcobalamin I and transcobalamin III, as well as in saliva, milk, and other body fluids. Transcobalamin I probably serves only as a backup transport system for endogenous cobalamin. Endogenous vitamin is synthesized in the human GI tract by bacterial action, but none is adsorbed.

Autoimmune Liver Disease

Autoimmune processes are believed to be the possible cause of chronic liver disease. Hypergammaglobulinemia, prominent lymphocyte and plasma cell inflammation of the liver, and the presence of one or more circulating tissue antibodies are commonly manifested. These manifestations suggest an organ-localized autoimmune pathogenesis.

Chronic active hepatitis, for example, is an inflammatory condition that is most common in young women. It is characterized by prominent lymphocyte and plasma cell inflammatory changes, which start in the portal tracts. In some cases, this condition results from a chronic viral infection or inflammation; but in other cases, a number of immunologic abnormalities are present to varying degrees, in addition to hypergammaglobulinemia and an elevated erythrocyte sedimentation rate. A defect in immunoregulation is commonly demonstrated, which possibly leads to unrestrained immunoglobulin production. These patients display antinuclear antibodies and antismooth muscle antibodies. A high and persistent titer of antismooth antibodies is suggestive of the autoimmune form of chronic active hepatitis or viral disorders such as infectious mononucleosis.

In some case, this disease is referred to as *lupoid hepatitis.* Patients with aggressive chronic active hepatitis have a poor prognosis, and a significant rate of mortality is reported 5 years after diagnosis.

Idiopathic Biliary Cirrhosis

Idiopathic biliary cirrhosis is a slowly progressive disease that starts as an apparently noninfectious inflammation in the bile ducts of young to middle-aged women. An increased familial incidence has been noted.

Patients exhibit increased serum IgM, depression of cellular immunity with prominent decreases in suppressor T cells common, and associated autoimmune disorders. It is believed that tissue damage results from an unmodulated attack against host tissue antigens. Antimitochondrial antibodies directed against the cellular ultrastructures, mitochondria, can be displayed. A high titer of these strongly suggests primary biliary cirrhosis (PBC); the absence of mitochondrial antibodies is strong evidence against PBC. Other forms of liver disease, however, frequently exhibit low mitochondrial antibody titers.

Inflammatory Bowel Disease

Antibodies directed against colon components are commonly found in the serum of patients with chronic ulcerative colitis, Crohn's disease of the colon, and in some cases of regional ileitis. There is evidence that lymphocytes from some patients with inflammatory bowel disease are cytotoxic for human fetal colon tissue. It is not clear, however, whether antibody-dependent cellular cytotoxicity plays a role in the disease. Other manifestations of uncertain significance are the presence of circulating immune complexes and the depressed capacity to express delayed hypersensitivity (anergy), which occurs commonly but not consistently in inflammatory bowel disease.

Cardiac Disorders

The immunologic basis for rheumatic heart disease has been suspected for a long time. Patients who have rheumatic heart disease (RHD) exhibit antimyocardial antibodies that bind in vitro to foci in the myocardium and heart valves. These antibodies may be responsible for the deposition of immunoglobulin and complement components found in the same area of RHD tissues at autopsy.

Antimyocardial antibodies appears to be strongly cross-reactive with streptococcal antigens, but they are not toxic to heart tissue unless the latter is damaged previously by some other cause. Because antimyocardial antibodies are commonly found in patients who have recently suffered a myocardial infarction or who have had a recent streptococcal infection (see Chapter 15) without cardiac sequela, detection of these antibodies has not been a particularly useful differential diagnostic test for cardiac injury. The presence of myocardial antibodies, however, is diagnostic of Dressler's (cardiac injury) syndrome or rheumatic fever.

Neuromuscular Disorders

Several important neurologic disorders are related to the immune system. The immune system may play an important role in the pathogenesis and/or etiology of myasthenia gravis and multiple sclerosis.

Myasthenia Gravis

Myasthenia gravis is a disorder of the neuromuscular junction characterized by neurophysiologic and immunologic abnormalities (see box). In this disease, a postsynaptic defect is caused by a de-

---

Abnormalities Associated with Myasthenia Gravis

1. Thymic hyperplasia with germinal follicles
2. Increase in thymic B cells
3. Thymoma
3. Expression of acetylcholine receptor (AchR) binding antibody and acetylcholine receptor (AcHR) blocking antibody
4. Associated with other autoimmune diseases

crease in receptors for acetylcholine and frequently an anatomic defect in the neuromuscular junction plate. Acetylcholine receptor (AcHR) binding antibody is an antibody directed against acetylcholine receptors at neuromuscular junctions of skeletal muscle and acetylcholine receptor (AcHR) blocking antibodies. The ligand bungarotoxin or acetylcholine is important in producing a neuromuscular block. About one third of patients with myasthenia gravis demonstrate AcHR blocking antibodies.

The role of these antibodies in producing disease is unclear. Complement-mediated antibody-determined damage may be an important mechanism in myasthenia gravis because IgG, C3, and C9 can be demonstrated at the neuromuscular junction and the motor endplate is often abnormal. This suggests that antibody to acetylcholine receptor is capable of increasing the normal rate of degradation resulting in less available receptors.

Multiple Sclerosis

Multiple sclerosis (MS) is a common demyelinating disease of the central nervous system (CNS) related to abnormalities of the immune system. It is characterized by regions of demyelinization of varying size and age scattered throughout the white matter of the CNS. Demyelinization "plaques" have a propensity to form in the cerebrum, optic nerves, brain stem, spinal cord, and cerebellum.

Immunologic manifestations. The immunologic manifestations of this disease that are suggestive of its autoimmune nature are presented in the box below. Antimyelin antibodies directed against components of the myelin sheath of nerves or myelin basic protein can be demonstrated in patients with MS or other neurologic diseases. Myelin antibodies, however, are not detectable in the cerebrospinal fluid (CSF) of MS patients.

Detection of oligoclonal bands. Oligoclonal immunoglobulins may be seen in both serum and cerebrospinal fluid. An oligoclonal immunoglobulin pattern consists of multiple homogeneous, narrow, and probably faint bands in the gamma zone on electrophoresis.

Electrophoresis on cellulose acetate will rarely resolve an oligoclonal pattern. Therefore, electrophoretic media with greater resolution such as agar or agarose gel are required, and both require the use of concentrated CSF. It is important to electro-

phorese a serum specimen concurrently with the CSF specimen to ensure that the demonstrated homogeneous bands are present only in the CSF, which implies endogenous synthesis rather than serum band that might appear secondarily in the CSF. Uncommonly, if a prominent CSF band is present, it may appear in the serum as a homogeneous band. This situation is most frequently encountered in subacute sclerosing panencephalitis (SSPE).

High-resolution electrophoresis attempts to achieve better resolution of proteins beyond the classic five band pattern. The primary reason for performing high-resolution protein electrophoresis is for the detection of oligoclonal bands in CSF to increase the diagnostic usefulness of protein patterns. About 80% of CSF proteins originate from the plasma. The electrophoretic pattern of normal CSF is similar to a normal serum protein pattern; however, several differences are detectable. The differences include a prominent prealbumin band and two transferrin bands.

Immunofixation has been used in some research studies to show that the oligoclonal bands seen in CSF protein patterns are made up primarily of IgG. Although this may be of academic interest, characterization of the immunoglobulin bands does not significantly improve the diagnostic usefulness of the procedure. Isoelectric focusing, however, is becoming the method of choice for oligoclonal band detection.

Significance of oligoclonal bands. If oligoclonal bands are present in CSF but not in the serum, they are the result of increased production of IgG by the central nervous system (CNS). CNS production of IgG occurs in the subarachnoid space of the brain in conjunction with the local accumulation of immunocytes. Each has its own specificity that gives rise to oligoclonal bands. Although the immunoglobulin is IgG, it is polyclonal in nature with several groups of cells producing the immunoglobulin. Oligoclonal bands are therefore defined as discrete populations of IgG with restricted heterogeneity

---

Immunologic Manifestation of Multiple Sclerosis

1. Antimyelin antibodies
2. Myelinotoxicity and glial toxicity of serum and cerebrospinal fluid in vitro
3. In vitro cell-mediated immunity by blood and cerebrospinal fluid cells to myelin components
4. Oligoclonal increase in cerebrospinal fluid immunoglobulin
5. Increase in certain HLA and Ia antigens (HL-A A3, B7, DW2, and DRW2)

Condition Associated with Oligoclonal Cerebrospinal Fluid Gammaglobulins

1. Multiple sclerosis (MS)
2. Neurosyphilis-paresthesia
3. Paraneoplastic syndrome—subacute sclerosing panencephalitis
4. Chronic mycobacterial and fungal meningitis
5. Chronic viral meningitis and meningoencephalis (uncommon)
6. Acute viral meningitis (uncommon)
7. Primary optic neuritis
8. Acute disseminated encephalomyelitis
9. Peripheral neuropathy
10. Guillain-Barré syndrome
11. Burkitt's lymphoma
12. Psychoneurosis
13. Cerebral infarction

demonstrated by electrophoresis.

One procedure for confirming local CNS production of oligoclonal IgG is to assay a matched serum specimen diluted 1:100 concurrently with an unconcentrated CSF sample. Oligoclonal bands present in CSF but not in the serum indicate CNS production. This matched sample procedure is especially useful if damage to the blood-brain barrier is suspected because of acute or chronic inflammations, such as meningitis, intracranial tumor, or cerebral vascular disease.

Serum oligoclonal bands may represent immune complexes and are associated with diseases such as Hodgkins or a nonspecific early immune response to a number of diseases (see box on p. 292).

Findings in multiple sclerosis. Total CSF protein in patients with MS is usually normal or slightly elevated. In general, patients with no neurologic disease have IgG concentration of less than 10% of the total CSF proteins. Almost 70% of MS patients typically have IgG concentration of 11% to 35% of total CSF proteins.

Oligoclonal bands in serum are not absolutely indicative of MS and their presence should be used in conjunction with other information available from clinical evaluation and other diagnostic procedures. Although oligoclonal bands can be present in more than 90% of MS patients at some time during the course of the disease, their presence does not correlate with the activity of the disease. The exact number of bands present in MS is variable. Some studies have demonstrated 7 to 15 bands.

Autoimmune Renal Disorders

It is generally accepted that most immunologically mediated renal diseases fall into several categories (see box below).

Categories of Immunologic Renal Disease

Associated with circulating immune complexes
Systemic lupus erythematosus (SLE)
Certain vasculites
Infections
Tumors (possibly)
Immunoglobulins and antiimmunoglobulins

Membranoproliferative glomerulonephritis
Activation of the alternate complement pathway
Possible genetic factors

Associated with antiglomerular basement membrane antibody
Most cases of Goopasture's syndrome
Some rapidly progressive glomerulonephritis
Membrane altered by a virus or drugs (possibly)

Tubulo-interstitial nephritis
Associated with immune complex-mediated disease
Drugs and possibly infection
Involvement of transplanted kidneys

Renal Disease Associated With Circulating Immune Complexes

Renal diseases associated with circulating immune complexes are caused by nonrenal antigens and their corresponding antibodies (see box). These complexes are deposited in one or more of several loci in the glomerulus. Deposition may be dependent on the size and other characteristics of the complex. Recent evidence suggests that potentially damaging immune complexes may be formed in situ and involve antigens already present or fixed in the glomerulus. In addition, immune complex activation of complement in the glomerular basement membrane may be augmented by the presence of cells with receptors for C3 located in that area. The result of activation probably involves the release of biologically active products, such as chemotactic substances, and causes an inflammatory type of tissue injury. A renal complication of this type can be manifested in systemic lupus erythematosus.

Membranoproliferative Glomerulonephritis

Another type of glomerular disease, membranoproliferative glomerulonephritis, is believed to be caused by nonimmunologically activated complement. Activation is thought to be analogous to the alternate pathway activation of C3 by certain bacterial products and polysaccharides.

Renal Disease Associated with Antiglomerular Basement Membrane Antibody

Glomerular basement membrane antibodies (anti-GBM) are antibodies directed against the glomerular basement membrane of the glomerulus of the kidney (Fig. 25-2). These antibodies are induced in vivo against the basement membrane of the glomerulus and possibly the renal tubule or lung basement membrane. The factors that stimulate antibody production are not well defined, but it appears likely that binding of drugs such as methicillin, certain infectious agents, or renal damage caused by other immune mechanisms may lead to an immune antibody response. The end result may be direct damage to the bone marrow with or without complement activation. Production of anti-bone marrow antibodies, however, appears to be self-limited and lasts for several weeks to months after removal of the inciting agent, i.e., the kidney.

High antibody titers of anti-GMB are suggestive of Goodpasture's disease, early systemic lupus erythematosus, or anti-GBM nephritis. The absence of antibodies, however, does not rule out Goodpasture's disease. This type of renal disease represents less than 5% of glomerular disorders.

Tubulo-interstitial Nephritis

Tubulo-interstitial nephritis involving the renal tubules has been associated with a variety of causes. In addition to being associated with immune complex-mediated disease, precipitating fac-

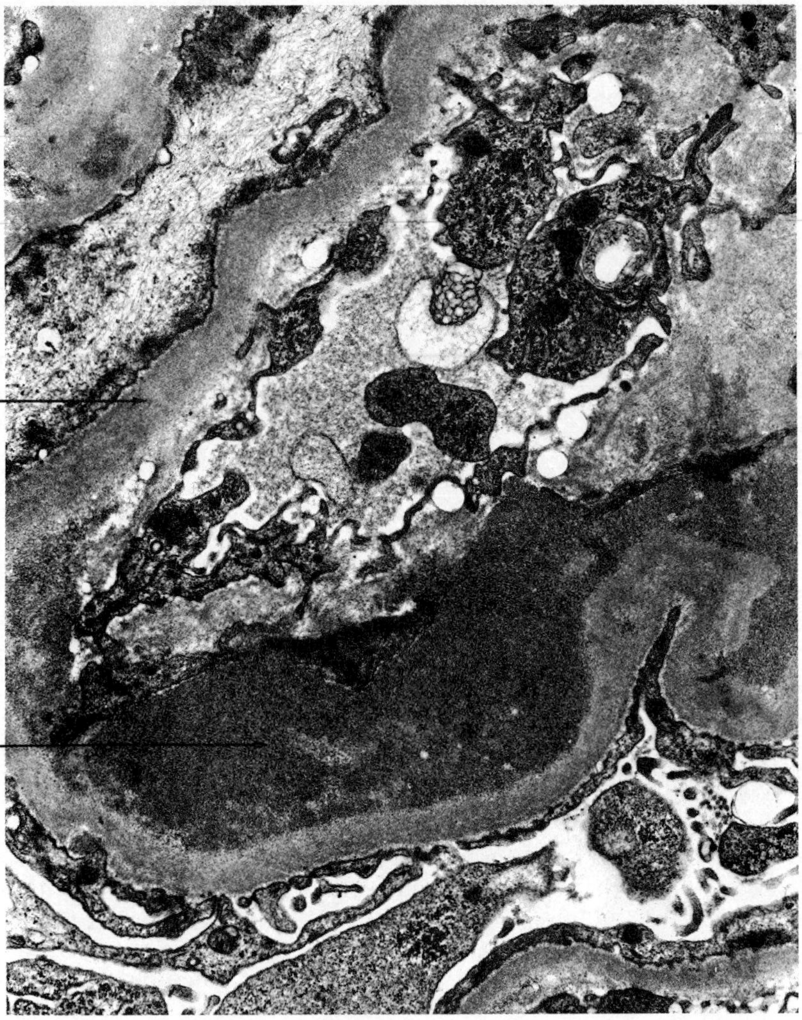

Normal membrane thickness

Heavy immunoglobulin deposit

FIGURE 25-2

An electron-photomicrograph demonstrating an immunoglobulin deposit in the basement membrane of a patient with systemic lupus erythematosus (SLE).
(From Barrett JT: Textbook of immunology, ed 5, St. Louis, 1988, The CV Mosby Co.)

Autoimmunity and the Skin

> Discoid lupus
> Bullous pemphigoid
> Pemphigus group
> Dermatitis herpetiformis
> Skin may be involved in the autoimmune reaction in at least three ways:
> 1. Inflammatory involvement of cutaneous vessels with secondary effects, e.g., some lesions in systemic lupus erythematous, hypersensitivity angiitis, and the syndrome of urticaria and palpable purpura with or without mixed cryoglobulinemia
> 2. Deposition of putative circulating immune complexes in the skin, e.g., systemic lupus erythematosus
> 3. Localized autoreactivity against skin components, e.g., primary skin disorders

tors can include drugs and possibly infection as well as the involvement of transplanted kidneys.

Skin Disorders (Bullous Disease and Other Conditions)

A wide variety of autoimmune disorders is associated with skin manifestations (see box at left).

Two immunologic assays that can be used in conjunction with other clinical information include measurement of antibodies to the basement membrane area of the skin and antibodies to intercellular substance of the skin.

Anti-skin (dermal-epidermal) antibodies are present in more than 80% of patients with bullous pemphigoid but the absence of antibodies does not rule out the disorder. Anti-skin (inter-epithelial) antibodies can be detected in most (90%) of patients with pemphigus. A rising antibody titer may indicate an impending relapse of pemphigus, and a falling titer is suggestive of effective control of the disease. The absence of demonstrable antibody usually excludes the diagnosis.

Chapter Review

HIGHLIGHTS

Autoimmunity represents a breakdown of the immune system in its ability to discriminate between self and non-self. The term *autoimmune disease* is used in those cases where demonstrable immunoglobulins, autoantibodies, or cytotoxic (T) cells display a specificity for self-antigens and contribute to the pathogenesis of the disease. Many disorders are believed to be related to immunologic abnormalities that manifest a full spectrum of tissue reactivity. At one extreme are organ-specific diseases such as Hashimoto's disease of the thyroid; at the other end of the spectrum are diseases that manifest themselves as non-organ–specific diseases such as systemic lupus erythematosus and rheumatoid arthritis. In organ-specific diseases both the lesions produced by tissue damage and the autoantibodies are directed at a single target organ, e.g., the thyroid. Midspectrum disorders are characterized by localized lesions in a single organ and autoantibodies that are non-organ specific. Non-organ specific disorders are characterized by the presence of both lesions and autoantibodies not confined to any one organ.

The potential for autoimmunity, if given appropriate circumstances, is constantly present in every immunocompetent individual because lymphocytes that are potentially reactive with self-antigens exist in the body. Antibody expression appears to be regulated by a complex set of interacting factors. These influences include genetic factors, age, and exogenous factors. Autoimmune disease is usually prevented by the normal functioning of immunologic regulatory mechanisms. When these controls dysfunction, antibodies to self-antigens may be produced and bind to antigens in the circulation to form circulating immune complexes or bind to antigens deposited in specific tissue sites. The mechanisms that govern the deposition in one organ or another are unknown; however, several mechanisms may be operative in a single disease. Wherever antigen-antibody complexes accumulate, complement can be activated with the subsequent release of mediators of inflammation that increase vascular permeability and attract phagocytic cells to the reaction site and cause local tissue damage. Alternatively, cytotoxic T cells can directly attack body cells bearing the target antigen, which releases mediators that amplify the inflammatory reaction. Autoantibody and complement fragments coat cells bearing the target antigen, which leads todestruction by phagocytes or by antibody-seeking K type lymphocytes.

An individual may develop an autoimmune response in a variety of immunogenic stimuli. These responses may be caused by antigens that do not normally circulate in the blood, altered antigens, a foreign antigen that is shared or cross-reactive with self-antigens or tissue components, mutation of immunocompetent cells to acquire a responsive to self-antigens, and loss of the immunoregulatory function by T cell subsets. Self-recognition of membrane idiotypic receptors and the major histocompatibility complex (MHC) antigens appear to be fundamental to facilitating the regulatory interactions between cells. Many of these interactions are mediated through the production of highly specific soluble fraction that contains Ia and idiotypic determinants and transmits signs from one cell to another. Whether the immunologic response to any given antigen will be expressed as immunity or tolerance is probably determined by a regulatory equilibrium, primarily established by the balance between helper and suppressor T cells. This equilibrium appears to be controlled by Ir genes linked to the MHC and expressed on the surface of lymphocytes and macrophages as the Ia antigens. In addition, aberrant Ia expression on inflamed cells may lead to inappropriate antigen presentation by these cells, immune cell activation, and ultimately, to organ-specific autoimmune disease.

Self-tolerance is induced by at least two mechanisms involving contact between antigen and immunocompetent cells: elimination of the small clone of immunocompetent cells programmed to react with the antigen (Burnet's clonal selection theory) or induction of unresponsiveness in the immunocompetent cells through excessive antigen binding to them and/or through triggering of a suppressor mechanism. The normal immune response is modulated by both antigen-specific and nonspecific suppressor cell activity. The major mechanism in antigen-specific suppression of antibody response appears related to an anti-idiotypic immune response induced by the antigen-binding site (idiotype) unique for a particular antibody. In the opposite situation, prolonged antigen stimulation leads to polyclonal activation of the B cell response with a resultant polyclonal hypergammaglobulinemia.

Major autoantibodies can be detected in different diseases. Many diagnostic laboratory tests are based on detecting these autoimmune responses. Commonly encountered autoantibodies include thyroid, gastric, adrenocortical, striated muscle, acetylcholine receptor, smooth muscle, salivary gland, mitochondrial, reticulin, myelin, islet cell, and skin antibodies. Antibodies to antinuclear antibodies include DNA, histone, and nonhistone protein antibodies.

REVIEW QUESTIONS

1. All of the following characteristics are common to organ-specific and non-organ-specific disorders *except:*
   A. Autoantibody tests are of diagnostic value
   B. Antibodies may appear in each of the main immunoglobulin classes
   C. Antigens are available to lymphoid system in low concentrations
   D. Circulatory autoantibodies react with normal body constituents
   E. Disease processes are not always progressive

2. Antibody expression in the development of autoimmunity is regulated by all of the following factors *except:*
   A. Genetic predisposition
   B. Increasing age
   C. Environmental factors, e.g., UV radiation
   D. Drugs
   E. Active infectious disease

3. The mechanism responsible for autoimmune disease is:
   A. Circulating immune complexes
   B. Antigen excess
   C. Antibody excess
   D. Antigen deficiency
   E. Antibody deficiency

4. One of the mechanisms believed to induce self-tolerance is:
   A. Induction of responsiveness in immunocompetent cells
   B. Elimination of clone programmed to react with antigen
   C. Decreased suppressor cell activity
   D. Stimulation of clones of immunocompetent cells
   E. Either A or B

Match the following (use an answer only once):

5. Acetylcholine receptor blocking antibodies
6. Anticardiolipin antibody
7. Anti-DNA antibodies
8. Antiglomerular basement membrane antibodies
   A. Helpful in monitoring Addison's disease
   B. Found in one third of patients with myasthenia gravis
   C. Useful in monitoring the activity and exacerbations of SLE
   D. Suggestive of Goodpasture's disease
   E. Present in SLE and associated with arterial and venous thrombosis

9. Antinuclear ribonucleoprotein
10. Anti-Scl
11. Anti-Sm
12. Antismooth muscle
    A. Antibody to basic nonhistone nuclear protein, diagnostic of systemic sclerosis
    B. Present in bullous pemphigoid
    C. Presence of antibody confirms diagnosis of SLE
    D. Seen in viral disorders
    E. Characteristic of mixed connective tissue disease

13. Anti SS-A
14. Histone reactive antinuclear antibody
15. PM-I antibody
    A. Detectable in patients with myasthenia gravis
    B. Demonstrable in Sjögren's syndrome-Sicca complex

C. Highly suggestive of drug-induced lupus erythematosus
D. Found in one third of patients with uncomplicated polymyositis and some patients with dermatomyositis
E. Found in majority of patients with polymyositis

Answers

1. C 2. E 3. A 4. B 5. B 6. E 7. C 8. D 9. E 10. A 11. C 12. D 13. B 14. C 15. E

BIBLIOGRAPHY

Ashman RF: Rheumatic diseases. In Lawlor GJ and Fischer TJ, editors: Manual of allergy and immunology, ed 2, Boston, 1988, Little, Brown & Co.

Barrett J: Textbook of immunology, St Louis, 1988, The CV Mosby Co.

Bottazzo GF and Doniach D: Autoimmune thyroid disease, Ann Rev Med 37:353-359, 1986.

Caroscio JT: Quantitative CSF IgG measurements in multiple sclerosis and other neurologic diseases," Arch Neurol 40:409-413, 1983.

Chaplin H: Clinical usefulness of specific antiglobulin reagents in autoimmune hemolytic anemia, vol 8, Progress in Hematology, New York, 1973, Grune & Stratton, Inc.

Freedman J and others: Hemolytic warm Ig M autoagglutinins in autoimmune hemolytic anemia, Transfusion 27(6):464-467, 1987.

Gerson B, Orr JD, and Orr JM: Oligoclonal bands and quantitation of IgG in cerebrospinal fluid as indicators of multiple sclerosis, Am J Clin Pathol, 75:1, 87-91, Jan 1980.

Henry JB, editor: Clinical diagnosis and management, Philadelphia, 1982, WB Saunders Co.

Internal medicine, Jay Stein, editor: Boston, 1987, Little, Brown & Co.

Keshgegian AA, editor: Oligoclonal immunoglobulins in cerebrospinal fluid in multiple sclerosis, Clin Chem 26:9, 1340-1345, 1980.

Killingsworth LM: Deciphering cerebrospinal fluid patterns," Diag Med, March/April, 1-7, 1982.

Killingsworth LM: Clinical applications of protein determination in biological fluids other than blood, Clin Chem 28(5):1093-1258, 1982.

Link H and Kostulas V: Utility of IEF of CSF and serum on agarose evaluated from neurological patients, Clin Chem 2915:810-815, 1983.

Papadopoulos NM and others: A unique protein in normal human cerebrospinal fluid, Clin Chem 29:10, 1842-1844, 1983.

Peter JB: Thyroid autoimmunity, Diagnostic medicine, July/Aug, 19-25, 1981.

Rees-Smith B: Autoantibodies to the thyrotropin receptor, Endocr Rev 9(1):106-121, 1988.

Roitt IM: Essential immunology, ed 5, Oxford, England, 1984, Blackwell Scientific Publications Inc.

Salama AB and others: Immune complex-mediated intravascular hemolysis due to IgM cephalosporin-dependent antibody, Transfusion 27(6):460-463, 1987.

Talal N: In Stein J, editor: Internal medicine, Boston, 198, Little, Brown & Co.

Tsieh S and others: Synthesis of immunoglobulin within the central nervous system in multiple sclerosis and other neurological diseases, detection by analysis of CSF/serum IgG ratio, Am J Clin Pathol, 76:4, 458-461, 1981.

Turgeon ML: Fundamentals of immunohematology, Philadelphia, 1989, Lea & Febiger, 1989.

Turgeon ML Clinical hematology, Boston, 1988, Little, Brown & Co.

Systemic Lupus Erythematosus

Systemic lupus erythematosus (SLE) is the classic model of autoimmune disease. It is a *systemic rheumatic disorder. Systemic rheumatic disorders* is the most commonly used term for the group of disorders that includes SLE and other abnormalities that involve the joints, connective tissue, and collagen-vascular system in the disease process.

ETIOLOGY

The cause of SLE is unknown. Although no single etiologic agent has been identified, a primary defect in the regulation of the immune system is regarded as being of importance in the pathogenesis of the disorder. Other influences include the effect of estrogens, genetic predisposition, and extraneous factors. A combination of these factors, however, may be synergistic.

Hormonal Influences

A disproportionate number of females between puberty and menopause suffer from SLE. There is, in addition, a propensity for the disease to worsen during pregnancy and the immediate postpartum period. These observations suggest that estrogens may play a potentially harmful role in disease development or progression. Sex hormones are known to influence both humoral and cellular immunity.

Genetic Predisposition

Because there is an increased familial incidence of SLE, a primary genetic relationship to the disease is suspected. Although SLE patients have an increased frequency of histocompatibility antigens HLA-B8, HLA-DRw2, HLA-DRw3, and of select B cell alloantigens, as compared to the general population, none of these antigens is absolute for SLE. Therefore two or more of these genes may be involved in increased disease susceptibility, or these antigens may be associated with other specific disease-associated genes.

Environmental Factors

A variety of factors, including ultraviolet light and bacterial and viral infections, is capable of inducing or exacerbating the signs and symptoms of lupus erythematosus. These factors may act in different ways. For example, ultraviolet light may cause DNA to form thymine dimers. This significantly alters the antigenicity of DNA and could result in the formation of anti-DNA.

Drug-Induced Lupus

A reversible drug-induced lupus syndrome is caused by a number of chemically diverse drugs (see box on p. 298). In rare cases, contraceptives and phenothiazines have been suspected to produce symptoms. The physiologic mechanism of drug-induced SLE is unknown. Factors such as the rate of metabolism of the drug, the influence of the drug on immune regulation, and the host's genetic composition are all considered to influence pathogenesis. Lupus-inducing drugs, however, do not appear to exacerbate idiopathic SLE.

Drugs That Can Produce Clinical and Serologic Features of Systemic Lupus Erythematosus

Antiarrhythmics
  Practolol
  Procainamide hydrochloride
  Hydrochloride
Anticonvulsants
  Ethosuximide
  Mephenytoin trimethadione
  Phenytoin
  Primidone
Antihypertensives
  Hydralazine hydrochloride
  Methyldopa
Miscellaneous
  Chlorprothixene
  Chlorthalidone
  Chlorpromazine
  Isoniazid
  Methylthiouracil
  Penicillamine
  Penicillin
  Propylthiouracil
  Sulfonamides

Implicated drugs are capable of producing serologic abnormalities and clinical manifestations resembling SLE. The drugs procainamide hydrochloride and hydralazine hydrochloride are extremely potent inducers of antinuclear (ANA), antierythrocyte, and antilymphocyte antibodies. In these cases high antibody titers may exist for months without the development of any clinical symptoms. Even with discontinuation of the drug, antibody titers usually remain elevated for months or years. A small percent of patients who develop drug-related antibodies manifest a clinical syndrome that is similar to SLE. Drug-related SLE patients suffer from a predominance of pulmonary and polyserositis signs and symptoms. Other disorders, such as renal and neurologic abnormalities, do not usually occur.

EPIDEMIOLOGY

The overall incidence of SLE is estimated to be 50 to 70 new cases per year per million of population. Racial groups such as American blacks and Native Americans, Puerto Ricans, and Orientals (particularly Chinese) demonstrate an increased frequency of SLE. In addition, this disorder is approximately eight times more common in females than in males. It is most common in females during the reproductive years and may be present for years before diagnosis.

Survival is estimated to be greater than 90% at 10 years after diagnosis. The highest mortality is in patients with progressive renal involvement or central nervous system disease. The two most frequent causes of death are renal failure and infectious complications.

SIGNS AND SYMPTOMS

SLE is a disease of acute and chronic inflammation. Manifestations of the disease range from a typical mild illness that is limited to a photosensitive facial rash and transient diffuse arthritis to life-threatening involvement of the renal, cardiac, respiratory, or central nervous systems. In the early phases it is often difficult to distinguish SLE from several of the other systemic rheumatic disorders, such as progressive systemic sclerosis, polymyositis, primary Sjögren's syndrome, primary Raynaud's phenomenon, and rheumatoid arthritis.

The course of the disease is highly variable. It usually follows a chronic and irregular course with periods of exacerbations and remissions. Clinical signs and symptoms can include fever, weight loss, malaise, arthralgia (joint pain) and arthritis (inflammation of the joints), and the characteristic erythematous, maculopapular (butterfly) rash over the bridge of the nose. In addition, there is a tendency to increased susceptibility to common and opportunistic infections. Multiple organ systems may be affected simultaneously.

Cutaneous Features

Approximately 20% to 25% of patients with SLE develop dermal disorders as the initial manifestation of the disease. As many as 65% of patients will develop a cutaneous abnormality sometime during the course of the disease. The characteristic erythematous, maculopapular "butterfly rash" across the nose and upper cheeks is the cutaneous feature from which the disease gets its name, *lupus erythematosus*, the "red wolf" (Fig. 26-1). This rash may also be observed on the arms and trunk of the body. Exposure to ultraviolet light will worsen erythematous as well as other types of cutaneous lesions.

The spectrum of cutaneous abnormalities includes urticaria, angioedema, nonthrombocytopenic purpura associated with the presence of cryoglobulins, scale formation, and ulcerations of oral and genital mucous membranes. Although neither the collection of immunoglobulins and complement at the dermal-epidermal junction, nor the presence of specific antibody (nuclear ribonucleoprotein (RNP), Sm, native DNA, and single-stranded DNA appear to play a direct role in the pathogenesis of cutaneous lupus lesion, Ri (SS-A), and perhaps the La (SS-B) antibodies, may be prominent factors.

Diffuse or patchy alopecia is also a common cutaneous manifestation. Hair loss is caused by pustular lesions of the scalp and is most often related to the stress of the disease process. Although the cause of pustular lesions is unknown, these inflammatory infiltrates are characterized by the presence of predominantly Ia-positive (activated) T lymphocytes with both OKT4 and OKT8 phenotypes.

Approximately 2% or 3% of SLE patients demonstrate *lupus panniculitis*. This condition is char-

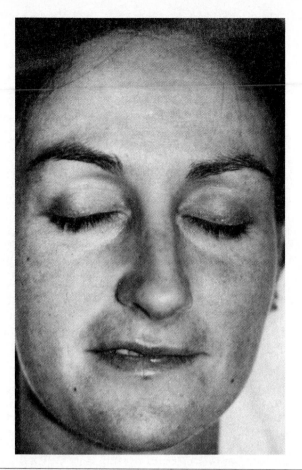

FIGURE 26-1
Facial rash over bridge of nose, upper lip, and chin in patient with active SLE.
(From Kaye D and Rose LF: Fundamentals of internal medicine, St Louis, 1983, The CV Mosby Co.)

acterized by tender or nontender subcutaneous nodules that sometimes ulcerate and discharge a yellowish lipid material. In addition, a variety of nonspecific skin changes are observable secondary to vascular insults. Raynaud's phenomenon is demonstrated by approximately one third of patients with SLE; this phenomenon appears to be increased in SLE patients who have antibodies to nuclear RNP in their serum.

The presence of lesions, however, does not distinguish between the limited cutaneous (discoid lupus erythematosus) and the cutaneous manifestation of SLE. The term *discoid lupus* is used to differentiate the benign dermatitis of cutaneous lupus from the cutaneous involvement of SLE. In discoid lupus the round lesion is an erythematous, inflammatory dermatosis. These lesions are primarily located in light-exposed areas of the skin.

Renal Characteristics
Deterioration of the renal system is a usual consequence of the high levels of immune complexes in the blood that are deposited in tissues such as the kidneys. Renal disease progression is highly unpre-

dictable. It may be acute, but more typically it progresses slowly. As the kidneys degenerate, the urinary sediment is typical of *acute glomerulonephritis* and later that of *chronic glomerulonephritis.* Acute glomerulonephritis is characterized by the presence of erythrocytes, leukocytes, and granular and red blood cell casts in urinary sediment. The presence of proteinuria may lead to *nephrotic syndrome.* If end-stage renal failure occurs, it can be managed by dialysis or allograft transplantation.

The systemic necrotizing vasculitis of SLE involves small blood vessels and leads to renal involvement. The most common method of classification of the renal involvement of SLE is the WHO system (Table 26-1), which is based on histopathologic criteria. The stages of renal disease range from the earliest and least severe form, class II, characterized by mesangial deposits of immunoglobulin and the C3 component of complement, to class V, the most severe form of involvement.

Lymphadenopathy
Enlargement of peripheral and axial lymph nodes and splenomegaly both occur in SLE patients; however, these conditions are usually transient. Patients with SLE may be at a greater risk of development of lymphoma than the general population, especially if there is an associated secondary Sjögren's syndrome.

Serositis in SLE
Serositis is an inflammation of the membrane consisting of mesothelium, a thin layer of connective tissue that lines enclosed body cavities. Mesothelium, a type of epithelium, is originally derived from the mesoderm lining the primitive embryonic body cavity. It becomes the covering of the serous membranes of the body surfaces such as the peritoneum, pleura, and pericardium. Inflammation of these serosal surfaces leads to sterile peritonitis, pleuritis, or pericarditis and is frequently accompanied by severe pain. In the presence of serositis an increased frequency of thrombophlebitis is observed and may lead to pulmonary embolization.

Cardiopulmonary Characteristics
Inflammation of the myocardium in SLE patients can produce persistent tachycardia and, occasionally, intractable congestive heart failure. Ischemic disease or, more commonly, atherosclerotic coronary disease may occur. Patients with severe nephrosis or those treated with corticosteroids for a prolonged time are at an increased risk for developing atherosclerosis.

Pulmonary function studies reveal occult diffusion and obstructive abnormalities in a high proportion of SLE patients, but clinical problems secondary to pulmonary involvement are unusual. Massive hemoptysis, however, may result from acute alveolar hemorrhage. This particular complication occurs in the absence of any detectable

TABLE 26-1

WHO Classification System for Renal Involvement in SLE

Histologic type	Class	Frequency (%)	Proteinuria	Nephrotic syndrome	Death (%)	Uremic death (%)
Normal	I	<5				
Mesangial	II	15	68	0	18	0
Focal proliferative	III	20	100	15	30	11
Diffuse proliferative	IV	50	100	87	58	36
Membranous	V	15	100	88	38	6

bleeding diathesis, and is associated with a high rate of mortality.

Gastrointestinal Manifestations

Nonspecific gastrointestinal symptoms are relatively frequent in cases of SLE, but acute abdominal crises due to visceral and peritoneal vasculitis are less common. Infarction and perforation of the bowel and viscera, however, are associated with a high rate of mortality. Acute and chronic pancreatitis may also develop as a secondary complication of acute lupus or as a complication during therapy.

Musculoskeletal Features

A characteristic arthritis of SLE is a transient and peripheral polyarthritis with symmetric involvement of both small and large joints. Chronic arthritis can result in disability and deformity in SLE patients. Rheumatoid-like hand deformities develop in about 10% of patients. Osteonecrosis develops in one fourth of all SLE patients. Arthropathy of osteonecrosis, or avascular necrosis, is often initially detected in weight-bearing joints such as the hips and knees.

Neuropsychiatric Features

In SLE various kinds of neurologic and psychiatric manifestations develop secondarily to the involvement of the central and peripheral nervous system. The most common abnormalities are disturbances of mental function ranging from mild confusion, with memory deficiency and impairment of orientation and perception, to psychiatric disturbances such as hypomania, delirium, and schizophrenia. Seizures of the grand mal type may be the initial manifestation of SLE and may be present long before the multisystem disease develops. In addition, some patients may suffer from epilepsy and severe headaches.

Effects of Pregnancy

The incidence of premature delivery and spontaneous abortion are increased in pregnant women with SLE. Both the developing fetus and pregnant mother with lupus are at increased risk of various complications during and after pregnancy. Pregnant women are at an increased risk of disease flare-ups during pregnancy as well as in the immediate postpartum period. Passive transfer of maternal antibodies across the placenta can produce transient abnormalities such as heptosplenomegaly, cytopenia, and a photosensitive rash in the newborn. These conditions do resolve themselves in the newborn after the antibody titer declines.

IMMUNOLOGIC MANIFESTATIONS
Cellular Aspects

SLE is a disease that results from defects in the regulatory mechanism of the immune system. Studies of the immunopathogenesis of lupus nephritis have demonstrated a variety of aberrations in T cell and B cell function. It is uncertain, however, if the disease represents a primary dysfunction of T cells or B cells, but alterations in function do result. Lymphocyte subset abnormalities are a major immunologic feature of SLE. Among the T cell subsets, a lack of, or reduced, generalized suppressor T cell function and/or hyperproduction of helper T cells occurs. The formation of lymphocytotoxic antibodies with a predominant specificity for T lymphocytes by SLE patients at least partially explains the interference with certain functional activities of T lymphocytes manifested by the patient with SLE. Lymphocytotoxic antibodies are capable of both destroying T lymphocytes in the presence of complement and coating peripheral blood T cells.

The regulation of antibody production by B lymphocytes, ordinarily a function of the subpopulation of T suppressor cells, appears to be defective in patients with SLE. Although no single cause can be implicated in the pathogenesis of SLE, patients exhibit a state of spontaneous B-lymphocyte hyperactivity with ensuing uncontrolled production of a wide variety of antibodies to both host and exogenous antigens. Host response to some antigens, however, such as vaccination with influenza, is normal in many instances, and the patient manifests a specific well-controlled humoral immune response.

Humoral Aspects

Circulating immune complexes are the hallmark of SLE. Patients with SLE exhibit multiple serum antibodies that react with native or altered self-antigens. Demonstrable antibodies include antibodies to:

1. Nuclear components
2. Cell surface and cytoplasm antigens of polymorphonuclear and lymphocytic leukocytes, erythrocytes, platelets, and neuronal cells
3. Immunoglobulin IgG

Antibodies to host antigens, particularly nuclear antigens such as DNA, are the principal type of antibody produced. Antinuclear antibodies (ANAs) are a heterogeneous group of antibodies produced against a variety of antigens within the cell nucleus. ANAs may be found in diseases other than SLE, as well as in some patients undergoing specific drug therapy and in normal persons such as the elderly. The absence of ANAs virtually excludes the diagnosis of SLE unless the patient is being chemically immunosuppressed. ANA titers and specific anti-DNA fluctuate during the course of the disease. In some cases a rise in titer may forewarn of an impending disease flare-up.

Antigens to which antibodies are formed are present on nucleic acid molecules (DNA and RNA) or proteins (histones and nonhistones), and on determinants consisting of both nucleic acid and protein molecules. Drug-induced cases of SLE have a high incidence of antibodies to histones. Some of these antibodies are directed against the double-stranded helical DNA (native DNA or DS-DNA). The presence of anti-native DNA (anti-n-DNA) antibodies was reported in 1957. High titers of DS-DNA are seen primarily in SLE and closely parallel disease activity. A majority of SLE patients demonstrate antibodies to nucleoprotein and native DNA simultaneously.

Other nuclear antibodies are directed at the determinants of single-stranded DNA (SS-DNA). Antibody titers of 1:32 or greater indicate a substantial concentration of antibody in an autoimmune response. Antibody to the Smith (Sm) antigen, a nuclear acidic protein extractable by aqueous solution, is considered to be a marker for SLE because anti-Sm has been found almost exclusively in patients with SLE. The presence of anti-Sm is seen in 25% to 30% of patients with SLE, but it rarely occurs in other systemic rheumatic (collagen) diseases.

The antinuclear antibody (anti-DNP) gives rise to the *LE cell*, which is found in more than 90% of untreated patients with active SLE. SLE patients with serositis may form LE cells in vivo. The LE cell testing procedure was the first method extensively developed to detect antibodies to nuclear antigens. LE cells have been shown to be an expression of the interaction between IgG antibodies and deoxyribonucleohistones (DNP). Anti-DNP is referred to as the *LE serum factor*.

Immunologic Consequences

Antibodies combine with their corresponding antigens to form immune complexes. When the mononuclear phagocytic system is unable to entirely eliminate these immune complexes, an accumulation of immune complexes results in the blood circulation. These circulating immune complexes are deposited in the subendothelial layers of the vascular basement membranes of multiple target organs and mediate inflammation. The sites of deposition are determined in part by the physiochemical properties of the particular antigens or antibodies involved. These properties include:

1. Size
2. Molecular configuration
3. Immunoglobulin class
4. Complement-fixing ability

Following deposition, the immune complexes seem to initiate a localized inflammatory response that stimulates neutrophils to the site of inflammation, activates complement, and results in the release of kinins and prostaglandins. These activities become the basis of antibody-dependent cell-mediated tissue injury.

DIAGNOSTIC EVALUATION

The manifestations of SLE that are expressed in laboratory findings are numerous. Histologic, hematologic, and serologic abnormalities reflect the multisystem nature of this disease.

Histologic Changes

The earliest pathologic abnormalities are those of acute vasculitis. Supportive tissue becomes edematous, initially infiltrated with neutrophils and later with plasma cells and lymphocytes. Persistent inflammation results in local deposition of a cellular homogeneous material, histologically similar to fibrin. Nuclear debris from resulting cellular necrosis reacts with antinuclear antibodies (discussed later in this section) to form hematoxylin bodies. The presence of immunoglobulins, predominantly IgM and IgG, in vascular lesions can be demonstrated by indirect immunofluorescence.

Renal pathology can also be observed in SLE. Two basic types of changes can be manifested. One type of change is proliferative glomerulonephritis, a condition that resembles the renal changes in immune complex nephritis. The other form of renal abnormality is membranous nephritis.

Hematologic and Hemostatic Manifestations

In SLE a moderate anemia (normocytic normochromic anemia) representing chronic disease is a consistent factor. Some patients display coating of erythrocytes, which can be demonstrated by a positive antihuman globulin (AHG), but actual hemolysis is infrequent. Lymphocytopenia is common and often reflects disease activity. Thrombocytopenia (50 to 100 × 10^9/L) may also be displayed.

Hemostatic Testing

Lupus anticoagulants can be commonly seen in association with SLE. They can be found in approximately 1% to 10% of SLE patients. Circulating anticoagulants are believed to be associated with the

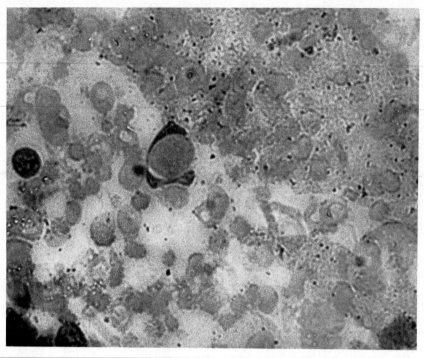

FIGURE 26-2

An LE cell in a peripheral blood specimen from a patient with systemic lupus erythematosus.
(From Bauer JD: Clinical laboratory methods, ed 9, St Louis, 1982, The CV Mosby Co.)

presence of false positive serologic test results for syphilis. Because of the presence of lupus anticoagulant, patients with SLE frequently demonstrate prolonged prothrombin (PT) and partial thromboplastin time (PTT) results, but lupus anticoagulant rarely causes hemostatic problems. Inhibitors are not necessarily associated with bleeding, unless some other defect is present. Because lupus anticoagulant is an inhibitor or a prothrombin activator, it is often associated with excessive thrombosis rather than bleeding. Patients with SLE have a high incidence of thrombotic episodes. Although less frequent, specific coagulation factor antibodies directed against coagulation factors VIII, IX, XI, and XII have also been described.

LE Cells

The classic test for SLE is the *LE cell test*. An LE cell is either a normal segmented neutrophil or other phagocytic cell (Fig. 26-2) with the engulfed homogeneous and swollen nucleus of either a neutrophil or lymphocyte. In order to demonstrate the LE phenomenon in vitro, the following factors need to be present:
1. The LE factor, an antinuclear antibody, found in the globulin portion of serum that acts as a nucleolytic agent
2. Viable phagocytic cells
3. Cell nuclei of either segmented neutrophils or lymphocytes

Rosette formation may be observed in an LE prep. Rosettes represent several phagocytic cells attempting to engulf one nucleus. Care must be taken to distinguish a "tart cell" from an LE cell. Tart cells usually represent monocytes that have phagocytized another whole cell or nucleus, often a lymphocyte. The ingested material is well preserved in contrast to the LE cell inclusion; it may even be found in normal persons. The significance of tart cells is unknown. The presence of rosettes does not constitute a positive reaction. Usually, two or more true LE cells must be seen in order for the test to be considered positive.

Cellular destruction within the marrow may lead to the phagocytosis of nuclear debris and, rarely, the formation of in vivo LE cells. In patients with serositis, LE cells that have been formed in vivo may be observed in aspirate fluid, e.g., pleural fluid.

Serologic Manifestations

Serologic testing frequently reveals high levels of anti-DNA antibodies, reduced complement levels, and the presence of complement breakdown products of C3 (C3d and C3c). In addition, cryoglobulins, which in some instances represent immune complexes, are frequently present in the serum of patients with SLE. Because monoclonal gammopathies have occasionally been described, a marked increase in gammaglobulins may result in a hyperviscosity syndrome or renal tubular acidosis. Serum

TABLE 26-2

Antibodies in Systemic Rheumatic Diseases

Systemic lupus erythematosus	Progressive systemic sclerosis	Polymyositis	Rheumatoid arthritis
Antinuclear antibodies	Antinuclear antibodies	Antinuclear antibodies	Antinuclear antibodies
Antinative DNA	Anti-Scl-1	Anti-Jo-1	Rheumatoid factors
Anti-Sm			

cryoglobulin of a mixed IgG-IgM type are found in patients with hypocomplementemia. The level of cryoglobulin correlates well with the severity of SLE.

Procedural results that are helpful in assessing renal disease include:
1. Antibody to double-stranded DNA
2. Levels of C3, C4, and CH_{50}, with C4 probably being the most sensitive
3. Cryoglobulin levels

A general correlation exists between abnormalities in each of these procedures and disease activity in many patients, but there is considerable disagreement about the usefulness of such measurements in predicting renal disease activity. The best laboratory procedures for monitoring the activity of renal disease are serum creatinine, urinary protein excretion, and careful examination of urinary sediment.

Complement

Inherited deficiencies of several complement components are associated with lupus-like illnesses. Some, but not all deficiencies, are coded for by autosomal recessive genes of the sixth chromosome, which are in linkage disequilibrium with HLA-DRw2. It is possible that the association of complement deficiencies with SLE represents the fortuitous association of linked HLA-D region genes, rather than some unusual susceptibility induced by the complement deficiency.

Serum levels of complement are commonly reduced, particularly during states of active disease. Deficiencies involving both the classic and alternative pathway complement components in patients with SLE have been noted as a result of consumption of components at the tissue sites of immune complex deposition and as a result of impaired synthesis. Levels of total hemolytic complement (CH_{50}), C3, and C4 are generally reduced in relationship to disease activity, and the fluctuation in these levels is often used to monitor disease activity. Persistent and markedly reduced levels of CH_{50} suggests the possible presence of an inherited complement deficiency, the most common being a deficiency of the second component (C2).

Antibodies

Nonspecific elevation in the levels of immunoglobulins, particularly IgM and IgG, are frequent in SLE. An actual deficiency of IgA appears to be more common in SLE than in normal individuals.

The antinuclear antibody (ANA) procedure (discussed in detail in the next section) is a valuable screening tool for SLE; it has virtually replaced the LE cell test because of its wider range of reactivity with nuclear antigens, as well as its greater sensitivity and quality-control characteristics.

Antinuclear Antibodies

Characteristics and implications of antinuclear antibodies. Antinuclear antibodies (ANAs; Table 26-2) are a heterogenous group of circulating immunoglobulins such as IgM, IgG, and IgA. These immunoglobulins react with the whole nucleus or nuclear components such as nuclear proteins, deoxyribonucleic acid (DNA), or histones in host tissues. They are, therefore, true **autoantibodies.** Generally, ANAs have no organ or species specificity and are capable of crossreacting with nuclear material from humans (e.g., human leukocytes) or various animal tissues (e.g., rat liver or mouse kidney).

Demonstration of ANAs in laboratory testing can be indicative of various systemic autoimmune connective tissue disorders. These disease states are characterized by antibodies that react with different nuclear components, such as double-stranded DNA, single-stranded DNA, and Sm antigen. The presence of ANAs is the serologic hallmark of patients with systemic lupus erythematosus (SLE), which is considered to be the classic multisystem autoimmune disorder. Other disorders of this type include mixed connective tissue disease (MCTD), progressive systemic sclerosis (PSS) or scleroderma, Sjögren's syndrome, polymyositis/dermatomyositis, and rheumatoid arthritis (RA). A small percentage of patients with neoplastic diseases may also demonstrate the presence of ANAs.

ANAs, however, can be exhibited by elderly individuals without disease and in a small percentage of healthy, nonelderly persons. These antibodies are also often detected in liver disease associated with autoimmunity such as chronic active hepatitis, primary biliary cirrhosis, and cryptogenic cirrhosis. In addition, varying levels of ANAs may be activated or induced by certain drugs, including procainamide hydrochloride, hydralazine hydrochloride, diphenylhydantoin, isoniazid, methyldopa, penicillin, tetracycline, streptomycin, and oral contraceptives. The significance of the presence of ANAs in a patient must be assessed in regard to the patient's age, sex, clinical signs and symptoms, and other laboratory findings.

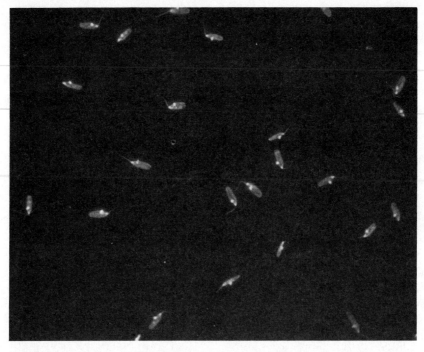

FIGURE 26-3

Anti-nDNA shown by indirect immunofluorescence. Staining of both the small kinetoplast and the adjacent larger nucleus of *Crithidia luciliae* occurs simultaneously.

Systematic classification of ANAs. It is possible to divide ANAs into different groups to provide a systematic classification. These groups are antibodies to DNA, antibodies to histone and nonhistone proteins, and antibodies to nuclear antigens.

Antibodies to DNA. Antibodies to DNA can be divided into two major groups: (1) antibodies that react with native (double-stranded) DNA, and (2) antibodies that recognize denatured (single-stranded) DNA only.

Antibodies that react with native DNA appear to interact with antigenic determinants that are present on the deoxyribose-phosphate backbone of the B (beta)-helix of DNA. These autoantibodies characteristically stain the kinetoplast of the hemoflagellate, *Crithidia luciliae*, a substrate that is used to detect anti-native DNA antibodies by indirect immunofluorescence (see Fig. 26-3). Antibodies that are reactive with denatured DNA probably react with the purine and pyrimidine bases of DNA. These bases are readily accessible on single-stranded DNA; they are buried within the B (beta)-helix of double-stranded DNA and are therefore inaccessible. Antidenatured DNA antibodies are unable to cross-react with native DNA. Conformational changes of the deoxyribose-phosphate backbone of denatured DNA appear to be important for antigenicity.

Antibodies to histone. Antibodies to histones have been shown to react with all major classes of histones—H1, H2A, H2B, H3, and H4. Antihistone antibodies can be induced by drugs such as procainamide and hydralazine. Procainamide-induced lupus erythematosus is characterized by the IgG class of antibodies against the histone complex H2A-H2B in symptomatic cases of SLE. In asymptomatic cases the antibody may be restricted to the IgM class. Antibodies specific to other nuclear antigens are usually absent in drug-induced lupus, in contrast with cases of SLE, which have ANAs of multiple specificity. Therefore demonstration of only antihistone antibodies may be useful in distinguishing drug-induced lupus from SLE.

Antibodies to nonhistone proteins. Another primary class of ANAs in systemic autoimmune disorders is characterized by reactivity with soluble nonhistone nuclear protein and RNA-protein complexes. Clinically important antibodies that react with nuclear nonhistone proteins are listed in Table 26-3.

Antibodies to nucleolar antigens. The antibodies to nucleolar antigens are:
1. U3-RNA-protein complex (the enzyme transcribing ribosomal genes in the nucleolus)
2. 7-2-RNP
3. RNA polymerase I
4. PM-Scl

These antinucleolar antibodies are primarily associated with polymyositis-scleroderma overlap, where they have the highest incidence and titers. They are, however, rarely demonstrated in progressive systemic sclerosis, dermatomyositis, and scleroderma.

TABLE 26-3

Antibodies to Nonhistone Proteins (NHP) and NHP-RNA Complexes in Systemic Rheumatic Diseases

Antibody	Disease	Incidence (%)
Centromere/kinetochore	CREST variant of progressive systemic sclerosis (PSS)	70-90
	Diffuse scleroderma	10-20
Jo-1	Polymyositis	31
Ki antigen	Systemic lupus erythematosus (SLE)	20
Ku	Polymyositis/scleroderma overlap	55
Ma antigen	Systemic lupus erythematosus	20
Mi-1	Dermatomyositis	11
NuMa (nuclear mitotic apparatus) antigen	Rheumatoid arthritis Sjögren's syndrome Carpal tunnel syndrome	
Proliferating cell nuclear antigen (PCNA)	Systemic lupus erythematosus	3
RANA (rheumatoid arthritis-associated nuclear antigen)	Rheumatoid arthritis	90
SCl-70	Progressive systemic sclerosis	20
Sm (Smith)	Systemic lupus erythematosus	30
SS-A/Ro	Sjögren's syndrome	70
	Systemic lupus erythematosus	50
	Other connective tissue diseases	
SS-B/La	Sjögren's syndrome	40-50
	Systemic lupus erythematosus	15
U1-RNP	Mixed connective tissue disease	>95
	Systemic lupus erythematosus	35

Modified from Reimer G and Tan E: Antinuclear antibodies. In Stein J, editor: Internal medicine, Boston, 1987, Little, Brown & Co, p 1202.

Laboratory Evaluation of ANAs

The ANA method provides the laboratory with a simple and sensitive technique for detection and measurement of these antibodies. Indirect immunofluorescence is the preferred initial screening procedure. If the ANA method is positive, additional immunologic evaluation is necessary to determine the specificity of the reaction. These evaluations include double immunodiffusion, counter immunoelectrophoresis, passive hemagglutination, enzyme-linked immunosorbent assay (ELISA), radioimmunoassay, and identification of nuclear antigens by immunoprecipitation or immunoblotting. These evaluations may demonstrate that more than one ANA specificity is present in the serum. An LE cell preparation, however, has limited usefulness.

Indirect Immunofluorescent Technique

Detection of autoantibodies by immunofluorescence has become an extremely valuable tool. This method is extremely sensitive and may be positive in cases where procedures for antinuclear antibodies, such as complement fixation or precipitation, are negative. At present the immunofluorescent method is the most widely used technique for ANA screening.

Principle of the procedure. The antigen in the substrate tissue is fixed to a slide for testing. ANA is not specific for a particular organ; therefore any tissue containing nuclei may be used as substrate. The most commonly used tissues are rat or mouse liver or kidney, or cell-cultured fibroblasts grown on slides. If antibody is present in a patient's serum, the unlabeled antibody will attach to the nuclei in the substrate. After the substrate is washed in buffer, it is incubated with fluorescein-tagged goat antihuman immunoglobulin (AHG). If patient antibodies have affixed themselves to the nuclear antigens of the substrate, the fluorescein-tagged goat AHG will attach to these antibodies. When the slide is examined microscopically, fluorescence will be visible with ultraviolet light.

Interpretation of staining patterns. Because ANAs react with the whole nucleus or with nuclear components such as nuclear proteins, DNA, or histone, reaction patterns reflect the distribution of the various antigens within the nuclei. Several patterns of reactivity can be observed when examining a slide in the ANA procedure.

Diffused or homogeneous pattern. The diffused or homogeneous pattern characterizes anti-deoxyribonucleic acid - nucleoprotein antibodies, i.e., antibodies to nDNA, dsDNA, ssDNA, DNP, or histones. Antibodies to DNP have been shown to have the same specificity as the LE factor. Although vacuoles may be seen, the whole nucleus fluoresces evenly. This pattern is typically seen in rheumatoid disorders. High titers of homogeneous ANA are suggestive of SLE, while low titers may be found in SLE, rheumatoid arthritis, Sjögren's syndrome, and mixed connective tissue diseases (MCTD).

Peripheral pattern. The peripheral (marginal or rim) pattern results from antibodies to deoxyribonucleic acid (DNA), i.e., nDNA, dsDNA, or DNP. The central protein of the nucleus is only lightly stained or not stained at all, but the nuclear margins fluoresce strongly and appear to extend into the cytoplasm. This pattern is associated with SLE in the active stage of the disease and in Sjögren's syndrome.

Speckled pattern. The speckled pattern occurs in the presence of antibody to any extractable nuclear antigen devoid of DNA or histone. The antibody is detected against the saline extractable nuclear antigens: anti-RNP and anti-Smith (Anti-Sm). A grainy pattern with numerous round dots of nuclear fluorescence, without staining of the nucleoli, are seen in this pattern type.

Antibodies to Sm antigen have been shown to be highly specific for patients with SLE and appear to be a "marker" antibody. Anti-RNP has been found in patients with a wide variety of rheumatic diseases including SLE, rheumatoid arthritis, Sjögren's syndrome, progressive systemic sclerosis, mixed connective tissue disease, and dermatomyositis.

Nucleolar pattern. The nucleolar pattern reflects an antibody to nucleolar RNA (4-6S RNP). A few round, smooth nucleoli that vary in size will fluoresce when examined with ultraviolet light. The nucleolar pattern is present in about 50% of patients with scleroderma (progressive systemic sclerosis), Sjögren's syndrome, and in SLE. This pattern can also be observed in undiagnosed illnesses manifesting Raynaud's phenomenon.

Anti-centromere antibody (ACA). The anti-centromere antibody reacts with centromeric chromatin of metaphase and interphase cells. The particular pattern on tissue culture cells is discrete and speckled. This antibody appears to be be highly selective for the CREST variant of progressive systemic sclerosis. The CREST syndrome is a variant of systemic sclerosis characterized by the presence of calcinosis, Raynaud's phenomenon, esophageal motility abnormalities, sclerodactyly, and telangiectasia. This antibody is found infrequently in the serum of patients with SLE, MCTD, and systemic sclerosis.

PROCEDURE

Antinuclear Antibody (ANA) Visible Method*

PRINCIPLE

This is an indirect immunoenzyme method that uses tissue culture cells (human epithelial cells) as a substrate for the detection and titration of circulating antinuclear antibodies in human serum. Patient serum samples are diluted in buffer and added to microscope slide wells with HEp-2 (human epithelial) cells cultured in them. HEp-2 cells are characterized by extremely large nuclei and the presence of mitotic figures to aid in detection. If specific antibodies are present, stable antigen-antibody complexes are formed that bind antihuman gamma globulin labeled with horseradish peroxidase (HRP). The presence of HRP is indicated by a reaction with 3, 3'-diaminobenzidine stain. The resulting dark brown to black staining patterns of the nuclei can be seen with a light microscope. The presence of one or more types of circulating autoantibodies is the hallmark of systemic rheumatic diseases.

SPECIMEN COLLECTION AND PREPARATION

The patient should be in a fasting state prior to specimen collection. The patient must be positively identified when the specimen is collected and the specimen is to be labeled at the bedside. Specimen labels must include the patient's full name, the date the specimen is collected, the patient's hospital identification number, and the phlebotomist's initials.

Blood should be drawn by an aseptic technique. A minimum of 5 mL to 8 mL of clotted blood (red-top evacuated tube) is required. Allow the blood to clot at room temperature. The specimen should be centrifuged promptly and the serum should be separated from the red cells *immediately.* Serum specimens may be stored at 2° to 8° C, if tested within 24 to 48 hours. If the specimen cannot be tested within this period of time, it should be stored frozen at −20° C or below. Do not freeze and thaw sera more than once. Allow serum specimens to reach room temperature before testing. Avoid the use of sera exhibiting a high degree of lipemia, hemolysis, or microbial growth, since these characteristics may result in increased background staining, a decrease in titers, and/or unclear staining patterns.

REAGENTS, SUPPLIES, AND EQUIPMENT

Warning: Sodium azide and thimerosol are used as preservatives. Sodium azide may react with lead and copper plumbing to form highly explosive metal azides. Upon disposal, flush with a large

---

*ISOLAB, Inc.

volume of water to prevent azide buildup. Sodium azide and thimerosol may be toxic, if ingested.

1. The following reagents and controls are supplied in the Visible Test ANA System from ISOLAB, Akron, Ohio:
   a. Substrate slides. Each HEp-2 slide well contains HEp-2 cells grown and fixed on the slide. The slides are stable until the labeled expiration date when stored at −20° C. Do not handle the flat surface of the slide or the foil envelope. *Protect the cells by handling the foil envelope by the edges.*
   b. HRP lyophilized conjugate is stable before reconstitution until the labeled expiration date when stored at 2° to 8° C. The reconstituted cojugate is stable for 90 days when stored at 2° to 8° C.
   c. HRP stain reagent. Each vial contain 0.4% diaminobenzidine-HCl and phosphate buffer. Thimerosal is added as a preservative. Reconstitute the stain reagent with deionized water as directed on the label. Add the contents of one vial of 0.3% H_2O_2 *immediately before use.* The unreconstituted stain reagent is stable until the labeled expiration date when stored at 2° to 8° C. *Caution:* Diaminobenzidine-HCl is a possible carcinogen. Avoid contact with the skin or ingestion.
   d. Hydrogen peroxide. Ready to use 0.3% hydrogen peroxide. The H_2O_2 is stable until the labeled expiration date when stored at 2° to 8° C.
   e. Phosphate-buffered saline (PBS). Each unit contains dry powder phosphate buffered saline blend. Dissolve contents in distilled or deionized water as directed by the label and store at 2° to 8° C.
   f. Mounting medium. Ready to use. Contains phosphate-buffered glycerol. Thimerosal is added as a preservative.
2. 12 × 75 mm test tubes and rack
3. Pasteur and calibrated pipettes
4. Staining dish or Coplin jar
5. Moist chamber for incubation
6. Volumetric flask for PBS
7. Distilled or deionized water: CAP Type 1 or equivalent, pH 6.0-7.0
8. Forceps
9. Coverslips
10. Wash bottle
11. Blotting or bibulous paper
12. Light microscope

QUALITY CONTROL

Note: These controls are commercially prepared by ISOLAB and included in the test kit.

Positive control serum. ANA (homogeneous) positive control serum is a ready-to-use human serum in a dropper vial containing antinuclear antibodies demonstrating a strong homogeneous staining reaction (1:40 dilution). Sodium azide (0.1% W/V) is added as a preservative. The positive control serum is stable until the labeled expiration date, when stored at 2° to 8° C.

The ANA positive control should demonstrate homogeneous staining in the nuclei of the HEp-2 cells.

Negative control serum. This is a ready-to-use human serum in a dropper vial containing no detectable autoantibodies (1:40 dilution). Sodium azide (0.1% w/v) is added as a preservative. The negative control serum is stable until the labeled expiration date when stored at 2° to 8° C.

The ANA negative control serum should demonstrate little or no nuclear staining.

The control serums must be examined before any patient specimens are examined. The control results must provide the correct positive and negative reactions to validate procedural results. Controls that do not give expected reactions are considered unsatisfactory, and patient test results should not be reported. If the controls do not produce the expected results, the test procedure must be repeated.

Caution: Because the control serum is derived from human sources, it should be handled in the same manner as clinical serum specimens (see *Universal blood and body fluid precautions* in Chapter 6).

PROCEDURE

Allow serum specimens to reach room temperature before testing. Do not interchange components from other sources.

1. Prepare sample by diluting each serum 1:40 in PBS. If a serum has previously tested positive, it should be titered to the endpoint.
2. Prepare slides by removing a sufficient number of slides from storage. Allow them to equilibriate to room temperature (15 to 30 minutes); remove from envelope and label. Handle envelope and slide by edges only.
3. Apply samples and controls. Use 1 drop of the screening dilution or titration dilution per well. Apply 1 drop of the positive control and 1 drop of the negative control to the appropriate wells on at least one slide of each test run. *Note:* From this step on, the slides must remain wet.
4. Incubate the slides in a covered moist chamber at room temperature for 30 minutes.
5. Remove the slides from the chamber and rinse briefly with a gentle stream of PBS. Direct the stream away from wells.
6. Place the slides in a Coplin or staining jar filled with PBS for 5 minutes to wash. Occasionally agitate the slides initially, at midpoint, and prior to removal. Repeat this wash process with fresh PBS.
7. Remove the slides one at a time from the wash solution; drain the excess PBS. If blotting is

preferred, blot gently around slide periphery only, with the edge of blotting or bibulous paper. Do not blot directly over the wells. Return to moist chamber.

8. Apply conjugate by dispensing 1 drop (approximately 20 to 30 μL) of conjugate to each well on each slide used.
9. Incubate the slides in a moist chamber at room temperature for 30 minutes. *Protect from excess light.*
10. Remove the slides from the moist chamber and rinse briefly with a gentle stream of PBS. Direct the stream away from the wells.
11. Place the slides in a Coplin or staining jar filled with PBS to wash. Leave the slides in the PBS for 5 minutes with occasional agitation (initially, at midpoint, and before removing the slides from the wash). Repeat this washing process once with fresh PBS.
12. Reconstitute with 10 mL of distilled water. Add the contents of one vial of 0.3% H_2O_2 immediately before use. Mix well by gentle inversion or agitation.
13. Remove the slides from the wash buffer, drain the excess PBS and return to the moist chamber. Flood the wells with the stain reagent. *Do not allow wells to dry.* Discard any unused reconstituted stain.
14. Incubate the slides for 15 minutes in a covered moist chamber at room temperature. *Protect from light.*
15. Remove the slides from the moist chamber and rinse with a gentle stream of PBS. Place the slides in a Coplin or staining jar filled with PBS for 10 minutes. Agitate at entry, midpoint, and prior to removal.
16. Remove the slides (one at a time) from the wash buffer and drain excess PBS by gently tapping the horizontal edge of the slide. If blotting is preferred, see directions in step 7.
17. Apply one small drop of mounting media in each specimen well. Gently apply coverslip without pressure.
18. Examine the slides with a light microscope using high (40x) magnification.

REPORTING RESULTS

Negative: No cytoplasmic or nuclear specific stain is observed. The cells may be slightly colored due to some nonspecific reaction of the peroxidase stain reagent.

Positive: A serum is considered to be positive if the nuclei of the cells stain more intensely than the negative control well and there is a clearly discernible pattern of colorations.

A grading scale similar to the one shown in the accompanying box may be helpful in establishing the criteria for each laboratory. Positive specimens should be confirmed by repeating the test with twofold dilutions of serum. All positive ANA patterns should be titered to endpoint dilution to detect possible mixed antinuclear reactions that may

Grading Reactions

Negative	No cytoplasmic or nuclear specific stain observed. The cells may be slightly colored due to some non-specific reaction of the peroxidase staining reagent.
Borderline (+/−)	Beige specific stain
Positive	
1+	Tan
2+	Light brown
3+	Medium brown
4+	Dark chocolate brown to black

not be apparent when interpreting a single screening dilution. The endpoint titer is the last serial dilution in which a 1+ coloration with a clearly discernible pattern is detected.

PROCEDURE NOTES

The indirect immunofluorescence test and the immunoenzyme methods are probably the most practical ways of screening for ANA in the clinical laboratory. The peroxidase enzyme-conjugated antibody method, which is comparable in sensitivity and patterns of reactivity to fluorescent methods, has certain advantages. The HRP technique has the advantages of resulting in a permanent slide and requires only a conventional light microscope with no special equipment.

SOURCES OF ERROR. **False negative** results can occur if the ANA happens to be specific for an antigen other than the one used in the procedure. False negative results may also occur if the substrate is fixed in acetone and is inadequately washed. Without fixation, however, some soluble nuclear antigen may be lost. False negative results may also be related to the binding of antinuclear factor to circulating immune complexes and to a low antibody titer.

False positive interpretations may occur because of nonspecific staining. Nonspecific staining may resemble a speckled pattern of reactivity. These staining reactions occur whenever the conjugate or the serum contains antibodies to other tissue antigens. Careful rinsing and removal of excess fluoresceinated conjugate minimizes the risk of some nonspecific staining reactions.

CLINICAL APPLICATIONS. In the evaluation of patients with connective tissue disease, the ANA must be interpreted with caution. Under proper testing conditions, a negative ANA generally rules out systemic lupus erythematosus. A negative ANA result, however, can result from autoimmune disease in remission or nuclear autoantibodies not detectable with indirect immunofluorescent or peroxidase immunoenzyme procedures.

The significance of a positive ANA depends on the titer and to a lesser extent on the observed pattern (Table 26-4). There is no general agreement on

TABLE 26-4

Antinuclear Antibody Patterns and Disorders

ANA staining pattern	Antibody specificities	Related disorders
Homogeneous	nDNA dsDNA ssDNA DNP Histones	Systemic lupus erythematosus (SLE) Rheumatoid arthritis Sjögren's syndrome Mixed connective tissue diseases (MCTD)
Peripheral or rim	nDNA dsDNA DNP	Active systemic lupus erythematosus Sjögren's syndrome
Speckled	Smith (Sm) RNP	Systemic lupus erythematosus Rheumatoid arthritis Sjögren's syndrome Progressive systemic sclerosis MCTD
Nucleolar	4-6S RNP	Scleroderma Sjögren's syndrome Undiagnosed illnesses manifesting Raynaud's phenomenon
Discrete, speckled	Centromere DNA, RNA ENA	CREST variant of progressive systemic sclerosis

the significance of the various patterns, and it should be noted that some patterns may mask other patterns in high concentration. Interpretation of ANA patterns, however, can provide additional information about the type of nuclear component reacting.

Because of the sensitivity of the HEp-2 cell substrate, some apparently normal individuals may show a low degree of staining at the 1:40 screening dilution. ANA titers of 1:10 to 1:80 usually have little significance but may be seen in patients with rheumatoid arthritis or scleroderma. Antinuclear antibodies are know to be sex and age dependent; therefore a positive low titer result may be "normal" for certain individuals in the absence of other clinical signs and symptoms. If a specimen is positive at a 1:10 dilution, it should be retested at dilutions from 1:20 to 1:320. The higher the antibody titer, the more likely is the diagnosis of connective tissue disorder. Changes in the antibody titer can also be used to observe disease activity.

If the ANA test is positive, additional immunologic evaluation is necessary to determine the specificity of the reaction. These evaluations include double immunodiffusion, counter immunoelectrophoresis, passive hemagglutination, radioimmunoassays, and identification of nuclear antigens by immunoprecipitation or immunoblotting. Such evaluations may demonstrate that more than one

ANA specificity is present in the serum. An LE cell preparation is not useful because it is positive in only 75% of patients with confirmed SLE.

LIMITATIONS. No diagnosis should be based solely on the results of laboratory testing. Clinical data, antibody titers, and other laboratory findings should all be reviewed before a definitive diagnosis is established.

REFERENCES

ISOLAB, Inc., Product Insert, 1985.

☐ PROCEDURE

Rapid Slide Test for Antinucleoprotein Factors Associated with Systemic Lupus Erythematosus (Qualitative)

PRINCIPLE

Systemic lupus erythematosus (SLE) reagent contains stabilized animal erythrocytes coated with a preparation of deoxyribonucleoprotein (DNP) from calf thymus, the antigen for detection of antinucleoprotein. When the reagent is mixed with serum containing nucleoprotein antibodies, macroscopic agglutination occurs. The procedure is positive in SLE and systemic rheumatic diseases such as rheumatoid arthritis, scleroderma, Sjögren's syndrome, mixed connective tissue disease, and drug-induced lupus erythematosus.

SPECIMEN COLLECTION AND PREPARATION

No special preparation of the patient is required prior to specimen collection. The patient must be positively identified when the specimen is collected and the specimen is to be labeled at the bedside. Specimen labels must include the patient's full name, the date the specimen is collected, the patient's hospital identification number, and the phlebotomist's initials.

Blood should be drawn by an aseptic technique. A minimum of 2 mL of clotted blood (red-top evacuated tube) is required. The specimen should be centrifuged promptly and an aliquot of serum removed.

Use fresh serum. If the test cannot be performed immediately, refrigerate the specimen between 2° and 8° C for no longer than 48 hours after collection. Freeze the serum if testing is postponed for more than 48 hours.

REAGENTS, SUPPLIES, AND EQUIPMENT

Systemic Lupus Erythematosus (SLE) Test Kit (available commercially from ICL Scientific, Fountain Valley, Calif.)

The following components are available in the kit:

1. Serascan SLE Reagent with dropper cap assembly. Contains deoxyribonucleoprotein extracted

from calf thymus and coated on stabilized animal erythrocytes. Refrigerate the latex reagent at 2° to 8° C. It is stable until the expiration date on the kit label. Do not use the reagent if it becomes grossly contaminated. Do not use the reagent if evidence of freezing is apparent.
2. Capillary pipettes
3. Applicator sticks
4. Glass slide. It is essential that the glass slide is clean. Before use, wash it thoroughly with mild detergent, rinse several times with distilled water, and dry.

Additional required equipment:
Timer or stopwatch

QUALITY CONTROL

Positive Control (human). Must be tested with each set of tests. The positive control and SLE reagent should form a visible agglutination pattern distinctly different from the slight granularity that may be observed with the negative control. If agglutination is not visible with the positive control, the patient's test is invalid.

Negative Control (human). The reaction between the negative control and SLE reagent should produce a smooth or slightly granular appearance at the end of the 2 minutes of testing. If agglutination is observed, the patient's test is invalid.

Caution: Because the control sera are derived from human sources, They should be handled in the same manner as clinical serum specimens (see *Universal blood and body fluid precautions* in Chapter 6).

Warning: The latex reagent and controls contain 0.1% sodium azide as a preservative. Sodium azide may react with lead and copper plumbing to form highly explosive metal azides. Upon disposal, flush with a large volume of water to prevent azide buildup.

PROCEDURE

Note: All reagents, controls, and test sera must be at room temperature prior to testing.
1. Check the slide for cleanliness.
2. Fill a capillary pipette provided in the kit. Hold the pipette perpendicular to the slide above the appropriate square. Deliver 1 free-falling drop onto the slide.
3. Repeat step 2, using both the positive and negative control.
4. Resuspend the latex reagent by gently mixing it. Replace the screw-top cap with the dropper assembly. Subsequent resuspension of the reagent should be done by dispelling reagent from the dropper and gently inverting the vial until the suspension is homogeneous.
5. Add 1 drop of the SLE reagent to each of the divisions containing a serum specimen and the positive and negative controls.
6. Using separate applicator sticks, mix each specimen and control serum with the SLE reagent in

a circular manner over the entire area within the division of the slide.
7. Slowly tilt the slide back and forth for *1 minute.* Place the slide on a flat surface and allow it to stand undisturbed for *1 minute. Do not move the slide.*
8. Observe for agglutination. Agglutination reactions with the SLE reagent are similar to those observed in blood grouping and typing reactions and should be read using a good source of indirect light.
9. Wash the glass slide thoroughly with mild detergent and rinse several times with distilled water.

REPORTING RESULTS

Positive = agglutination
Negative = no agglutination

PROCEDURE NOTES

SOURCES OF ERROR. Failure to observe the test mixture at the appropriate time can yield false results.

CLINICAL APPLICATIONS. Serum from patients with SLE have been shown to contain several antinuclear antibodies as determined by a wide variety of laboratory tests. A specific diagnosis depends on the evaluation of test results and clinical manifestations.

LIMITATIONS. No one test has been shown to be completely reliable for the diagnosis of SLE because many of the antinuclear antibodies accompanying this disease are also demonstrated in other systemic rheumatic diseases such as rheumatoid arthritis, Sjögren's syndrome, and progressive systemic sclerosis.

REFERENCES

Greenwals CA, Peebles CL, and Nakamura RM: Laboratory tests for antinuclear antibody (ANA) in rheumatic disease, Lab Med 9:19-27, 1978.

☐ PROCEDURE

Quantitative Determination of IgG and IgM Antibodies to Deoxyribonucleoprotein (DNP) in Human Serum*

PRINCIPLE

This procedure is an indirect enzyme-labeled immunoassay for determination of IgG and IgM antibodies to deoxyribonucleoprotein using antigen-coated microwells as a solid phase. Calf thymus-derived deoxyribonucleoprotein (DNP) antigen is coated onto the wells of the microplate. Diluted test samples are added to the coated wells and incu-

*Sigma Immunoassay.

bated. During incubation, antibodies to DNP present in the sample bind to the antigen-coated well. After washing to remove unbound material, antibodies to human IgG and IgM labeled with alkaline phosphatase (conjugate) are added. The conjugate binds to any antibodies bound to DNP. The well is washed to remove unbound conjugate and incubated with *p*-nitrophenyl phosphate. The *p*-nitrophenyl phosphate is hydrolyzed by alkaline phosphatase to form *p*-nitrophenol, a yellow-colored end product with an absorbance maximum at 405 nm>. The intensity of the absorbance at 405 nm is proportional to the amount of antibody to DNP present in the specimen.

SPECIMEN COLLECTION AND PREPARATION

No special preparation of the patient is required prior to specimen collection. The patient must be positively identified when the specimen is collected and the specimen is to be labeled at the bedside. Specimen labels must include the patient's full name, the date the specimen is collected, the patient's hospital identification number, and the phlebotomist's initials.

Blood should be drawn by an aseptic technique. A minimum of 2 mL of clotted blood (red-top evacuated tube) is required. The specimen should be centrifuged promptly and an aliquot of serum removed.

Serum specimens should be stored in the refrigerator (2° to 6° C) or frozen (−20° C) if kept for more than 7 days. Specimens containing visible particulate matter should be clarified by centrifugation prior to testing. Serum sample should not be heat-inactivated, as this may cause false positive results.

REAGENTS, SUPPLIES, AND EQUIPMENT

Reagents and controls are available commercially from Sigma Chemical Co.

Note: Store reagents at 2° to 6° C. The reagents are stable until the expiration date on the label.

Kit components include the following:

1. Antigen wells. Microplate wells coated with calf thymus DNP antigen. Store antigen wells with desiccant in the reusable plastic bag. Reseal the bag after opening.
2. Holder for wells.
3. Sample diluent. This buffered protein solution contains surfactant and blue dye, pH 7.5. It also contains absorbent (heat-aggregated human IgG) and 0.1% sodium azide as a preservative.
4. Calibrator. This is a human serum containing antibodies to DNP. The content (IU/mL) is indicated on the label. It contains 0.1% sodium azide as a preservative.
5. Conjugate. This solution contains goat antibodies to human IgG and IgM labeled with calf alkaline phosphatase. It contains a pink dye and 0.02% sodium azide as a preservative.
6. Substrate. This solution contains *p*-nitrophenyl phosphate, disodium, hexahydrate 1mg/mL, pH

9.6. The substrate may develop a slight yellow color upon storage. Do not use if absorbance of the undiluted substrate is greater than 0.4 at 405 nm when measured against water using a microplate reader or a spectrophotometer with a 1-cm lightpath.
7. Wash concentrate. This is a buffer solution concentrate with surfactant. It contains 0.1% sodium azide as a preservative. The wash solution is prepared by adding the contents of wash concentrate bottle to 1 liter of deionized water. Mix well.
8. Stop solution. Alkaline solution pH 12.0. Store at room temperature. Reagent is stable until expiration date on the label. *Warning:* Stop solution causes irritation. Avoid contact with eyes, skin and clothing. Avoid breathing vapor. Wash thoroughly after handling.

Note: Except for the wash, do not interchange reagents from different lots.

Warning: The reagents and controls contain sodium azide as a preservative. Sodium azide may react with lead and copper plumbing to form highly explosive metal azides. Upon disposal, flush with a large volume of water to prevent azide buildup. Sodium azide is also toxic. Care should be taken to avoid ingestion.

Additional required equipment and supplies

1. Spectrophotometer that accommodates a 1-mL volume, or microplate reader capable of accurately measuring absorbance at 405 nm
2. Pipetting device for the accurate delivery of 5 μL. 100 μL, and 200 μL
3. Timer
4. 1-liter measuring cylinder
5. Squeeze bottle for dispensing wash solution
6. Dilution plates or tubes
7. Test tubes or cuvettes, 1.0 mL

QUALITY CONTROL

Positive control: Human serum containing antibodies to DNP. Content (IU/mL) indicated on the label. This solution contains 0.1% sodium azide.

Negative control: Human serum containing no detectable antibodies to DNP. This solution contains 0.1% sodium azide.

Caution: Because the controls and calibrator sera are derived from human sources, they should be handled in the same manner as clinical serum specimens (see *Universal blood and body fluid precautions* in Chapter 6).

PROCEDURE

1. Dilute calibrator, positive and negative controls, and test samples by combining 5 μL of each of with 200 μL sample diluent in labeled tubes or dilution plates.
2. Place the desired number of antigen wells in a holder.
3. Using a pipette tip, mix the samples and diluent by drawing up and expelling 2 or 3 times.

Transfer 100 μL of each diluted specimen to the appropriate antigen well.

4. Include one well that contains only 100 μL sample diluent. This serves as the reagent blank and is used to zero the photometer.
5. Allow the plate to stand at room temperature (18° to 26° C) for 30 +/− 2 minutes.
6. Shake out or aspirate contents of wells. Wash the wells by filling them with wash solution from a squeeze bottle and shaking out or aspirating. Wash 3 times. Drain the wells on a paper towel to remove excess fluid.
   Note: Thorough washing is necessary to achieve accurate results. Avoid bubbles.
7. Place 2 drops (or 100 μL) conjugate into each well, including the reagent blank well.
8. Allow to stand at room temperature (18° to 26° C) for 30 minutes +/− 2 minutes.
9. Wash wells by repeating step 6.
10. Place 2 drops (or 100 μL) of substrate into each well, including the reagent blank well.
11. Allow to stand at room temperature (18° to 26° C) for 30 minutes +/− 2 minutes.
12. Place 2 drops (or 100 μL) of stop solution into each well.
13. Read and record absorbance of each test at 405 nm within 2 hours after the reaction has been stopped:
    MICROPLATE READER. Set absorbance at 405 nm to zero with water as a reference. Read and record absorbance of reagent blank (A blank). Then set absorbance to zero with the reagent blank as a reference. Read and record absorbance of samples (A sample) and calibrator (A calibrator).
    SPECTROPHOTOMETER. Completely remove contents of each well and transfer to cuvette or test tube. Add 800 μL of deionized water to each sample and mix. Set absorbance at 405 nm to zero with water as a reference. Read and record the absorbance of each sample including the reagent blank. Subtract the absorbance of the reagent blank for the absorbance of each sample.

CALCULATION

Concentration of IgG and IgM antibodies to DNP in samples is calculated as follows:

Antibody Concentration (IU/mL) in sample =

$$\frac{\text{A sample}}{\text{A calibrator}} \times \text{IU/mL of calibrator}$$

EXAMPLE:
Absorbance Measured Using a Microplate Reader

$$\text{A sample} = 0.924$$

$$\text{A calibrator} = 1.756$$

$$\text{IU/mL of calibrator} = 292$$

$$\text{Antibody concentration (IU/mL) in sample} = \frac{0.0924}{1.756} \times 292 = 154$$

Absorbance Measured Using a Spectrophotometer

$$\text{A blank} = 0.015$$

$$\text{A sample} = 0.186$$

$$\text{A calibrator} = 0.353$$

$$\text{A sample} - \text{A blank} = 0.186 - 0.015 = 0.171$$

$$\text{A calibrator} - \text{A blank} = 0.3530 - 0.015 = 0.338$$

$$\text{IU/mL of calibrator} = 292$$

$$\text{Antibody concentration (IU/mL) in sample} = \frac{0.171}{0.338} \times 292 = 148$$

REPORTING RESULTS

Results are reported in International Units (IU)/mL standardized to the World Health Organization antinuclear factor serum (homogeneous), human, First Reference Preparation, 1970.
Positive = equal to or >40 IU/mL
Negative = <40 IU/mL

PROCEDURE NOTES

The absorbance values will vary with the temperature of the room and incubation time. Absorbance value or reagent blank when read against water at 405 nm should be less than 0.4 using a microplate reader, or less than 0.09 using a spectrophotometer with a 1-cm lightpath. The absorbance value of the calibrator should be greater than or equal to 0.5 using a microplate reader when the assay is performed at 22° C. The assay value of the positive control should be within the range printed on the label. The negative control should be less than 40 IU/mL. If these requirements are not satisfied, the test results may be inaccurate and they should be repeated.

Specimens giving absorbance values above that of the calibrator should be diluted appropriately and reassayed. The value obtained should be multiplied by the dilution factor.

SOURCES OF ERROR. *Biological false positives.* Antibodies to DNP are the most common antinuclear antibodies found in SLE, but they also occur at low titers in other disorders such as chronic hepatitis, periarteritis nodosa, dermatomyositis, scleroderma, and drug sensitivities.

CLINICAL APPLICATIONS. Antibodies to nuclear components occur in many connective tissue disorders. Idiopathic systemic lupus erythematosus (SLE) is characterized by the presence of antibodies to double-stranded DNA and to deoxyribonucleoprotein (DNP). Patients with drug-induced lupus, however, usually lack antibodies to double-stranded DNA, although they do have antibodies to DNA and histones.

LIMITATIONS. This procedure serves as an aid to diagnosis and should not be interpreted as diagnostic in itself.

REFERENCES

Sigma Product Insert, May 1988, St Louis, Mo.

Chapter Review

HIGHLIGHTS

Systemic lupus erythematosus (SLE) is the classic model of autoimmune disease. It is a systemic rheumatic disorder. Although no single cause of SLE has been identified, a primary defect in the regulation of the immune system is regarded as being of importance in the pathogenesis of the disorder. Other influences include the affect of estrogens, genetic predisposition, and extraneous factors. A combination of these factors, however, may be synergistic.

SLE is a disease of acute and chronic inflammation. Manifestations of the disease range from a typical mild illness, which is limited to a photosensitive facial rash and transient diffuse arthritis, to life-threatening involvement of the renal, cardiac, respiratory, or central nervous systems. The manifestation of SLE results from defects in the regulatory mechanism of the immune system. Studies of the immunopathogenesis of lupus nephritis have demonstrated a variety of aberrations in T cell and B cell function. It is uncertain, however, if the disease represents a primary dysfunction of T cells or B cells. Lymphocyte subset abnormalities are a major immunologic feature of SLE. Among the T cell subsets, a lack of, or reduced, generalized suppressor T cell function and/or hyperproduction of helper T cells occurs. The formation of lymphocytotoxic antibodies with a predominant specificity for T lymphocytes by SLE patients at least partially explains the interference with certain functional activities of T lymphocytes manifested by the patient with SLE. Lymphocytotoxic antibodies are capable of both destroying T lymphocytes in the presence of complement and of coating peripheral blood T cells. The regulation of antibody production of B lymphocytes, ordinarily a function of the subpopulation of T suppressor cells, appears to be defective in SLE. Patients exhibit a state of spontaneous B-lymphocyte hyperactivity with ensuing uncontrolled production of a wide variety of antibodies to both host and exogenous antigens. Host response to some antigens, however, is normal in many instances, and patients manifest a specific well-controlled humoral immune response.

Circulating immune complexes are the hallmark of SLE. Patients with SLE exhibit multiple serum antibodies that react with native or altered self-antigens. Demonstrable antibodies include antibodies to nuclear components; cell surface and cytoplasmic antigens of polymorphonuclear and lymphocytic leukocytes, erythrocytes, platelets, and neuronal cells; and immunoglobulin, (Ig) G. The antinuclear antibody (anti-DNP) gives rise to the LE cell, which is found in the majority of untreated patients with active SLE. SLE patients with serositis may form LE cells in vivo. Antibodies also combine with their corresponding antigens to form immune complexes. When the mononuclear phagocytic system is unable to entirely eliminate these immune complexes, an accumulation of immune complexes result in the blood circulation. These circulating immune complexes are deposited in the subendothelial layers of the vascular basement membranes of multiple target organs and mediate inflammation. The sites of deposition are determined in part by the physiochemical properties of the particular antigens or antibodies involved.

The manifestations of SLE that are expressed in laboratory findings are numerous. Histologic, hematologic, and serologic abnormalities reflect the multisystem nature of this disease. Serologic testing frequently reveals high levels of anti-DNA antibodies, reduced complement levels, and presence of complement breakdown products of C3 (C3d and C3c). In addition, cryoglobulins, which in some instances represent immune complexes, are frequently present in the serum of patients with SLE. Because monoclonal gammopathies have occasionally been described, a marked increase in gammaglobulins may result in a hyperviscosity syndrome or renal tubular acidosis. Nonspecific elevation in the levels of immunoglobulins, particularly IgM and IgG, are frequent in SLE. An actual deficiency of IgA appears to be more common in SLE than in normal individuals.

The antinuclear antibody (ANA) procedure is a valuable screening tool for SLE. It has replaced the LE cell test because of its wider range of reactivity with nuclear antigens and its greater sensitivity and quality control characteristics. Antinuclear antibodies (ANAs) are a heterogenous group of circulating immunoglobulins (e.g., IgM, IgG, and IgA). These immunoglobulins react with the whole nucleus or nuclear components such as nuclear proteins, deoxyribonucleic acid (DNA), or histones in host tissues. They are, therefore, true autoantibodies. Generally, ANAs have no organ or species specificity and are capable of cross-reacting with nuclear material from humans (e.g., human leukocytes, or various animal tissues). Demonstration of ANAs in laboratory testing can be indicative of various systemic autoimmune connective tissue disorders. These disease states are characterized by antibodies that react with different nuclear components, such as double-stranded DNA, single-stranded DNA, and Sm antigen. ANAs can be found in SLE, mixed connective tissue disease (MCTD), progressive systemic sclerosis (PSS), or scleroderma, Sjögren's syndrome, polymyositis/dermatomyositis, and rheumatoid arthritis (RA). A small percentage of patients with neoplastic diseases may also demonstrate the presence of ANAs.

It is possible to divide ANAs into different groups to provide a systematic classification. These groups are antibodies to DNA, antibodies to histone and nonhistone proteins, and antibodies to nuclear antigens. Antibodies to DNA can be divided into two major groups: antibodies that react with native (double-stranded) DNA, and antibodies that recognize denatured (single-stranded) DNA only. Detection of autoantibodies by immunofluorescence has become an extremely valuable method. Immunofluorescence is extremely sensitive and may show positive results in cases where procedures for antinuclear antibodies, such as complement fixation or precipitation, give negative results. At present, the immunofluorescent method is the most widely used technique for ANA screening.

REVIEW QUESTIONS

1. Systemic lupus erythematosus (SLE) is more common in:
    A. Female infants
    B. Male infants
    C. Adolescent through middle-aged women
    D. Adolescent through middle-aged males
    E. Elderly females and males
2. One of the most potent inducers of abnormalities and clinical manifestations of SLE is:
    A. Hydralazine
    B. Procainamide
    C. Isoniazid
    D. Penicillin
    E. Propylthiouracil
3. The cellular aberrations in SLE include:
    A. B cell depletion
    B. Deficiency of T suppressor cell function
    C. Hyperproduction of helper T cells
    D. Depletion of macrophages
    E. Both B and C
4. The principal demonstrable antibody in SLE is antibody to:
    A. Nuclear antigen
    B. Cell surface antigens of hematopoietic cells
    C. Cell surface antigens to neuronal cells
    D. Lymphocytic leukocytes
    E. IgG
5. The sites of immune complex deposition in SLE is influenced by all of the following factors *except:*
    A. Molecular size
    B. Molecular configuration
    C. Immune complex specificity
    D. Immunoglobulin class
    E. Complement fixing ability
6. Renal disease secondary to SLE can be assessed by:
    A. Antibody to native DS-DNA
    B. Levels of C3 and C4
    C. Levels of CH50
    D. Cryoglobulin levels
    E. All of the above

Answers

1. C 2. B 3. E 4. A 5. C 6. E

BIBLIOGRAPHY

Couser WG: Glomerular involvement in systemic diseases. In Stein J, editor: Internal medicine, Boston, 1987, Little, Brown & Co, Inc, pp 856-859.

Fritzler MJ and Tan EM: Antibodies to histones in drug induced and idiopathic lupus erythematosus, J Clin Invest 62:560, 1978.

Greenwals CA, Peebles CL, and Nakamura RM: Laboratory tests for antinuclear antibody (ANA) in rheumatic disease, Lab Med 9:19-27, 1978.

Hidalgo C and Vladutiu AO: Lupus erythematosus cells in serum and pleural fluid of a patient with negative fluorescent antinuclear antibody test, AJCP 87(5):660-662, 1987.

Holborow EJ: Autoantibodies in rheumatic diseases. In Scott JT, editor: Copeman's textbook of the rheumatic diseases, New York, 1986, Churchill Livingstone, Inc, ed 6, pp 355-375.

Hughes GVR: Systemic lupus erythematosus. In Scott JT, editor: Copeman's textbook of the rheumatic diseases, ed 6, New York, 1986, Churchill Livingstone, Inc, pp 1325-1349.

Karsh J et al: Anti-DNA, anti-deoxyribonucleoprotein and rheumatoid factor measured by ELISA in patients with systemic lupus erythematosus, Sjögren's syndrome and rheumatoid arthritis, Int Arch Allergy Appl Immunol 68:60, 1982.

Klippel JH and Decker JL: Systemic lupus erythematosus. In Stein JH, editor: Internal medicine, Boston, 1987, Little, Brown & Co, Inc, pp 1270-1278.

Metzger AL et al, editors: In vivo LE cell formation in peritonitis due to systemic lupus erythematosus, J Rheum 1(1):130-133, 1974.

Pandya MR: In vivo L phenomenon in pleural fluid, Arthritis Rheum 19(5):962-963, 1976.

Persellin RH and Takeuchi A: Antinuclear antibody-negative systemic lupus erythematosusa: loss in body fluids, J Rheum 7(4):547-550, 1980.

Provost TT and Alexander EL: Cutaneous manifestations of connective tissue disease. In Stein JH, editor: Internal medicine, Boston, 1987, Little, Brown & Co, Inc, pp 1363-1366.

Rheumatoid Arthritis

ETIOLOGY

Because evidence exists that immunologic factors are involved in both the articular and extra-articular manifestations of the disease, rheumatoid arthritis (RA) may represent an unusual host response to one or perhaps many etiologic agents. An infectious etiology is possible, although it has not been established.

EPIDEMIOLOGY

The incidence of RA is 1% to 2% in most populations that have been studied. The disorder occurs worldwide, but no definite racial, geographic, or climatic variation in incidence has been established. Although no specific genetic relationship has been established, a small increase in incidence has been noted in first-degree relatives of patients with RA. Persons with the HLA DR4 haplotype do have a significantly higher incidence of RA.

Women are two to three times more likely than men to develop RA. It can begin at any age, but the disease initially occurs most frequently between the ages of 30 and 50 years. Complications due to an increased frequency of local or extra-articular infections in RA patients have been demonstrated. Mortality may result from conditions such as septicemia, pneumonia, lung abscess, or pyelonephritis.

SIGNS AND SYMPTOMS

RA is a chronic, usually progressive inflammatory disorder of the joints (Fig. 27-1). It is, however, a highly variable disease that ranges from a mild illness of brief duration to a progressive, destructive polyarthritis associated with a systemic vasculitis.

The pathogenesis of the disorder has three distinct stages:
1. Initiation of synovitis by the primary etiologic factor

2. Subsequent immunologic events that perpetuate the initial inflammatory reaction
3. Transition of an inflammatory reaction in the synovium to a proliferative destructive process of tissue

RA often begins with prodromal symptoms such as fatigue, anorexia, weakness, and generalized aching and stiffness that is not localized to articular

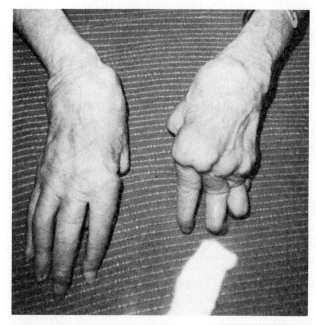

FIGURE 27-1

Swan-neck deformity, ulnar deviation, dorsal interosseous muscle atrophy, and swelling of wrist—characteristics of rheumatoid arthritis.
(From Kaye D and Rose LF: Fundamentals of internal medicine, St Louis, 1983, The CV Mosby Co.)

Extra-articular Manifestations of Rheumatoid Arthritis

> Constitutional manifestations, e.g., weight loss and fatigue
> Subcutaneous rheumatoid nodules
> Ocular abnormalities, e.g., inflammatory lesions of the episclera and sclera
> Vasculitis
> Neuropathy, e.g., mononeuritis multiplex
> Myopathy
> Cardiac manifestations, e.g., pericarditis
> Pulmonary manifestations, e.g., pleural effusion
> Osteoporosis
> Felty's syndrome—a complex of chronic rheumatoid arthritis, splenomegaly, anemia, thrombocytopenia, and neutropenia

American Rheumatism Association Criteria for Diagnosis of Rheumatoid Arthritis

> 1. Morning stiffness
> 2. Pain on motion or tenderness in at least one joint
> 3. Swelling of one joint, representing soft tissue or fluid
> 4. Swelling of at least one other joint (soft tissue or fluid)
> 5. Symmetrical joint swelling (simultaneous involvement of the same joint, right and left)
> 6. Subcutaneous nodules over bony prominences or extensor surfaces or near joints
> 7. Typical radiologic changes which must include demineralization in periarticular bone as an index of inflammation; degenerative changes do not exclude diagnosis of RA
> 8. Positive demonstration of rheumatoid factor in patient serum
> 9. A poor mucin clot formation on adding synovial fluid to dilute acetic acid
> 10. Synovial histopathology consistent with RA from a rheumatoid nodule biopsied from any site
> 11. Characteristic histologic changes of a rheumatoid nodule biopsied from any site

From Zvaifler N: Rheumatoid arthritis. In Stein J, editor: Intern Med, ed 2, Boston, 1987, Little, Brown & Co, p 1261.

structures. Joint symptoms usually appear gradually over weeks to months. A wide variety of extra-articular manifestations (see box above) can be manifested.

The American Rheumatism Association criteria for diagnosis of RA is presented in the box at right. If criteria 1 to 5 and two additional criteria of this group of signs, symptoms, and laboratory findings are demonstrated in a patient whose disease has been continuous for at least 6 weeks, the patient is designated as suffering from *classic rheumatoid arthritis.* The greater the number of criteria in the patient, the more likely the diagnosis of rheumatoid arthritis.

IMMUNOLOGIC MANIFESTATIONS

Two pathogenic mechanisms have been hypothesized in RA:

1. The extravascular immune complex hypothesis proposes an interaction of antigens and antibodies in synovial tissues and fluid. Antigens exist as complexes in collagen, cartilage, proteoglycans, fibrinogen or fibrin, partially digested IgG, and soluble nucleoproteins. These substances can be found in articular tissues or by-products of the inflammatory process. These complexes react with antibodies in joint tissues and initiate the complement cascade that generates various biologically active products. Subsequent initiation of phagocytosis, engulfment with the release of hydrolytic enzymes, and production of toxic O_2 and arachidonic acid metabolites are directly responsible for inflammation and tissue damage.

2. The alternate hypothesis is that RA results from cell-mediated damage because the accumulation of lymphocytes, primarily T cells, in the rheumatoid synovium resembles a delayed-type hypersensitivity reaction. The presence of lymphokines, which effect both articular inflammation and destruction, supports this hypothesis.

When the rheumatoid synovium is examined by the immunofluorescent technique, it can be seen to contain large amounts of IgG and IgM, alone or together. Immunoglobulins can also be seen in synovial lining cells, blood vessels, and interstitial connective tissues. B cells make immunoglobulin in the synovium of patients with RA. As many as half of the plasma cells that can be located in the synovium secrete an IgG rheumatoid factor that combines in the cytoplasm with similar IgG molecules (self-associating IgG).

The various vascular and parenchymal lesions of RA suggest that the lesions result from injury induced by immune complexes, especially those containing antibodies to IgG. The serum of most patients with RA has detectable soluble immune complexes. Anti-gamma globulins of the IgG and IgM classes are an integral part of these complexes.

Rheumatoid factor belongs to a larger family of antiglobulins that are usually defined as antibodies with specificity for antigen determinants on the Fc fragment of human or certain animal IgG. Rheumatoid factors have been associated with three major immunoglobulin classes: IgM, IgG, and IgA. IgM and IgG rheumatoid factors are the most common.

DIAGNOSTIC EVALUATION

Low serum iron and a normal or low iron-binding capacity is a common feature. The erythrocyte sedimentation rate (ESR) is elevated to a variable degree in most patients and roughly parallels the level of disease activity. Serum protein electrophoresis may demonstrate elevations in the alpha-2 and gamma globulin fractions, with a mild to moderate decrease in serum albumin. The gamma globulin increase is polyclonal.

Hemolytic complement levels are reduced in the serum of less than one third of patients, especially in patients with seropositive disease. Levels of C4 and C2 are most profoundly depressed in these patients.

Antibodies to native double-stranded DNA are very rare. Circulating immune complexes and cryprecipitable proteins consisting of immunoglobulins, complement components, and rheumatoid factors are demonstrable in the serum of some patients with RA. IgM rheumatoid factor is manifested in approximately 70% of adults, but it is not specific for RA. The determination of rheumatoid factor is important in the prognosis of RA.

Changes in the serologic activity in rheumatoid arthritis were initially observed in 1929 to 1931, when it was shown that sera from RA patients agglutinated various coccal organisms. In 1940 it was demonstrated that sera from RA patients agglutinated sheep cells "sensitized" with rabbit antibody against sheep cells. In 1953 it was found that Cohn fraction II, or gamma globulin in human sera, tended to inhibit the rheumatoid reaction. It was shown that tanned cells coated with human gamma globulin absorbed out all agglutinating activity from rheumatoid sera. This suggested that an antigen-antibody reaction occurred. It was later demonstrated that the addition of latex particles coated with gamma globulin to sera caused flocculation with about 70% of rheumatoid sera. Agglutination tests for rheumatoid factor, such as the sensitized sheep cell test, latex agglutination, and bentonite flocculation, generally detect IgM rheumatoid factors because these molecules are more potent than IgG in agglutinating appropriate antigen suspensions. Because conventional procedures are semiquantitative, they may be insensitive to changes in titer and may detect only those rheumatoid factors that agglutinate. Newer, more sensitive methods, such as nephelometric and turbidometric assays, radioimmunoassays, and enzyme-linked immunoassays have been developed.

Rheumatoid factor (RF) has been associated with some bacterial and viral infections such as hepatitis and infectious mononucleois and some chronic infections such as tuberculosis, parasitic disease, subacute bacterial endocarditis, and cancer. Elevated values may also be observed in the normal elderly population.

JUVENILE RHEUMATOID ARTHRITIS

Juvenile rheumatoid arthritis (JRA) is a condition of chronic synovitis beginning during childhood. The etiologic hypotheses are similar to those proposed for adult RA. The incidence of JRA in pediatric populations is between 0.1 and 1.1 per 1000 children in the United States. Diagnostic criteria include onset before the age of 16, presence of arthritis (i.e., joint swelling for 6 consecutive weeks or longer), and exclusion of other conditions known to cause or

TABLE 27-1

Apparent Subgroups of JRA

Subgroup	Age at onset	Immunologic manifestations
Systemic onset (Still's disease)	Any	ANA = negative RF = negative
RF negative polyarthritis	Any	ANA = 25% positive RF = negative
RF positive polyarthritis	Older	ANA = 50% positive RF = 100% positive HLA-DR4
Pauciarticular I	Younger	ANA = 60% positive HLA-DR5, HLA-DRw6, and HLA-DRw8
Pauciarticular II	Older	HLA-B27

mimic childhood arthritis. Several distinct subgroups of JRA (Table 27-1) vary in signs and symptoms and immunologic manifestations.

DIAGNOSTIC PROCEDURES
Rapid Latex Agglutination

☐ PROCEDURE

Rheumatoid Arthritis Test*

PRINCIPLE

The rheumatoid arthritis agglutination test is based on the reaction between patient antibodies in the serum, known as the "rheumatoid factor," and an antigen derived from gamma globulin. Latex reagent consists of a stabilized latex suspension coated with albumin and chemically bonded with denatured human gamma globulin. This reagent serves as an antigen in the procedure. If rheumatoid factors are present in the serum, macroscopic agglutination will be visible when the latex reagent is mixed with the serum. The determination of rheumatoid factors is important in the prognosis and therapeutic management of rheumatoid arthritis; however, positive test results may be observed in a variety of disorders such as lupus erythematosus, Sjögren's syndrome, syphilis, and hepatitis.

SPECIMEN COLLECTION AND PREPARATION

No special preparation of the patient is required prior to specimen collection. The patient must be positively identified when the specimen is collected and the specimen is to be labeled at the bedside. Specimen labels must include the patient's full name, the date the specimen is collected, the

*Modified from Rheuma-Fac Rheumatoid Arthritis Test (Latex) Product Insert, ICL Scientific, Fountain Valley, Calif, July 1987 (with permission).

patient's hospital identification number, and the phlebotomist's initials.

Blood should be drawn by an aseptic technique. A minimum of 2 mL of clotted blood (red-top evacuated tube) is required. The specimen should be centrifuged promptly and an aliquot of serum removed.

If the test cannot be performed immediately, the specimen should be refrigerated (2° to 8° C) for no longer than 72 hours. If additional delay occurs, the serum should be frozen at −18° C or below. Frozen serum should be thawed rapidly at 37° C.

PRELIMINARY SPECIMEN PREPARATION. Serum must be at room temperature. Prepare a 1:5 dilution of patient serum by pipetting 0.1 mL of serum into a test tube and adding 0.4 mL of the commercially prepared glycine-saline buffer diluent. Mix the contents thoroughly.

REAGENTS, SUPPLIES, AND EQUIPMENT

The following components are commercially available in kit form, such as the ICL RA Kit:

1. Latex reagent with dropper assembly. This is a suspension of stabilized polystyrene latex particles coated with human albumin and chemically bonded with denatured human gamma globulin. *Note:* Store at 2° to 8° C. *Do not freeze latex reagent.*

   Properly stored reagent is stable until expiration date indicated on the label. Reagent that does not produce appropriate quality control results should be discarded after verification by repeat testing.
2. Glycine-saline buffer (pH 8.2 =/− 0.1)
   Note: Store at 2° to 8° C. Properly stored reagent is stable until expiration date indicated on the label. Reagent that does not produce appropriate quality control results should be discarded after verification by repeat testing. Discard if contaminated, i.e., evidence of cloudiness or particulate material in solution.
3. Capillary pipettes
4. Applicator sticks
5. Glass slide

Additional required equipment and supplies:

1. Stopwatch or timer
2. 12 × 75 mm test tubes
3. Serologic pipettes (1 mL graduated) and safety pipettor
4. Light source

QUALITY CONTROL

Positive Control Serum (human). This prediluted serum is provided in the ICL RA Kit. The value of the control in International Units/mL (IU/mL) is printed on the vial label and is established by comparison to a reference preparation that was calibrated using the World Health Organization International Reference Preparation of Rheumatoid Arthritis Serum. The positive control should not be used as a standard for titration because the predilution varies from lot to lot. Store at 2° to 8° C.

Note: Failure to observe a positive reaction (agglutination) with this serum is indicative of deterioration of the latex reagent and/or positive control.

Negative control serum (human). This prediluted serum is provided in the ICL CRP Kit. Store at 2° to 8° C.

Note: A smooth reaction must be observed with the negative control. If agglutination is exhibited with this control, the test should be repeated. If repeat testing produces the same results, the reagents should be replaced.

A positive and negative control must be tested with each unknown patient specimen. *Caution:* Because the control sera are derived from human sources, they should be handled in the same manner as clinical serum specimens (see *Universal blood and body fluid precautions* in Chapter 6).

PROCEDURE

Note: All reagents and specimens must be at room temperature prior to testing.

QUALITATIVE SLIDE TEST

1. Prepare a 1:20 dilution of patient serum in glycine saline buffer, i.e., 0.1 mL of serum and 1.9 mL of diluent, and thoroughly mix the tube contents.
2. Using one of the capillary pipettes provided, fill approximately two thirds of the pipette with diluted serum. Deliver 1 free falling drop of the diluted serum from the perpendicularly held pipette to the center of one of the oval divisions of the slide.
3. Add 1 drop of positive control and 1 drop of negative control to the appropriately labeled divisions of the slide.
4. Mix the latex reagent and add 1 drop of reagent to the patient specimen and to each of the controls.
5. Mix each specimen with a separate applicator stick. All the contents of the mixtures are to spread evenly over the entire area of their respective division on the slide.
6. Tilt the slide back and forth, slowly and evenly, for 2 minutes.
7. Place the slide on a flat surface and observe immediately for macroscopic agglutination, using a direct light source.

Warning: The latex reagent, controls, and buffer contain 0.1% sodium azide as a preservative. Sodium azide may react with lead and copper plumbing to form highly explosive metal azides. Upon disposal, flush with a large volume of water to prevent azide buildup.

REPORTING RESULTS

Positive Reaction: Agglutination of the latex suspension is a positive result that indicates the presence of rheumatoid factor (RF) in the specimen.

Negative Reaction: The absence of visible agglutination and the presence of opaque fluid constitutes a negative reaction.

PROCEDURE NOTES

Latex slide and tube tests demonstrate slightly greater sensitivity than sensitized sheep cells. The specificity of latex tube tests is comparable to sensitized sheep cell procedures.

Specimen collection and handling are important to the quality of the test. Strict adherence must be paid to technique with a special emphasis on drop size, complete mixing, reaction time, and temperature of reagents.

The strength of a positive reaction may be graded as follows:

1+ Very small clumping with an opaque fluid background

2+ Small clumping with slightly opaque fluid in the background

3+ Moderate clumping with fairly clear fluid in the background

4+ Large clumping with a clear fluid background

It is recommended that a quantitative titer be established for all RA positive samples.

QUANTITATIVE TUBE TEST. If a patient serum exhibits a positive reaction, the serum may be serially diluted with glycine-saline buffer to determine a quantitative estimate of the RA level.

1. Label 10 12 × 75 mm test tubes (1 to 10) for the reference preparation. *Note:* The reference preparation is to be used to establish a unit value in International Units (IU/mL) for quantitative determinations of serum specimens. The value assigned to the RA Reference Preparation is derived from the World Health Organization International Reference Preparation of Rheumatoid Arthritis Serum.

2. Label 10 12 × 75 mm test tubes (1 to 10) for the patient serum.

3. Pipette 1.9 mL of glycine-saline buffer diluent into the first tube of each set of tubes.

4. Pipette 1.0 mL of glycine-saline buffer diluent into the each of the remaining tubes in each set.

5. Pipette 0.1 mL of the reference preparation to the first tube of the reference set of tubes. Mix and transfer 1.0 mL from tube 1 to tube 2 and continue this procedure through tube 9. Mix and discard 1.0 mL of the dilution from tube 9. Tube 10 is a reagent negative control.

6. Pipette 0.1 mL of the patient serum to the first tube of the reference set of tubes. Mix and transfer 1.0 mL from tube 1 to tube 2 and continue this procedure through tube 10. Mix and discard 1.0 mL of the dilution from tube 10.

CONCENTRATION OF DILUTIONS

Tube Number	Dilution
1	1:20
2	1:40
3	1:80
4	1:160
5	1:320
6	1:640
7	1:1280
8	1:2560
9	1:5120
10	1:10,240 (patient specimen only)

7. To each tube of both sets of tubes, add 1 drop of well-mixed latex reagent.

8. Mix all tubes thoroughly and incubate at 37° C for 15 minutes.

9. Following incubation, centrifuge all tubes at 600-900 rcf for 2 minutes, or for 5 to 10 minutes at a lower rcf. The rcf can be calculated by using the following formula:

$$rcf = 28.38 \ (R) \left(\frac{N}{1000}\right)2$$

R = radius of rotor in inches

N = revolutions per minute

10. Gently shake each tube to resuspend the precipitate until an even suspension is achieved. Examine each tube for the presence of macroscopic agglutination by observing against a dark or back background under an oblique light.

In reporting results as a titer, use the same lot of latex reagent to establish the titer range. Any change in the reagent lot will necessitate re-establishment of the titer in order to be assured of reproducible results. It is necessary to run the RA reference preparation only once with each series of specimens.

CALCULATIONS. To calculate the results of the quantitative method in International Units (IU/mL) based on the value of a reference preparation, the following formula is used.

IU/mL of patient's serum =

$$\frac{IU/mL \text{ of RA reference} \times \text{titer of patient's serum}}{\text{titer of RA reference}}$$

EXAMPLE:

If the IU/mL value of the RA reference preparation is 1000 IU/mL and the last tube to demonstrate agglutination in the serial dilution was tube 6 (dilution 1:640), the IU/mL of the patient's serum that exhibited agglutination up to tube 5 (dilution 1:320) is calculated as follows:

$$\text{IU/mL of patient's serum} = \frac{1000 \times 320}{640}$$

$$= 500 \text{ IU/mL}$$

REPORTING RESULTS. Titers of less than 1:20 are considered to be negative for rheumatoid factors. Positive reactions have been shown to be present in RA patients with titers ranging from 1:20 to 1:40,950.

SOURCES OF ERROR. **False positive** results may be observed if serum specimens are lipemic, hemolyzed, or heavily contaminated with bacteria. If the reaction time is longer than 2 minutes, a false positive result may also be produced due to a drying effect.

False negative results may be observed in undiluted serum specimens because of high levels of CRP (antigen excess). A 1:5 dilution of serum is also tested for this reason. Under these testing conditions there is a low probability of false negatives.

CLINICAL APPLICATIONS. Although the latex agglutination procedure has a 95% correlation with a clinical diagnosis of probable or definite rheumatoid arthritis, rheumatoid factor is not exclusively limited to patients with rheumatoid arthritis. Biological false positives can be manifested by disorders such as lupus erythematosus, Sjögren's syndrome, syphilis, and hepatitis. A low rate of positive reactions have been observed in abnormalities such as periarteritis nodosa, rheumatic fever, osteoarthritis, tuberculosis, cancer, some diseases of viral origin, osteoarthrosis, arthritis type undetermined, myositis, and polymyalgia rheumatica.

LIMITATIONS.

1. Parallel titrations must be performed under similar conditions. Variations in any one set of titrations may affect the values obtained.
2. Since tube dilution methods are more sensitive than slide methods, there is a possibility of differences between slide qualitative tests. Use of the RA reference preparation will compensate for this difference by standardizing the test results through the assignment of IU/mL to each specimen.

REFERENCES

Jones WL and Wiggins GL: A study of rheumatoid arthritis latex kits, Amer J Clin Pathol 60:703-706, 1973.

Galen RS and Gambino SR: Beyond normality: the predictive value and efficiency of medical diagnosis, New York, 1975, John Wiley & Sons, pp 9-14.

Mackay IR and Burnett FM, editors: Autoimmune disease: serologic reactions in rheumatoid arthritis, Springfield, Ill, 1964, Charles C Thomas, Publisher, pp 138-143.

Rheuma-Fac Rheumatoid Arthritis Test (Latex) Product Insert, ICL Scientific, Fountain Valley, Calif, July 1987

Singer JM, Plotz CM, and Goldberg R: The detection of antiglobulin factors utilizing pre-coated latex particles, Arth Rheum 8:194-201, 1965.

Quantitative Determination of IgM Rheumatoid Factor in Human Serum

☐ PROCEDURE*

PRINCIPLE

The following procedure is an indirect enzyme-labeled immunoassay using microwells as a solid phase. Human immunoglobulin G (IgG) is coated onto wells of microplates. Diluted test samples are added to the coated wells and incubated. During incubation, rheumatoid factor present in the sample will bind to the IgG-coated well. After washing to remove unbound material, antibodies to human IgM labeled with alkaline phosphatase (conjugate) are added. The conjugate binds to the rheumatoid factor bound to IgG. The well is washed to remove unbound conjugate and incubated with p-nitrophenyl phosphate. The p-nitrophenyl phosphate is hydrolyzed by alkaline phosphatase to form p-nitrophenol, a yellow-colored end product with absorbance maximum at 405 nm. The intensity of absorbance at 405 nm is proportional to the amount of IgM rheumatoid factor present in the specimen. Results are reported in international units (IU/mL) standard to the World Health Organization (WHO).

Establishing the presence of rheumatoid factor is useful in supporting the differential diagnosis of rheumatoid arthritis from other chronic inflammatory arthritides. The frequency of IgM rheumatoid factor is 70% to 80% in patients with clinical features of rheumatoid arthritis. Determination of rheumatoid factor is also important in the prognosis and therapeutic management of this disease. Rheumatoid factor, however, has been associated with some bacterial and viral infections, such as hepatitis and infectious mononucleosis and some chronic infections such as tuberculosis, parasitic disease, subacute bacterial endocarditis, and cancer. Elevated values may also be observed in the normal elderly population.

SPECIMEN COLLECTION AND PREPARATION

No special preparation of the patient is required prior to specimen collection. The patient must be positively identified when the specimen is collected and the specimen is to be labeled at the bedside. Specimen labels must include the patient's full name, the date the specimen is collected, the patient's hospital identification number, and the phlebotomist's initials.

Blood should be drawn by an aseptic technique. A minimum of 2 mL of clotted blood (red-top evacuated tube) is required. The specimen should be centrifuged promptly and an aliquot of serum removed.

*Modified from Sigma Diagnostics Product Brochure, Procedure No. SIA 107.

If the test cannot be performed immediately, the specimen should be refrigerated (2° to 8° C) for no longer than 72 hours. If additional delay occurs, the serum should be frozen at −20° C or below. Frozen serum should be thawed rapidly at 37° C. Specimens containing visible particulate matter should be clarified by centrifugation prior to testing. The serum sample should not be heat-inactivated prior to testing.

REAGENTS, SUPPLIES, AND EQUIPMENT

SIA Rheumatoid Factor Kit Reagents available commercially from Sigma Chemical Co, St. Louis, Mo.

Note: Store reagents at 2° to 6° C. The reagents are stable until the expiration date on the label.

1. Antigen wells. Microplate wells coated with human IgG. Store antigen wells with dessicant in the reusable plastic bag. Reseal the bag after opening.
2. Holder for wells.
3. Sample dilutent. Buffered protein solution containing surfactant and blue dye, pH 7.5. Contains 0.1% sodium azide as a preservative.
4. Calibrator. Human serum containing IgM rheumatoid factor. Content (IU/mL) indicated on the label. This constituent contains 0.1% sodium azide as a preservative.
5. Conjugate. Goat antibodies to human IgM labeled with calf alkaline phosphatase. This solution contains a pink dye and 0.02% sodium azide as a preservative.
6. Substrate. Contains *p*-nitrophenyl phosphate, disodium, hexahydrate 1 mg/mL, pH 9.6. The substrate may develop a slight yellow color upon storage. Do not use if absorbance of the undiluted substrate is greater than 0.4 at 405 nm when measured against water using a microplate reader or a spectrophotometer with a 1-cm lightpath.
7. Wash concentrate. Buffer solution concentrate with surfactant. This solution contains 0.1% sodium azide as a preservative. The wash solution is prepared by adding the contents of wash concentrate bottle to 1 liter of deionized water. Mix well.
8. Stop solution. This is an alkaline solution pH 12.0. Store at room temperature. Reagent is stable until expiration date on the label. *Warning:* Stop solution causes irritation. Avoid contact with eyes, skin, and clothing. Avoid breathing vapor. Wash thoroughly after handling.

Note: Do not interchange reagents from different lots.

Warning: The latex reagent, controls, and buffer contain 0.1% sodium azide as a preservative. Sodium azide may react with lead and copper plumbing to form highly explosive metal azides. Upon disposal, flush with a large volume of water to prevent azide buildup. Sodium azide is also toxic. Care should be taken to avoid ingestion.

Additional required supplies and equipment:

1. Spectrophotometer or microplate reader capable of accurately measuring absorbance at 405 nm
2. Pipetting device for the accurate delivery of volumes required for the assay
3. Timer
4. 1-liter measuring cylinder
5. Squeeze bottle for dispensing wash solution
6. Dilution plates or tubes
7. Test tubes or cuvettes, 1.0 mL

QUALITY CONTROL

Positive control. Human serum containing IgM rheumatoid factor. Content (IU/mL) indicated on the label. This serum contains 0.1% sodium azide.

Negative control. Human serum containing no detectable IgM rheumatoid factor. This serum contains 0.1% sodium azide.

Caution: Because the antigen wells and control and calibrator sera are derived from human sources, it should be handled in the same manner as clinical serum specimens (see *Universal blood and body fluid precautions* in Chapter 6).

PROCEDURE

1. Dilute calibrator, positive and negative controls, and test samples by combining 2 μL of each of with 200 μL sample diluent in labeled tubes or dilution plates.
2. Place the desired number of antigen wells in holder.
3. Using a pipette tip, mix the samples and diluent by drawing up and expelling 2 or 3 times. Transfer 100 μL of each diluted sample to the appropriate antigen well.
4. Include one well that contains only 100 μL sample diluent. This serves as the reagent blank and is used to zero the photometer.
5. Allow the plate to stand at room temperature (18° to 26° C) for 20 +/− 2 minutes.
6. Shake out or aspirate contents of wells. Wash wells by filling them with wash solution from a squeeze bottle and shaking out or aspirating. Wash 3 times. Drain wells on paper towel to remove excess fluid.

Note: Thorough washing is necessary to achieve accurate results. Avoid bubbles.

7. Place 2 drops (or 100 μL) conjugate into each well, including the reagent blank well.
8. Allow to stand at room temperature (18° to 26° C) for 20 minutes +/− 2 minutes.
9. Wash wells by repeating step 6.
10. Place 2 drops (or 100 μL) substrate into each well, including the reagent blank well.
11. Allow to stand at room temperature (18° to 26° C) for 20 minutes +/− 2 minutes.
12. Place 2 drops (or 100 μL) stop solution into each well.
13. Read and record absorbance of each test at 405 nm within 2 hours after reacton has been stopped.

MICROPLATE READER. Set absorbance at 405 nm to zero with water as a reference. Read and record absorbance of reagent blank (A blank). Then set absorbance to zero with a reagent blank as a reference. Read and record absorbance of samples (A sample) and calibrator (A calibrator).

SPECTROPHOTOMETER. Completely remove contents of each well and transfer to cuvette or test tube. Add 800 µL of deionized water to each sample and mix. Set absorbance at 405 nm to zero with water as a reference. Read and record the absorbance of each sample including the reagent blank. Subtract the absorbance of the reagent blank for absorbance of each sample.

CALCULATION

IgM rheumatoid factor concentration

(IU/mL) in specimen

$$= \frac{A \text{ sample}}{A \text{ calibrator}} \times \text{IU/mL of calibrator}$$

EXAMPLE:
Absorbance Measured Using a Microplate Reader

A sample = 1.292

A calibrator = 1.823

IU/mL of calibrator = 106

IgM Rheumatoid factor concentration

(IU/mL) in sample $= \frac{1.292}{1.823} \times 106 = 75$

Absorbance Measured Using a Spectrophotometer

A blank = 0.074

A sample = 0.570

A calibrator = 0.829

A sample − A blank = 0.570 − 0.074 = 0.496

A calibrator − A blank = 0.829 − 0.074 = 0.755

IU/mL of calibrator = 106

IgM Rheumatoid factor concentration (IU/mL) in

sample $= \frac{0.496}{0.775} \times 106 = 68$

REPORTING RESULTS

Reference ranges should be established by each laboratory to reflect the characteristics of the populations of the area in which it is located.

IgM rheumatoid factor value

(IU/mL)	Interpretation
< 20	Negative for IgM rheumatoid factor
> 20	Positive for IgM rheumatoid factor
>60	Indicative of rheumatoid arthritis

PROCEDURE NOTES

Specimens giving absorbance values above that of the calibrator should be diluted appropriately with sample diluent and reassayed. The value obtained should be multiplied by the dilution factor.

SOURCES OF ERROR. Biologic false positive results may be manifested in a variety of disorders, such as systemic lupus erythematosus (SLE).

The absorbance values will vary with room temperature and incubation time. The absorbance value of the reagent blank when read against water at 405 nm should be less than 0.4 using a microplate reader, or less than 0.09 using a spectrophotometer with a 1-cm lightpath. The absorbance value of the calibrator should be greater than or equal to 0.5 using a microplate reader when the assay is performed at 22° C. The assay value (IU/mL) of the positive control should be within the range shown on label. The negative control should be less than 15 IU/mL. If these requirements are not satisfied, test results may be inaccurate and the assay should be repeated.

CLINICAL APPLICATIONS. Determination of the presence of rheumatoid factor is important to physicians in the diagnosis, prognosis, and therapeutic management of patients with rheumatoid arthritis.

LIMITATIONS. The results obtained with the assay should serve only as an aid to diagnosis and should not be interpreted as diagnostic in itself.

REFERENCES

Borque L et al: Turbidimetry of rheumatoid factor in serum with a centrifugal analyzer, Clin Chem 32:124, 1986.

Holborow EJ: Autoantibodies in the rheumatic diseases, In Scott JT, editor: Copeman's textbook of the rheumatic diseases, ed 6, New York, 1986, Churchill Livingstone, Inc, pp 355-375.

Linker JB III and Williams Jr RC: Tests for detection of rheumatoid factors, In Rose NR, Friedman H, and Fahey JL, editors: Manual of clinical laboratory immunology, ed 3, Washington, DC, 1986, American Society for Microbiology, pp 759-761.

Sigma Diagnostics Product Brochure, SIA Rheumatoid Factor, 1987 St Louis, Mo.

Wernick R et al: IgG and IgM rheumatoid factors in rheumatoid arthritis: quantitative response to penicillamine therapy and relationship to disease activity, Arthritis Rheum 26:593, 1983.

Chapter Review

HIGHLIGHTS

Evidence exists that immunologic factors are involved in both the articular and extra-articular manifestations of the disease rheumatoid arthritis (RA). RA may represent an unusual host response to one or perhaps many etiologic agents. An infectious etiology is possible. RA is a chronic, usually progressive inflammatory disorder of the joints. It is, however, a highly variable disease that ranges from a mild illness of brief duration to a progressive, destructive polyarthritis associated with a systemic vasculitis.

Two pathogenic mechanisms have been hypothesized in RA. The extravascular immune complex hypothesis proposes an interaction of antigens and antibodies in synovial tissues and fluid. The alternate hypothesis is that RA results from cell-mediated damage because of the accumulation of lymphocytes, primarily T cells, in the rheumatoid synovium, resembling a delayed-type hypersensitivity reaction. The presence of lymphokines, which effect both articular inflammation and destruction, supports this hypothesis.

If the rheumatoid synovium is examined by an immunofluorescent technique, it can be seen to contain large amounts of IgG and IgM, alone or together. Immunoglobulins can also be observed in synovial lining cells, blood vessels, and in the interstitial connective tissues. B cells make immunoglobulin in the synovium of patients with RA. As many as half of the plasma cells that can be located in the synovium secrete an IgG rheumatoid factor that combines in the cytoplasm with similar IgG molecules (self-associating IgG). The cause of the various vascular and parenchymal lesions of RA suggests that the lesions result from injury induced by immune complexes, especially those containing antibodies to IgG. The serum of most patients with RA has detectable soluble immune complexes. Anti-gamma globulins of the IgG and IgM classes are an integral part of these complexes. Rheumatoid factor belongs to a larger family of antiglobulins that are usually defined as antibodies with specifity for antigen determinants on the Fc fragment of human or certain animal IgG. Rheumatoid factors have been associated with three major immunoglobulin classes: IgM, IgG, and IgA.

Juvenile rheumatoid arthritis (JRA) is a condition of chronic synovitis, beginning during childhood. The etiologic hypotheses are similar to those proposed for adult RA.

REVIEW QUESTIONS

1. Rheumatoid arthritis most frequently develops in:
   A. Adolescent females
   B. Adolescent males
   C. Middle-aged females
   D. Middle-aged males
   E. Elderly females and males
2. Rheumatoid factor is defined as:
   A. Antigens with specificity for antibody determinants on the Fc fragment of human or certain animal IgG

   B. Antibodies with specificity for antigen determinants on the Fc fragment of human or certain animal IgG
   C. Antigens with specificity for antibody determinants on the Fc fragment of human or certain animal IgD
   D. Antibodies with specificity for antigen determinants on the Fc fragment of human or certain animal IgD
   E. Antibodies with specificity for antigen determinants on the Fc fragment of human or certain animal IgE

3. and 4. The principle of the latex agglutination test is based on the reaction of patient ____(3)____ and ____(4)____ derived from gamma globulin.

(3).		(4).	
A.	Antigen	A.	Antigen
B.	Antibody	B.	Antibody
C.	Complement levels	C.	Complement levels
D.	Leukocytes	D.	Leukocytes
E.	Serum	E.	Serum

Answers

1. C   2. B   3. B   4. A

BIBLIOGRAPHY

Ashman RF: Rheumatic disease. In Lawlor GJ and Fischer TJ, editors: Manual of allergy and immunology, ed 2, Boston, 1988, Little, Brown & Co, Inc, pp 284-285.

Borque L et al: Turbidimetry of rheumatoid factor in serum with a centrifugal analyzer, Clin Chem 32:124, 1986.

Galen RS and Gambino SR: Beyond normality: the predictive value and efficiency of medical diagnosis, New York, 1975, John Wiley & Sons, pp 9-14.

Holborow EJ: Autoantibodies in the rheumatic diseases. In Scott JT, editor: Copeman's textbook of the rheumatic diseases, ed 6, New York, 1986, Churchill Livingstone, Inc, pp 355-375.

Jones WL and Wiggins GL: A study of rheumatoid arthritis latex kits, Am J Clin Pathol 60:703-706, 1973.

Linker JB III and Williams RC Jr: Tests for detection of rheumatoid factors. In Rose NR, Friedman H, and Fahey JL, editors: Manual of clinical laboratory immunology, ed 3, Washington, DC, 1986, American Society for Microbiology, pp 759-761.

Mackay IR and Burnett FM, editors: Autoimmune disease: serologic reactions in rheumatoid arthritis, pp 138-143, Springfield, Ill, 1964, Charles C Thomas, Publisher.

Rheuma-Fac Rheumatoid Arthritis Test (Latex) Product Insert, ICL Scientific, Fountain Valley, Calif, July 1987.

Sigma Diagnostics Product Brochure, SIA rheumatoid factor, St Louis, Mo., 1987.

Singer JM, Plotz CM, and Goldberg R: The detection of antiglobulin factors utilizing precoated latex particles, Arthritis Rheum 8:194-201, 1965.

Wernick R et al: IgG and IgM rheumatoid factors in rheumatoid arthritis: quantitative response to penicillamine therapy and relationship to disease activity, Arthritis Rheum 26:593, 1983.

Zvaiflere NJ: In Stein J, editor: Evaluation of joint complaints. In Internal medicine, Boston, 1987, Little, Brown & Co, Inc, pp 1251-1264.

CHAPTER 28

Transplantation and Tumor Immunology

INTRODUCTION

At the present time a variety of tissues and organs are transplanted in humans, including bone marrow, bone matrix, skin, kidneys, liver, cardiac valves, heart, pancreas, corneas, and lungs. Transplantation is one of the areas in addition to hypersensitivity (see Chapter 23) and auto-immunity (see Chapter 25) in which the immune system functions in a detrimental way.

Early in the history of transplantation, tissue antigens were recognized as important to successful grafting. If significantly different foreign antigens were introduced into an immunocompetent host, the transplanted tissue or organ would undoubtedly fail. Today, tissue (histocompatibility) matching with concomitant immunosuppression of the host in many cases is used to enhance the probability of success in organ and tissue transplantation.

HISTOCOMPATIBILITY ANTIGENS
General Characteristics

All vertebrates capable of acute rejection of foreign skin grafts possess a localized complex involving-

many genes that exerts major control over the organism's immune reactions. Many nucleated cells possess cell-surface-protein antigens, which are part of this complex that readily provokes an immune response if transferred into a genetically different (allogeneic) individual of the same species. Some of these antigens are much more potent than others in provoking an immune response and are, therefore, called the *major histocompatibility complex (MHC)*.

In humans, the MHC is referred to as *human leukocyte antigen* (HLA). It is the most complex immunogenetic system presently known in man and is controlled by a MHC, or supergene, which includes several loci closely linked on the short arm of chromosome 6. Each of these loci involves numerous alleles having at least 10 to 40 alleles per locus that control the production of their corresponding antigens. The MHC is divided into four major regions: D, B, C, and A. The A, B, and C regions code for class I molecules, whereas the D region codes for class II molecules.

Class I includes the main HLA-A, B, and C antigens. The three principle loci A, B, and C, and their respective antigens are numbered 1, 2, 3, etc. The three specificities of class I are composed of a single heavy chain and a light chain, β-2 microglobulin, which is controlled by a gene on chromosome 15. The class II gene region antigens are encoded in the HLA-D region and can be subdivided into three families, HLA-DR, -DC(DQ), and -SB(DP).

Multiple alleles occur at each locus and are followed by an Arabic number, e.g., HLA-A1 or HLA-B27. If there is not yet collective agreement, the number of the allele is preceded by a "w," e.g., HLA-A2 (w69) or HLA-Cw7. Genes of class I, II, and III antigens at each locus are inherited as codominant alleles. Inheritance within families closely follows simple Mendelian dominant characteristics. Conservation of entire haplotypes through generation after generation is the general rule. Very strong linkage disequilbrium is displayed between several HLA loci, creating super or extended haplotypes that may differ from race to race. For example, the most frequent Caucasoid superextended haplotype, AL, Xw7, BB, BfS, C2-1, C4AQOB1, DR3, is virtually absent in Orientals.

The class I major transplantation antigens have been serologically defined. Class I and class II antigens can be found on body cells (Table 28-1) and in body fluids. Class I and class II molecules are surface membrane proteins. Class I molecules are transmembrane glycoproteins, but the class II dimer molecule differs from class I in that both dimers span the cell membrane. Class I and class II gene products are biochemically distinct, although they appear to be distantly related through evolution. Class III gene products, such as C2, C4A, C4B, and Bf complement components, are incomplete; but these structures are defined by genes lying between or very near the HLA-B and -DR loci.

The Role of MHC/HLA

The histocompatibility complex that encodes cell surface antigens was first discovered in graft rejection experiments with mice. When the antigens were matched between donor and recipient, the ability of a graft to survive was remarkably improved. A comparable genetic system of alloantigens was subsequently identified in man. The presence of HLA was first recognized when multiply transfused patients experienced transfusion reactions despite proper crossmatching. It was discovered that these reactions resulted from leukocytes' antibodies rather than antibodies directed against erythrocyte antigens. These same antibodies were subsequently discovered in the sera of multiparous women.

The MHC gene products have an important role in clinical immunology. For example, tranplants are rejected if performed against MHC barriers, thus immunosuppressive therapy is required. These antigens are of primary importance and are second only to the ABO antigens in influencing the genetic basis of survival or rejection of transplanted organs.

TABLE 28-1

Expression of HLA Antigens on Surface Membranes

Class I	
Not expressed	Erythrocytes, corneal endothelium, villus of trophoblast, exocrine pancreas, patoid acinar cells, and some duodenal Bruner's glands
Weakly expressed	Endocrine thyroid, parathyroid, pituitary, pancreatic islet cells, myocardial, skeletal muscle, gastric mucosa, and mature granulocytes
Variably expressed	Hepatocytes
Expressed	All other body cells
Class II	
Not expressed	Erythrocytes; all resting endocrine cells; hepatocytes and biliary epithelium; myocardial, skeletal, and smooth muscle cells; epithelial cells of the esophagus; stomach; Brunner's glands; colon and rectum; parotid acinar and ductal epithelium; spermatozoa; bladder; prostate and ureter epithelium; neurons; platelets; mature granulocytes; and resting T cells
Expressed	B cells, activated T cells, and immature granulocytes; epithelium of the epiglottis; trachea, tonsils, and epididymis; renal glomeruli and tubules; dura; Langerhans cell; skin; dendritic cells; and epithelial cells of the deeper layers of the duodenum, ileum, and appendix
HLA-DR expressed	Monocytes, macrophages, and vascular endothelial cells
HLA-DQ weakly expressed or absent	

From Thompson J: The human leukocyte antigen system. In Stein J, editor: Internal medicine, ed 2, Boston, 1987, Little, Brown & Co.

Although HLA was originally identified by its role in transplant rejection, it is now recognized that the products of HLA genes play a crucial role in our immune system. T cells do not recognize antigens directly but do so when the antigen is presented on the surface of an antigen-presenting cell, the macrophage. In addition to presentation of the antigen, the macrophage must present another molecule for this response to occur. This molecule is a cell-surface glycoprotein that is coded in each species by the MHC. T cells are able to interact with the histocompatibility molecules only if they are genetically identical (MHC restriction).

Both class I and class II antigens function as targets of T lymphocytes that regulate the immune response. Class I molecules regulate interaction between cytolytic T cells and target cells, and class II molecules restrict the activity of regulatory T cells (helper, suppressor, and amplifier subsets). Hence, class II molecules regulate the interaction between helper T cells and antigen-presenting cells. Cytotoxic T cells directed against class I antigens are inhibited by OKT8 cells; cytotoxic T cells directed against class II antigens are inhibited by OKT4 cells. Many of the genes in both class I and class II gene families have no known functions.

Class III molecules bear no clear relation to class I and II molecules aside from their genetic linkage (the presence of the gene in or near the MHC complex). Class III molecules are involved in immunologic phenomenon because they represent components of the complement pathways.

HLA Applications

HLA matching is of value in organ transplantation as well as in the transplantation of bone marrow. In kidney allografts, the method of organ preservation, time elapsed between harvesting and transplanting, the number of pretransplantation blood transfusions, recipient age, and primary cause for kidney failure are all important determinants of early transplant success or failure. HLA compatibility, however, exerts the strongest influence on long-term kidney survival. The one-year survival for kidneys transplanted from an HLA identical sibling approaches 95%. Approximately 50% to 65% of cadaver kidneys that are mismatched for all four HLA-A and B antigens function for 6 months but deteriorate thereafter with time. Only 15% to 25% of these mismatched cadaver kidneys remain functioning 4 years after transplantation.

It is obligatory to select HLA identical donors for bone marrow transplantation to reduce the frequency of graft versus host disease (GVHD) (discussed later in this chapter). A new method, however, that depletes donor marrow T cells capable of recognizing foreign host antigens has markedly reduced the incidence of GVHD.

HLA matched platelets are useful to patients who are refractile to random donor platelets. In paternity testing, HLA typing, along with the determination of ABO, Rh, MNSs, Kell, Duffy, and Kidd erythrocyte antigen, is used. In the past, most laboratories involved in testing individuals in disputed parentage cases used only the ABO, Rh, and MNSs systems. The chances of identifying a falsely accused man with these tests was 58%. Additional testing for Kell, Duffy, Kidd erythrocyte antigens, and HLA typing offers an exclusion rate estimated at 92%.

HLA typing is also useful in forensic medicine, anthropology, and basic research in immunology. In studies of racial ancestry and migration, some antigens are virtually excluded or confirmed to a

Relationship of Certain HLA Antigens and Disease

Ankylosing spondylitis	B27
Reiter's syndrome	B27
Psoriasis vulgaris	Cw6
Rheumatoid arthritis	DR4
Behçet's disease	B5 (Bw51)
Type I diabetes	DR3
Gold-induced nephropathy	DR5
Congenital adrenal hyperplasia	B47
Chronic lymphatic leukemia	DR 5
Kaposi's sarcoma (Mediterranean)	DR5

From Thompson J: The human leukocyte antigen system. In Stein J, editor: Internal medicine, ed 2, Boston, 1987, Little, Brown & Co.

race, e.g., A1 and B8 are rarely detected in Mongoloids and Bw57 is uncommon in whites and blacks. These distinctions allow for precise conclusions to be drawn regarding origin and ancestry.

HLA testing is increasingly being used as a diagnostic and genetic counseling tool. Knowledge of HLA antigens and their linkage is becoming important because of the recognized association of certain antigens (see box) with distinct immunologic mediated reaction, autoimmune diseases, some neoplasms, and other disorders which, although nonimmunologic, are influenced by non-HLA genes also located within the major MHC region.

The estimated relative risks or chances of developing a disease if a given antigen is present (Table 28-2) may be elevated in individuals bearing certain HLA antigens compared to individuals who lack the antigen. The HLA-B27 antigen, however, is the only HLA antigen with a disease association strong enough to be useful in differential diagnosis. Although the degree of association between HLA antigens and other diseases may be statistically significant, it is not strong enough to be of diagnostic or prognostic value.

Although only 8% of normal whites carry HLA-B27 antigen, 90% of patients with either ankylosing spondylitis (AS) or spondylitis in association with Reiter's syndrome are positive for the antigen. An elevated percentage of HLA-B27 positive patients is also observed in juvenile chronic arthritis with spinal involvement. Therefore, the major indication for screening for HLA-B27 test is to rule out AS when back pain develops in relatives of patients with the disease and to help to distinguish incomplete Reiter's syndrome from gonoccocal arthritis, or chronic or atypical Reiter's syndrome from rheumatoid arthritis. A negative test for HLA-B27, however, does not exclude the diagnosis of AS or Reiter's syndrome.

Methods of Detection

Because different individuals in a species carry different HLA antigens on their cell surfaces, introduction of foreign antigens can stimulate T cells.

TABLE 28-2

Relationship of HLA Antigens to Risk of Disease

Antigen present	Related disease	Increased risk of developing the disease over a lifetime (×-times)
B27	Ankylosing spondylitis	100× *
	Reiter's syndrome	40×
	Anterior uveitis	25×
	Arthritic infection with *Yersinia* or *Salmonella*	20×
	Psoriatic arthritis with spinal involvement	11×
	Spondylitis associated with inflammatory bowel disease	9×
	Juvenile chronic arthritis with spinal involvement	5×
B8	Celiac disease	9×
	Addison's disease	6×
	Myasthenia gravis	5×
	Dermatitis herpetiformis	4×
	Chronic active hepatitis	4×
	Sjögren's syndrome	3×
	Diabetes mellitus (insulin dependent)	2×
	Thyrotoxicosis	2×
B5	Behcet's syndrome	6×
BW 38	Psoriatic arthritis	7×
BW 15	Diabetes mellitus (insulin dependent)	3×
DR2	Goodpasture's syndrome	16×
	Multiple sclerosis	4×
DR3	Gluten-sensitive enteropathy	21×
	Dermatitis herpetiformis	14×
	Subacute cutaneous lupus erythematosus	12×
	Addison's disease	11×
	Sjögren's syndrome (primary)	10×
DR4	Pemphigus[†]	32×
	Giant-cell arthritis	8×
	Rheumatoid arthritis	6×
	Juvenile diabetes mellitus	5×
DR5	Pauciarticular juvenile arthritis	5×
	Scleroderma	5×
	Hashimoto's thyroiditis	3×

*Varies with ethnic group, e.g., 3× for Pima Indians and 300× for Japanese

[†]In Jewish persons

From Ashman RF: Rheumatic diseases. In Lawlor GJ and Fischer TJ, editors: Manual of allergy and immunology, ed 2, Boston, 1988, Little, Brown & Co.

These T cells are prominently implicated in graft rejection, and they can also stimulate antibody formation under certain circumstances. Human sera containing these antibodies can be obtained from some multiply transfused patients or multiparous women for use as reagents to detect different HLA antigens.

Class I antigens are determined by several techniques; the most popular and reproducible method is the lymphocyte microcytotoxicity method (complement-mediated cytoxicity). With this technique, a battery of reagent antisera and isolated target cells are incubated with a source of complement under oil to prevent evaporation. If a specific alloantibody and cell membrane antigen combine, complement-mediated damage to the cell wall allows for penetration of a vital dye and the cells are killed. Cell death is determined by staining. A stain such as trypan blue will penetrate dead cells but not living ones. Unaffected cells remain brilliantly refractile when observed microscopically. Other methods of analysis include leukocyte agglutination and complement fixation on platelets in suspension.

Class II HLA-DR and HLA-DQ specificities are also recognized by similar serologic methods, except that isolated B cells are the usual target cells because their surface is rich in these molecules as well as class I determinants. At the present time, HLA-Dw and -DP cannot be serologically defined, and their detection relies on the ability of these molecules to stimulate newly synthesized DNA when added to primary mixed lymphocyte (HLA-Dw) or when re-added to secondary primary lymphocyte (HLA-DP) in vitro cultures. Class III complement specificities are recognized by the availability of diagnostic reagents, but reagents remain scarce.

TABLE 28-3

Transplantation Terms

Term	Definition
Autograft	Graft transferred from one position to another in the same individual, e.g., skin, hair, bone
Syngraft	Graft transplanted between different but identical recipient and donor, e.g., kidney transplant between monozygous twins
Allograft (homograft)	Graft between genetically different recipient and donor of the same species; the grafted donor tissue or organ contains antigens not present in the recipient
Xenograft (heterograft)	Graft between individuals of different species, e.g., a pig heart valve to a human heart

TRANSPLANTATION TERMINOLOGY

The transplanting or grafting of an organ or tissue ranges from self-transplantation, such as skin grafts from one part of the body to another to correct burn injuries, or hair transplants from one area of the scalp to another to correct patterned balding, to the grafting of a body component from one species to another, such as the transplanting of a pig's heart valve to a human. The most recent terms used in transplantation are presented in Table 28-3.

TYPES OF TRANSPLANTS
Kidney

The first successful human kidney transplant was performed in 1954 between monozygotic twins. Induction of tolerance (discussed later in this chapter) was attempted through the use of sublethal total body irradiation and allogeneic bone marrow transplantation, followed by renal transplantation. By 1960, renal transplantation was firmly established as a viable treatment for end-stage renal disease. Because of the continuing problems associated with total body irradiation, chemical immunosuppression became the mode of treatment. The criteria for recipients of renal allografts generally excludes elderly patients and those with a history of malignancy. In addition, the presence of active sepsis or patients in whom chronic infection may be reactivated by treatment with steroids or immunosuppressive therapy are also not considered as transplant candidates.

Kidney donations are not accepted from individuals who are over 65 years of age because of a decreased likelihood of recipient survival. Donors are excluded if chronic renal disease or sepsis is present. Donations are additionally not accepted from individuals with generalized or systemic diseases such as diabetes mellitus, hypertension, tuberculosis, or other infections. Young trauma victims are the most desirable source of cadaver organ transplants, including the kidneys. Cadaver organs are not accepted from donors with a history of any malignancy other than that involving the central nervous system.

In addition to compatibility of ABO blood group systems, newer methods of harvesting kidneys have reduced the sensitizing effect related to "passenger" leukocytes against transplantation antigens borne on these cells. HLA-A and -B loci matches have the best chance for long-term survival of the graft and the recipient. The increased survival rate with HLA-A and -B matches is determined not as much by class I compatibility as by the HLA-D related region antigens that are associated with these regions. The strongest association between transplant survival and tissue antigens is with the D-region related antigens (-DR, -MB, -MT). Lewis antigens on the erythrocytes and H-Y antigens associated with X and Y chromosomes are among the other antigen systems that demonstrate a reasonably significant association with graft survival.

Heart Valves

Xenogenic valve replacements are a standard modality for the treatment of aortic and mitral valve defects. Sources of these xenogenic valves are either bovine (cow) or porcine (pig), and the valves are chemically or physically modified to reduce antigenicity.

Patients receiving xenoallografts of heart valves are not immunosuppressed postoperatively because only minimal or nonexistent graft-rejection reactions take place in these modified valves.

Heart

The first successful allograft cardiac transplant was performed in 1967 by Dr. Christiaan Barnard in Cape Town, South Africa. The criteria for selecting the donor and recipient combination for cardiac transplantation are essentially the same as those used for cadaver renal transplantation. The most significant exclusion for cardiac transplantation, however, is the presence of an active infection. Cardiac transplantation donors must have sustained irreversible brain death, but nearly normal cardiac function must be maintained. Prophylactic antibiotics and cytotoxic drugs are given to the donor just before harvesting the heart. Because of the urgency of most situations, most grafts are performed despite multiple HLA incompatibilities. Transplantation recipients are maintained on immunosuppressive therapy, anticoagulants, and antithrombotic agents as well as low lipid diets.

Cornea

Corneal transplants have been a common form of therapy for many years. The first human corneal eye bank was established in New York City in 1944. This type of transplantation has an extremely high success rate because of the ease in obtaining and storing viable corneas.

Corneal grafts are generally performed for the replacement of nonhealing corneal ulcerations. Because of the avascularity (lack of blood vessels) of this tissue, a reasonably low concentration of class I transplantation antigens, and an essential absence of class II antigens, graft rejection is minimal. To avoid rejection, grafts are made as small as possible and are placed centrally to avoid contact with the highly vascularized limbic region. Eccentrically placed grafts are subject to a high rate of immunologic failure because vascularity will allow for lymphocyte contact. Immunosuppression is not routinely administered.

Skin

The development of nonimmunogenic skin replacement materials has lowered the demand for allografts of skin. Skin allografts elicit the rejection phenomenon because skin has an extremely high density of class I histocompatibility antigens. Therefore, sensitization and recognition of antigenic differences are very likely with resultant rejection of the grafted skin. If done, skin allografts are performed and supported with immunosuppressive therapy.

Liver

Potential liver transplant recipients must have no extrahepatic disease or infection present. The largest group of transplanted patients have been those suffering from congenital biliary atresia. Patients with cirrhosis may also be good candidates. HLA crossmatching appears to increase the rate of graft survival, but the influence of tissue typing is somewhat unclear. Immunosuppressive regimens such as azathioprine and corticosteroids or cyclosporine-A increases survival. Major complications of this procedure have been biliary tract fistulae or leaks, which have occurred in 30% to 50% of patients.

Lung

Successful lung transplants have been difficult to achieve because of technical, logistic, and immunologic problems. Technically, lung donor and recipient must have essentially identical bronchial circumferences to obtain a good match. An additional technical problem is that the lungs are extremely sensitive to ischemic damage, and successful preservation after harvesting has been unsuccessful. Occasional lung and heart combination transplants have been attempted. The combined procedure is less difficult than single organ tranplant.

The lungs are very susceptible to infection; sepsis is very common among potential donors. Severe rejection is common because of the high density of Ia positive cells in the vasculature and the high concentration of passenger leukocytes trapped in the alveoli and blood vessels. Intensive immunosuppressive therapy is needed to maintain the graft. Many lung recipients have died from massive infection and sepsis.

Pancreas

New modes of transplantion include full pancreatic or isolated islet cell transplantation. Pancreatic grafts have been successful for only a short period because of a high rate of technical failure or irreversible rejection. Transplantation of small quantities of isolated islet cells into the retroperitoneal space, however, has demonstrated a reasonably good success rate.

Bone

Bone matrix autografts or allografts are common. Transplantation of bone matrix is used after certain limb-sparing tumor resections and to correct congenital bone abnormalities. The major criteria for bone donation are a lack of infection, no history of IV drug use, and no history of prolonged steroid therapy or human growth hormone treatment. Bone can be easily harvested and frozen. Freezing not only preserves the bone but offers the additional benefit of concomitant diminuition of histocompatibility antigens.

The major technical requirement for allograft transplantation is maintaining the periosteal sheath of the recipient bone in order to strip the donor bone completely of all periosteal elements. Tranplantation of bone is an easy procedure. Processed bone lacks significant quantities of immunogenic substances; therefore, the need for immunosuppression is almost completely eliminated.

Bone Marrow

Bone marrow transplantation is used for the treatment of patients with severe aplastic anemia, acute leukemia, and dangerous immunodeficiency states in cases where the defect in hematopoietic stem cells is responsible for the underlying disease state. The technical aspects of harvesting bone marrow are quite simple. Marrow cells are aspirated aseptically from a donor at multiple sites in the iliac crest. The aspirate is heparinized and filtered to disperse the cells into a suspension. This preparation is then immediately transfused intravenously into the patient or processed with depletion or enrichment techniques. The patient receives a dose of approximately 10^9 nucleated cells per kg.

When human bone marrow transplants were initially attempted in the early 1960s, the results were poor. Recipients and donors were selected based on ABO blood group compatibility. Subsequent therapy consisted of administering potentially lethal radiation followed by plasma exchange or plasmaphereis or both to rid the recipient of circulating autoreactive antibodies.

The importance of matching the HLA-D related region became increasingly apparent. Patients who were matched for the D region but who were incompatible for the HLA-A, HLA-B, and HLA-C regions began to be transplanted with increasing success if the patient was appropriately pretreated. Antithymocyte or antilymphocyte globulin appears to decrease the probability of the major complication of bone marrow transplantation, *graft versus host disease* (GVHD). Although cyclosporine-A is helpful, it does not appear to prevent in vivo expression of T cell activation antigens following allogeneic bone marrow transplation. It does, however, suppress the development of cytotoxic T cells. In addition, patients with leukemia may require more intense pretreatment conditioning or immunosuppression in order to destroy resident leukemia cells.

GRAFT-VERSUS-HOST DISEASE

In instances such as bone marrow transplantation host immunity to the donor can cause *graft-versus-host disease (GVHD)*. This condition is believed to result from the patient being sensitized to unshared HLA antigen before transplant.

Etiology

When allogenic T lymphocytes are transfused from donor to recipient with a graft, the patient can develop acute or chronic GVHD. GVHD occurs in immunodeficient or immunosuppressed patients. Engraftment and multiplication of donor lymphocytes can also be caused by transfused blood because lymphocytes capable of mitosis can be found in stored blood products. Where the donor and recipient differ at HLA or H-2 loci, the reaction can be fatal. The stronger the antigen difference, the more severe the reaction.

Epidemiology

It is now accepted that GVHD can occur whenever immunologically competent allogeneic lymphocytes are transfused into a severely immunocompromised host. Patients at risk include those who are immunodeficient or immunosuppressed with severe lymphocytopenia and bone marrow suppression. Despite chemotherapy at the time of bone marrow transplantation, 20% to 50% of patients will develop acute GVHD, and 20% to 40% of these patients will die of GVHD or associated infections.

Chronic GVHD affects 20% to 40% of patients within more than 6 months after tranplantation. Two factors closely associated with the development of chronic GVHD are increasing age and a preceding episode of acute GVHD.

Cases of transfusion-related GVHD have increased significantly in the past two decades. This reaction has been reported subsequent to blood transfusion in bone marrow transplant recipients following total body irradiation and adults receiving intensive chemotherapy for hematologic malignancies. GVHD has also occurred in infants with severe congenital immunodeficiency and those who have received intrauterine transfusions followed by exchange transfusion. Nearly 90% of patients with posttransfusion GVHD will die of acute complications of the disease. The usual cause of death is generalized infection.

Signs and Symptoms

In bone marrow transplant patients, acute GVHD develops within the first 3 months of tranplantation. The initial manifestations are lesions of the skin, liver, and gastrointestinal tract. An erythematous maculopapular skin rash, particularly on the palms and soles is usually the first sign of GVHD. Disease progression is characterized by diarrhea, often with abdominal pain, and liver disease. Other signs and symptoms of complications related to therapy include fever, granulocytopenia, and bacteremia. Interstitial pneumonia, frequently associated with cytomegalovirus (CMV), can also occur.

Chronic GVHD resembles a collagen vascular disease with skin changes, such as erythema and cutaneous ulcers, and liver dysfunction, which is characterized by bile duct degeneration and cholestasis. Patients with chronic GVHD are suspectible to bacterial infections. For example, increasing age and preexisting lung disease increase the incidence of interstitial pneumonia.

GVHD causes an inflammatory response. Posttransfusion signs and symptoms begin within 3 to 30 days after transfusion. Because of lymphocytic infiltration of the intestine, skin, and liver, mucosal destruction including ulcerative skin and mouth lesions, diarrhea, and liver destruction results. Other clinical symptoms include jaundice, fever, anemia, weight loss, skin rash, and splenomegaly.

Immunologic Manifestation

In immunocompromised patients, the transfused or grafted lymphocytes recognize the antigens of the host as foreign and react immunologically against them. Instead of the usual transplantation reaction of host against graft, the reverse GVHD occurs.

In a normal lymphocyte-transfer reaction, the results of GVHD are usually not serious because the recipient is capable of destroying the foreign lymphocytes. If the recipient, however, cannot reject the transfused lymphocytes, the grafted lymphocytes may cause uncontrolled destruction of the host's tissues and death.

Diagnostic Evaluation

Laboratory evidence of immunosuppression or immunodeficiency, such as a decreased total lymphocyte concentration, suggest that a patient may develop GVHD. Evidence of inflammation such as an increased C-reactive protein, elevated leukocyte count with granulocytosis, and increased erythrocyte sedimentation rate may suggest that GVHD has developed in GVHD candidates. Complications of anemia and liver disease, characterized by increased bilirubin and blood enzymes (such as transaminases and alkaline phosphatase) and the presence of opportunistic pathogens, e.g., CMV, can further support the diagnosis.

Pathologic features include lymphocytic and monocytic infiltration into perivascular spaces in the dermis and dermoepidermal junction of the skin and into the epithelium of the oropharynx, tongue, and esophagus. Infiltration can also be observed into the base of the intestinal crypts of the small and large bowel and into the periportal area of the liver with secondary necrosis of cells in infiltrated tissues.

Prevention

Although a minimal number of bone marrow transplant patients actually develop GVHD disease, the incidence of GVHD can be minimized by depletion of mature lymphocytes from the marrow by using monoclonal antibodies or physical methods. The risk of graft versus host disease, however, can be minimized if not eliminated by irradiation of the marrow transplant or blood products. Blood product irradiation is believed to be the most efficient and probably the most economical method available for prevention of posttransfusion GVHD. No cases of posttransfusion GVHD have been reported following administration of blood products irradiated with at least 1500 rad. The recommended radiation dose ranges from a minimum of 1500 to 3000 rad as an effective and appropriate radiation dose.

Several categories of patients possess the clinical indications for irradiated products:

High-Risk Patients

Patients at the highest risk with an absolute need for irradiated blood products include:
1. Recipients of autologous or allogeneic bone marrow grafts. Recipients of autologous bone marrow may be expected to have the same risk of post-transfusion GVHD as patients receiving allogeneic bone marrow.
2. Children with severe congenital immune deficiency syndromes involving T lymphocytes. The degree of immunodeficiency in the host, rather than the number of transfused immunocompetent cells, determines whether GVHD will occur.

Intermediate-Risk Patients

Patients considered to be at less of a risk of developing GVHD include:
1. Infants receiving intrauterine transfusions followed by exchange transfusions, and possibly infants receiving only exchange transfusions. The immune mechanism of the fetus and newborn infant may not be sufficiently mature to reject foreign lymphocytes, and prior transfusions may induce a state of immune tolerance in the newborn. Transfused lymphocytes may continue to circulate for a prolonged time in some immunologically tolerant hosts without the development of GVHD. There is insufficient evidence to recommend irradiation of blood given to all premature infants.
2. Patients receiving total body radiation or immunosuppressive therapy for disorders such as lymphoma and acute leukemia. Although routine irradiation of blood products given to these patients can be justified, it cannot be regarded as absolutely indicated since the risk of developing GVHD is so small. Blood product irradiation, however, is advised for selected patients with hematologic malignancies, especially when transfusions are given in or near the time of sustained and severe therapy-induced immunosuppression.

Low-Risk Patients

Patients who are also at risk but are considered to be the least susceptible include:
1. Patients with solid tumors. The incidence of the development of GVHD is difficult to determine. However, in nonhematologic malignancies, such as neuroblastoma, the disease has developed. In one case, the disease developed after the infusion of a single unit of packed red cells.
2. Patients with aplastic anemia receiving anti-thymocyte globulin theoretically may be at increased risk of posttransfusion GVHD during therapy-induced periods of lymphocytopenia.
3. Although a theoretical risk of posttransfusion GVHD may exist in patients with acquired immune deficiency syndrome (AIDS), the disease has not actually been observed in this disorder. The routine use of irradiated blood is not recommended.

Effects of Radiation on Specific Cellular Components

Lymphocytes. Ionizing radiation is known to inhibit lymphocyte mitotic activity and blast transformation. Irradiation of normal donor lymphocytes with 1500 rad from a cesium^{-137} source results in a 90% reduction in mitogen-stimulated ^{14}C-thymidine incorporation. An 85% reduction in mitogen-induced blast transformation after exposure to 1500 rad and a 97% to 98.5% reduction in mitogenic response have been noted after exposure to 5000 rads.

Granulocytes. Ionizing radiation may impair granulocyte function; this impairment is dose dependent. The degree of actual damage to granulocytes is controversial. Chemotactic activity decreased linearly with increasing doses of irradiation from 500 to 120,000 rads, but the reduction only reached statistical significance at 10,000 rad. A linear dose-response curve demonstrates that granulocyte locomotion is affected by very small doses of irradiation. A dose of 2000 rads is likely to eliminate lymphocytic mitotic activity and to prevent GVHD without causing significant damage to granulocytes or altering their chemotactic or bactericidal ability. Irradiation before transfusion has been demonstrated to contribute to defective oxidative metabolism, but this effect is highly variable.

Mature red blood cells. Mature red cells appear to be highly resistant to radiation damage. After exposure to 10,000 rad, ^{52}Cr-labeled in vivo red cell survival was the same as that of untreated controls. It has been demonstrated that stored erythrocytes could be treated with up to 20,000 rads without changing their viability or in vitro properties including adenosine triphosphate (ATP) and 2,3 diphosphoglycerate (2,3 DPG) levels, plasma hemoglobin, and potassium ions.

Platelets. Ionizing radiation may impair platelet function. Although this impairment is dose dependent, the effects of irradiation on platelets have been difficult to characterize. Several studies have demonstrated unchanged in vivo platelet survival after exposure to 5000 to 75,000 rad. A 33% decrease in the expected platelet count increase was noted after transfusion of platelets exposed to 5000 rad, and similarly irradiated autologous platelets had a diminished ability to correct the bleeding times in a small number of volunteers who had consumed aspirins. In one study, platelet aggregation was not affected by exposure to 5000 rad, but an impaired response to collagen was noted.

FACTORS IN GRAFT REJECTION

Organs vary with respect to their susceptibility to rejection based on inherent immunogenicity (see the box below) which is influenced by factors such as vascularity.

Types of Graft Rejection

The role of sensitized lymphocytes and antibodies in graft rejection differs and is influenced by the type of organ transplanted. Lymphocytes, particularly recirculating small lymphocytes, are effective in shortening graft survival. Cell-mediated immunity is responsible for the rejection of skin and solid tumors. Humoral antibodies, however, can be also be involved in the rejection process. The complexity of the action and interaction of cellular and humoral factors in grafts is considerable. Five possible categories of graft rejection (Table 28-4) have been demonstrated in human kidney transplant rejection: hyperacute, accelerated, acute, chronic, and immunopathologic.

Examples of the Immunogenicity of Different Transplant Tissues

Most immunogenic	Bone marrow
	Skin
	Islets of Langerhans
	Heart
	Kidney
	Liver
	Bone
	Xenogenic valve replacements
Least immunogenic	Cornea

First and Second Set Rejection

Skin transplantation (Fig. 28-1) is the most common experimental model for transplantation research. Rejection of skin and solid tumors can be divided into first and second set rejection. Activation of cellular immunity by T cells is the predominant cause of the first set allograft rejection. Lymphocytes can directly attack cellular antigens to which they are sensitized by previous exposure or by cytotoxic lymphokines. The primary role of lymphocytes in first set rejection would be consistent with the histology of early reaction showing infiltration by mononuclear cells with very few polymorphonuclear leukocytes or plasma cells. Sensitization occurs within the first few days of transplantation and the tissue is lost in 10 to 20 days.

When sensitized lymphocytes are already present as the result of prior graft rejection, an accelerated rejection of tissue results from regrafting-second set rejection. Lymphocytes from a sensitized animal transferred to a first graft recipient will accelerate rejection of the graft. Graft rejection is primarily a T cell function with some assistance from antibodies.

Hyperacute Rejection

Hyperacute reactions are caused entirely by the presence of preformed humoral antibodies within the host, which react with donor tissue cellular antigens. These antibodies are usually anti-A or anti-B related to the ABO blood group systems or antibodies to class I MHC antigens (hypersensitivity type II). Potential recipients harboring antibodies to HLA-A, -B, and -C (class I) but not HLA-DR (class II) antigens are at high risk for this process.

The interaction of cellular antigens with antibodies activates the complement system and leads to grafted cell lysis and clotting within the grafted tissue. Kidney allografts can be rejected by the hyperacute rejection process within minutes of transplantation. The irreversible kidney damage of hyperacute rejection is characterized by sludging of erythrocytes, development of microthrombi in the small arterioles and glomerular capillaries, and infiltration of phagocytic cells.

Accelerated Rejection

Accelerated rejection is comparable to the second set rejection phenomenon observed in animal models. In these cases, retransplantation is less severe than hyperacute rejection and is considered to be accelerated rejection. Accelerated rejection is due to activation of the T-cell—mediated response.

Acute Rejection

Acute rejection can result after the first exposure to alloantigens. In this reaction, donor antigens select reactive T cell clones and initiate visible manifestation of rejection within 6 to 14 days. The early processes in acute rejection appear to be T-

TABLE 28-4

Categories and Characteristics of Graft Rejection Based on Immune Destruction of Kidney Grafts

Type	Time of tissue damage	Predominant mechanism	Cause
Hyperacute	Within minutes	Humoral	Preformed cytotoxic antibodies to donor antigens
Accelerated	2 to 5 days	Cell-mediated	Previous sensitization to donor antigens
Acute	7 to 21 days	Cell-mediated (possibly antibody cell-mediated cytotoxicity [ADCC])	Development of allogeneic reaction to donor antigens
Chronic	Later than 3 months	Cell-mediated	Disturbance of host/graft tolerance
Immunopathologic damage to the new organ	Later than 3 months	1. Immune complex disorder 2. Complex formation with soluble antigens	Immunopathologic mechanisms related to circumstances necessitating transplant

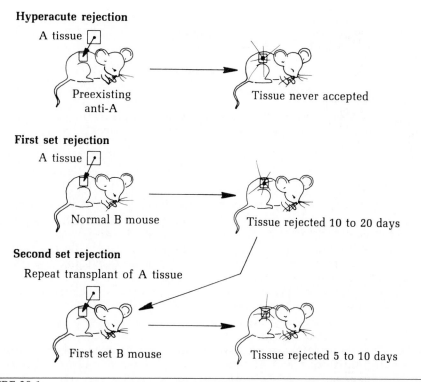

Hyperacute rejection

A tissue

Preexisting anti-A

Tissue never accepted

First set rejection

A tissue

Normal B mouse

Tissue rejected 10 to 20 days

Second set rejection

Repeat transplant of A tissue

First set B mouse

Tissue rejected 5 to 10 days

FIGURE 28-1

Hyperacute rejection results from placement of tissue in an animal already possessing antibodies to antigens of grafted tissue. Second-set rejection is an accelerated first-set reaction and is seen in animals that have already rejected tissue at least once.
(From Barrett JT: Textbook of immunology, ed 5, St Louis, 1988, The CV Mosby Co.)

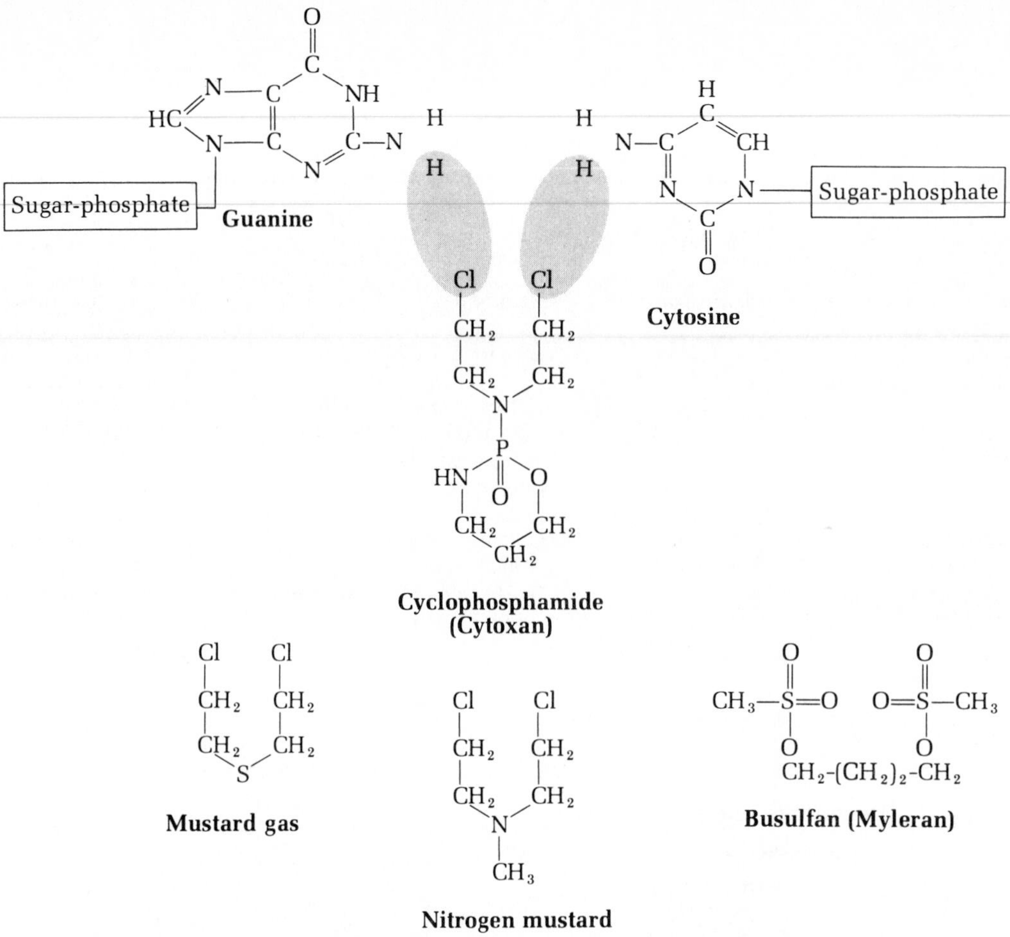

FIGURE 28-2

Structures of cyclophosphamide and busulfan, which are alkylating immunosuppressants, clearly are related to the structure of mustard gas. The alkylating reaction of cyclophosphamide with nucleic acids also is illustrated.
(From Barrett JT: Textbook of immunology, ed 5, St Louis, 1988, The CV Mosby Co.)

cell mediated; however, later aspects may involve antibodies and complement.

Acute rejection is equivalent to a first set allograft rejection in experimental animals, and an accelerated rejection is equivalent to second set rejection. Both are primarily mediated by cells. Immunopathological changes include the presence of immune complex deposition and other hypersensitivity reactions already present in the recipient.

Acute early rejection, which occurs up to about 10 days after transplantation, is histologically characterized by dense cellular infiltration and rupture of peritubular capillaries. It appears to be a cell-mediated hypersensitivity reaction involving T cells. In comparison, acute late rejection occurs 11 days or more after transplantation in patients suppressed with prednisone and azathioprine. In kidney allografts, acute-late rejection is probably caused by the binding of immunoglobulin, presumably antibody and complement, to the arterioles and glomerular capillaries where they can be visualized by immunofluorescent techniques. These immunoglobu-lin deposits on the vessel walls include platelet aggregates in glomerular capillaries, which causes acute renal shutdown. The possibility of damage to antibody-coated cells through antibody-dependent, cell-mediated cytotoxicity (ADCC) may also take place.

Chronic Rejection

Chronic rejection occurs in most graft recipients. The process results in a slow but continual loss of organ function over months or years. Chronic rejection, however, is often responsive to various immunosuppressive therapies.

In kidney allografts, this insidious rejection is associated with subendothelial deposits of immunoglobulin and the C3 component of complement on the glomerular basement membranes. This may occasionally be an expression of an underlying immune complex disorder, which may have originally necessitated the transplant, or it may possibly result from complex formation with soluble antigens derived from the grafted kidney.

Immunologic Tolerance

The importance of tolerance to self-antigens was recognized very early in the study of immunology. Immunologic tolerance is the acquisition of non-reactivity toward particular antigens. Self-tolerance is a critical process, and the failure to recognize self antigens can result in autoimmune disease (see Chapter 25).

Various pathways to immunologic tolerance have been recognized. It has been suggested that both T and B cells are affected independently and differently and may be tolerated under certain circumstances. Several mechanisms may operate simultaneously in a single host. During fetal development of the immune system and during the first few weeks of neonatal life, none of the cells of the immune system has reached maturity. For this reason, the entire immune system is particularly susceptible to tolerance induction at this stage of development.

T Cell Tolerance

T cells do not show a marked difference in tolerance at different stages of maturation. The antigen required to produce tolerance and the circumstance of its presentation is specific for each individual T cell subset. At least three pathways have been recognized for T cell tolerance:
1. Clonal abortion. Immature T cell clones may be aborted in a manner similar to B cells.
2. Functional deletion. The subsets of a mature T cell may be individually deleted leading to the loss of only one of the functions of the T cell group.
3. T cell suppression. T cell suppressors actively suppress the actions of other T cell subsets or B cells.

B Cell Tolerance

As a B cell matures, it becomes less susceptible to tolerization. In addition, during B cell maturation the forms of antigen presentation which will produce tolerance also varies. Four pathways have been established for the induction of B cell tolerance. The mode of tolerance, therefore, is dependent on the maturity of the cell, the antigen, and the manner of antigen presentation to the immune system.

The pathways of B cell tolerance are as follows:
1. Clonal abortion. A low concentration of multivalent antigen may cause the immature clone to abort. Tolerance of immature B cells by this mechanism is high.
2. Clonal exhaustion. Repeated antigen challenge with a T independent antigen may remove all mature functional B cell clones. Tolerance of mature B cells is moderate.
3. Functional deletion. The absence of the T helper subset and the presence of T dependent antigen (or with T suppressor cells) or an excess of T independent antigen prevents mature B cells from functioning normally. The ability to tolerize B cells by this mechanism is moderate.
4. Antibody forming cell blockade. An excess of T independent antigen interferes with the secretion of antibody by antibody forming cells. B cell tolerance by this mechanism is low.

Immune Response Gene-Associated Antigens

The specific immune responses to a variety of antigenic substances are now known to be regulated by an immune response (Ir) gene. Ir gene control is considered to be genetically dominant. The homology of the HLA-D region with the animal I-region suggests that the human Ir gene might be found to be linked to the HLA complex. Evidence for the existence of the Ir gene is obtained from family and population studies. Additional evidence for the presence of Ir genes comes from HLA-linked disease susceptibility genes and HLA-disease associations. It is believed that individuals who lack that gene are unresponsive.

The generally accepted concept is that the Ir gene is responsible for the interaction of T cells with both B cells and macrophages, which are necessary for T cell activation. Activation of T cells is necessary for:
1. Conversion to active helper function
2. Production of lymphokines
3. Mediation of delayed and contact hypersensivity
Because the proliferative response to antigen depends on the interaction of T cell with an antigen-presenting cell, usually macrophage-monocytes. Helper function also depends on T cell interaction with precursors of antibody-secreting cells. T cells interact with these cells by recognizing specific antigen bound to macrophages or B cells and the I-region gene products expressed on the surface of these cells. T cells are able to recognize the precise details of antigen structure and distinguish between two closely related immune response gene-associated molecules expressed on the surface of these antigen-presenting cells as well as the B cell.

MECHANISMS OF REJECTION
General Characteristics

Variations in the expression of class II histocompatibility antigens by different tissues and the presence of antigen-presenting cells in some tissues highly influence the success of a transplant. Antigen-presenting cells that enter the graft through the donor's circulation are very likely to elicit graft rejection. If these "passenger lymphocytes" leave the graft after transplantation and enter the draining lymphatic system, they are particularly effective in sensitizing the host.

Rejection of a graft displays the two key features of adaptive immunity:
1. Memory
2. Specificity
Only sites that are accessible to the immune system in the recipient are susceptible to graft rejection. Certain "privileged" sites in the body allow allogeneic grafts to survive indefinitely.

The Role of T Cells

Graft rejection is primarily regulated by the interaction of the host's T cells with the antigens of the graft. Unmodified rejection, however, results from the destructive effects of cytotoxic T cells, activated macrophages, and antibody.

In tissue transplants, the graft consists of tissue cells that carry class I (HLA-A, HLA-B, and HLA-C antigens) and lymphocytes that carry both class I and class II (HLA-D and related antigens of the associated immune response gene). Activated T cells specific for class I antigens have the potential to express cytotoxic activity, which damages both the endothelium and the parenchymal cells of the graft. Binding of these cells to the class I antigens on target cells of the donor organ triggers the release of lymphokines and subsequently activates a nonspecific inflammatory response in the allograft.

T cells specific for class II antigens of the donor tissue are unable to react directly with the parenchymal cells of the graft not expressing class II antigens. These cells, however, can activate lymphocytes in the transplant through lymphokine release. Therefore, damage to the graft can result from a cytotoxic reaction directed against cells of the transplanted organ or from a severe nonspecific inflammatory response or both.

Activation of T helper cells by class II antigens such as HLA-DR probably stimulates the release of interleukin-1 (IL-1). IL-1 subsequently stimulates the release of a variety of lymphokines from helper T cells, which in turn activate macrophages, cytotoxic T cells, and antibody-releasing B cells, as well as increase the immunogenicity of the graft. In addition, macrophages and other accessory cells are subsequently stimulated by T cell products and release IL-1, which in turn stimulates the formation of interleukin-2 (IL-2) receptors as well as the release of IL-2 by T helper cells. IL-2 interacts with specific IL-2 receptors expressed on activated helper and cytotoxic T cells. This interaction stimulates the initiation of DNA synthesis and the eventual clonal proliferation of IL-2 receptor-bearing cells. IL-2 also causes the release of gamma-interferon, which activates macrophages and stimulates the release of B cell differentiation factors required for the proliferation of antigen-activated B cells. The release of IL-2 dependent gamma-interferon by activated T cells may initiate a vicious circle as gamma-interferon induces the expression of class II molecules on endothelial cells as well as the expression of certain class II negative macrophages.

Histologic examination of an allogenic skin graft during the process of rejection demonstrates that the dermis becomes infiltrated by mononuclear cells, many of which are small lymphocytes. This accumulation of lymphocytes precedes the destruction of the graft by several days. Although this graft rejection process is caused by cytotoxic T cells, in some cases the helper cells are also elicited by MHC gene differences. Graft rejection may be a special form of response related to delayed hypersensitivity reactions, in which case the ultimate effectors of graft destruction are the monocytes and macrophages recruited to the site. It is debatable whether the macrophages seen in grafts are effectors of graft destruction or arrive as a consequence of the inflammatory process and cell damage.

Antibody Effects

Cell-mediated immunity is the major effector mechanism in graft rejection. Antibodies, however, can also be involved in graft rejection. Antibodies can cause rapid (hyperacute) graft rejection, but they are usually less significant than cell-mediated immunity. Exceptions include cases where the recipient has been previously sensitized to a particular antigen, in reactions to hematopoietic cells, and where the graft is directly connected to the host's blood circulation, e.g., a kidney allograft.

In dispersed cellular grafts such as infusion of erythrocytes, leukocytes, and platelets, antibodies (humoral immunity) may dominate the rejection process because antigens are fully exposed to a preexisting or a developing antibody response. Cells are highly susceptible to complement activated membrane damage. If cytolysis does not occur immediately, antibodies may function as opsonins to encourage phagocytic destruction of transfused cells.

Humoral immunity is suspected of playing a major role in the rejection of xenografts. Xenografts possess a large number of antigens shared between donor and recipient. One species can possess agglutinins for cells of distantly related species, which can attack the xenogenic tissue as soon as it is transplanted.

Immunosuppression

Immunosuppression is usually necessary to modify or suppress immune responses to allow the recipient to accept an allogenic graft. Forms of immunosuppression can or have included chemical, biologic, or irradiation of the lymphoid system or the donated organ. The immunosuppressive activities of therapeutic agents used in transplantation directly interferes with the allograft rejection response. The problem arising from all immunosuppressive techniques is that the individual is more susceptible to infection. If infection occurs, immunosuppression has to be suspended, at which time allogeneic reactions frequently develop.

Immunosuppressive measures may be antigen-specific or antigen-nonspecific (Table 28-5). Antigen-nonspecific immunosuppression includes drugs and other methods of specifically altering T cell function. Many cytotoxic drugs are primarily active against dividing cells and therefore have some functional specificity for any cells activated to divide by donor antigens. The use of these drugs is limited by the toxic effects they may have on other dividing cells or on the physiologic functioning of organs such as the liver. Antigen-specific immunosuppression is an ideal form of immunosuppression. Antigen-specific tolerance is that induced by the infusion of donor cells. This is generally impractical in transplantation, but it may be useful in the phenomenon of immunologic enhancement. Enhancement of tolerance has been attempted in renal allograft patients. In a donor-specific blood transfusion program, the patient is transfused several times before elective transplantion with blood from the prospective kidney donor. The overall effect of these transfusions appears to be a tolerance of the recipient to donor transplantation antigens other than the HLA-linked regions, such as minor histo-

TABLE 28-5

Types of Immunosuppressive Treatments

Drugs	Antigen nonspecific	Antigen specific
	Azathioprine	Neonatal
	Steroids	tolerization
	Cyclosporine A	
	Antilymphocyte globulin	Enhancing (antiallogenic) antibodies
	Radiation	Antiidiotype antibodies to receptors on T cells
		Blood transfusion in human kidney transplant

compatibility loci, red blood cell loci, and leukocyte surface antigens. This treatment has prolonged graft survival markedly in these patients.

Cytotoxic Drugs

Cytotoxic drugs are the most common form of therapy and most frequently include alkylating agents (Fig. 28-2), purine and pyrimidine analogs (Fig. 28-3), folic acid analogs (Fig. 28-4), or the alkaloids. The drugs of choice, excluding alkylating drugs, are azathioprine, 6-mercaptopurine, 6-thioguanine, 5-fluorouracil, cytosine arabinoside, methotrexate and aminopterin, and vinblastine and vincristine.

Most immunosuppressive drugs administered alone, however, cannot produce antigen-specific tolerance because they act equally on all susceptible clones. With the exception of certain immunosuppressive drugs, such as cyclosporine A, most immunosuppressive drugs can only be rendered antigen specific by including an antigen-specific element in the tolerizing regime. In these cases, the drugs act as cofactors in tolerogenesis. Experimental evidence suggests that these regimes may act by:
1. Lowering the threshold for tolerance induction
2. Blocking the differentiation sequence in cells triggered by antigen

Azathioprine

Since its introduction in 1961, azathioprine, an oral purine analog that is an antimetabolite with multiple activities, has been the mainstay of antire-

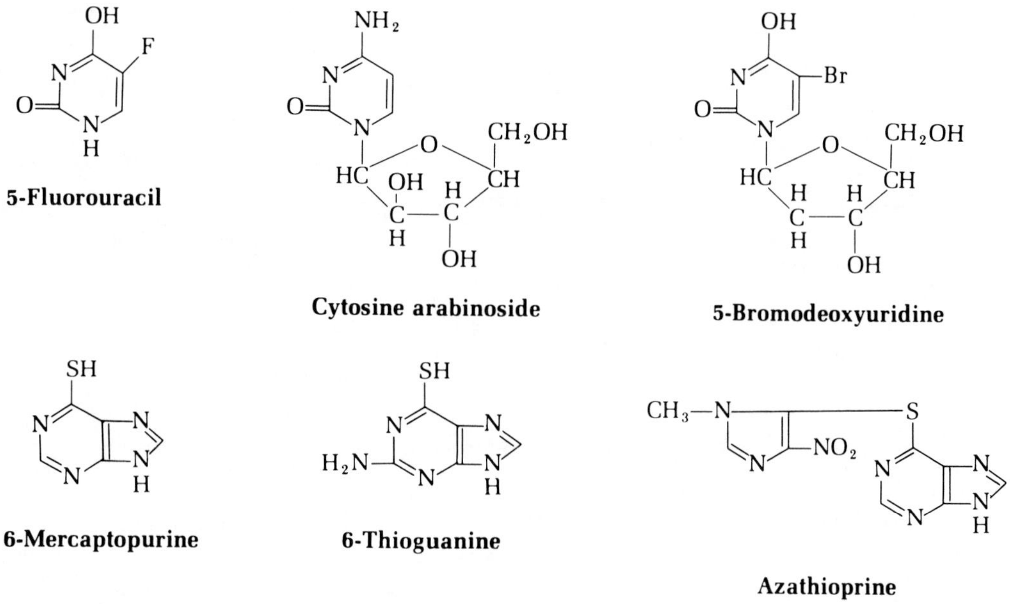

FIGURE 28-3

Pyrimidine analogs (upper row) and purine analogs (lower row) with B and T cell-suppressing activity. A large number of similar compounds are available for human use.
(From Barrett JT: Textbook of immunology, ed 5, St Louis, 1988, The CV Mosby Co.)

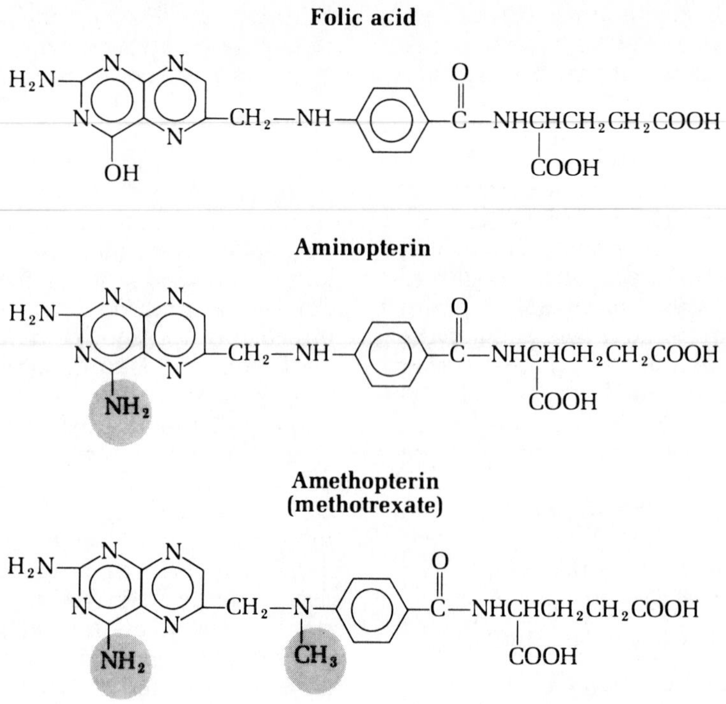

Folic acid

Aminopterin

**Amethopterin
(methotrexate)**

FIGURE 28-4

Structural analogs of folic acid-aminoptrine and methotrexate differ from the vitamin by the substituents in the stippled circles. These differences confer an immunosuppressant function on the analogs.

(From Barrett JT: Textbook of immunology, ed 5, St Louis, 1988, The CV Mosby Co.)

Cortisone   **Corticosterone**   **Cortisol
(hydrocortisone)**

Triamcinolone   **6α-Methylprednisolone**   **Prednisolone**

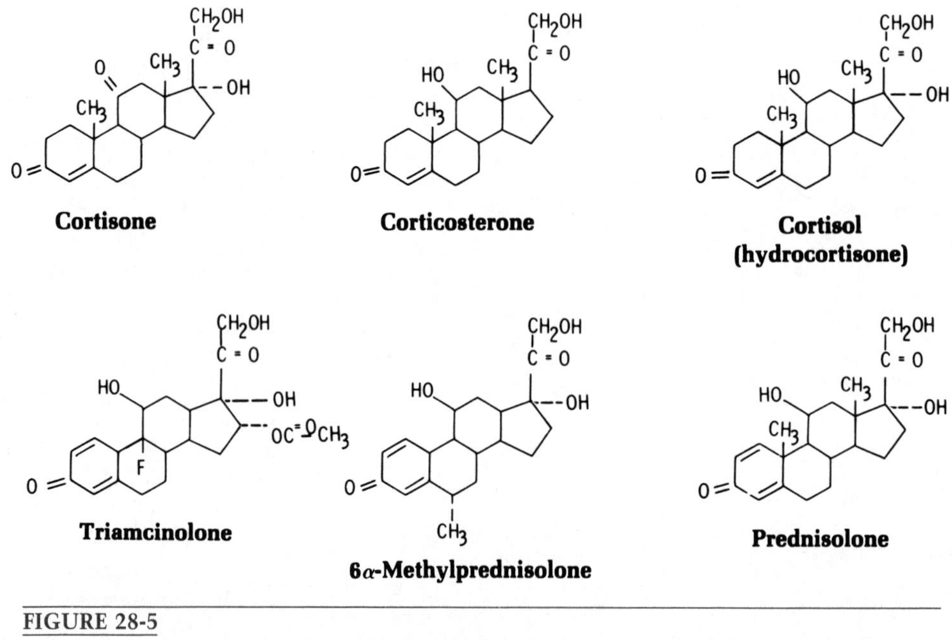

FIGURE 28-5

Chemical structures of some steroidal immunosuppressants. The differences in structure reside primarily in the side chains and the oxidation state of carbon 11 in the C ring.

(From Barrett JT: Textbook of immunology, ed 5, St Louis, 1988, The CV Mosby Co.)

jection therapy. Metabolites of azathioprine, such as the in vivo metabolite, 6-mercaptopurine, are incorporated into cellular DNA. This causes inhibition of purine nucleotide synthesis and metabolism and alters the synthesis and function of RNA. Therefore, azathioprine acts at an early stage in either T or B cell activation during the proliferative cycle of effector lymphocyte clones. Azathioprine is useful in preventing acute rejection because it inhibits the primary immune response. It has, however, little or no effect on secondary responses.

Corticosteroids

Corticosteroids can be used in conjunction with azathioprine or another immunosuppressant such as cyclosporin. Corticosteroids directly inhibit antigen-driven T cell proliferation. Steroids (Fig. 28-5) do not directly act on the IL-2 producing T cell. They do, however, inhibit production of lymphokines by preventing monocytes from releasing IL-1, thereby blocking IL-1 dependent release of IL-2 from antigen-activated T cells. Other activities of monocytes, such as inhibition of chemotaxis, are also likely to be important in the immunosuppressive process.

High doses of corticosteroids are used to treat acute rejection. In addition, steroids probably reverse in vivo rejection episodes by preventing the production of IL-2, which would inhibit activated T cells as an essential trophic factor.

Cyclosporine A

Cyclosporine-A affects T cells preferentially by inhibiting the induction of cytotoxic T cells. Unlike corticosteroids, cyclosporine does not inhibit the capacity of all accessory cells to release IL-1. Cyclosporine does prevent activation of IL-2 gene in activated helper T cells and the release of certain other lymphokines, such as gamma-interferon.

The secretion of B cell growth and differentiation factors by activated T cells is also inhibited by cyclosporine. Therefore, under the influence of cyclosporine, helper T cell-dependent B cells are not fully activated because of a lack of necessary helper T cell stimulation. In pharmacologic doses, however, cyclosporine does not grossly interfere with the activation and proliferation of suppressor T cells. Recent data indicates prolonged renal allograft survival with the use of cyclosporine-A despite potential mismatches of the HLA system.

Antilymphocyte Globulin and Other Immunosuppressive Measures

Other immunosuppressive measures directed at T cells include the use of antilymphocyte globulin at the time of transplantation and lymphoid irradiation before transplantation. Use of antilymphocyte antibody in preventing or reversing rejection in renal allograft recipients is well established. Monoclonal antibody (OKT3) is used because the T3 surface membrane marker is found on all mature postthymic T cells. Its use reverses almost all acute renal transplant rejection.

Immunologic Evaluation of Potential Transplant Recipients

Systems developed to ascertain compatibility between donor and recipient include screening the potential recipient's serum for the presence of a positive lymphocytotoxic crossmatch, which is associated with hyperacute or accelerated rejection in kidney allografts. Antibody-dependent, cell-mediated cytotoxicity (ADCC) is another sensitive method for the detection of antibodies important in graft rejection. The target cells from the donor are incubated with serum from the recipient to detect donor-specific antibodies. Graft failure is correlated with the presence of a positive ADCC crossmatch.

TUMOR IMMUNOLOGY
Introduction

Oncology is that branch of medicine devoted to the study and treatment of tumors. The term tumor is commonly used to describe a proliferation of cells, which produces a mass rather than a reaction or inflammatory condition. Tumors are neoplasms frequently described as benign or malignant. A benign neoplasm is usually a nonspreading tumor; a malignant neoplasm is a growth that usually infiltrates tissues, metastasizes and often recurs after attempts to eradicate it by surgery, radiation, or chemotherapy. A malignant neoplasm is referred to as cancer, which is characterized by the rapid proliferation or abnormal growth of cells, which will ultimately destroy the host.

Etiologic Factors in Human Cancer

The factors that cause the majority of neoplasms are unknown. The incidence of cancer, however, has been correlated with certain environmental factors, such as occupational exposure to known carcinogenic agents, and host susceptibility considerations, such as heredity, sex, or age.

Environmental factors, such as aerosols and industrial pollutants, drugs, radiation, and infectious agents, that have been definitely linked with cancer are cited in Table 28-6. A variety of host factors has been linked to a higher-than-expected incidence of cancer. For example, the presence of certain genetic disorders, such as Down's syndrome, is associated with an increased incidence of leukemia. The incidence of cancer is extremely increased (10,000 times greater than expected) in patients suffering from immunodeficiency syndromes. The link between certain genetic abnormalities and leukemia is consistent with a germinal or somatic mutation in a stem cell line; the increased incidence of lymphomas in congenital, acquired, and drug-induced immunosuppresion is consistent with the failure of normal immune mechanisms or antigen overstimulation with a loss of normal feedback control.

TABLE 28-6

Selected Environmental Factors Associated With Cancer

	Factor	Type of cancer
Aerosol and/or industrial pollutants		
	Asbestos (silica)	Mesothelioma
	Lead, copper, zinc, arsenic, cyclic aromatics, tobacco	Lung cancer
	Vinyl chloride	Liver angiosarcoma
	Benzene	Leukemia
	Aniline dyes, coal	Skin and bladder carcinoma
Drugs		
	Androgenic steroids	Hepatocellular carcinoma
	Stilbestrol (prenatal)	Vaginal adenocarcinoma
	Estrogen (postmenopausal)	Endometrial carcinoma
	Hydantoins	Lymphoma
	Chloramphenicol, alkylating agents	Leukemias, lymphomas
Infectious agents		
	Herpesvirus (Epstein-Barr virus)	Burkitt's lymphoma, nasopharyngeal carcinoma
	Herpes virus type 2	Cervical cancer
	Human immunodeficiency virus (HIV)	Kaposi's sarcoma Non-Hodgkin's lymphoma Primary lymphoma of the brain Bladder cancer

Modified from Zeltzer PM: In Lawlor GJ and Fischer TJ, editors: The immune system and neoplasia. In Manual of allergy and immunology ed 2, Boston, 1988, Little, Brown & Co.

TABLE 28-7

Examples of Tumors Associated with Homozygous Loss of Specific Chromosomal Loci

Tumor Type	Chromosomal linkage
Multiple endocrine neoplasia, type 2	1
Renal cell carcinoma	3
Lung carcinoma	3
Colon carcinoma, familial polyposis	5
Multiple endocrine neoplasia, type 2a	10
Wilms' tumor, hepatoblastoma, rhabdomyosarcoma	11
Retinoblastoma	13
Ductal breast carcinoma	13
Colon carcinoma	17
Acoustic neuroma, meningioma	22

Stages of Carcinogenesis

A single oncogene produced through mutation in a target cell does not suffice to convert these cells into fully developed tumor cells. Tumor cells typically carry multiple genetic changes that act together. Cancer predisposing genes may act in several ways:

1. They may affect the rate at which exogenous precarcinogens are metabolized to actively carcinogenic forms that can damage the cellular genome directly
2. A gene may affect a host's ability to repair resulting damage to DNA.
3. They may alter the immune ability of the body to recognize and eradicate incipient tumors.
4. Some genes may affect the function of the apparatus responsible for the regulation of normal cell growth and associated proliferation of tissue.

Relatively few cancer-predisposing genes have been described. An absence of functional alleles at specific loci, however, allows the genesis of the malignant process (Table 28-7). For example, ductal breast carcinomas are associated with a specific deletion on chromosome 13. In addition, a predisposition to the malignant embryonal retinal tumor of childhood, retinoblastoma, is governed by mutant alleles mapping to a single locus on chromosome 13. Retinoblastoma develops in 80% to 90% of children carrying a tumor predisposing allele at this locus.

The Role of Oncogenes

The malignant proliferation of cells is controlled by genes. Cancer often begins when a carcinogenic agent such as a chemical or ionizing radiation damages the DNA of a critical gene in a cell. The mutant cell multiplies and the succeeding generations of cells aggregate to form a malignant tumor.

Proto-oncogenes act as central regulators of the growth in normal cells and are antecedents of *onco-*

Examples of Oncogenes Formed by Somatic Mutation of Normal Genetic Loci

Oncogene	Disorder
abl	Chronic myelogonous leukemia
myc	Burkitt's lymphoma
N-myc	Neuroblastoma
neu/erbB2	Mammary carcinoma
ras type	Wide variety of tumors

Oncogenic Viruses

RNA-Leukemia, carcinoma viruses, mammary tumor viruses
DNA-Herpes viruses, adenoviruses, papilloma viruses

genes. Not one of the proto-oncogenes, however, has yet been linked to genes that are thought to increase the risk of cancer. The rare involvement of these genes in the cancer process is a consequence of somatic mutation that takes place in specific target tissues with conversion of these genes into oncogenic alleles. Because oncogene alleles arise somatically, they cannot be used to explain genetic susceptibilities to cancer that exist at the moment of conception.

The genetic targets of carcinogens are known to be oncogenes. Oncogenes have been associated with various tumor types that stem in a large part from pre-existing genes present in the normal human genome. Therefore, oncogenes are considered to be altered versions of normal genes. In the course of a lifetime, a variety of mutations can convert a normal gene into a malignant oncogene. Once an oncogene is activated by mutation, it promotes excessive or inappropriate cell proliferation. Oncogenes have been detected in about 15% to 20% of a variety of human tumors and appear to be responsible for specifying many of the malignant traits of these cells. More than 30 distinct oncogenes, some of which are associated with specific tumor types, have been identified (see box above). Each gene has the ability to evoke many of the phenotypes characteristic of cancer cells.

Viral Oncogenes

A variety of RNA and DNA viruses has been associated with human malignancies (see box above, right). Some viral agents have a clear causative role, such as the Epstein-Barr virus (EBV) and certain papilloma viruses that are the etiologic agents in Burkitt's lymphoma and cervical carcinoma, respectively.

Viruses carry viral oncogenes into target cells, where they become firmly established. Clonal descendants then carry the viral genes, which maintain the malignant phenotype of the cell clones.

Tumor-Suppressing Genes

A very different class of cancer genes has recently been discovered. These tumor-suppressing genes in normal cells appear to regulate the proliferation of cell growth When this type of gene is inactivated, a block to proliferation is removed and cells begin a program of deregulated growth or the genetically depleted cell itself may proliferate uncontrollably. Thus, tumor-suppressing genes are referred to as *antioncogenes*. In time their discovery will lead to the reformulation of ideas about how the growth of normal cells is regulated.

Much speculation exists concerning the operation of tumor-suppressing genes in normal tissue. It is known that normal cells exert a negative growth influence on each other within a tissue. Normal cells also secrete factors that are negative regulators of their own growth and that of adjacent cells. Diffusible factors may also be released by normal cells to induce the end-stage differentiation of other cells in the immediate environment. Examples of such factors include:
1. Beta-interferon
2. Tumor growth factor
3. Tumor necrosis factor

Normal gene products appear to prevent malignant transformation in some way. It is speculated that normal cells must have receptors that detect the presence of these growth-inhibiting and differentiation-inducing factors, which allow them to process the signals of negative growth and respond with appropriate modulation of growth. Genes may specify proteins that are necessary to detect and respond to the negative regulators of growth. If this process becomes dysfunctional due to inactivation or the absence of a critical component, such as the loss of chromosomal loci, a cell may continue to respond to mitogenic stimulation but lose its ability to respond to negative feedback to cease proliferation. Animal experiments suggest that humans carry a repertoire of genes, each of which is involved in the negative regulation of the growth of specific cell types. Somatic inactivation of these genes may be involved in the initiation of tumor-cell growth or the transformtion of benign tumors into malignant ones. Therefore, the somatic inactivation of tumor-suppressing genes may be as important to carcinogenesis as the somatic activation of oncogenes.

Immunologic Surveillance

Clinical immunologists regard the immune response as a means of diagnosing and treating malignancy. Although no single satisfactory explanation exists to explain the success of tumors in escaping the immune rejection process, it is believed that

TABLE 28-8

Tumor Markers in Neoplasms

Tumor markers	Clinical value
Carcinoembryonic antigen (CEA)	Monitors response to therapy of patients with various types of cancer
Alpha$_1$-fetoprotein	Diagnosis of germ-cell and hepatic tumors
CA 125	Diagnosis of ovarian cancer
Chorionic gonadotropin (B-HCG)	Diagnosis of germ cell tumors
Prostate acid phosphatase	Diagnosis of prostate cancer

TABLE 28-9

Examples of Nonneoplastic Conditions in Which Elevated Serum/Plasma Concentrations of Tumor Markers Occur

Tumor Marker	Concentration in normal serum	Nonneoplastic conditions
Carcinoembryonic antigen (CEA)	< 2.5 ng/mL	Inflammatory bowel disease, pancreatitis, gastritis, smoker's chronic bronchitis, alcoholic liver disease, hepatitis
Alpha-fetoprotein (AFP)	<40 ng/mL	Pregnancy, regenerating liver tissue after viral hepatitis, chemically-induced liver necrosis, partial hepatectomy, cystic fibrosis, ataxia-telangiectasia, premature infants, and tyrosinemia
Human chorionic gonadotropin B-subunit (B-HCG)	Negative	Pregnancy
Serum acid phosphatase	Negative	Pregnancy
Placental alkaline phosphatase	Negative	Pregnancy

early clones of neoplastic cells are eliminated by the immune response. Cells such as the large granular lymphocytes (LGLs), ADCC effector cells, and cytotoxic T cells, dominate the rejection process that leads to the elimination of foreign tissue. Therefore, cells, rather than immunoglobulins, are believed to dominate tumor immunity. The functions of normal antitumor mechanisms and the failure of these mechanisms in the pathogenesis of cancer are incompletely understood at the present time.

In tumor immunology, a fundamental tenet is that when a normal cell is transformed into a malignant cell, it develops unique antigens not normally present on the mature normal cell. A controversial hypothesis is that the development of these new antigens in conjunction with HLA antigens makes them prime targets for immune rejection. Consequently, the rejection of allografts is a modern application of tumor rejection. Supporters of this hypothesis further claim that the emergence of tumors is evidence of the failure of the immune surveillance system.

Tumor Antigens

Tumor cells manifest tumor antigens as well as self-HLA antigens. The four types of tumor antigens that have been identified are the following:
1. Tumor-specific antigens on chemically induced tumors
2. Tumor-associated antigens on virally induced tumors
3. Carcinofetal antigens
4. Spontaneous tumor antigens

Tumor-Specific Antigens

Chemically induced tumors are known to develop antigens called *tumor-specific antigens (TSA)*, which are uniquely associated with each tumor. These antigens are not found in normal cells. They demonstrate little or no cross-reactivity between different tumors caused by the same carcinogen, perhaps because every tumor caused by chemical agents has unique surface characteristics.

Tumor-Associated Antigens

Tumor-associated antigens (TAA) are cell surface molecules that are coded for by tumorogenic viruses. These antigens are not expressed on the virion but are synthesized by the host cell. In contrast to TSA antigens, TAA antigens are virus specific. Therefore, each specific virus induces the same antigens irrespective of the tissue of origin or the animal species.

Carcinofetal Antigens

Well-differentiated tissue produces and secretes little or no fetal gene products. The abnormal behavior of malignant cells is believed to derepress genes normally only expressed during fetal life. Because the products of these fetally active genes are

TABLE 28-10

Examples of Serum Markers

Type of cancer	Alphafetoprotein	Carcinoembryonic antigen	Beta subunit of human chorionic gonadotropin	Neuronal enolase	Other hormones
Adrenocortical	–	–	–	–	+
Breast	–	+	–	–	–
Choriocarcinoma	–	–	+	–	+
Colorectal	rare	+	–	–	–
Esophageal	–	+	–	–	+
Gastric	rare	+	–	–	–
Ovarian	–	rare	–	–	+
Pancreatic	rare	+	–	–	rare
Parathyroid	–	–	–	+	+
Pheochromocytoma	–	–	–	+	+
Pulmonary (oat-cell)	–	–	+	+	+
Pulmonary (squamous)	–	+	+	–	+
Seminoma	–	–	+	–	–
Teratocarcinoma	+	–	+	–	–
Thyroid (colloid)	–	–	–	–	+
Thyroid (medullary)	–	–	–	+	+

recognized as *self,* they do not elicit either humoral or cell-mediated responses.

During malignant transformation, however, gene derepression is responsible for the production of increased concentrations of these gene products, which are known as oncofetal proteins. Carcinoembryonic antigen (CEA) is an example of this type of antigen.

Spontaneous Tumor Antigens

Tumors caused by no known mechanism are thought to produce antigens. Disagreement exists regarding whether or not these tumors are similar to those produced experimentally by chemical, viral, or physical agents. Although substantial evidence supports the contention that these tumors do not produce unique antigens, some evidence exists that refutes this contention. The importance of these findings remains unclear.

Tumor Markers

A tumor marker is a characteristic of a neoplastic cell that can be detected in plasma or serum (Table 28-8). Although these markers are not tumor specific and may be detected in nonneoplastic conditions (Table 28-9), markers may be useful in diagnosis (Table 28-10). and selection of different treatment approaches, monitoring therapy, or prognosis. Examples of tumor markers include:
1. Carcinoembryonic antigen (CEA)
2. Alpha-fetoprotein (AFP)
3. Beta subunit of human chorionic gonadotropin (B-hcG)
4. Neuron-specific enolase
5. Prostatic acid phosphatase
6. Placental alkaline phosphatase

Oncofetal Proteins

Carcinoembryonic antigen (CEA) is a cell-surface protein found predominantly on normal fetal endocrine tissues in the second trimester of gestation. If CEA is detected in mature individuals, it is of limited diagnostic value, but it is helpful in differentiating between benign and malignant pleural and ascites effusions. Plasma levels greater than 12 ng/mL are strongly correlated with malignancy. Elevated neoplastic states frequently associated with an increased CEA level are endodermally derived gastrointestinal neoplasms and neck and breast carcinomas. Also, 20% of smokers and 7% of former smokers have elevated CEA levels.

CEA is used clinically to monitor tumor progress in patients who have diagnosed cancer with a high blood CEA level. If treatment leads to a decline to normal levels (<2.5 ng/mL), a rise in CEA may indicate a cancer recurrence to the clinician. Blood specimens should be obtained 2 to 4 weeks apart to detect a trend.

Alpha-fetoprotein (AFP) is normally synthesized up to birth in humans. It is secreted in the serum in nanogram to milligram quantities in the following conditions: hepatocarcinoma, endodermal sinus tumors, nonseminomatous testicular cancer, teratocarcinoma of the testis or ovary, and malignant tumors of the mediastinum and sacrococcyx. In addition, a small percentage of patients with gastric and pancreatic cancer with liver metastasis may have elevated AFP levels. Both AFP and B-hCG should be quantitated initially in all patients with teratocarcinoma because one or both markers may be secreted in 85% of patients. The concentration of AFP may be elevated in nonneoplastic conditions such as hepatitis and cystic fibrosis.

Alpha-fetoprotein is a very reliable marker for following a patient's response to chemotherapy and radiation therapy. Levels should be obtained every 2 to 4 weeks (metabolic half-life in vivo is 4 days).

Ectopic Proteins

The beta subunit of human chorionic gonadotropin is a sensitive tumor marker with a metabolic half-life in vivo of 16 hours. A serum level of B-hCG greater than 1 ng/mL is strongly suggestive of pregnancy or a malignant tumor such as endodermal sinus tumor, teratocarcinoma, choriocarcinoma, molar pregancy, testicular embryonal carcinoma, or oat cell carcinoma of the lung.

Enzymes

Neuron-specific enolase is an isoenzyme specific for all tumor cells derived from the neural crest. An enzyme increase has been detected in neuroblastoma, pheochromocytoma, oat cell carcinomas, medullary thyroid and C-cell parathyroid carcinomas, and other neural crest-derived cancers. Serum levels are frequently elevated in disseminated disease.

Prostatic acid phosphatase is a serum enzyme exclusively diagnostic of prostatic carcinoma.

Placental alkaline phosphatase can be detected during pregnancy. It is also associated with the neoplastic conditions of seminoma and ovarian cancer.

Hormones

Elevated or inappropriate serum levels of hormones can function as tumor markers. Adrenocorticotropic hormone (ACTH), calcitonin, and catecholamines may be secreted by differentiated tumors of endocrine organs and squamous cell lung tumors. Oat cell carcinomas may produce B-hCG, antidiuretic hormone (ADH), serotonin, calcitonin, parathyroid hormone, and ACTH. These hormones can be used to follow a patient's response to therapy.

In addition, some breast cancers demonstrate progesterone and/or estradiol (estrogen) receptors, which are strongly correlated with a positive response to antihormone therapy. Patients with neuroblastomas and pheochromocytomas secrete catecholamine metabolites that can be detected in the urine. Neuroblastomas also release neuron-specific enolase and ferritin; these markers can be used for diagnosis and prognosis.

Modalities for Treating Cancer

Until recently, three modalities were used to treat cancer—surgery, radiation, and chemotherapy. The biologic response modifiers, such as interferon (IFN), are now the newest or fourth modality. Many different modes of therapy have demonstrated effectiveness in the treatment of cancer (Table 28-11); however, drug-induced immunosuppression and interferon therapy alone or in combination with drugs are the most frequent forms following surgery or in cases where surgery is not appropriate, e.g., hematologic disorders.

TABLE 28-11

Immunotherapy in Malignant Disease

Approach	Agent	Proposed mechanism
Active		
Specific	Modified or unmodified tumor cells, cell extract	Cellular and/or humoral response
Nonspecific systemic	Calmette-Guérin bacillus (BCG)	General immunocompetence
	Methanol-extracted residue (MER) of mycobacteria skeletal wall, *Corynebacterium parvum*, *Pseudomonas* vaccine	Increased mononuclear phagocyte system activity
	Levamisole, interferon	Restores immunocompetence
Local	BCG	Macrophage activation; killing of tumor with bystander effect
	Virus, Hapten, dinitrochlorobenzene (DNCB)	
Passive	Allogeneic or xenogeneic antibody	Removes soluble antigen or directly kills target cell
	Targeted monoclonal antibody	Conjugated with antitumor drug or radioisotope
Adoptive specific	Lymphocytes, Lymphocyte extract, i.e., immune RNA, transfer factor	Transfer of immunity
	Lymphokine-activated killer cells	Cytolysis of tumor cells

Chemotherapeutic Agents

Drugs are used in cancer therapy for curing, palliation, and research to develop more effective therapy. The categories of chemotherapeutic agents include:

1. Alkylating agents
2. Antimetabolites
3. Plant alkaloids
4. Antibiotics
5. Steroids
6. Miscellaneous agents

Alkylating agents. The alkyl groups of alkylating agents form covalent bonds with DNA and thus interfere with cellular replication. This interference is not only cytotoxic, but also potentially mutagenic and carcinogenic. The many drugs that are alkylating agents include:

TABLE 28-12

Examples of the Effects of Chemotherapy on the Immune Response

	Antibody		Delayed hypersensitivity	
	Primary response	*Secondary response*	*Primary response (initial)*	*Secondary response (recall)*
Corticosteroid	0	0	+ +	+
Methotrexate	+ +	+	+	0
6-Mercaptopurine	0	+	+	0
Azathioprine	0	+	+	0
6-Thioguanine	0	+	+	0
Cytosine arabinoside	+	+ +	0	0
Cyclophosphamide	+ +	0	+	0
L-Asparaginase	+	0	0	0
Daunomycin	+	0	+	0

Mustard derivatives: mechlorethamine (Mustargen), cyclophosphamide (Cytoxan), Chlorambucil (Leukeran), and melphalan (Alkeran)

Alkyl sulfonates: busulfan (Myleran)

Ethylenimine: triethylenethiophosphoramide (Thiotepa)

Triazene: dacarbazine (DTIC)

Nitrosoureas: carmustine (BiCNU) and lomustine (CeeNU)

Platinum analogs: cisplatin (Platinol), carboplatin

Antimetabolites. Antimetabolites are structural analogs of normal metabolites that compete with normal metabolites in the synthesis of DNA and RNA. This competition interferes with normal cellular replication. Examples of antimetabolites include:

Folate analogs: methotrexate

Purine analogs: 6-mercaptopurine (Purinethol), thioguanine 6-TG (Tabloid)

Pyrimidine analogs: 5-fluorouracil (5-FU), cytosine arabinoside (Cytosar)

Plant alkaloids. The chemotherapeutic agents classified as plant alkaloids interfere with mitotic spindle formation in the dividing cell. Examples of plant alkaloids are vincristine (Oncovin) and vinblastine (Velban).

Antibiotics. Antibiotics, substances derived from living microorganisms, can function as chemotherapeutic agents. The antibiotics used in cancer therapy include dactinomycin actinomycin D (Cosmegen), doxorubicin (Adriamycin), daunorubicin, daunomycin, rubidomycin (Cerubidine), bleomycin (Blenoxane), mitomycin (Mutamycin), and mithramycin (Mithracin).

Steroids. Steroids, organic compounds containing the perhydrocyclopentanophenanthrene in their nucleus, can be used as chemotherapeutic agents. The steroids used in cancer oncology include glucocorticoids (prednisone), estrogens (diethylstilbestrol), androgens (testosterone proprionate), and progestational agents (medroxyprogesterone, megestrol acetate).

Miscellaneous agents. Several compounds classified as miscellaneous agents are useful in the treatment of cancer. These compounds include L-asparaginase (Elspar), procarbazine (Matulane), and hydroxyurea (Hydrea).

The Effects of Drug-Induced Immunosuppression

Drugs used to treat malignancies such as solid tumors or leukemia have profoundly suppressive effects on the inflammatory response, delayed hypersensitivity, and/or specific antibody production (Table 28-12). Examples of the immune depression induced by drugs include depletion of T cells by corticosteroids because of the blocking of egress from the bone marrow into the circulation and dysfunction of the antibody response caused by folate antagonists and purine analogs. For this reason, infection secondary to immune suppression is a major cause of death in cancer patients beginning therapy and those who are in clinical remission.

Interferon

The clinical development of recombinant alpha-interferon represents the most rapid development of any antineoplastic drug in the United States. Interferon was first recognized as a naturally occurring antiviral substance in 1957 and identified for its antineoplastic properties. In 1981 large amounts of highly purified alpha-interferon became available because of recombinant DNA technology. Prior to that time, interferon preparations were produced by purification of supernatants harvested from virally stimulatd leukocytes. The Food and Drug Administration approved interferon for clinical use in the United States in June, 1986 without the benefit of animal studies. Research scientists were unable to study interferon in animal models because it is a species-specific molecule.

Alpha-interferon appears to have activity in a wide range of malignancies. Beginning in 1982, alpha-interferons were demonstrated to inhibit tumor growth in the absence of effector cells, such as monocytes or lymphocytes. The most notable responses to interferon have been in certain hematologic malignancies, including diseases of presumptive B cell, T cell, and myeloid origin. High rates of activity have also be seen in patients with Kaposi's sarcoma associated with acquired immunodeficiency syndrome (AIDS). The response of most solid tumors, however, has not been as dramatic.

Interferon has been used as a sole therapeutic agent, but it has been clearly demonstrated that an additive effect or synergy in various cell lines can occur with several cytotoxic drugs and different forms of interferons. For example, patients with malignant hematologic disease who had demonstrated resistance to standard agents have had positive responses to simultaneous or sequential treatments with alpha-interferon and the cytotoxic agent to which resistance had occurred.

The ultimate role of interferons in the management of malignant disease has not yet been fully explored. Interferon alone or in combination with cytotoxic agents, radiation therapy, or other lymphokines may prove to be the most effective form of therapy for many patients with malignancies.

Chapter Review

HIGHLIGHTS

All vertebrates capable of acute rejection of foreign skin grafts possess a localized complex involving many genes that exert major control over the organism's immune reactions. Many nucleated cells possess cell-surface-protein antigens that are part of this complex that readily provokes an immune response if transferred into an allogeneic individual of the same species. Some of these antigens are much more potent than others in provoking an immune response and are, therefore, called the major histocompatibility complex (MHC). In humans, the MHC is referred to as human leukocyte antigen (HLA). It is the most complex immunogenetic system presently known in man and is controlled by a MHC, or supergene, which includes several loci closely linked on the short arm of chromosome 6. The MHC is divided into four major regions: D, B, C, and A. The A, B, and C regions code for class I molecules, whereas the D region codes for class II molecules. Class I and class II antigens can be found on surface membrane proteins of body cells and in body fluids. The presence of HLA was first recognized when multiply transfused patients experienced transfusion reactions despite proper crossmatching. It was discovered that these reactions resulted from leukocyte's antibodies rather than antibodies directed against erythrocyte antigens. The MHC gene products have an important role in clinical immunology. For example, transplants are rejected if performed against MHC barriers; thus, immunosuppressive therapy is required. These antigens are of primary importance in influencing the genetic basis of survival or rejection of transplanted organs.

Although HLA was originally identified by its role in transplant rejection, it is now recognized that the products of HLA genes play a crucial role in our immune system. T cells do not recognize antigens directly but do so when the antigen is presented on the surface of an antigen-presenting cell, the macrophage. In addition to presentation of the antigen, the macrophage must present another molecule for this response to occur. This molecule is a cell surface glycoprotein that is coded in each species by the MHC. T cells are able to interact with the histocompatibility molecules only if they are genetically identical (MHC restriction). Both class I and class II antigens function as targets of T lymphocytes that regulate the immune response. Class I molecules regulate interaction between cytolytic T cells and target cells, and class II molecules restrict the activity of regulatory T cells (helper, suppressor, and amplifier subsets). Hence, class II molecules regulate the interaction between helper T cells and antigen-presenting cells. HLA matching is of value in organ transplantation as well as in the transplantation of bone marrow. HLA matched platelets are useful to patients who are refractile to random donor platelets. In paternity testing, HLA typing and selected erythrocyte antigens is used. HLA testing is also increasingly being used as a diagnostic and genetic counseling tool. Knowledge of HLA antigens and their linkage is becoming important because of the recognized association of certain antigens with distinct immunologic mediated reaction, autoimmune diseases, some neoplasms, and other disorders which, although nonimmunologic, are influenced by non-HLA genes also located within the major MHC region.

A variety of tissues and organs are transplanted in humans. Transplantation is one of the areas in addition to hypersensitivity and autoimmunity in which the immune system functions in a detrimental way. The transplanting or grafting of an organ or tissue ranges from self-transplantation to the grafting of a body component from one species to another. Tissues and organs transplanted include bone marrow, bone matrix, skin, kidneys, liver, cardiac valves, heart, pancreas, corneas, and lungs.

In instances such as bone marrow transplantation, host immunity to the donor can cause graft verus host disease (GVHD). This condition is believed to result from the patient being sensitized to unshared HLA antigens before transplantation or transfusion. When allogenic T lymphocytes are transfused from donor to recipient with a graft or blood transfusion, the patient can develop acute or chronic GVHD. Engraftment and multiplication of donor lymphocytes can also be caused by transfused blood because lymphocytes capable of mitosis can be found in stored blood products. Where the donor and recipient differ at HLA or H-2 loci, the reaction can be fatal. It is now accepted that GVHD can occur whenever immunologically competent allogeneic lymphocytes are transfused into a severely immunocompromised host. Patients at risk include those who are immunodeficient or immunosuppressed with severe lymphocytopenia and bone marrow suppression. In bone marrow transplant patients, acute GVHD develops within the first 3 months of tranplantation. Chronic GVHD resembles a collagen vascular disease with skin changes, such as erythema and cutaneous ulcers, and liver dysfunction, which is characterized by bile duct degeneration and cholestasis. Patients with chronic GVHD are suspectible to bacterial infections. In immunocompromised patients, the transfused or grafted lymphocytes recognize the antigens of the host as foreign and react immunologically against them. Instead of the usual transplantation reaction of host against graft, the reverse GVHD occurs. The risk of graft-versus-host disease, however, can be minimized if not eliminated by irradiation of the marrow or blood products. Radiation has an effect on specific cellular components, such as lymphocytes. In these cells, ionizing radiation is known to inhibit lymphocyte mitotic activity and blast transformation.

The role of sensitized lymphocytes and antibodies in graft rejection differs and is influenced by the type of organ transplanted. Lymphocytes, particularly recirculating small lymphocytes, are effective in shortening graft survival. Cell-mediated immunity is responsible for the rejection of skin and solid tumors. Humoral antibodies, however, can be also be involved in the rejection process. The complexity of the action and interaction of cellular and humoral factors in grafts is considerable. Five possible categories of graft rejection have been demonstrated in human kidney transplant rejection: hyperacute, accelerated, acute, chronic, and immunopathological.

The importance of tolerance to self-antigens was recognized very early in the study of immunology. Immunologic tolerance is the acquisition of non-reactivity toward particular antigens. Self-tolerance is a critical process and the failure to recognize self antigens can result in autoimmune disease. The specific immune responses to a variety of antigenic substances are now known to be regulated by an immune response (Ir) gene. Ir gene control is considered to be genetically dominant. The homology of the HLA-D region with the animal I-region suggests that the human Ir gene might be found to be linked to the HLA complex.

Immunosuppressive measures may be antigen specific or antigen nonspecific. Antigen-nonspecific immunosuppression includes drugs and other methods of specifically altering T cell function. Many cytotoxic drugs are primarily active against dividing cells and therefore have some functional specificity for any cells activated to divide by donor antigens. Other immunosuppressive measures directed at T cells include the use of antilymphocytes globulin at the time of transplantation and lymphoid irradiation before transplantation.

Tumors are neoplasms described as benign or malignant. A benign neoplasm is a nonspreading tumor; a malignant neoplasm is a growth that infiltrates tissues, metastasizes and often reoccurs after attempts to remove it surgically. The presence of a malignant neoplasm can be referred to as *carcinoma* or *cancer*. The factors that cause the majority of neoplasms are unknown. The incidence of cancer, however, has been correlated with certain environmental factors, such as occupational exposure to known carcinogenic agents, and host susceptibility considerations, such as heredity, sex, or age. Malignant proliferation of cells is also related to genes. Cancer often begins when a carcinogenic agent damages the DNA of a critical gene in a cell. The mutant cell multiplies and the succeeding generations of cells aggregate to form a malignant tumor. Proto-oncogenes act as central regulators of the growth in normal cells and are antecedents of oncogenes. The genetic targets of carcinogens are known to be oncogenes. Oncogenes have been associated with various tumor types that stem in a large part from preexisting genes present in the normal human genome. Therefore, oncogenes are considered to be altered versions of normal genes. In the course of a lifetime, a variety of mutations can convert a normal gene into a malignant oncogene. Once an oncogene is activated by mutation, it promotes excessive or inappropriate cell proliferation. A variety of RNA and DNA viruses have been associated with human malignancies. Some viral agents have a clear causative role such as the Epstein-Barr virus and certain papilloma viruses that are the etiologic agents in Burkitt's lymphoma and cervical carcinoma, respectively.

Viruses carry viral oncogenes into target cells, where they become firmly established. Clonal descendants then carry the viral genes which maintain the malignant phenotype of the cell clones. A very different class of cancer genes has been recently discovered. These tumor-suppressing genes in normal cells appear to regulate the proliferation of cell growth. When this type of gene is inactivated, a block to proliferation is removed and cells begin a program of deregulated growth or the genetically depleted cell itself may proliferate uncontrollably. Thus, tumor-suppressing genes are referred to as *antioncogenes*; their discovery will probably lead to the reformulation of ideas about how the growth of normal cells is regulated.

Although no single satisfactory explanation exists to explain the success of tumors in escaping the immune rejection process, it is believed that early clones of neoplastic cells are eliminated by the immune response. Cells such as the large granular lymphocytes (LGLs), ADCC effector cells, and cytotoxic T cells, dominate the rejection process that leads to the elimination of foreign tissue; therefore, cells rather than immunoglobulins are believed to dominate tumor immunity. Tumor cells manifest tumor antigens as well as self-HLA antigens. The four types of tumor antigens that have been identified are the following: tumor-specific antigens on chemically induced tumors, tumor-associated antigens on virally induced tumors, carcinofetal antigens, and spontaneous tumor antigens. A tumor marker is a characteristic of a neoplastic cell that can be detected in plasma or serum. Although these markers are not tumor specific and may be detected in nonneoplastic conditions, markers may be useful in diagnosis and selection of different treatment approaches, monitoring therapy, or prognosis. Tumor markers include carcinoembryonic antigen (CEA), alpha-fetoprotein (AFP), the beta subunit of human chorionic gonadotropin (B-hcG), neuron-specific enolase, prostatic acid phosphatase, and placental alkaline phosphatase.

Until recently, three modalities were used to treat cancer—surgery, radiation, and chemotherapy. The biologic response modifiers, such as interferon (IFN), are now the newest or fourth modality. Many different modes of therapy have been demonstrated in the treatment of cancer; however, drug-induced immunosuppression and interferon therapy alone or in combination with drugs are the most frequent forms of therapy following surgery or in cases where surgery is not appropriate, e.g., hematologic disorders.

REVIEW QUESTIONS

Match the following items:
1. Autograft
2. Syngraft
3. Allograft (hemograft)
4. Xenograft
   A. Graft transplanted between different but identical recipient and donor
   B. Graft transferred from one position to another in the same individual
   C. Graft between genetically different recipient and donor of the same species
   D. Graft between individuals of different species
5. Graft versus host disease is most frequently associated with transplant.
   A. Corneal
   B. Bone marrow
   C. Bone matrix
   D. Lung
   E. Heart valve

Match the following types of graft rejection:
6. Hyperacute
7. Accelerated
8. Acute
9. Chronic
   A. Caused by performed cytotoxic antibodies
   B. An immunopathologic mechanism
   C. Caused by previous sensitization to donor antigens
   D. Disturbance of host/graft tolerance
   E. Development of allogeneic reaction to donor antigens

10. Oncogenes are:
    A. Altered versions of normal genes.
    B. Central regulators of the growth in normal cells.
    C. Not related to an increased risk of cancer.
    D. Can be detected in all human tumors.
    E. Both A and E.

Match the following:
11. CEA
12. Alpha-fetoprotein
13. Beta-HCG
14. Prostatic acid phosphatase
    A. Of diagnostic value in germ-cell tumors and hepatic tumors
    B. Diagnosis of ovarian cancer
    C. Diagnostic of germ-cell tumors
    D. Useful for monitoring response to therapy of patients with various types of cancer
    E. Diagnostic of cancer of the prostrate

Answers

1. B 2. A 3. C 4. D 5. B 6. A 7. C 8. E 9. D 10. A 11. D 12. A 13. C 14. E

BIBLIOGRAPHY

Aloisi RM: Principles of immunology and immunodiagnostics, Philadelphia, Lea & Febiger, 1988.

Ashman RF: Rheumatic diseases. In Lawlor GJ and Fischer TJ, editors: Manual of allergy and immunology, ed 2, Boston, 1988, Little, Brown & Co.

Barrett J: Textbook of immunology, St Louis, 1988, The CV Mosby Co, 1988.

Bennett WM and Norman DJ: Action and toxicity of cyclosporine, Ann Rev Med 37:215-224, 1986.

Bonnem EM: Alpha interferon: combinations with other antineoplastic modalities, Semin Oncol 14(2):48-60, June 1987.

Friend SH, Dryja TP and Weinberg RA: Oncogenes and tumor-suppressing genes, New Engl J Med 318(10):618-623, March 1988.

Nehlsen-Cannarella SL: HLA and disease, Complements 3(1):2, 1983.

Roitt IM: Essential immunology, ed 5, Oxford, England, 1984, Blackwell Scientific Publications Inc.

Roitt IM: Immunology, London, 1985, Gower Medical Publishing Ltd.

Russell PS, Colvin RB, and Cosimi AB: Monoclonal antibodies for the diagnosis and treatment of transplant rejection, Ann Rev Med 37:63-79, 1986.

Solinger AM: Organ transplantation and the immune response gene. In Symposium on clinical immunology I, Med Clin North Am 69(3):565-577, May 1985.

Spiegel RJ: The alpha interferons: clinical overview, Semin Oncol 14(2):1-12, June 1987.

Stein JH: Internal medicine, ed 2, Boston, 1987, Little, Brown & Co.

Thompson J: The human leukocyte antigen system. In Stein J, editor: Internal medicine, ed 2, Boston, 1987, Little, Brown & Co.

Tizard IR: Immunology: an introduction, Philadelphia, 1984, Saunders College Publishing.

Turgeon ML: Fundamentals of immunohematology, 1989, Philadelphia, Lea & Febiger.

Weinberg RA: Finding the anti-oncogene, Scientific American Books, 259(3):44-51, Sept 1988.

Zeltzer PM: In Lawlor GJ and Fischer TJ, editors: The immune system and neoplasia. In Manual of allergy and immunology, ed 2, Boston, 1988, Little, Brown & Co.

Lyme Disease

During the writing of this book, the incidence of Lyme disease has increased dramatically. It has spread to most states in the United States and is therefore no longer a regionally limited disease. Although serologic testing for Lyme disease is being conducted chiefly by reference laboratories at this time, a discussion of this disease has been added to *Immunology and Serology in Laboratory Medicine* in order to achieve completeness in the scope of topics included in the book.

ETIOLOGY

Lyme disease is an infectious disease caused by the spirochete *Borrelia burgdorferi* and is transmitted by certain ixodes ticks that are part of the *I. ricinus* complex. These include *I. dammini* in the northeastern and midwestern United States, *I. pacificus* in the western United States, *I. ricinus* in Europe, and *I. persulcatus* in Asia. The vector has not been identified in Australia. Although ixodid ticks are also indigenous to Africa and South America, it is not clear whether Lyme borreliosis occurs on these continents.

In the United States, the preferred host for both the larval and nymphal states of *I. dammini* is the white-footed mouse, *Peromyscus leucopus.* White-tailed deer, which are not involved in the life cycle of the spirochete, are the preferred host for *I. dammini's* adult stage, and they seem to be critical to tick survival. Ixodes ticks have also been found on at least 30 types of wild animals and 49 species of birds. Illness is not known to develop in wild animals but clinical Lyme disease does occur in domestic animals, including dogs, horses, and cattle.

Spirochetes are transmitted from the gut of the tick to human skin at the site of a bite, and then they migrate outwardly into the skin causing the unique expanding skin lesion, *erythema migrans* (EM). Subsequent dissemination of spirochetes to secondary sites may cause major organ system involvement in humans. In dogs, the most common symptom is arthritis.

EPIDEMIOLOGY

Retrospectively, it appears that the first symptom of Lyme disease was recognized as early as 1908 in Sweden. In the decades that followed, the rash produced by the disease (*erythema chronicum migrans* ECM) was noted elsewhere in Europe as were other symptoms that seemed to follow ECM's eruption. Secondary symptoms such as impairment of the nervous system were described in France, Germany, and again in Sweden. In the United States, the European rash was virtually unknown until 1969 when a case of a physician who was bitten by a tick while hunting in Wisconsin was reported. Although a few ECM cases were seen in Americans who had traveled to Europe, there were no further native American cases until 1975 when physicians at the U.S. Navy base in Groton, Connecticut reported seeing four patients with a rash similar to EM. At the same time an epidemiologist at the Connecticut State Department of Health and a rheumatologist at Yale were notified of an unusual cluster of cases of arthritis occurring in children in Lyme, Connecticut. It was not until 1982 that Burgdorfer and Barbour isolated a previously unrecognized spirochete, now called *Borrelia burgdorferi*, from *I. dammini* ticks and Lyme disease became a recognized infectious disease.

In 1988, the overall incidence of Lyme disease in Connecticut residents was 22 per 100,000. These case rates demonstrated a three to eightfold increase compared to 1977. The average annual incidence of reported Lyme disease in the United States in 1987-1988 was 1.4 per 100,000. New York led the nation in reported cases in 1988 with 57% of the cases reported nationally. Eight states: New York, New Jersey, Pennsylvania, Connecticut, Massachusetts, Rhode Island, Wisconsin, and Minnesota, reported 92% of the nation's cases. Only seven states, all located west of the 100th meridian, have not reported any cases of Lyme disease.

In 1987 and 1988, 6876 cases of Lyme disease from 43 states were reported to the Centers for Disease Control (CDC). The 4507 cases reported in 1988 was nearly double the number of cases reported in 1987, and ninefold the number reported in 1982 when a systematic system of national surveillance was established.

SIGNS AND SYMPTOMS

The Centers for Disease Control case definition for Lyme disease acquired in endemic areas includes the presence of erythema migrans (EM) regardless of serologic results or neurologic, cardiac, or arthritic manifestations characteristic of Lyme disease, and a positive serologic test for antibody to *Borrelia burgdorferi.*

Lyme borreliosis is a multisystem illness that primarily involves the skin, nervous system, heart, and joints. Clinically, this borrelial infection is comparable to syphilis because of its multisystem involvement, occurrence in stages, and mimicry of other diseases. Lyme disease usually begins during the summer months with EM and flu-like symptoms and may be accompanied by right upper-quadrant tenderness and a mild hepatitis (stage 1). This stage is followed weeks to months later by acute cardiac or neurologic disease in a minority of untreated individuals (stage 2), and then is followed by arthritis and chronic neurologic disease (stage 3) in many untreated patients weeks to years after the onset of the disease. There is considerable overlap between these stages; however, Lyme disease is best characterized as an illness that evolves from early to late disease without reference to an arbitrary staging system. A patient may have one or all of the stages, and the infection may not become symptomatic until stage 2 or 3. The majority of affected patients have EM, 1 to 4 patients manifest arthritis, and neurologic manifestations and cardiac involvement is infrequent.

Cutaneous Manifestations

Cutaneous manifestations can be demonstrated as early (EM), secondary (disseminated lesions and lymphocytoma) and late lesions (acrodermatitis chromica atrophicans). With the exception of the late lesions, cutaneous manifestations generally resolve spontaneously over weeks to months. The red papule at the site of the tick bite is most commonly located on the thigh, groin, or axilla. Facial EM is more commonly seen in children.

Several days to weeks after the onset of EM, nearly one-half of untreated patients develop secondary skin lesions. A rare early manifestation of Lyme disease is a borrelia lymphocytoma, a tumor-like violaceous swelling or nodule at the base of the earlobe or the nipple, caused by a dense lymphocytic infiltrate of the dermis. This lesion occurs at the site of a tick bite, and, in conjunction with other symptoms, it may be confused with lymphoma. *Acrodermatitis chronica atrophican (ACA)* is a late skin manifestation of Lyme disease that is more prevalent in Europe than the United States.

Cardiac Manifestations

Lyme carditis occurs in approximately 8% of untreated patients within two to six weeks following initial infection, and may be the initial manifestation of Lyme disease. The cardiac conduction abnormalities of Lyme disease are usually brief, lasting days to weeks, and generally do not require permanent cardiac pacing. A less common cardiac manifestation is arrhythmia, which may be mistaken for acute rheumatic fever.

Neurologic Manifestations

Neurologic abnormalities occur in approximately 15% of untreated patients. These manifestations usually appear two to eight weeks after the onset of the disease and may include aseptic meningitis, cranial nerve palsies, peripheral radiculoneuritis, and peripheral neuropathy. The predominant symptoms of Lyme meningitis are severe headache and mild neck stiffness, which may fluctuate for weeks after a post-erythema migrans latent period.

Other Manifestations

Arthralgia and myalgia are common features of early Lyme disease, but frank arthritis during EM is unusual.

Ocular manifestations may occur in Lyme disease, and include cranial nerve palsies, optic neuritis, panophthalmitis with loss of vision, and choroiditis with retinal detachment.

A uniform pattern of congenital malformations has not been identified in maternal-fetal transmission of Lyme disease.

Immunologic Manifestations

Specific IgM or IgG antibodies against *B. burgdorferi* are usually not detectable in a patient's serum unless symptoms have been present for at least two to four weeks. In cases of Lyme arthritis, tests for serum antinuclear antibodies, rheumatoid factor, and the VDRL (Venereal Disease Research Laboratories) test are generally negative. However, anti-*B. burgdorferi* antibodies of the IgG type should be present in the serum of patients with Lyme arthritis.

DIAGNOSTIC EVALUATION

Numerous laboratory techniques are available for the diagnosis of Lyme disease. In the early phase of Lyme disease, laboratory findings are nonspecific and typically may include an elevated sedimentation rate (ESR), elevated serum IgM levels, and mildly elevated hepatic transaminase (SGPT/ALT) levels.

Assays for the detection of antibodies to *Borrelia burgdorferi* are the most practical means of confirming infection. Several commercial antibody test kits, including a recently introduced latex agglutination procedure, are available for verifying *B. burgdorferi* infection. The most common procedures include indirect fluorescent antibody (IFA) staining methods and enzyme-linked immunosorbent assays (ELISA) for total immunoglobulins (Ig) or IgM and IgG antibodies. Immunoblotting techniques can be used along with ELISA to characterize immune response and for diagnosis. Western blot analysis can verify reactivity of antibody to major surface or flagellar proteins of *B. burgdorferi*.

The sensitivities of IFA and ELISA methods are usually low during the initial three weeks of infection; therefore, negative results are common. The most serious disadvantages of current techniques are low sensitivity and lengthy processing times. In addition, false-positive reactions resulting from cross-reactivity can occur in tests for Lyme disease. For example, tick-borne relapsing fever spirochetes, *Borrelia hermsii*, are closely related to *B. burgdorferi*. Antibodies to *B. hermsii*, an agent that coexists with the Lyme disease spirochete in portions of the western United States strongly cross-react with *B. burgdorferi* in IFA staining and ELISA testing. Common antigens are shared among the *Borrelia* and even with the Treponemes. Serum from syphilitic patients reacts positively in assays for Lyme disease. Therefore, serologic test results for antibodies to *B. burgodorferi* should be considered along with clinical data and epidemiologic information when evaluating a patient for Lyme disease.

BIBLIOGRAPHY

Cartter ML, Mshar P, and Hadler JL: The epidemiology of Lyme disease in Connecticut, Conn Med 53:6, 1989.

Lang J: Catching the bug: how scientists found the cause of Lyme disease and why we're not out of the woods yet, Conn Med 53:6, 1989.

Magnarelli LA: Laboratory analyses for Lyme disease, Conn Med 53:6, 1989.

Steere AC: Lyme disease N Engl J Med 321:9, 1989.

Trock DH, Craft JE, and Rahn DW: Clinical manifestations of Lyme disease in the United States, Conn Med 53:6, 1989.

Tsai TF, Bailey RE, and Moore PS: National surveillance of Lyme disease, Conn Med 53:6, 1989.

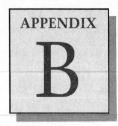

Diagnostic Tests in Medical Laboratory Immunology

ACETYLCHOLINE RECEPTOR (AchR) BINDING ANTIBODY

Measures antibody to acetylcholine receptors at neuromuscular junctions of skeletal muscle. Useful in the diagnosis of myasthenia gravis. Negative in ocular myasthenia, Eaton-Lambert syndrome, and in generalized myasthenia gravis if treated or inactive.

ACETYLCHOLINE RECEPTOR (AcHR) BLOCKING ANTIBODY

Measures antibody to acetylcholine receptors that block binding of 125_I-(alpha)-bungarotoxin. Found in about one third of patients with myasthenia gravis.

ALBUMIN INDEX

Measures albumin in cerebrospinal fluid and serum. Elevated values suggest blood-brain barrier damage as seen in Guillain-Barré syndrome and similar conditions or possibly a traumatic tap. This test is of value in the interpretation of CNS IgG synthesis rates.

ALPHA-1-ANTITRYPSIN

Measures the quantity of alpha-1-antitrypsin, an acute-phase inflammatory reactant, in the blood. A deficiency of this protein is found if the alleles Z and S are present; moderate reduction is exhibited by the MS and MZ phenotypes are increased in chronic or recurrent anterior uveitis and rheumatoid arthritis. The MZ phenotype is also associated with hepatoma and chronic hepatitis in adults. The ZZ phenotype predisposes an individual to the development of severe, early-onset pulmonary emphysema and to liver disease in infancy and childhood.

ANTIADRENAL ANTIBODY

Measures antibody to adrenal cortex cells. High antibody titers are characteristic of autoimmune hypoadrenalism in about three fourths of cases but are not found in tuberculous Addison's disease.

ANTICENTRIOLE ANTIBODY

Measures antibody to the cellular ultrastructures, centrioles. The appearance of these antibodies is unusual but can be demonstrated in systemic sclerosis.

ANTICARDIOLIPIN ANTIBODY

Measures antibody directed to cardiolipin. The presence of antibody in systemic lupus erythematosus (SLE) is associated with arterial and venous thromboses, and in patients with placental infarcts in early pregnancy with or without SLE. Elevation of anticardiolipin antibody may be predictive of the risk of thrombosis or recurrent spontaneous abortions of early pregnancy.

ANTICENTROMERE ANTIBODY

Measures anticentrome (antikinetocore) to chromosomal centromeres. The majority of patients with CREST syndrome demonstrate these antibodies. These antibodies are seen in about one third of patients with Raynaud's disease and approximately 10% of patients with systemic sclerosis.

ANTI-DNA ANTIBODY

Measures antibody to double-stranded deoxyribonucleic acid (DNA). Increased amounts (>25% by membrane assay) and decreased quantities of the C4 complement component confirm the diagnosis of systemic lupus erythematosus (SLE). These tests are useful in monitoring the activity and exacerbations of SLE. The absence of anti-DNA is demonstrated in about one fourth of SLE patients; therefore a negative test does not rule out SLE.

ANTIGLOMERULAR BASEMENT MEMBRANE ANTIBODY

Measures the amount of antibody to glomerular basement membrane (anti-GBM). High titers are suggestive of Goodpasture's disease or anti-GBM nephritis. The test is useful for monitoring anti-GBM nephritis. Negative results, however, do not rule out Goodpasture's disease.

ANTI-INTRINSIC FACTOR

Measures antibodies to intrinsic factor (IF). The presence of IF-blocking antibodies is diagnostic of pernicious anemia and occurs in about 60% of cases.

ANTI-ISLET-CELL ANTIBODY

Measures antibodies to the islet cells of the pancreas. This test is useful as an early marker of beta pancreatic cell destruction.

ANTI-LKM ANTIBODY

Measures antibodies to components of renal and hepatic microsomes. The presence of a high titer is diagnostic of hepatic illness and suggests aggressive disease.

ANTIMITOCHONDRIAL ANTIBODY

Measures antibodies to the cellular ultrastructures, mitochondria. A high titer strongly suggests primary biliary cirrhosis (PBC); the absence of mitochondrial antibodies is strong evidence against PBC. Other forms of liver disease frequently exhibit low mitochondrial antibody titers.

ANTIMYELIN ANTIBODY

Measures antibody to components of the myelin sheath of nerves or myelin basic protein. Antibodies to myelin are associated with multiple sclerosis (MS) or other neurologic diseases. Myelin antibodies are not detectable in the cerebrospinal fluid of multiple sclerosis patients.

ANTIMYOCARDIAL ANTIBODY

Measures antibody to components of the myocardium. The presence of myocardial antibodies is diagnostic of Dressler's syndrome (cardiac injury) or rheumatic fever.

ANTINUCLEAR ANTIBODY

Measures antibody to nuclear antigens. Antinuclear antibodies are found in 99% of patients with untreated systemic lupus erythematosus.

ANTIPARIETAL CELL ANTIBODY

Measures antibody to parietal cells (large cells on the margin of the peptic glands of the stomach). The majority (80%) of patients with pernicious anemia have parietal cell antibodies. In the presence of these antibodies, gastric biopsy almost always demonstrates gastritis. Low antibody titers to parietal cells are often found with no clinical evidence of pernicious anemia or atrophic gastritis and are sometimes seen in elderly patients.

ANTIPLATELET ANTIBODY

Measures immunologically attached IgG on platelets. The presence of platelet antibodies, measured indirectly, is associated with immune thrombocytopenia (ITP) and systemic lupus erythematosus (SLE).

ANTIRETICULIN ANTIBODY

Measures antibody to reticulin, an albuminoid or scleroprotein substance present in the connective framework of reticular tissue. The majority (80%) of cases of childhood gluten-sensitive enteropathy demonstrate reticulin antibodies. These antibodies can also be found in dermatitis herpetiformis and adult gluten-sensitive enteropathy and in about one fifth of patients suffering from chronic heroin addiction.

ANTI-RHEUMATOID ARTHRITIS NUCLEAR ANTIGEN (ANTI-RANA) ANTIBODY
(also called Rheumatoid Arthritis Precipitin-RAP)

Measures antibody to a component of the Epstein-Barr virus. Antibody is found in the majority of patients with rheumatoid arthritis and in about 15% of patients with systemic lupus erythematosus (SLE). Anti-RANA is not useful in diagnosis or differential diagnosis of arthritis.

ANTIRIBOSOME ANTIBODY

Measures the presence of antibodies to the cellular organelles, ribosomes. Ribosomal antibodies are found in about 10% of patients with systemic lupus erythrematosus.

ANTINUCLEAR RIBONUCLEOPROTEIN (ANTI-nRNP) ANTIBODY

Measures an antinuclear antibody (ANA), nuclear ribonucleoprotein. A high titer of this antibody is characteristic of mixed connective tissue disease (MCTD) or undifferentiated connective tissue disease. In MCTD, anti-nRNP is found in the absence of various other ANAs. Low titers of anti-nRNP are seen in about one third of patients with systemic lupus erythematosus and are typically found in association with other ANAs, such as anti-DNA or anti-Sm.

ANTI-ScL OR ANTI-SCL-70 ANTIBODY

Measures an antibody to a basic nonhistone nuclear protein. The presence of anti-Scl is diagnostic of systemic sclerosis; however, it is demonstrable in only about one fifth of the patients suffering from systemic sclerosis.

ANTI-SKIN (DERMAL-EPIDERMAL) ANTIBODY

Measures antibody to the basement membrane area of the skin. Antibodies are present in more than 80% of patients with bullous pemphigoid, but the absence of antibodies does not rule out the disorder.

ANTI-SKIN (INTER-EPITHELIAL) ANTIBODY

Measures antibody to intercellular substance of the skin. Antibodies can be detected in most (90%) of patients with pemphigus. The absence of demonstrable antibody usually excludes the diagnosis. The presence of antibodies is also useful in evaluating "blistering" disease. A rising antibody titer may indicate an impending relapse of pemphigus; a falling titer is suggestive of effective control of the disease.

ANTI-SM ANTIBODY

Measures Sm (Smith) antibody to acidic nuclear protein. Sm antibody is demonstrated by about one third of patients with systemic lupus erythematosus (SLE). Presence of the antibody confirms the diagnosis of SLE, but the absence of antibody does not exclude the diagnosis.

ANTISMOOTH MUSCLE ANTIBODY

Measures antibody to components of smooth muscle. A high and persistent titer is suggestive of the autoimmune form of chronic active hepatitis. Antismooth muscle antibodies are also seen in viral disorders such as infectious mononucleosis.

ANTISPERM ANTIBODY

Evaluates the presence of reproductive cell, or sperm, antibodies. Half of vasectomized males and 40% of males and females with fertility problems demonstrate the antibody.

ANTI-SS-A (SS-A PRECIPITIN, ANTI-Ro) ANTIBODY

Detects the presence of antibody to acidic nucleoprotein of human spleen extract. SS-A precipitins are demonstrable in more than 70% of patients with Sjögren's syndrome—Sicca complex and are often found in a subset of these patients who are at risk for vasculitis. The antibody is also found in one third of patients with systemic lupus erythematosus or Sjögren's rheumatoid arthritis, or the annular variety of subacute cutaneous lupus erythematosus (LE). In neonatal LE, autoantibodies to SS-A, discoid skin lesions, and congenital heart blocks are common.

ANTI-SS-B (SS-B PRECIPITIN, ANTI-La) ANTIBODY

Detects antibody to acidic nucleoprotein of rubbati thymus. Anti-SS-B is demonstrated by the majority of patients with Sjörgren's syndrome—systemic lupus erythematosus. One half to three fourths of patients with Sjögren's syndrome—sicca complex have the antibody; it is frequently found in a subset of these patients at risk for vasculitis.

ANTISTRIATIONAL ANTIBODY

Measures antibody to components of striated muscle. Antibodies to striated muscle may be detected in patients with myasthenia gravis, thymoma, or with penicillamine treatment. Absence of the antibody in patients with myasthenia gravis generally rules out the presence of thymoma.

ANTITHYROGLOBULIN AND ANTITHYROID MICROSOME ANTIBODY

Evaluates the presence of antibody to the thyroid components: thyroglobulin, an iodine-containing protein secreted by the thyroid gland and stored within its colloid substance; and thyroid microsomes, particles derived from the endoplasmic reticulum. The presence of microsome antibodies is considered to be predictive of an elevated thyroid-stimulating hormone (TSH) level. A positive thyroid antibody test and an elevated TSH titer are associated with a risk of hypothyroidism. Absence of both antibodies is strong evidence against autoimmune thyroiditis.

BETA-GLUCURONIDASE

Measures the enzyme activity of the enzyme, beta-glucuronidase, in cerebrospinal fluid. Increased levels of enzyme activity are associated with bacterial or fungal meningitis; extremely elevated enzyme levels are encountered in untreated leptomenigeal (pia or arachnoid) metastases. Treated cases of leptomeningeal carcinoma may demonstrate decreased enzyme levels. Normal enzyme levels are usually seen in primary brain tumors and parenchymal metastases.

BETA$_2$-MICROGLOBULIN

Measures the quantity of beta$_2$-microglobulin in either serum or cerebrospinal fluid. Elevated levels of this protein are associated with central nervous system (CNS) involvement in patients suffering from leukemia or lymphoma. Determination of beta$_2$-microglobulin levels in both serum and cerebrospinal fluid (CSF) are of value in the early diagnosis of CNS involvement and in monitoring intrathecal (within the spinal canal) therapy.

C1 ESTERASE INHIBITOR (C1 INHIBITOR)

Measures the activity and/or concentration of C1 inhibitor in serum. A deficiency of this protein is characteristic of hereditary angioedema (HAE). Some patients demonstrate catalytically inactive protein.

C1q

Evaluates the complement component, C1q, in serum. Decreased levels can be demonstrated in patients who are suffering from hypocomplementemic urticarial vasculitis, severe combined immunodeficiency or X-linked hypogammaglobulinemia.

C1q BINDING

Measures the binding of immune complexes containing IgG$_1$, IgG$_2$, IgG$_3$, and/or IgM to the complement component, C1q. High values of C1q binding are associated with the presence of circulating immune complexes of the type that interact with the classic pathway of complement activation. This test can be useful as a prognostic tool at diagnosis and during remission of acute myelogenous leukemia.

C2

Measures the second component of complement. An extremely low level of C2 component is suggestive of a lupus-like disease that may be caused by a genetic deficiency associated with HLA-A25, B18, or DR2. Approximately half of the individuals with decreased levels of C2 have autoimmune disease; the other half are apparently normal but have an increased susceptibility to bacterial infection.

C3

Measures the third component of complement. Extremely decreased levels are seen in patients with poststreptoccocal glomerulonephritis or inherited (C3) complement deficiency. This component is also decreased in cases of severe liver disease and in systemic lupus erythematosus (SLE) patients with renal disease.

C3b INHIBITOR (C3b INACTIVATOR)

Measures the C3b component of complement. This component causes low complement C3 levels, the absence of C3PA in serum, and high C3b levels. A deficiency of C3b inhibitor is associated with an increased predisposition to infection.

C3PA (C3 PROACTIVATOR, PROPERDIN FACTOR B)

Evaluates the level of the factor B component, which is consumed by activation of the alternative complement pathway. Assessment of C3PA indicates whether or not a decreased level of C3 is due to the classic or alternate pathways of complement activation. A decreased level of complement components C3 and C4 demonstrates activation of the classic pathway. Decreased levels of C3 and C3PA with a normal level of C4 is indicative of complement activation via the alternative pathway.

Activation of the classic pathway (sometimes with accompanying alternative pathway activation) is associated with disorders such as immune complex diseases, various forms of vasculitis, and acute glomerulonephritis.

Activation of the alternative pathway is associated with many disorders. These disorders include chronic hypocomplementemic glomerulonephritis, diffuse intravascular coagulation, septicemia, subacute bacterial endocarditis, paroxysmal nocturnal hemoglobinuria (PNH), and sickle cell anemia.

In systemic lupus erythematosus, both the classic and alternative pathways are activated.

C4

Measures the level of component C4 of the classic complement activation pathway. A decreased C4 level with elevated anti-DNA and ANA titers confirms the diagnosis of systemic lupus erythematosus (SLE) in a patient. In cases of SLE, the periodic assessment of C4 can be useful in monitoring the progress of the disorder. Patients with extremely low C4 and CH50 levels in the presence of normal levels of the C3 component may be demonstrating the effects of a genetic deficiency of C1 inhibitor or C4.

C4 ALLOTYPES

Evaluates the antigenically distinct forms of C4A and C4B, alleles located on the sixth chromosome in the major histocompatibility complex. Identification of C4 allotypes in conjunction with specific HLA antigens are markers for disease susceptibility.

C5

Measures the concentration of the C5 complement component. A genetic deficiency of the C5 component is associated with increased susceptibility to bacterial infection and is expressed as an autoimmune disorder, e.g., systemic lupus erythematosus. In the case of dysfunction of C5 (Leiner's disease), the patient is predisposed to infections of the skin and bowel and the disease is characterized by eczema. In such a patient the level of C5 is normal, but the C5 component fails to promote phagocytosis.

C6

Measures the level of the C6 complement component. A decreased quantity of C6 predisposes an individual to significant *Neisseria* (bacteria) infections.

C7

Measures the quantity of the C7 complement component. A decreased level of this component is associated with severe bacterial infections caused by *Neisseria* species, Raynaud's phenomenon, sclerodactyly, and telangiectasia.

C8

Measures the level of the C8 complement component. A decreased quantity of this component is associated with systemic lupus erythematosus. A deficiency of C8 makes patients highly susceptible to *Neisseria* infections.

CARCINOEMBRYONIC ANTIGEN (CEA)

Detects the presence of CEA in spinal fluid. An increased level of CEA in cerebrospinal fluid (CSF) is very suggestive of primary or secondary intradural malignancy. The level of CEA may decline with effective therapy.

CERULOPLASMIN

Detects the level of the protein ceruloplasmin in blood. Although increased or decreased levels of this protein are associated with a variety of clinical conditions, a severe decrease or complete absence of ceruloplasmin can be demonstrated in most homozygous patients suffering from Wilson's disease. The absence or gross deficiency of ceruloplasmin in heterozygous carriers of the gene responsible for Wilson's disease is infrequent.

CH$_{50}$

Assesses the hemolytic activity of the complement system, a series of proteins found in the blood. Monitoring CH$_{50}$ is useful in following the course of immune complex disease, in screening for genetic deficiencies of the complement system, and in diagnosing hereditary angioneurotic edema.

COLD AGGLUTININS

Evaluates the ability of antibodies to agglutinate group O erythrocytes at 4° C. The presence of an elevated titer of cold-reacting antibodies can cause acrocyanosis or hemolysis. These antibodies can be demonstrated in patients with primary (chronic) or secondary cold agglutinin syndromes due to bacterial or viral disease, such as *M. pneumoniae* or Epstein-Barr virus, or neoplasms such as lymphoma or histiocytic lymphoma.

COMPLEMENT ACTIVATION PRODUCTS

Measures the protein fragments of C3 and C4 to reflect in vivo or in vitro activation. In vivo activation of complement, e.g., immune complex diseases, or in vitro activation, e.g., complement degradation, causes proteolytic digestion of these components and altered electrophoretic mobility. Assessment of these components is not considered to be of reliable diagnostic value.

COMPLEMENT COMPONENTS (C1r, C1s, C2, C3, C4, C5, C6, C7, C8)

Assesses various components of complement. These components are often elevated in certain inflammatory conditions; acute illnesses, such as myocardial infarction; trauma; or some infectious diseases, such as typhoid fever. Homozygous component deficiencies predispose an individual to autoimmune diseases, such as systemic lupus erythematosus, chronic glomerulonephritis, infections, arthritis, and vasculitis. Determination of complement levels in synovial (joint) fluid is of value. Increased levels may been demonstrated in Reiter's syndrome; decreased levels (relative to plasma concentrations) may be observed in rheumatoid arthritis.

COMPLEMENT DECAY RATE

Assesses the decrease of CH_{50} activity in plasma at 37° C. A rate greater than 50% is consistent with, but not diagnostic of, a C1 esterase inhibitor deficiency.

CONGLUTININ SOLID PHASE (Kg SP) ASSAY FOR IMMUNE COMPLEXES

Measures the quantity of immune complexes binding to the protein, conglutinin. If circulating immune complexes, which are capable of activating the classic or alternative complement pathways, are present, large quantities of conglutinin binding activity are demonstrated. The majority of circulating immune complexes can be detected by combining the Kg SP, C1q binding, Raji cell, and polyethylene glycol (PEG) assays.

C REACTIVE PROTEIN (CRP)

Assesses one of the acute-phase inflammatory proteins, C reactive protein. This protein is increased in rheumatoid arthritis and bacterial meningitis.

CRYOFIBRINOGEN

Evaluates cold precipitable fibrinogen and other similar plasma proteins. The presence of cryofibrinogen is suggestive of primary or secondary disorders. Secondary disorders include acute and chronic inflammation, lymphoproliferative and connective tissue disorders, necrosis, or tumors.

CRYOGLOBULINS

Detects the presence of cold precipitable immunoglobulins in serum. The major types of cryoglobulins and associated conditions include:
1. Monoclonal IgM, IgG, or IgA without known antibody specificity or monoclonal Bence Jones protein associated with disorders such as Raynaud's phenomenon, myeloma, and macroglobulinemia.
2. Monoclonal IgM, IgG, or IgA antibodies directed against polyclonal IgG associated with disorders such as Sjögren's disease, lymphoproliferative disorders, purpura, vasculitis, and macroglobulinemia.
3. Mixed (usually IgM and IgG) polyclonal immunoglobulins associated with disorders such as Sjögren's disease, systemic lupus erythematosus (SLE), vasculitis, or purpura.

DIPHTHERIA ANTIBODIES

Measures the quantity of antibody present after the administration of diphtheria toxoid. The absence of antibody after immunization confirms a patient's inability to form new antibody, i.e., abnormal humoral immunity.

FERRITIN

Evaluates the concentration of the storage form of iron, ferritin, in serum. In conjunction with abnormalities of erythrocyte, e.g., mean corpuscular volume and mean corpuscular hemoglobin, this assay is useful in establishing the diagnosis of iron deficiency anemia.

HISTONE REACTIVE ANTINUCLEAR ANTIBODY (HRANA)

Measures the presence of HRANA. A high titer of HRANA is highly suggestive of drug-induced (e.g., hydralazine) lupus erythematosus. HRANA may occasionally be demonstrated in patients with systemic lupus erythematosus (SLE).

HLA-B27

Assesses one of the human leukocyte antigens (HLA) on the surface of lymphocytes. Detection of HLA-B27 is useful in establishing the diagnosis of ankylosing spondylitis (AS). The majority of white patients with AS are antigen positive, and about half of black patients with AS are antigen positive.

HLA-DR

Assesses one of the human leukocyte antigens (HLA) on the surface of lymphocytes. Detection of

HLA-DR is useful in predicting a person's susceptibility to disease and also in estimating adverse reactions to certain drugs, e.g., hydralazine.

Identification of combinations of HLA alleles at various loci, such as HLA-A, B, C, and DR antigens, together with the inheritance of allotypes of C4 and allelic forms of C2 and properdin factor B (referred to as supratypes), are becoming useful tools in diagnosing immunoregulatory abnormalities, as well as different types of clinical diseases and susceptibility to infection.

HLA-DR3

Evaluates one of the human leukocyte antigens (HLA) on the surface of lymphocytes. Detection of HLA-DR3 and an elevated titer of thyroid stimulating hormone (TSH) is prognostic for forms of Graves' disease that will not respond or will relapse with antithyroid medication.

IMMUNOGLOBULINS

Measures the total immunoglobulin concentration in the serum. Increased concentration is representative of hyperglobulinemia. A major decrease in concentration, immunodeficiency, is the cause of recurrent infections, atypical arthritis, or persistent diarrhea.

IMMUNOGLOBULIN A (IgA)

Quantitates the concentration of the immunoglobulin, IgA. Normal concentrations rule out agammaglobulinemias in childhood and selective IgA deficiency. Selective deficiencies of IgA are the most common type of immunodeficiency.

IMMUNOGLOBULIN D (IgD)

Quantitates the concentration of the immunoglobulin IgD. It is found in very low concentrations in serum and its functional role is not well characterized.

IMMUNOGLOBULIN E (IgE)

Measures the immunoglobin, IgE. Markedly increased values can be found in patients with immunodeficient states, especially cell-mediated immunodeficiency and atopic eczema; systemic fungal infections such as allergic bronchopulmonary aspergillosis, and invasive parasitic infections.

IMMUNOGLOBULIN G (IgG)

Quantitates the concentration of the immunoglobulin IgG. It is the major antibacterial, antifungal, and antiviral antibody. A severe deficiency is manifested by repeated infections.

IMMUNOGLOBULIN G (IgG) INDEX

Compares the relative ratio of IgG to albumin in serum and cerebrospinal fluid (CSF). If the IgG index is increased (<0.7) and the IgG synthesis rate is increased in a specimen without oligoclonal immu-

noglobulins, the possibility exists that plasma contamination is present due to a leaky blood-brain barrier or a traumatic spinal tap.

IMMUNOGLOBULIN G (IgG) RHEUMATOID FACTORS

Measures the quantity of IgG antibodies that are reacting with human IgG. The role of IgG rheumatoid factor is considered to be of major pathogenic importance in rheumatoid arthritis.

IMMUNOGLOBULIN G (IgG) SUBCLASSES

Quantitates the subclasses IgG_1, IgG_2, IgG_3, and IgG_4 in serum.

Increased levels of IgG_4 can be demonstrated by patients with allergies who have normal IgE levels. A deficiency of IgG_4 can be associated with severe, recurrent sinopulmonary infections, symptomatic IgA deficiency and common variable immunodeficiency (with pneumonia and/or bronchiectasis). In addition, elevated IgG_4 is found in some highly allergic patients who have normal IgE concentrations.

IMMUNOGLOBULIN G (IgG) SYNTHESIS RATE

Measures the rate of IgG synthesis in cerebrospinal fluid (CSF). Elevated rates are associated with demyelinating disease. Conditions associated with increased rates include multiple sclerosis, bacterial meningitis, subacute sclerosing panencephalitis, lupus-related central nervous system involvement, presenile dementia (Alzheimer's disorder), IgG-synthesizing neoplasms, syphilis, cryptococcosis, chronic relapsing polyneuropathy, and acute cerebrovascular disease. If the IG synthesis rate and IgG index are elevated, contamination of the specimen with plasma protein should be suspected.

IgM ANTIBODIES (ANTIGEN SPECIFIC)

Provides identification of antigen-specific IgM antibodies in the presence of antigen-specific IgG and rheumatoid factor. The separation of IgM and IgG antibodies is important in the serodiagnosis of congenital infections.

IgM RHEUMATOID FACTORS

Measures IgM antibodies to human IgG fixed to latex particles. Elevated levels of rheumatoid factor are associated with rheumatoid arthritis, but such elevations may also be seen in other disorders. Increased levels of rheumatoid factors in combination with high levels of c-reactive protein are predictive of aggressive rheumatoid disease. In the case of a negative rheumatoid factor assay, a patient may be diagnosed through clinical signs and symptoms as suffering from seronegative rheumatoid disease.

Jo-1 ANTIBODY

Detects precipitins to an acidic nuclear protein from calf thymus. Approximately one third of patients with uncomplicated polymyositis, and some patients with dermatomyositis, demonstrate this antibody.

Ku ANTIBODY

Detects precipitins to an acidic nuclear protein from calf thymus. About one half of patients with overlapping signs and symptoms of scleroderma and polymyositis demonstrate Ku precipitins.

LYMPHOCYTE MITOGEN STIMULATION

Measures the rate of DNA synthesis by isolated lymphocytes. Decreased proliferation and DNA synthesis is diagnostic of a defect in cellular immunity. Cellular immunity is frequently defective in immunodeficiency disorders, infectious diseases, carcinoma, and occasionally in autoimmune disorders.

LYMPHOCYTE TYPING

Differentiates and measures (using monoclonal antibodies to identify cell surface markers) the quantities of T cells and B cells in the circulating blood. Useful in distinguishing T and B cell leukemias and lymphomas. Determination of T cell subsets (helper/inducer, suppressor/cytotoxic) is helpful in monitoring treatment in patients with immunodeficiencies such as HIV infection or transplant patients.

Mi-1-ANTIBODY

Detects antibodies to an acidic nuclear protein from calf thymus. Some patients with dermatomyositis and polymyositis demonstrate Mi-1-antibodies.

MYELIN BASIC PROTEIN

Measures the concentration of myelin basic protein in cerebrospinal fluid. Elevated values indicate extensive and active demyelination of the central nervous system. Disorders in which the level of myelin basic protein can be increased include multiple sclerosis, subacute sclerosing panencephalitis, transverse myelitis, and optic neuritis. Increased values can also be observed in conditions producing damage to nervous tissue but in which demyelination is not the primary process, e.g., radiation or chemotherapy of neoplasms in or near the central nervous system.

NITROBLUE TETRAZOLIUM (NBT)

Measures the reduction of nitroblue tetrazolium dye by polymorphonuclear leukocytes. Failure to reduce the dye demonstrates that the neutrophilic leukocytes are unable to effectively destroy bacteria. Patients with this defect suffer from chronic granulomatous disease and have increased susceptibility to bacterial infections.

OLIGOCLONAL IMMUNOGLOBULINS

Evaluates the presence of abnormal bands of immunoglobulins in cerebrospinal fluid. Abnormal bands of mini-monoclonal immunoglobulins are associated with disorders such as multiple sclerosis, subacute sclerosing panencephalitis, paraprotein disorders, and infections.

POLYETHYLENE GLYCOL (PEG)

Measures the amount of IgG precipitated in the chemical, polyethylene glycol. Increased amounts of precipitated IgG are associated with immune complexes and with aggregates of immunoglobulins found with paraproteins.

PLATELET-ASSOCIATED IGG (PAIgG)

Detects IgG found on the surface of platelets after thorough washing. Elevated levels of PAIgG with inversely proportional platelet counts are found in patients with immune thrombocytopenic purpura (ITP). Increased values can also be found in patients suffering from systemic lupus erythematosus.

PLATELET ANTIBODY

Evaluates the quantity of platelets with immunologically attached IgG by the use of fluorescein-tagged antihuman immunoglobulin specific for the Fc portion of IgG. Antibodies can be demonstrated by this indirect test in less than half of patients with immune thrombocytopenia (ITP) and the majority (82%) of patients with systemic lupus erythematosus (SLE).

PM-1 ANTIBODY

Detects antibodies to an acidic nuclear protein from calf thymus. These precipitins are found in the majority (87%) of patients with polymyositis-scleroderma. More than half of the patients suffering from polymyositis demonstrate the antibody, but the antibody is detected in less than one fifth of patients with dermatomyositis.

PNEUMOCOCCAL ANTIBODIES

Measures the antibody response to 12 pneumococcal serotypes. Postimmunization concentrations of antibody in babies who were immunized at 6 months of age should persist until at least 1 year of age and then decline.

PROPERDIN FACTOR B

Measures the level of properdin factor B in serum. A decreased concentration of factor B demonstrates activation of the alternative pathway of complement.

RADIO ALLERGO SORBENT TEST (RAST)

Detects IgE antibodies to various allergens. Increased levels are useful in identifying allergens in patients who have skin diseases or other problems that make skin testing difficult and in assessing patients with suspected food allergies or penicillin hypersensitivity.

RAJI CELL ASSAY
Measures the binding of immune complexes to complement receptors on a lymphoblastoid cell line, Raji cells.

SHEEP CELL AGGLUTINATION TITER (SCAT)
Measures IgM antibodies to rabbit IgG fixed to sheep or turkey erythrocytes. Elevated titers of IgM antibodies are associated with rheumatoid arthritis.

SKIN TESTING
Evaluates delayed hypersensitivity reactivity. The inability to respond to an antigenic challenge strongly suggests that cell-mediated immunity is depressed.

TETANUS ANTIBODY
Measures antibody to tetanus toxoid. If a patient has a history of immunization and antibodies are not demonstrable, abnormal humoral immunity is suspected.

THYROID-STIMULATING IMMUNOGLOBULINS (TSI)
Measures the concentration of antibody stimulating triiodothyronine (T_3) synthesis in thyroid tissue. The majority of patients with Graves' disease have elevated TSI levels.

TRANSFERRIN
Measures the quantity of iron transport protein in serum. Increased levels of transferrin are classically associated with iron deficiency anemia; decreased levels are associated with hemochromatosis. Other conditions, however, may express altered quantities of transferrin.

Immunologic Assays

EXAMPLES OF IMMUNOLOGIC ASSAYS PERFORMED BY RADIOIMMUNOASSAY

Acetylcholine Receptor (AchR) Binding Antibody
Acetylcholine Receptor (AcHR) Blocking Antibody
Anti-DNA Antibody
Antiglomerular Basement Membrane Antibody
Anti-intrinsic Factor Antibody
Antimyelin Antibody
Antisperm Antibody
Beta$_2$-Microglobulin
C1q Binding
Carcinoembryonic Antigen (CEA)
Conglutinin Solid Phase (Kg SP) Assay for Immune
   Complexes
Diphtheria Antibody
Ferritin
Immunoglobulin E (IgE)
Immunoglobulin G (IgG) Rheumatoid Factors
Immunoglobulin G (IgG) Subclasses
Myelin Basic Protein
Platelet-Associated IgG (PAIgG)
Platelet Antibody
Pneumococcal Antibody
Radio Allergo Sorbent Test (RAST)
Raji Cell Assay
Thyroid-Stimulating Immunoglobulins (TSI)

EXAMPLES OF IMMUNOLOGIC ASSAYS PERFORMED BY NEPHELOMETRY

Albumin Index
Alpha-1-Antitrypsin
C1 Esterase Inhibitor (C1 Inhibitor)
C3
C3b Inhibitor (C3b Inactivator)
C3PA (C3 ProActivator, Properdin Factor B)
C4
C6
C7
C8

Ceruloplasmin
Complement Components (C1r, C1s, C2, C3, C4,
   C5, C6, C7, C8)
C Reactive Protein (CRP)
Cryofibrinogen
Cryoglobulins
Immunoglobulins
Immunoglobulin G (IgG) Index
Properdin Factor B
Transferrin

EXAMPLES OF IMMUNOLOGIC ASSAYS PERFORMED BY INDIRECT FLUORESCENCE ANTIBODY TECHNIQUE

Antiadrenal Antibody
Anticentriole Antibody
Anticentromere Antibody
Antiglomerular Basement Membrane Antibody
Anti-islet-cell Antibody
Anti-LKM Antibody
Antimitochondrial Antibody
Antimyelin Antibody
Antimyocardial Antibody
Antinuclear Antibody
Antiparietal Cell Antibody
Antiplatelet Antibody
Antireticulin Antibody
Antiribosome Antibody
Anti-Skin (Dermal-Epidermal) Antibody
Anti-Skin (Inter-Epithelial) Antibody
Antismooth Muscle Antibody
Antistriational Antibody
Histone Reactive Antinuclear Antibody
Antibody (HRANA)
IgM Antibodies (Antigen Specific)
Lymphocyte Typing

EXAMPLES OF IMMUNOLOGIC ASSAYS PERFORMED BY FLOW CYTOMETRY

Antiplatelet Antibody
Lymphocyte Typing

EXAMPLES OF IMMUNOLOGIC ASSAYS PERFORMED BY INDIRECT HEMAGGLUTINATION

Antinuclear Ribonucleoprotein (Anti-nRNP) Antibody
Anti-Sm Antibody
Antithyroglobulin and Antithyroid Microsome Antibody
Sheep Cell Agglutination Titer (SCAT)

EXAMPLES OF IMMUNOLOGIC ASSAYS PERFORMED BY COUNTERIMMUNOELECTROPHORESIS

Antinuclear Ribonucleoprotein (Anti-nRNP) Antibody
Anti-Sm Antibody

EXAMPLES OF IMMUNOLOGIC ASSAYS PERFORMED BY DOUBLE DIFFUSION

Anti-Rheumatoid Arthritis Nuclear Antigen (Anti-RANA)
Antinuclear Ribonucleoprotein (Anti-nRNP) Antibody
Anti-Scl or Anti-SCl-70 Antibody
Anti-Sm Antibody
Anti-SS-A (SS-A Precipitin, Anti-Ro) Antibody
Anti-SS-B (SS-B Precipitin, Anti-La) Antibody
Jo-1 Antibody
Ku Antibody
Mi-1-Antibody
PM-1 Antibody

EXAMPLES OF IMMUNOLOGIC ASSAYS PERFORMED BY SPECTROPHOTOMETRY (ULTRAVIOLET OR VISIBLE)

Beta-Glucuronidase Assay

EXAMPLES OF IMMUNOLOGIC ASSAYS PERFORMED BY ELECTROIMMUNODIFFUSION

C1q
C2
Immunoglobulin G (IgG) Subclasses

EXAMPLES OF IMMUNOLOGIC ASSAYS PERFORMED BY AGAROSE ELECTROPHORESIS

C4 Allotypes
Oligoclonal Immunoglobulins
C4 Allotypes

EXAMPLES OF IMMUNOLOGIC ASSAYS PERFORMED BY RADIAL IMMUNODIFFUSION

C5
Polyethylene Glycol (PEG)

EXAMPLES OF IMMUNOLOGIC ASSAYS PERFORMED BY HEMOLYTIC ASSAY

CH_{50}
Complement Decay Rate
Cold Agglutinins

EXAMPLES OF IMMUNOLOGIC ASSAYS PERFORMED BY IMMUNOELECTROPHORESIS

Complement Activation Products

EXAMPLES OF IMMUNOLOGIC ASSAYS PERFORMED BY LATEX PARTICLE AGGLUTINATION

c Reactive Protein (CRP)
IgG Rheumatoid Factors
IgM Rheumatoid Factors
Tetanus Antibodies

EXAMPLES OF IMMUNOLOGIC ASSAYS PERFORMED BY LYMPHOCYTE MICROCYTOTOXICITY

Assay	Method
HLA-B27	
HLA-DR	
HLA-DR3	
Immunoglobulin A (IgA)	
Immunoglobulin D (IgD)	
Immunoglobulin G (IgG)	
IgM Antibodies (antigen specific)	Ultracentrifugation
Lymphocyte Mitogen Stimulation	Cell culture
Lymphocyte Typing	Rosettes
Nitroblue Tetrazolium (NBT)	Light microscope
Skin Testing/INTRADERMAL	

TABLE C-1

Examples of Serologic Diagnosis of Infectious Diseases

Organism or disease	Method	Comments
Adenovirus	Direct electron microscopy	
	Complement fixation	Antibody to group common antigens
	Complement fixation	Antibody to types 3 and 5
Arboviruses	Complement fixation	Antibody
	Indirect fluorescent antibody	IgG and IgM
	Enzyme immunoassay	IgG and IgM in serum and CSF*
Ascaris sp.	Indirect hemagglutination†	
	Gas-liquid chromatography†	Fatty acids
Aspergillus spp.	Complement fixation	
	Enzyme immunoassay	Antigen or antibody
	Immunodiffusion	Antibody
	Radioimmunoassay	Antigen
Babesia microti	Indirect fluorescent antibody	Antibody
Blastomyces dermatitidis	Complement fixation	Antibody
	Complement fixation	Antibody to "A" Ag
	Immunodiffusion	Antibody to "A" Ag
	Enzyme immunoassay	Antibody to "A" Ag
Bordetella pertussis and *Bordetella parapertussis*	Direct agglutination	Antigen
	Direct fluorescent antibody	IgG, IgM, and IgA
	Enzyme immunoassay	
Borrelia burgdorferi	Enzyme immunoassay	IgG and IgM
Borrelia hermsii	Indirect fluorescent antibody	IgG and IgM
Branhamella catarrhalis	Enzyme immunoassay‡	Antibody
Brill-Zinsser disease	Complement fixation	Antibody to typhus group antigen
	Indirect fluorescent antibody	Total and IgM antibody
Brucella sp.	Complement fixation	Antibody
	Direct agglutination	
	Direct agglutination	
	Enzyme immunoassay	2-ME-treated serum (antibody)
	Direct agglutination	IgG, IgM, and IgA *B. canis* antibody
Campylobacter sp.	Complement fixation	Antibody to *C. jejuni*
		Antibody to *C. fetus*
IgG *Candida* sp.	Latex agglutination	Antibody
	Latex agglutination	Antigen
	Latex agglutination	Mannan antigen
	Immunodiffusion	Antibody
	Countercurrent immunoelectrophoresis	Antibody
	Enzyme immunoassay	Antibody to mannan
	Electrophoresis	Mannan antigen
	Enzyme immunoassay	Mannan antigen
Chlamydia psittaci	Complement fixation	Antibody
	Indirect fluorescent antibody	IgG
	Enzyme immunoassay	IgG and IgM
Chlamydia trachomatis	Enzyme immunoassay	IgG and IgM
	Direct fluorescent antibody	Antigen
	Enzyme immunoassay	Antigen
Clostridium difficile	Latex agglutination	Toxin
	Countercurrent immunoelectrophoresis	Toxin
	Tissue culture assay	Toxin A and B
	Enzyme immunoassay	
Clostridium tetani	Latex agglutination	Antibody
	Enzyme immunoassay	Antibody

* Cerebrospinal fluid.
† Method not considered to be reliable.
‡ Research method.

TABLE C-1

Examples of Serologic Diagnosis of Infectious Diseases—cont'd

Organism or disease	Method	Commets
Coccidioides immitis	Latex agglutination	Serum antibody
	Complement fixation	Serum and cerebrospinal fluid antibody
	Immunodiffusion	Serum and cerebrospinal fluid antibody
	Enzyme immunoassay	Serum antigen
	Radioimmunoassay	Serum antigen
Colorado tick fever	Complement fixation	Antibody
	Indirect fluorescent antibody	Antibody
	Enzyme immunoassay	Antibody
	Neutralization	Antibody
	Direct fluorescent antibody	Antigen (RBCs)
Coronaviruses	Indirect fluorescent antibody	Antibody to strains OC-43 229E
Corynebacterium diphtheriae	Enzyme immunoassay	Antitoxin
	Radioimmunoprecipitation	Antitoxin
Coxiella burnetti	Complement fixation	Antibody
	Complement fixation	Antibody to phase 1 and 2
	Indirect fluorescent antibody	IgM, IgG, and IgA antibody to phase 1 and 2
Coxsackie virus	Complement fixation	Antibody to Coxsackie A and B types
Cryptococcus neoformans	Latex agglutination	Serum and cerebrospinal fluid antigen
	Indirect fluorescent antibody	Antigen
	Direct agglutination	Antibody
Cryptosporidia	Light microscopy	Antigen
	Indirect fluorescent antibody	Antibody
Cysticercus cellulosae	Enzyme immunoassay	IgM, IgG, and IgA
	Enzyme immunoassay	Antigen
Dengue viruses	Indirect fluorescent antibody	IgM and IgG
	Complement fixation	Antibody
Echinococcus sp.	Countercurrent immunoelectrophoresis	Antibody
	Enzyme immunoassay	Species-specific antibody
	Indirect hemagglutination	Antibody to *E. granulosus*
Echoviruses	Complement fixation	Antibody
	Hemagglutination	
	Hemagglutination	
	Inhibition	
	Neutralization	
Entamoeba	Countercurrent	
	Immunoelectrophoresis	Antibody
	Enzyme immunoassay	Antibody
	Indirect fluorescent antibody	Antibody
	Indirect hemagglutination	Antibody
	Enzyme immunoassay	Antigen
Escherichia coli	Indirect hemagglutination	Antibody
	Enzyme immunoassay	IgM, IgG, and IgA
	Enzyme immunoassay	Enterotoxin
	DNA hybridization (cDNA probe)	Entertoxin DNA
Fasciola sp.	Countercurrent immunoelectrophoresis	Antibody
	Complement fixation	Antibody
	Enzyme immunoassay	Antibody
	Indirect fluorescent antibody	Antibody
Filariasis	Countercurrent immunoelectrophoresis	Antibody
	Enzyme immunoassay	Antibody
	Indirect fluorescent antibody	Antibody
	Indirect hemagglutination	Antibody

Continued.

TABLE C-1

Examples of Serologic Diagnosis of Infectious Diseases—cont'd

Organism or disease	Method	Commets
Francisella tularensis	Complement fixation	Antibody
	Direct agglutination	Antibody
	Enzyme immunoassay	IgM Antibody
	Enzyme immunoassay	IgG Antibody
	Enzyme immunoassay	IgA Antibody
Giardia lamblia	Complement fixation	Antibody
	Enzyme immunoassay	IgM antibody
	Enzyme immunoassay	IgG antibody
	Indirect fluorescent antibody	Antibody
	Counterimmunoelectrophoresis	Antibody
	Enzyme immunoassay	Antigen
Haemophilus ducreyi	Western Blot (immunoblot)	Antibody
	Indirect fluorescent antibody (MoAb)	Antigen
Herpes simplex viruses (HSV)	Complement fixation	Antibody
	Enzyme immunoassay	HSV-1 and HSV-2; IgG
	Indirect fluorescent antibody	HSV-1 and HSV-2; IgM
	Neutralization	HSV-1 and HSV-2
Histoplasma capsulatum	Complement fixation	Antibody
	Countercurrent immunoelectrophoresis	Antibody
	Immunodiffusion	Antibody in serum or cerebrospinal fluid
	Latex agglutination	Antibody
	Enzyme immunoassay	Antigen
Influenza A, B, C	Complement fixation	Antibody to types A, B, and C
	Enzyme immunoassay	IgM, IgG, and IgA antibody to types A, B, and C
Interferon	Inhibition of viral nucleic acid synthesis	
	Plaque reduction assay	
Japanese encephalitis virus	Complement fixation	Antibody
	Enzyme immunoassay	IgM and IgG
Legionella pneumophilia	Enzyme immunoassay	Antibody
	Indirect fluorescent antibody	Antibody
	Direct fluorescent antibody	Antigen
	Enzyme immunoassay	Antigen in urine
	cDNA probe	RNA in *L. pneumophilia*
Leishmania sp.	Complement fixation	Antibody
	Indirect fluorescent antibody	Antibody
	Indirect hemagglutination	Antibody
Leptospira	Complement fixation	Antibody
	Direct agglutination	Antibody
	Enzyme immunoassay	IgM and IgG antibody
	Indirect hemagglutination	Antibody
Listeria monocytogenes	Complement fixation	Antibody
	Latex particle agglutination	Antibody
Lymphocytic choriomeningitis virus	Complement fixation	Antibody
	Indirect fluorescent antibody	IgM and IgG antibody
	Indirect fluorescent antibody in cerebrospinal fluid	IgM antibody
Measles (rubella) virus	Complement fixation	Antibody
	Enzyme immunoassay	IgM and IgG antibody
	Hemagglutination inhibition	Antibody
	Latex particle agglutination	Antibody
Mumps virus	Complement fixation	Antibody to soluble antigen
	Complement fixation	Antibody to viral antigen
	Enzyme immunoassay	IgM and IgG

TABLE C-1

Examples of Serologic Diagnosis of Infectious Diseases—cont'd

Organism or disease	Method	Commets
Mycobacterium avium-intracellulare	Enzyme immunoassay	Antibody
	Immunodiffusion	Antibody
Mycobacterium leprae	Enzyme immunoassay	IgM and IgG
Mycobacterium tuberculosis	Enzyme immunoassay	IgG
	Enzyme immunoassay	Antigen
Mycoplasma hominis	Enzyme immunoassay	Antibody
Mycoplasma pneumoniae	Complement fixation	
	Enzyme immunoassay	IgM and IgG
	Indirect fluorescent antibody	IgM and IgG
	cDNA probe	RNA of *M. pneumoniae*
Neisseria gonorrhoeae	Complement fixation	Antibody
	Enzyme immunoassay	IgM, IgG, and IgA
	Latex agglutination	Antibody
	Enzyme immunoassay	Antigen
Neisseria meningitidis	Enzyme immunoassay	Antibody to outer membrane complex
	Indirect hemagglutination	Antibody to capsular polysaccharide antigen
	Counterimmunoelectrophoresis	Antigen
	Coagglutination	Antigen
	Latex particle agglutination	Antigen
Nocardia sp.	Complement fixation	Antibody
	Immunodiffusion	Antibody
Norwalk virus	Enzyme immunoassay	IgM and IgG
	Immune electron microscopy	Antigen
	Radioimmunoassay	Antigen
Papillomaviruses	cDNA probe	Human papillomaviruses
Paracoccidioides brasiliensis	Complement fixation	Antibody
	Immunodiffusion	Antibody
	Direct fluorescent antibody	Antigen
Paragonimus westermani	Complement fixation	Antibody
	Enzyme immunoassay	Antibody
Parainfluenza	Hemadsorption immunosorbent technique	IgM antibody
Parvoviruses	Radioimmunoassay	Antibody
Plasmodium sp.	Indirect fluorescent antibody	IgG
Pneumocystis carinii	Enzyme immunoassay	Antibody
	Indirect fluorescent antibody	Antibody
	Counterimmunoelectrophoresis	Antigen
	Flow cytometry	Antigen
	Indirect fluorescent antibody	Antigen
Poliovirus types 1, 2, 3	Complement fixation	Antibody
	Neutralization	Antibody
Polyomaviruses	Enzyme immunoassay	IgG
	Hemagglutination inhibition	Antibody
	Enzyme immunoassay	BK virus
Prions	Western Blot	Proteinase-K-resistant antigen
	2DE	Cerebrospinal fluid electrophoresis
Proteus mirabilis	Indirect hemagglutination	
	Agglutination	Antibody
Pseudomonas pseudomallei	Enzyme immunoassay	IgM and IgG
	Indirect fluorescent antibody	IgM and IgG
Pseudomonas sp.	Complement fixation	Antibody
	Indirect hemagglutination	Antibody
	Counterimmunoelectrophoresis	Antibody

Continued.

TABLE C-1

Examples of Serologic Diagnosis of Infectious Diseases—cont'd

Organism or disease	Method	Commets
Reovirus	Complement fixation	Antibody
	Hemagglutination inhibition	Antibody
Respiratory syncytial virus	Complement fixation	Antibody
	Enzyme Immunoassay	IgM and IgG
	Direct fluorescent antibody	Antigen
	Enzyme immunoassay	Antigen
Rickettsia akari	Complement fixation	Antibody to spotted fever group
	Indirect fluorescent antibody	Total and IgM antibody
Rickettsia prowazekii	Complement fixation	Antibody to typhus group antigen
	Indirect fluorescent antibody	IgM and IgG
	Direct agglutination	Antibody to *Proteus* OX-19 and OX-2
Rickettsia rickettsii	Complement fixation	Antibody to spotted fever group antigen
	Indirect fluorescent antibody	Total and IgM antibody
	Direct immunofluorescence	Antigen
Rickettsia tsutsugamushi	Indirect fluorescent antibody	Total and IgM antibody
	Direct agglutination	Antibody to *Proteus* OX-19 and OX-2
Rickettsia typhi	Complement fixation	Antibody to typhus group
	Indirect fluorescent antibody	Total and IgM antibody
	Direct agglutination	Antibody to *Proteus* OX-19 and OX-2
Rotavirus	Enzyme immunoassay	IgM and IgG
	Direct electron microscopy	
	Enzyme immunoassay	Antigen
	Latex particle agglutination	
Salmonella sp.	Widal test	Antibody to O
	Direct agglutination	Antigen group D (typhoid O)
		Antibody to H antigen *a* (paratyphoid A)
		Antibody to H antigen *b* (paratyphoid B)
		Antibody to H antigen *d* (typhoid H)
	Indirect hemagglutination	Antibody to Vi antigen
Schistosoma sp.	Enzyme immunoassay	Antibody
	Enzyme immunoassay	IgM and IgG
	Indirect fluorescent antibody	Antibody
	Indirect hemagglutination	Antibody

TABLE C-1

Examples of Serologic Diagnosis of Infectious Diseases—cont'd

Organism or disease	Method	Commets
Shigella sp.	Complement fixation	Antibodies to specific species
Sporothrix schenkii	Immunodiffusion	Antibody
	Latex particle agglutination	Antibody
	Periodic acid-Schiff stain	Antigen
	Light microscopy	Antigen
Staphylococcus sp.	Counterimmunoelectrophoresis	Antibody to teichoic acid
	Enzyme immunoassay	IgG to anti-*S. aureus* lipase
Streptococcus pneumoniae	Radioimmunoprecipitation	Antibodies to four serotypes
	Counterimmunoelectrophoresis	Antigen
	Coagglutination	Antigen
	Latex particle agglutination	Antigen
Strongyloides stercoralis	Enzyme immunoassay	IgG and IgE
Toxocara canis	Enzyme immunoassay	IgM, IgG, and IgA
Trichinella spiralis	Counterimmunoelectrophoresis	Antibody
	Latex particle agglutination	Antibody
	Enzyme immunoassay	IgM, IgG, and IgA
Trichomonas vaginalis	Enzyme immunoassay	IgM, IgG, and IgA
Trypanosoma cruzi	Complement fixation	Antibody
	Indirect fluorescent antibody	Antibody
	Indirect hemagglutination	Antibody
	Enzyme immunoassay	Total IgM in cerebrospinal fluid
Ureaplasma urealyticum	Indirect fluorescent antibody	IgM and IgG
Varicella-zoster virus	Complement fixation	Antibody
	Enzyme immunoassay	IgM and IgG
Vibrio cholerae	Direct agglutination	Antibody
	Enzyme immunoassay	IgG antitoxin
Visna virus	Neutralization	Antibody
Weil-Felix agglutinins	Direct agglutination	Antibodies to *Proteus vulgaris* strains OX-19, 2, and K
Yersinia enterocolitica	Complement fixation	Antibodies to types 0:3 and 0:9
	Direct agglutination	Antibodies to type 0:8
	Enzyme immunoassay	Antibodies to types 0:3, 0:4, 0:5, and 0:8
Yersinia pseudotuberculosis	Direct agglutination	Antibodies
	Complement fixation	Antibodies
Zygomycetes sp.	Immunodiffusion	Antibodies
	Enzyme immunoassay	Antibodies

TABLE C-2

Procedures in Microbial Immunology: Bacteria

Organism	Method	Comments
Bordetella pertussis and *Bodetella parapertussis*	Direct agglutination	
	Direct fluorescent antibody	Antigen
	Enzyme immunoassay	IgG, IgM, and IgA
Borrelia burgdorferi	Enzyme immunoassay	IgG and IgM
Borrelia hermsii	Indirect fluorescent antibody	IgG and IgM
Branhamella catarrhalis	Enzyme immunoassay*	Antibody
Brucella sp.	Complement fixation	Antibody
	Direct agglutination	
	Direct agglutination	2-ME-treated serum (antibody)
	Enzyme immunoassay	IgG, IgM, and IgA
	Direct agglutination	*B. canis* antibody
Campylobacter sp.	Complement fixation	Antibody to *C. jejuni*
		Antibody to *C. fetus*
Clostridium difficile	Latex agglutination	Toxin
	Countercurrent immunoelectrophoresis	Toxin
	Tissue culture assay	Toxin
	Enzyme immunoassay	Toxins A and B
Clostridium tetani	Latex agglutination	Antibody
	Enzyme immunoassay	Antibody
Corynebacterium diphtheriae	Enzyme immunoassay	Antitoxin
	Radioimmunoprecipitation	Antitoxin
Escherichia coli	Indirect hemagglutination	Antibody
	Enzyme immunoassay	IgM, IgG, and IgA
	Enzyme immunoassay	Enterotoxin
	DNA Hybridization (cDNA probe)	Entertoxin DNA
Francisella tularensis	Complement fixation	Antibody
	Direct agglutination	Antibody
	Enzyme immunoassay	IgM antibody
	Enzyme immunoassay	IgG antibody
	Enzyme immunoassay	IgA antibody
Haemophilus ducreyi	Western Blot (immunoblot)	Antibody
	Indirect fluorescent antibody (MoAb)	Antigen
Legionella pneumophilia	Enzyme Immunoassay	Antibody
	Indirect fluorescent antibody	Antibody
	Direct fluorescent antibody	Antigen
	Enzyme immunoassay	Antigen in urine
	cDNA probe	RNA in *L. pneumophilia*
Leptospira	Complement fixation	Antibody
	Direct agglutination	Antibody
	Enzyme immunoassay	IgM and IgG Antibody
	Indirect hemagglutination	Antibody
Listeria monocytogenes	Complement fixation	Antibody
	Latex particle agglutination	Antibody
Mycobacterium avium-intracellulare	Enzyme immunoassay	Antibody
	Immunodiffusion	Antibody
Mycobacterium leprae	Enzyme immunoassay	IgM and IgG
Mycobacterium tuberculosis	Enzyme immunoassay	IgG
	Enzyme immunoassay	Antigen

*Research method.

TABLE C-2

Procedures in Microbial Immunology: Bacteria—cont'd

Organism	Method	Comments
Neisseria gonorrhoeae	Complement fixation	Antibody
	Enzyme immunoassay	IgM, IgG, and IgA
	Latex agglutination	Antibody
	Enzyme immunoassay	Antigen
Neisseria meningitids	Enzyme immunoassay	Antibody to outer membrane complex
	Indirect hemagglutination	Antibody to capsular polysaccharide antigen
	Counterimmunoelectrophoresis	Antigen
	Coagglutination	Antigen
	Latex particle agglutination	Antigen
Proteus mirabilis	Indirect hemagglutination	
	Agglutination	Antibody
Pseudomonas pseudomallei	Enzyme immunoassay	IgM and IgG
	Indirect fluorescent antibody	IgM and IgG
Pseudomonas sp.	Complement fixation	Antibody
	Indirect hemagglutination	Antibody
	Counterimmunoelectrophoresis	Antibody
Salmonella sp.	Widal test	Antibody to 0
	Direct agglutination	Antigen
		Group D (typhoid 0)
		Antibody to H antigen *a* (paratyphoid A)
		Antibody to H antigen *b* (paratyphoid B)
		Antibody to H antigen *d* (typhoid H)
	Indirect hemagglutination	Antibody to Vi antigen
Shigella sp.	Complement fixation	Antibodies to specific species
Staphylococcus sp.	Counterimmunoelectrophoresis	Antibody to teichoic acid
	Enzyme immunoassay	IgG to anti-*S. aureus* lipase
Streptococcus pneumoniae	Radioimmunoprecipitation	Antibodies to four serotypes
	Counterimmunoelectrophoresis	Antigen
	Coagglutination	Antigen
	Latex particle agglutination	Antigen
Vibrio cholerae	Direct agglutination	Antibody
	Enzyme immunoassay	IgG antitoxin
Weil-Felix agglutinins	Direct agglutination	Antibodies to *Proteus vulgaris* strains OX-19, 2, and K
Yersinia enterocolitica	Complement fixation	Antibodies to types 0:3 and 0:9
	Direct agglutination	Antibodies to type 0:8
	Enzyme immunoassay	Antibodies to types 0:3, 0:4, 0:5, and 0:8
Yersinia pseudotuberculosis	Direct agglutination	Antibodies
	Complement fixation	Antibodies
Chlamydia psittaci	Complement fixation	Antibody
	Indirect fluorescent antibody	IgG
	Enzyme immunoassay	IgG and IgM
Chlamydia trachomatis	Enzyme immunoassay	IgG and IgM
	Direct fluorescent antibody	Antigen
	Enzyme immunoassay	Antigen

TABLE C-3

Procedures in Microbial Immunology: Sexually Transmitted Diseases

Organism	Method	Comments
Bacteria		
Chlamydia trachomatis	Enzyme immunoassay	IgG and IgM
	Direct fluorescent antibody	Antigen
	Enzyme immunoassay	Antigen
Haemophilus ducreyi	Western Blot (immunoblot)	Antibody
	Indirect fluorescent antibody (MoAb)	Antigen
Mycoplasma hominis	Enzyme immunoassay	Antibody
Neisseria gonorrhoeae	Complement fixation	Antibody
	Enzyme immunoassay	IgM, IgG, and IgA
	Latex agglutination	Antibody
	Enzyme immunoassay	Antigen
Neisseria meningitidis	Enzyme immunoassay	Antibody to outer membrane complex
	Indirect hemagglutination	Antibody to capsular polysaccharide antigen
	Counter immunoelectrophoresis	Antigen
	Coagglutination	Antigen
	Latex particle agglutination	Antigen
Ureaplasma urealyticum	Indirect fluorescent antibody	IgM and IgG
Fungi		
Candida sp.	Latex agglutination	Antibody
	Latex agglutination	Antigen
	Latex agglutination	Mannan antigen
	Immunodiffusion	Antibody
	Countercurrent immunoelectrophoresis	Antibody
	Enzyme immunoassay	Antibody to mannan
	Electrophoresis	Mannan antigen
	Enzyme immunoassay	Mannan antigen
Viruses		
Cytomegalovirus		
Herpes simplex viruses (HSV)	Complement fixation	Antibody
	Enzyme immunoassay	HSV-1 and HSV-2; IgG
	Indirect fluorescent antibody	HSV-1 and HSV-2; IgM
	Neutralization	HSV-1 and HSV-2
Human immunodeficiency virus (HIV)		
Protozoans		
Trichomonas vaginalis	Enzyme immunoassay	IgM, IgG, and IgA

TABLE C-4

Procedures in Microbial Immunology: Bacteria Infections

Organism	Method	Comments
Bordetella pertussis and Bordetella parapertussis	Direct agglutination	
	Direct fluorescent antibody	Antigen
	Enzyme immunoassay	IgG, IgM, and IgA
Borrelia burgdorferi	Enzyme immunoassay	IgG and IgM
Borrelia hermsii	Indirect fluorescent antibody	IgG and IgM
Branhamella catarrhalis	Enzyme immunoassay	Antibody
Brucella sp.	Complement fixation	Antibody
	Direct agglutination	
	Direct agglutination	2-ME-treated serum (antibody)
	Enzyme immunoassay	IgG, IgM, and IgA
	Direct agglutination	B canis antibody
Campylobacter sp.	Complement fixation	Antibody to C. jejuni
		Antibody to C. fetus
Chlamydia psittaci	Complement fixation	Antibody
	Indirect fluorescent antibody	IgG
	Enzyme immunoassay	IgG and IgM
Chlamydia trachomatis	Enzyme immunoassay	IgG and IgM
	Direct fluorescent antibody	Antigen
	Enzyme immunoassay	Antigen
Clostridium difficile	Latex agglutination	Toxin
	Countercurrent immunoelectrophoresis	Toxin
	Tissue culture assay	Toxin
	Enzyme immunoassay	Toxins A and B
Clostridium tetani	Latex agglutination	Antibody
	Enzyme immunoassay	Antibody
Corynebacterium diphtheriae	Enzyme immunoassay	Antitoxin
	Radioimmunoprecipitation	Antitoxin
Coxiella burnetti	Complement fixation	Antibody
	Complement fixation	Antibody to phase 1 and 2
	Indirect fluorescent antibody	IgM, IgG, and IgA antibody to phase 1 and 2
Escherichia coli	Indirect hemagglutination	Antibody
	Enzyme immunoassay	IgM, IgG, and IgA
	Enzyme immunoassay	Enterotoxin
	DNA hybridization (cDNA probe)	Entertoxin DNA
Francisella tularensis	Complement fixation	Antibody
	Direct agglutination	Antibody
	Enzyme immunoassay	IgM antibody
	Enzyme immunoassay	IgG antibody
	Enzyme immunoassay	IgA antibody
Haemophilus ducreyi	Western Blot (immunoblot)	Antibody
	Indirect fluorescent antibody (MoAb)	Antigen
Legionella pneumophilia	Enzyme immunoassay	Antibody
	Indirect fluorescent antibody	Antibody
	Direct fluorescent antibody	Antigen
	Enzyme immunoassay	Antigen in urine
	cDNA probe	RNA in L. pneumophilia
Leptospira	Complement fixation	Antibody
	Direct agglutination	Antibody
	Enzyme immunoassay	IgM and IgG antibody
	Indirect hemagglutination	Antibody
Listeria monocytogenes	Complement fixation	Antibody
	Latex particle agglutination	Antibody
Mycobacterium avium-intracellulare	Enzyme immunoassay	Antibody
	Immunodiffusion	Antibody
Mycobacterium leprae	Enzyme immunoassay	IgM and IgG
Mycobacterium tuberculosis	Enzyme immunoassay	IgG
	Enzyme immunoassay	Antigen

Continued.

TABLE C-4

Procedures in Microbial Immunology: Bacteria Infections—cont'd

Organism	Method	Comments
Mycoplasma hominis	Enzyme immunoassay	Antibody
Mycoplasma pneumoniae	Complement fixation	
	Enzyme immunoassay	IgM and IgG
	Indirect fluorescent antibody	IgM and IgG
	cDNA probe	RNA of *M. pneumoniae*
Neisseria gonorrheae	Complement fixation	Antibody
	Enzyme Immunoassay	IgM, IgG and IgA
	Latex agglutination	Antibody
	Enzyme immunoassay	Antigen
Neisseria meningitidis	Enzyme immunoassay	Antibody to outer membrane complex
	Indirect hemagglutination	Antibody to capsular polysaccharide antigen
	Counterimmunoelectrophoresis	Antigen
	Coagglutination	Antigen
	Latex particle agglutination	Antigen
Proteus mirabilis	Indirect hemagglutination agglutination	Antibody
Pseudomonas pseudomallei	Enzyme immunoassay	IgM and IgG
	Indirect fluorescent antibody	IgM and IgG
Pseudomonas sp.	Complement fixation	Antibody
	Indirect hemagglutination	Antibody
	Counterimmunoelectrophoresis	Antibody
Rickettsia akari	Complement fixation	Antibody to spotted fever group
	Indirect fluorescent antibody	Total and IgM antibody
Rickettsia prowazekii	Complement fixation	Antibody to typhus group antigen
	Indirect fluorescent antibody	IgM and IgG
	Direct agglutination	Antibody to *Proteus* OX-19 and OX-2
Rickettsia rickettsii	Complement fixation	Antibody to spotted fever group antigen
	Indirect fluorescent antibody	Total and IgM antibody
	Direct immunofluorescence	Antigen

TABLE C-4

Procedures in Microbial Immunology: Bacteria Infections—cont'd

Organism	Method	Comments
Rickettsia tsutsugamushi	Indirect fluorescent antibody	Total and IgM antibody
	Direct agglutination	Antibody to *Proteus* OX-19 and OX-2
Rickettsia typhi	Complement fixation	Antibody to typhus group
	Indirect fluorescent antibody	Total and IgM antibody
	Direct agglutination	Antibody to *Proteus* OX-19 and OX-2
Salmonella sp.	Widal test	Antibody to 0
	Direct agglutination	Antigen group D (typhoid O)
		Antibody to H antigen *a* (paratyphoid A)
		Antibody to H antigen *b* (paratyphoid B)
		Antibody to H antigen *d* (typhoid H)
	Indirect hemagglutination	Antibody to Vi antigen
Shigella sp.	Complement fixation	Antibodies to specific species
Staphylococcus sp.	Counterimmunoelectrophoresis	Antibody to teichoic acid
	Enzyme immunoassay	IgG to anti-*S. aureus* lipase
Streptococcus pneumoniae	Radioimmunoprecipitation	Antibodies to four serotypes
	Counterimmunoelectrophoresis	Antigen
	Coagglutination	Antigen
	Latex particle agglutination	Antigen
Ureaplasma urealyticum	Indirect fluorescent antibody	IgM and IgG
Vibrio cholerae	Direct agglutination	Antibody
	Enzyme immunoassay	IgG antitoxin
Weil-Felix agglutinins	Direct agglutination	Antibodies to *Proteus vulgaris* strains OX-19, 2, and K
Yersinia enterocolitica	Complement fixation	Antibodies to types 0:3 and 0:9
	Direct agglutination	Antibodies to type 0:8
	Enzyme immunoassay	Antibodies to types 0:3, 0:4, 0:5, and 0:8
Yersinia pseudotuberculosis	Direct agglutination	Antibodies
	Complement fixation	Antibodies

TABLE C-5

Procedures in Microbial Immunology: Viral Infections

Organism	Method	Comments
Adenovirus	Direct electron microscopy	
	Complement fixation	Antibody to group common antigens
	Complement fixation	Antibody to types 3 and 5
Arborviruses	Complement fixation	Antibody
	Indirect fluorescent antibody	IgG and IgM
	Enzyme immunoassay	IgG and IgM in serum and CSF*
Coronaviruses	Indirect fluorescent antibody	Antibody to strains OC-43 229E
Coxsackie virus	Complement fixation	Antibody to Coxsackie A and B types
Cytomegalovirus		
Echoviruses	Complement fixation	Antibody
	Hemagglutination	
	Hemagglutination	
	Inhibition	
	Neutralization	
Hepatitis		
Herpes simplex viruses (HSV)	Complement fixation	Antibody
	Enzyme immunoassay	HSV-1 and HSV-2; IgG
	Indirect fluorescent antibody	HSV-1 and HSV-2; IgM
	Neutralization	HSV-1 and HSV-2
Influenza A, B, C	Complement fixation	Antibody to types A, B, and C
	Enzyme immunoassay	IgM, IgG, and IgA antibody to types A, B, and C
Japanese encephalitis virus	Complement fixation	Antibody
	Enzyme immunoassay	IgM and IgG
Lymphocytic choriomeningitis virus	Complement fixation	Antibody
	Indirect fluorescent antibody	IgM and IgG antibody
	Indirect fluorescent antibody in cerebrospinal fluid	IgM antibody

*Cerebrospinal fluid.

TABLE C-5

Procedures in Microbial Immunology: Viral Infections—cont'd

Organism	Method	Comments
Measles (rubella) virus	Complement fixation	Antibody
	Enzyme immunoassay	IgM and IgG antibody
	Hemagglutination inhibition	Antibody
	Latex particle agglutination	Antibody
Mumps virus	Complement fixation	Antibody to soluble antigen
	Complement fixation	antibody to viral antigen
	Enzyme immunoassay	IgM and IgG
Norwalk virus	Enzyme immunoassay	IgM and IgG
	Immune electron microscopy	Antigen
	Radioimmunoassay	Antigen
Papillomaviruses	cDNA probe	Human papillomaviruses
Parainfluenza	Hemadsorption immunosorbent technique	IgM antibody
Parvoviruses	Radioimmunoassay	Antibody
Poliovirus types 1, 2, 3	Complement fixation neutralization	Antibody
Polyomaviruses	Enzyme immunoassay	Antibody
	Hemagglutination	IgG
	Inhibition	Antibody
	Enzyme immunoassay	BK virus
Reovirus	Complement fixation	Antibody
	Hemagglutination inhibition	Antibody
Respiratory syncytial virus	Complement fixation	Antibody
	Enzyme immunoassay	IgM and IgG
	Direct fluorescent antibody	Antigen
	Enzyme immunoassay	Antigen
Rotavirus	Enzyme immunoassay	IgM and IgG
	Direct electron microscopy	
	Enzyme immunoassay	Antigen
	Latex particle agglutination	
Varicella-zoster virus	Complement fixation	Antibody
	Enzyme immunoassay	IgM and IgG
Visna virus	Neutralization	Antibody

TABLE C-6

Procedures in Microbial Immunology: Parasitic Infections

Organism	Method	Comments
Ascaris sp.	Indirect hemagglutination	
	Gas-liquid chromatography	Fatty acids
Babesia microti	Indirect fluorescent antibody	Antibody
Cryptosporidia	Light microscopy	Antigen
	Indirect fluorescent antibody	Antibody
Cysticercus cellulosae	Enzyme immunoassay	IgM, IgG and IgA
	Enzyme immunoassay	Antigen
Echinococcus sp.	Countercurrent immunoelectro-phoresis	Antibody
	Enzyme immunoassay	Species-specific antibody
	Indirect hemagglutination	Antibody to *E. granulosus*
Entamoeba	Countercurrent immunoelectro-phoresis	Antibody
	Enzyme immunoassay	Antibody
	Indirect fluorescent antibody	Antibody
	Indirect hemagglutination	Antibody
	Enzyme immunoassay	Antigen
Fasciola sp.	Countercurrent immunoelectro-phoresis	Antibody
	Complement fixation	Antibody
	Enzyme immunoassay	Antibody
	Indirect fluorescent antibody	Antibody
Filariasis	Countercurrent immunoelectro-phoresis	Antibody
	Enzyme immunoassay	Antibody
	Indirect fluorescent antibody	Antibody
	Indirect hemagglutination	Antibody
Giardia lamblia	Complement fixation	Antibody
	Enzyme immunoassay	IgM antibody
	Enzyme immunoassay	IgG antibody
	Indirect fluorescent antibody	Antibody
	Counterimmunoelectrophoresis	Antibody
	Enzyme immunoassay	Antigen
Leishmania sp.	Complement fixation	Antibody
	Indirect fluorescent antibody	Antibody
	Indirect hemagglutination	Antibody
Paragonimus westermani	Complement fixation	Antibody
	Enzyme immunoassay	Antibody
Plasmodium sp.	Indirect fluorescent antibody	IgG
Pneumocystis carinii	Enzyme immunoassay	Antibody
	Indirect fluorescent antibody	Antibody
	Counterimmunoelectrophoresis	Antigen
	Flow cytometry	Antigen
	Indirect fluorescent antibody	Antigen
Schistosoma sp.	Enzyme immunoassay	Antibody
	Enzyme immunoassay	IgM and IgG
	Indirect fluorescent antibody	Antibody
	Indirect hemagglutination	Antibody
Strongyloides stercoralis	Enzyme immunoassay	IgG and IgE
Toxocara canis	Enzyme immunoassay	IgM, IgG, and IgA
Toxoplasma gondii		
Trichinella spiralis	Counterimmunoelectrophoresis	Antibody
	Latex particle agglutination	Antibody
	Enzyme immunoassay	IgM, IgG, and IgA
Trichomonas vaginalis	Enzyme immunoassay	IgM, IgG, and IgA
Trypanosoma cruzi	Complement fixation	Antibody
	Indirect fluorescent antibody	Antibody
	Indirect hemagglutination	Antibody
	Enzyme immunoassay	Total IgM in cerebrospinal fluid

TABLE C-7

Procedures in Microbial Immunology: Mycotic Infections

Aspergillus spp.	Complement fixation	
	Enzyme immunoassay	Antigen or antibody
	Immunodiffusion	Antibody
	Radioimmunoassay	Antigen
Blastomyces dermatitidis	Complement fixation	Antibody
	Complement fixation	Antibody to "A" Ag
	Immunodiffusion	Antibody to "A" Ag
	Enzyme immunoassay	Antibody to "A" Ag
Candida sp.	Latex agglutination	Antibody
	Latex agglutination	Antigen
	Latex agglutination	Mannan antigen
	Immunodiffusion	Antibody
	Countercurrent immunoelectro- phoresis	Antibody
	Enzyme immunoassay	Antibody to mannan
	Electrophoresis	Mannan antigen
	Enzyme immunoassay	Mannan antigen
Coccidioides immitis	Latex agglutination	Serum antibody
	Complement fixation	Serum and cerebrospinal fluid an- tibody
	Immunodiffusion	Serum and cerebrospinal fluid an- tibody
	Enzyme immunoassay	Serum antigen
	Radioimmunoassay	Serum antigen
Cryptococcus neoformans	Latex agglutination	Serum and cerebrospinal fluid an- tigen
	Indirect fluorescent antibody	Antigen
	Direct agglutination	Antibody
Histoplasma capsulatum	Complement fixation	Antibody
	Countercurrent immunoelectro- phoresis	Antibody
	Immunodiffusion	Antibody in serum or cerebrospi- nal fluid
	Latex agglutination	Antibody
	Enzyme immunoassay	Antigen
Nocardia sp.	Complement fixation	Antibody
	Immunodiffusion	Antibody
Paracoccidioides brasiliensis	Complement fixation	Antibody
	Immunodiffusion	Antibody
	Direct fluorescent antibody	Antigen
Sporothrix schenkii	Immunodiffusion	Antibody
	Latex particle agglutination	Antibody
	Periodic acid-schiff stain	Antigen
	Light microscopy	Antigen
Candida sp.	Latex agglutination	Antibody
	Latex agglutination	Antigen
	Latex agglutination	Mannan antigen
	Immunodiffusion	Antibody
	Countercurrent immunoelectro- phoresis	Antibody
	Enzyme immunoassay	Antibody to mannan
	Electrophoresis	Mannan antigen
	Enzyme immunoassay	Mannan antigen
Zygomycetes sp.	Immunodiffusion	Antibodies
	Enzyme immunoassay	Antibodies

Glossary

abruptio placentae The premature separation of a normally situated placenta.

acquired Incurred because of external factors; not inherited.

acquired immunodeficiency syndrome (AIDS) An immune disorder affecting T4 lymphocytes. This disorder is caused by the human immunodeficiency virus, (HIV) which was previously called HTLV III (Human T cell leukemia virus), or LAV virus.

acquired immunity (*see* Adaptive immunity)

acquired or secondary immunodeficiency A defect in the normal immune response caused by external factors or as the result of an existing disease or condition.

acute A condition of sudden and short duration.

acute glomerulonephritis A sudden inflammation of the small convoluted mass of capillaries of the kidney, primarily the capsule.

acute phase proteins (acute phase reactants) A group of glycoproteins associated with nonspecific inflammation of body tissues.

adaptive immunity The augmentation of body defense mechanisms in response to a specific stimulus, which can cause the elimination of micro-organisms and recovery from disease. This response frequently leaves the host with specific memory (acquired resistance), which enables the body to respond effectively if reinfection with the same micro-organism occurs.

adenocarcinoma A malignant new growth derived from glandular tissue or from recognizable glandular structures.

adenopathy Swelling or enlargement of the lymph nodes.

adrenal medulla The inner core of the small endocrine gland that rests on top of each kidney.

afferent lymphatic duct The vessel that carries transparent liquid and antigens into the lymph node.

affinity Propensity; the bond between a single antigenic determinant and an individual combining site.

agammaglobulinemia The absence of plasma gammaglobulin because of either a congenital or acquired condition.

agglutination The clumping or aggregation of particles that have antigens on their surface, e.g., erythrocytes, by antibody molecules that form bridges between the antigenic determinants.

agglutinin The older term for *antibody*.

agglutinogen The older term for antigen.

aggregation (*see* Agglutination)

allergic rhinitis Inflammation of the mucous membrane of the nose caused by a hypersensitivity reaction to environmental substances such as pollen or mold.

alloantibodies Immunoglobulins (antibodies) produced in response to exposure of foreign antigens of the same species.

allogenic Genetically different individuals of the same species.

allograft A graft of tissue from a genetically different member of the same species, e.g., human kidney.

alopecia Loss of hair; baldness.

alveolar The thin-walled chambers of the lungs are referred to as *pulmonary alveoli*.

amniocentesis The process of removing fluid from the amniotic sac for study, e.g., biochemical analysis.

amyloidosis A condition of intercellular deposition of an abnormal protein with a waxy, translucent appearance in various tissues.

anaerobic metabolism (also referred to as the *Embden-Meyerhof glycolytic pathway* or the *TCA cycle*). It is the major, non-oxygen–associated, energy-yielding pathway connected with the breakdown of glucose (glycolysis) in body cells.

anamnestic antibody response An antibody "memory" response. This secondary type of response occurs on subsequent exposure to a previously encountered and recognized foreign antigen and is characterized by the rapid production of IgG antibodies.

anaphylactic reaction A severe allergic reaction that can develop in IgA deficient patients who have developed anti-IgA antibodies.

anaphylactic shock A severe allergic reaction.

anaphylactoid reaction A severe reaction to soluble constituents in donor plasma which produces edema.

anaphylatoxins The complement components, C3a and C5a, which stimulate release by mast cells of their vasoactive amines.

anaphylaxis An immediate (type I) hypersensitivity reaction characterized by local reactions, such as urticaria (hives) and angioedema (redness and swelling) or systemic reactions in the respiratory tract, cardiovascular system, gastrointestinal tract, and skin.

angioedema Redness and swelling.

anicteric Without icterus or lacking a yellow discoloration of the skin and sclera.

anomalies Marked deviations from normal.

anorexia nervosa An eating disorder prevalent in adolescent females.

antenatal Before birth.

antibodies (antibody) Specific glycoproteins (immunoglobulins) produced in response to an antigenic challenge. Antibodies can be found in blood plasma and body fluids, e.g., tears, saliva, and milk. These serum globulins have a wide range of specificities for different antigens and can bind to and neutralize bacterial toxins or bind to the surfaces of bacteria, viruses, or parasites.

antibody affinity (*see* Affinity)

antibody-dependent cell-mediated cytotoxicity reaction (adcc) A cellular activity exhibited by both K cells and phagocytic and non-phagocytic myelogenous type leukocytes. The target cell in ADCC is coated with a low concentration of IgG antibody.

antibody titer (*see* Titer)

anti-core window The period of time in which antigen cannot be detected in the circulating blood, such as in hepatitis B testing.

antigen (immunogen) A foreign substance that can stimulate the production of antibodies (immune response).

antigenic determinant(s) The combining site or sites with which antibodies react.

antigenicity The ability of an antigen to stimulate an immune response.

antistreptolysin O (ASO) An antibody produced against

378

streptolysin O, a hemolysin produced by streptococci, particularly group A.

aplastic anemia A deficiency of blood cells such as erythrocytes caused by the lack of cell production (hematopoiesis) in the bone marrow. This form of anemia may result from exposure to toxic chemicals or drugs, such as chloramphenicol.

APTT Activated partial thromboplastin time.

artherosclerotic (also referred to as *arteriosclerosis).* This is a condition of loss of elasticity (hardening) of the walls of the blood vessels, i.e., arteries.

arthralgia Pain in a joint.

arthritis Inflammation of a joint.

arthropathy Joint disease.

aseptic technique Handling of materials or specimens without the introduction of extraneous microorganisms.

ASO (*see* Antistreptolysin O)

asthma A respiratory condition characterized by recurrent attacks of dyspnea (difficult or painful breathing) and wheezing caused by spasmodic constriction of the bronchi (larger air passages to or within the lungs).

astrocyte A nerve cell characterized by fibrous or protoplasmic processes. Collectively these cells are called macroglia or astroglia tissue.

asymptomatic Exhibiting no symptoms of a disease or disorder.

ataxia Irregularity of muscular action or faulty muscular coordination.

atopic eczema Inflammation of the epidermis (skin) characterized by redness, itching, and weeping, which is caused by a hypersensitivity reaction.

atrophy Wasting or lack of growth of tissues or organs.

autoantibody An Immunoglobulin produced against a self-antigen.

autoimmune hemolytic anemia A condition of destruction of erythrocytes by antibodies to self-antigens.

autoimmunity A condition in which the body's own antigenic structures stimulate an immune response and react with self-antigens in a manner similar to the destruction of foreign antigens. This process may cause autoimmune disease.

autologous A synonym for *self* or part of the same individual.

autonomic nervous system The branch of the nervous system that functions without conscious control.

autosomal dominant gene A genetic trait that expresses itself, if present, and is carried on one of the 1 through 22 pairs of (autosomal) chromosomes.

autosomal recessive gene A genetic trait carried on one of the 1 through 22 pairs of chromosomes that is only expressed if present in a homozygous state.

avascular necrosis The death of nonvascular cells or tissues.

avidity The strength with which a multivalent antibody binds to a multivalent antigen.

bacteremia An infection of the blood caused by bacterial microorganisms.

bare lymphocyte syndrome An infrequent cause of severe combined immunodeficiency (SCID).

Bence Jones (BJ) protein The abnormal protein frequently found in the urine of patients with multiple myeloma. It precipitates at 50° C, disappears at 100° C, and reappears upon cooling to room temperature.

benign Nonmalignant or noncancerous.

bilirubin A breakdown product of erythrocyte catabolism. If increased levels of this substance accumulate in the circulation, it will be deposited in lipid-rich tissues, such as the brain, and will be manifested by the skin and sclera as jaundice/icterus.

blast transformation The conversion of a B lymphocyte into a plasma cell.

B lymphocyte A lymphocyte subset type that secretes antibody, the humoral element of adaptive immunity.

bone marrow The structure that contains hematopoietic (blood-forming) tissues.

Burkitt's lymphoma An undifferentiated malignant neoplastic disorder of the lymphoid tissues.

bursa of Fabricius An outgrowth of the cloaca in birds that becomes the site of formation of lymphocytes with B cell characteristics.

C3 The most abundant and important component of complement that produces a small (C3a) and a large peptide (C3b) when activated.

C5 The complement component that is split by C3b into C5a and C5b.

C6789 The lytic complement sequence that is activated by C5b and terminates in lysing the cell membrane.

carrier state The asymptomatic condition of harboring an infectious organism. The term may also refer to a heterozygous individual or the carrier of a recessive gene.

catarrhal symptoms An older term used to describe the manifestations of inflammation of the mucous membranes, particularly of the head or throat, with an accompanying discharge.

catecholamines Biologically active amines, including epinephrine and norepinephrine, that have a marked effect on the nervous and cardiovascular systems, metabolic rate and temperature, and smooth muscle.

CD4 The protein receptor on the surface of a target cell to which the gp 120 protein of the HIV viral envelope binds.

cell-mediated immunity The type of immunity dependent on the link between T cells and macrophages.

cellulitis Inflammation within solid tissues, usually loose tissues beneath the skin, that is manifested by redness, pain, swelling (edema), and interference with function.

centromere The constricted portion of a chromosome.

cerebrospinal fluid (CSF) The fluid formed by the choroid plexus in the ventricles of the brain and found within the subarachnoid space, the central canal of the spinal cord and the four ventricles of the brain.

cerebrovascular accident Stroke.

chancre A lesion that begins as a papule and erodes into a red ulcer. It is the primary wound of syphilis that occurs at the site of entry of the spirochete.

Chediak-Higashi syndrome A rare inherited autosomal recessive trait characterized by the presence of large granules and inclusion bodies in the cytoplasm of leukocytes.

chemotaxis The release of substances that attracts phagocytic cells as the result of traumatic or microbial damage.

cholestasis The blockage or suppression of the flow of bile.

choreoathetosis A condition characterized by rapid, jerky, involuntary movements or slow, irregular, twisting, snake-like movements seen mostly in the upper extremities, e.g., hands and fingers.

chorioretinitis Inflammation of the choroid (the middle layer) and the retina (the innermost layer) of the eye.

chronic   A condition of long duration.

chronic glomerulonephritis   An inflammation of long duration of the small convoluted mass of capillaries of the kidney, primarily the capsule.

circulating immune complex   An antigen-antibody in the blood flow.

clone   Cells descended from the same single cell.

coalesce   A fusion of components.

collagen   A protein found in skin, tendons, bone, and cartilage.

collagen disease   Diseases of the skin, tendons, bone, and cartilage, such as systemic lupus erythematosus and rheumatoid arthritis.

collecting tubule   A small duct that receives urine from several renal tubules.

combining site   The portion of the Fab molecule that possesses specificity.

common immunocyte   Any cell of the lymphoid series that can react with an antigen to produce an antibody or participate in cell-mediated reactions.

common thymocyte   Lymphocytes arising in the thymus which precede mature (OKT 10, OKT6 surface antigen) thymocytes in development.

complement   A group of proteins (enzymes) present in the blood that can produce inflammatory effects and lysis of cells when activated. Some bacteria activate complement directly, while others only do so with the help of antibody. If this cascading sequence of proteins is activated directly, it follows the alternate pathway; if it is activated by antigen-antibody interaction, it follows the classic pathway.

complement cascade   The sequential activation of plasma proteins that causes lysis of a cell.

complete antibody   An older term for an IgM antibody.

congenital rubella syndrome   (*see* Rubella syndrome)

conjugate   A laboratory substrate prepared by joining two substances together such as fluorescein to an immunoglobulin molecule.

convalescence period   The time of recovery from conditions such as illness, injury, or surgery.

Coombs Test   The older term for the antiglobulin test.

cortical-hypothalmic-pituitary axis   The interrelated association between the outer layer of the brain, the structure located at the base of the cerebrum, and a small endocrine gland.

corticosteroid   Any of the hormones produced by the outer layer of the gland located on top of each kidney.

cosmopolitan distribution   Widely distributed.

cranial nerve neuritis   An inflammation of any of the nerves that are attached to the brain and pass through the openings of the skull.

C-reactive protein   A nonspecific, acute phase reactant glycoprotein.

cross-reactivity   A condition when some of the determinants of an antigen are shared by similar antigenic derminants on the surface of apparently unrelated molecules and a proportion of these antigens interact with the other kind of antigen.

cryoglobulin   An abnormal protein that precipitates at cold temperatures but redissolves at warm temperatures.

cryptogenic cirrhosis   A condition of the liver that has an obscure or doubtful cause.

cutaneous   Refers to the skin (epidermis).

cutaneous T cell lymphoma   A malignant neoplasm with epidermal manifestations that involves the T subset of lymphocytes.

cytomegalovirus   A herpes-family virus that can cause congenital infections in the newborn and a clinical syndrome resembling infectious mononucleosis.

cytopenia   A severe decrease in hematologic cells.

cytotoxic T cell   A subset type of lymphocyte.

cytotoxicity   A condition in which macrophages can kill some targets (possibly tumor cells) without phagocytizing them.

Dane particle   The intact, double-shelled hepatitis B virus.

DAT   (*see* direct antiglobulin test)

Davidsohn differential test   The classic laboratory reference test for the diagnosis of infectious mononucleosis.

delta agent   An RNA virus that causes hepatitis but requires the coexistence of hepatitis B infection.

dementia   An irreversible condition of organic loss of mental function.

dendritic cells   The weakly phagocyte Langerhans cell of the epidermis, and similar, nonphagocytic cells in the lymphoid follicles of the spleen and lymph nodes. These cells may be the main agent of T cell stimulation, but the precise region of these dendritic cells is not yet certain.

deoxyribonucleic acid (DNA)   The nucleic acid that forms the main structure of the genes.

dermatomyositis   An inflammatory condition included in the collage disorders in which the skin, subcutaneous tissues, and muscles are involved. Necrosis of the muscles is characteristic.

diagnosis   Determination of the nature of a disorder or disease.

diapedesis   Ameboid movement of cells.

DIC   (*see* Disseminated intravascular coagulation)

direct antiglobulin test   A test performed to detect the coating of erythrocytes with antibodies.

discoid lupus   The term used to differentiate the benign dermatitis of cutaneous lupus from the cutaneous involvement of systemic lupus erythematosus (SLE).

disease   A pathologic condition characterized by a specific and unique set of signs and symptoms.

disorder   An abnormality of body function.

disseminated intravascular coagulation (DIC)   A serious coagulation disorder that consumes platelets and blood coagulation factors. DIC is an example of a major breakdown of the hemostatic mechanism that occurs when the procoagulant factors outweigh the anticoagulant system. This type of secondary fibrinolysis is clinically characterized by excessive clotting and fibrinolytic activity.

distal tubules   Ducts in the kidney located farthest from the center of the structure.

DNA amplification   An ultrasensitive polymerase chain reaction technique for the detection of HIV-1 that amplifies minute amounts of viral nucleic acid in the DNA of lymphocytes.

domain   The basic unit of an antibody structure. Variations between the domains of different antibody molecules are responsible for differences in antigen binding and in biological function.

D^u   A phenotype of the Rh blood group system.

D^u Rosette Test   A procedure that uses D-positive indicator erythrocytes to form identifiable rosettes around individual D positive fetal cells that may be in the maternal circulation.

dysplastic   Faulty or abnormal development of body tissue.

dyspnea Difficulty in breathing.
dysproteinemia An abnormality of the protein content of the blood.

early antigen (EA) A "new" antigen expressed by B lymphocytes infected with Epstein-Barr virus in infectious mononucleosis. EA consists of early antigen-diffuse (EA-D), which is found in both the nucleus and cytoplasm of B cells, and early antigen-restricted (EA-R), which is usually found as a mass only in the cytoplasm.
early thymocyte Immature T cell in the thymus (cell surface antigen markers OKT10, OKT9) that precedes the common thymocyte in maturational development.
ectopic pregnancy The gestation of a fertilized egg outside of the uterus, most commonly in the fallopian tube.
eczema An inflammatory condition of the skin (epidermis) characterized by redness, weeping, and itching.
edema (edematous) Accumulation of fluid in the tissues that produces swelling.
efferent lymphatic duct The tubule through which semitransparent fluid (lymph) and possibly antigens exit the lymph node.
electrophoresis (*see* Serum electrophoresis)
ELISA (see Enzyme-linked immunosorbent assay)
eluate The product of purposely manipulating a red cell suspension to break an antigen-antibody complex with the subsequent release of the antibody into the surrounding medium.
embryogenesis The growth and development of a living organism. In humans, this period is from the second to approximately the eighth week of gestation.
encephalopathy Any degenerative disease of the brain.
endemic Present at all times, such as the continual existence of a specific microorganism in a population of individuals or geographic location.
endocarditis An inflammation of the inner lining of the heart (endocardium).
endothelial cell The type of epithelial cell that lines body cavities such as the serous cavities, the heart, and blood and lymphatic vessels.
endotoxemia A condition of having bacterial cell wall heat-stable toxins in the circulation. These toxins are pyrogenic and increase capillary permeability.
end-stage renal disease An irreversible, pathologic condition of the kidneys.
enterocolitis An inflammation of the small intestine and colon.
env gene A gene of a retrovirus, such as HIV, that encodes for a polyprotein that contains numerous glycosylation sites.
enzyme-linked immunosorbent assays (ELISA) A method of laboratory analysis.
epidemiology (epidemiologic) Pertains to the study of infectious diseases or conditions in many individuals in the same geographic location at the same time.
epilepsy A transient disturbance of nervous system function caused by abnormal electrical activity in the brain.
episomal DNA An accessory, extrachromosomal replicating genetic element.
epithelial cell Cell of a type of body tissue that forms the covering of external and internal surfaces or composes a body structure, such as glandular epithelium.
epitope A single antigenic determinant. It is functionally the portion of an antigen that combines with an antibody paratope (the part of the antibody molecule that makes contact with the antigenic determinant).
Epstein-Barr virus A human herpes DNA virus found in association with leukocytes and B lymphocytes. It is the causative agent of infectious mononucleosis in western countries and Burkitt's lymphoma in Africa.
erysipelas A febrile disease caused by group A streptococci. The disease is manifested by inflammation and redness of the skin and subcutaneous tissues and fever, vomiting, or headache.
erythema Redness of the skin caused by inflammation, infection, or injury.
erythematosus Characterized by erythema (*see* Erythema).
erythrocyte The scientific term for a red blood cell.
erythropoiesis The process of producing red blood cells.
estrogen The term for the female sex hormones including estradiol, estriol, and estrone.
etiology A synonym for the study of or the cause(s) of disease.
exchange transfusion The replacement of an infant's coated erythrocytes with donor blood until a one or two total blood volume transfer is accomplished.
extramedullary hematopoiesis Production of erythrocytes outside the bone marrow, which can produce enlargement of the liver and spleen.
extravascular destruction The destruction of an erythrocyte through phagocytosis and digestion by macrophages of the mononuclear-phagocytic system.
extravascular hemolysis The phagocytizing and catabolizing of erythrocytes by the mononuclear-phagocytic system.

Fab fragments Two of the three fragments formed, if a typical monmeric IgG is digested with a proteolytic enzyme such as papain. These fragments retain the ability to bind antigen and are called the antigen-binding fragments.
Fc portion The third fragment formed in addition to the two Fab fragments, if a typical monomeric IgG is digested with a proteolytic enzyme such as papain. This fragment is relatively homogeneous and sometimes crystallizable.
Fc receptor The portion of an antibody responsible for binding to antibody receptors on cells and the C1q component of complement.
Fd fragment The fragment consisting of a light chain and half of a heavy chain if the interchain disulfide bonds in the Fab fragment is disrupted.
febrile agglutinin An antibodies demonstrated in microbial diseases that are manifested by a high fever.
febrile disease A pathologic process in which an extremely high fever is a characteristic manifestation.
femur The bone of the leg that extends from the pelvic girdle to the knee (the thigh bone).
fibrin A meshy protein clot formed by the action of thrombin on fibrinogen.
fibroblast An immature fiber-producing cell of connective tissue capable of differentiating into a cartilage-forming cell (chondroblast), a collagen-forming cell (collagenoblast), or a bone-forming cell (osteoblast).
fimbriae Fringed or fingerlike.
flocculation The clumping together of particles to form visible masses.
Forssman antibody A heterophil type of immunoglobulin that is stimulated by one antigen and reacts with an

entirely unrelated surface antigen present on cells from different mammalian species. It can be absorbed from human serum by guinea pig kidney cells.

Franklin's disease   A dysproteinemia that is synonymous with gamma heavy chain disease. This abnormality is characterized by the presence of monoclonal protein composed of the heavy chain portion of the immunoglobulin molecule.

fulminant   To occur suddenly with great intensity such as lightening-like flashes of pain.

gag gene   A gene of a retrovirus, such as HIV, that encodes for the major core structural protein.

GALT   (*see* Gut-associated lymphoid tissue)

gamma heavy chain disease   (*see* Franklin's disease)

gastroenteritis   An inflammation of the lining of the stomach and intestine.

genitalia   The female and male reproductive organs and associated external structures such as the penis.

genome   The complete set of hereditary factors contained in the haploid set of chromosomes; the complete set of chromosomes contributed by one of the male-female pair.

gestation   The period of development and growth of the unborn in viviparous animals, e.g., humans, from fertilization of the ovum to birth.

giant cell; epithelioid cell   Macrophage-derived cells typically found at sites of chronic inflammation. A giant multinucleated cell is formed by the coalescing of cells into a solid mass, or granuloma.

giardiasis   A parasitic infection associated with the unicellular *Giardia* species.

glial cell   Also known as neuroglial cell. It is the nonnervous or supportive tissue of the brain and spinal cord known to produce minute amounts of CD4 or an alternate receptor molecule, which allows it to be infected with HIV virus.

glomerulonephritis   (*see* Acute glomerulonephritis or Chronic glomerulonephritis)

glomerulus (pl. glomeruli)   The small structure in the malpighian body of the kidney that is composed of a cluster of capillary blood vessels in a cluster and enveloped in a thin wall.

goodness of fit   The complementary matching of antigenic determinants and the antigen-binding sites of corresponding antibodies that influences the strength of bonding between antigens and antibodies.

grafting   The transfer of cells or organs from one individual to another or from one site to another in the same individual.

graft-versus-host disease   An intense and frequently fatal immunologic reaction of engrafted cells against the host caused by the infusion of immunocompetent lymphocytes into individuals with impaired immunity.

grand mal seizures   A major epileptic attack with or without loss of consciousness.

granulocyte   A type of leukocytic white blood cell.

granuloma   A macrophage-derived lesion containing sequestered noxious agents such as foreign bodies, some types of bacteria, etc., which cannot be eliminated.

granulomatous lesion   A wound composed of granuloma.

Guillain-Barré syndrome   A relatively rare disease of the nerves. Also called acute idiopathic polyneuritis.

gummas   A granuloma that may result from delayed hypersensitivity. It is the soft tumor of the tissues characteristic of the tertiary stage of syphilis.

gut-associated lymphoid tissue (GALT)   The GALT and bone marrow may play a role in the differentiation of stem cells into B lymphocytes and functions as the bursal equivalent in humans.

haptene(s)   Very small molecules that can bind to a larger carrier molecule and behave as an antigen.

helper/inducer subset   (also referred to as *T4* or *Leu 3*). A major phenotypic lymphocyte subset of T lymphocytes.

hemagglutination   A laboratory technique for the detection of antibodies that involves the agglutination of red blood cells.

hemagglutination inhibition technique (hai)   A laboratory technique for the detection of antibodies that involves the blocking of agglutination of red blood cells.

hematopoiesis (hematopoietic tissues)   Blood-producing structures of the body, such as the liver, spleen, and bone marrow.

hemodynamic shock   A physiologic condition such as decreased blood pressure, resulting from the rapid loss of 15% to 20% or more of blood volume.

hemoflagellate   A protozoan parasite found in the blood and/or body tissues.

hemolysin   A substance, such as streptolysin O and streptolysin S, produced by most group A strains of *Streptococci* that disrupts the membrane integrity of red blood cells, which causes the release of hemoglobin.

hemolysis   The rupturing of the cell membrane, e.g., an erythrocyte, with the subsequent dumping of cytoplasmic contents.

hemolytic anemia   A severe decrease in circulating erythrocytes and associated findings caused by the rupturing of circulating erythrocytes.

hemolytic disease of the newborn   (previously referred to as *erythroblastosis fetalis*). An immunologic incompatibility between mother and fetus that can produce severe or fatal consequences in the unborn or newborn because of destruction of erythrocytes and the accumulation of breakdown products.

hemolyzed   Ruptured erythrocytes.

hemoptysis   Coughing and spitting up of blood as the result of bleeding from any part of the respiratory system.

hemostatic   Stoppage of bleeding.

hepatitis   Inflammation of the liver caused by a virus or other agents such as drugs.

hepatomegaly   Excessive enlargement of the liver.

hepatosplenomegaly   An enlarged liver and spleen.

herpes virus   Any of a large group of DNA viruses such as *Herpes simplex* and varicella.

heterogeneous   Different; not originating in the body.

heterosexual disease   A pathologic condition transmitted between individuals of the opposite sex.

heterozygous   The genetic state of having two dissimilar genes for the same trait.

histamine   An amine produced by the catabolism of histidine, which causes dilation of blood vessels.

histiocyte   A large phagocytic interstitial cell of the mononuclear phagocytic system, a macrophage.

histocompatibility (hla) antigen   Cell surface protein antigen found on blood and body cells, e.g., leukocytes and platelets, that readily provokes an immune response if transferred into a genetically different (allogenic) individual of the same species.

histone A simple protein found in combination with acidic substances such as nucleic acids.

Hodgkin's lymphoma or Hodgkin's disease A major form of malignant lymphoma.

homogeneous Uniform; the same.

homozygous In genetics, when the genes for a trait on homologous chromosomes are the same.

HTLV III (human T cell leukemia virus) A type of retrovirus also known as LAV or HIV; a causative agent of acquired immunodeficiency syndrome (AIDS).

human B-cell lymphotropic virus (HBLV) A herpes virus that can interact with human immunodeficiency virus (HIV) in a way that may increase the severity of HIV infection.

human herpes virus 6 (HHV-6) A herpes virus that can interact with human immunodeficiency virus (HIV) in a way that may increase the severity of HIV infection.

human immunodeficiency virus (HIV) (also referred to as human T-lymphotropic virus type III, HTLV-III, LAV, or human immunodeficiency virus [HIV-1]). This virus is a causative agent of acquired immunodeficiency syndrome (AIDS).

human T-lymphotropic virus type III Also referred to as HTLV-III, LAV, or human immunodeficiency virus. This virus is a causative agent of acquired immunodeficiency syndrome (AIDS).

humoral Any fluid or semifluid in the body.

humoral immunity A form of body defense against foreign substances represented by antibodies and other soluble, extracellular factors in the blood and lymphatic fluid.

Hutchinsonian triad The characteristic manifestation of congenital syphilis. The three major features are notched teeth, interstitial keratitis, and nerve deafness.

hyaluronidase (also called spreading factor). An enzyme that breaks down hyaluronic acid found in connective tissue.

hybridoma Cell lines created in vitro by fusing two different cell types. A hybridoma is usually formed from a lymphocyte or plasma cells, one of which is a tumor cell.

hydrophilic Water loving.

hydrophobic Water hating.

hypercalcemia A marked increase in ionized calcium in the circulating blood.

hypergammaglobulinemia An increased gammaglobulin fraction of plasma protein.

hyperkeratosis A condition of increased growth of the upper layer of the skin (epidermis) or overgrowth of the cornea.

hypersensitivity An unpleasant or damaging condition of the body tissues caused by antigenic stimulation. Hypersensitivity reactions include allergies such as hay fever.

hyperviscosity An increase in the thickness (viscosity) of substances such as blood plasma.

hyperviscosity syndrome A collection of symptoms resulting from increased resistance (viscosity) of the flow of blood in the circulation.

hypervolemia An increase of total blood volume.

hypogammaglobulinemia A decreased in the gammaglobulin fraction of plasma protein.

hypoplastic Defective or incomplete development of a tissue or organ.

hypothalamus The portion of the brain beneath the thalamus at the base of the cerebrum that forms the floor and part of the walls of the third ventricle.

icterus (icteric) A synonym for jaundice or the yellow appearance of the skin and mucous membranes because of bilirubin (a product of red cell breakdown) accumulation.

idiopathic A disorder or disease that is without an identifiable external cause or self-originated.

idiotype The antigenic characteristic of the antibody variable region.

Ig (*see* Immunoglobulin)

iliac nodes Small rounded structure located in the lower three-fifths of the small intestines from the jejunum to the ileocecal valve or in the inguinal region.

immature B cell The receptor cell which is finally programmed for insertion of specific IgM molecules into the plasma membrane.

immune complex The noncovalent combination of an antigen with its specific antibody. An immune complex can be small and soluble or large and precipitating, depending on the nature and proportion of the antigen and antibody.

immune deficiency disease A condition in which a defect exists in the ability to detect antigens and/or to produce antibodies against foreign antigens.

immune status The ability of a host (an individual) to recognize and respond to foreign (non-self) substances, e.g., antigens.

immune system The structures, e.g., the bone marrow, thymus, and lymph nodes; cells, e.g., macrophages and lymphocytes; and soluble constituents of the circulating blood such as complement, that allow the host to recognize and respond to foreign (non-self) substances such as antigens.

immunity The process of being protected against foreign antigens.

immunocompetent The ability to mount an immune response; a host who is able to recognize a foreign antigen and build specific antigen-directed antibodies. The term specifically refers to lymphocytes that acquire thymus-dependent characteristics, which allow them to function in an immune response.

immunodeficiency A dysfunction in body defense mechanisms that causes a failure in detection of foreign antigens and production of antibodies against these foreign (non-self) substances.

immunodiffusion A laboratory method for the quantitative study of antibodies, e.g., radial immunodiffusion (RID) or qualitative identity of antigens, e.g., Ouchterlony technique.

immunofluorescent assay (IFA) A laboratory method that employs a fluorescent substance in immunologic studies. For example, particular antigens can be identified microscopically in tissues or cells by the binding of a fluorescent (light-emitting) antibody conjugate.

immunogenic (*see* Antigen)

immunogen A large organic molecule that is either protein or large polysaccharide and rarely, if ever, lipid.

immunoglobulin A synonym for antibody. The term describes all globulins with antibody activity and has replaced the term *gammaglobulin* because not all antibodies have gamma electrophoretic mobility. Immunoglobulins are divided into five classes with IgG being the most abundant.

immunologic dysfunction (*see* Immune deficiency disease)

immunology The study of all aspects of body defenses, such as antigens and antibodies, allergy, and hypersensitivity.

immunosuppression Repressing the normal adaptive immune response through the use of drugs, chemicals, or other means. This process is frequently necessary subsequent to organ transplantation or to alter a hypersensitivity reaction.

immunosuppressive agent Drug, chemical, or other mechanism that prevents the immune system from recognizing and responding to non-self.

impetigo A skin infection caused by *Streptococci* that begins as a papule.

incomplete antibody An older term that refers to IgG type antibodies.

indirect hemagglutination technique (also called *passive hemagglutination technique*). This laboratory method uses erythrocytes that are passively coated with substances such as extracts of bacterial cells, rickettsiae, pathogenic fungi, protozoa, purified polysaccharides, or proteins for the detection of antibody.

infarction An area of tissue, such as heart muscle, that undergoes necrosis (tissue breakdown) because of the lack of oxygen from the circulating blood. A condition of oxygen deprivation may be caused by a narrowing of blood vessels (stenosis) or a blockage of the blood circulation in the vessel (occlusion).

infection A pathogenic condition caused by microorganisms, e.g., viruses, bacteria, that produce injurious effects.

infectious material Body fluids or excretory products, or nonhuman substances contaminated with body fluids that contain disease-causing microorganisms.

infectious mononucleosis A benign lymphoproliferative disorder.

inflammation Tissue reaction to injury caused by physical or chemical agents, including microorganisms. Symptoms include redness, tenderness, pain, and swelling.

inflammatory response (*see* Inflammation)

inguinal adenopathy Enlarged lymph nodes in the region of the groin.

in situ hybridization A laboratory technique for demonstrating the presence of HIV-1 in lymphocytes in primary lymph nodes and peripheral blood from HIV infected patients.

interferon An antiviral substance.

interleukin-1 (IL-1) A lymphokine produced by activated macrophages, which activates T cells, B cells, NK cells, and other macrophages.

interleukin-2 (IL-2) Also known as *T cell growth factor*. A lymphokine that is important in cell-mediated immunity. It is produced by activated OKT4 cells, which initiates B cell proliferation and also activates cytotoxic T cells.

interstitial pneumonitis An inflammation situated between or in the interspaces of the lung tissue.

intraperitoneal fetal transfusion (IPT) The administration of blood to a fetus (unborn infant) via the abdominal cavity.

intrarenal obstruction A blockage within the kidney.

intratubular precipitation The formation of a solid mass from soluble substances within the tubules of the kidney.

intrauterine Within the uterus.

intravascular coagulation The formation of a clot within a vessel, i.e., blood vessels of the circulatory system.

intravascular destruction An alternate pathway for erythrocyte breakdown, which normally accounts for less than 10% of red cell destruction.

intravascular hemolysis An alternate pathway of red cell destruction in which the cells are lysed in the vessels of the circulatory system.

intravenous urography The radiologic study of any part of the urinary tract by the administration through a vein of an opaque medium, which is rapidly excreted in the urine.

intrinsic coagulation mechanism The initial stage of blood coagulation that can be activated by antigen-antibody complexes.

intrinsic factor (IF) A substance secreted by the parietal cells of the mucosa in the fundus region of the stomach.

in vitro A term used to designate outside the body, i.e., in the test tube.

in vivo A term used to designate in the living organism.

isoelectric focusing Separation of molecules on the basis of their charge. Each molecule migrates to the point in a pH gradient where it has no net charge.

isoimmune Possessing antibodies to antigens of the same system.

isotype A term that refers to genetic variation within a family of proteins or peptides so that every member of the species will have each isotype of the family represented in its genome, e.g., immunoglobulin classes.

isotypic varion The heavy chain constant region structure associated with the different classes and subclasses. Isotopic variants are present in all healthy members of a species.

jaundice (*see also* Icterus). A yellow appearance of the skin, sclerae, and body excretions.

Kahler's disease An alternate term for multiple myeloma.

Kaposi's sarcoma A rare, malignant, metastasizing disorder chiefly involving the skin. An increased incidence of this malignancy has been observed in patients suffering from acquired immunodeficiency syndrome.

keratinization The development of or conversion into keratin (an extremely tough scleroprotein found in structures such as hair and nails).

kernicterus The deposition of increased bilirubin, a red cell breakdown product, in lipid-rich nervous tissue, such as the brain, which can produce mental retardation or death in the newborn. This condition can occur when circulating plasma bilirubin levels reach 20 mg/dL in a full-term infant and at lower levels in a premature infant.

kinetochore A term for the centromere (the constricted area of the chromosome that demarcates the upper and lower arms of the structure).

kinetoplast A structure that may also be called the micronucleus. It is an accessory body found in many protozoa.

kinin A small, biologically active peptide.

kinin system A series of serum peptides sequentially activated to cause vasodilation and increased vascular permeability.

Kleihauer-Betke test A testing method based on the differences in solubility between adult and fetal hemoglobin. The test is performed on a maternal blood specimen for the detection of fetal-maternal hemorrhage.

Kupffer cell A phagocytic type of cell that lines the minute blood vessel (sinusoids) of the liver.

lag period The period of time between a stimulus, i.e., antigenic stimulation, and a reaction, i.e., immunoglobulin response.

Langerhans cell A macrophage found in the skin.

large granular lymphocyte (LGL) This term can synonomously refer to a NK cell. About 75% of LGLs function as NK cells and appear to account fully for the NK activity in mixed cell populations.

latent Hidden or inactive.

latent infection Persistent infections characterized by periods of reactivation of the signs and symptoms of the disease.

lattice formation The establishment of crosslinks between sensitized particles such as erythrocytes.

leukocyte A type of leukocyte that functions in antigen recognition and antibody formation.

leukocytosis A marked increase in the total circulating white blood cell concentration.

leukopenia A marked decrease in the total circulating white blood cell concentration.

leukotrine A term for the newly identified class of compounds that mediate the inflammatory functions of leukocytes. These substances are a collection of metabolites of arachidonic acid, which have powerful pharmacologic effects.

ligand A linking or binding molecule.

light chain disease (LCD) A dysproteinemia of the monoclonal gammopathy type. In LCD only kappa or lambda monoclonal light chains, or Bence Jones proteins, are produced.

lipopolysaccharide (LPS) The major component of some gram-negative bacterial cell walls which protects them from phagocytosis but activates C3 directly. LPS can also act as a B cell mitogen.

liposome A particle of fat-like substance held in suspension in tissues.

localized Confined to a specific area.

localized inflammatory response A tissue reaction confined to a specific area. This response is caused by physical or chemical agents, including microorganisms. The manifestations of the response include redness, tenderness, pain, and swelling.

long terminal redundancy (LTR) A structure that exists at each end of the proviral genome and plays an important role in the control of viral gene expression and the integration of the provirus into the DNA of the host.

LPS (*See* Lipopolysaccharide)

lymphadenopathy Disease of the lymph nodes.

lymph node Any of the accumulations of lymphoid tissue organized as definite lymphoid organs along the course of lymphatic vessels.

lymphoblast The most immature stage of the lymphocyte type of leukocyte.

lymphocyte A small white blood cell found in lymph nodes and the circulating blood. Two major populations of lymphocytes are recognized: T and B cells.

lymphocyte recirculation This process enables lymphocytes to come in contact with processed foreign antigens and to disseminate antigen-sensitized memory cells throughout the lymphoid system.

lymphocytopenia A severe decrease in the total number of lymphocytes in the peripheral blood.

lymphocytosis A significant increase in the total number of lymphocytes in the peripheral blood.

lymphokine (*see* Soluble mediator). This soluble protein mediator is released by sensitized lymphocytes on contact with an antigen.

lymphoma Solid, malignant tumor of the lymph nodes and associated tissues or bone marrow.

lymphoproliferative disorder A group of diseases characterized by the proliferation of lymphoid tissues and/or lymphocytes.

lymphosarcoma Malignant neoplastic disorders of the lymphoid tissues, excluding Hodgkin's disease.

lyse To break apart or dissolve.

lysis Irreversible leakage of cell contents following membrane damage.

lysozyme (muramidase) An enzyme secreted by macrophages, which attacks the cell walls of some bacteria.

macroglobulin A high-molecular-weight protein of the globulin type.

macrophage A large mononuclear phagocytic cell of the tissues that exists as either a wandering type or a fixed type that lines the capillaries and sinuses of organs such as the bone marrow, spleen, and lymph nodes. This cell phagocytizes, processes, presents antigens to T cells, and is also responsible for removing damaged tissue, cells, bacteria, etc., from the host.

macrophage migration inhibitory factor (MIF) A lymphocyte product which is chemotactic for monocytes. Other similar factors stimulate monocyte and macrophage functions.

macular lesion A discolored, unraised spot on the skin.

maculopapular A lesion with both macular and papular characteristics.

malaise A general feeling of tiredness or discomfort.

malignant (malignancy) Cancerous.

manifestation The development of the signs and symptoms of a disease or disorder.

mast cell A large tissue cell with basophilic granules containing vasoactive amines and heparin. When the cell is damaged, the granules release these inflammatory mediators which increase vascular permeability and allow complement and phagocytic cells to enter damaged tissues from the circulating blood.

mature B cell Concerned with synthesis of circulating antibodies.

mediastinum The tissues and organs, such as the heart, trachea, esophagus, and lymph nodes, that separate the sternum in the front (ventral side) from the vertebral column in the back (dorsal side) of the body.

megakaryocytic thrombocytopenic purpura A severe deficiency of the cells (thrombocytes/platelets) related to blood clotting that causes large, purple discolorations of the skin.

melanocyte A cell that produces melanin (the dark pigment normally found in structures such as the hair, eyes, and skin). It can also occur abnormally in certain tumors, melanomas.

memory cell Also called a memory B cell. These cells are lymphocytes that recall prior antigen exposure.

meningoencephalitis An inflammation of the brain and its membranous covering (the meninges).

meningovascular A term that refers to the blood vessels of the covering of the brain and spinal cord (meninges).

mesothelium A type of epithelium originally derived from the mesoderm lining the primitive embryonic body cavity that becomes the serous membrane of body surfaces, such as the peritoneum (the membrane viscera and lining of the abdominal cavity, except the kidneys), the pleura (the membrane covering the lungs), the walls of the thoracic cavity (the chest and diaphragm), and pericardium (the sac enclosing the heart).

microencephaly Abnormally small brain.

microglia The phagocytic cells of the brain, thought to be derived from incoming blood monocytes.

microplate A compact plate of rigid or flexible plastic with multiple wells.

MIF (*see* macrophage migration inhibitory factor)

mitogen A substance that stimulates cell division (mitosis).

monoclonal antibody Purified immunoglobulins produced by cells that are cloned from a single fusion-type hybridoma cell. Monoclonal antibodies are directed against antigens derived from a single cell line.

monoclonal gammopathy A dysproteinemia in which a single type of immunoglobulin is increased. This immunoglobulin is secreted by a single clone of plasma cells.

monoclonal protein (M protein, paraprotein) A protein characterized by a narrow peak or a localized band on electrophoresis, by a thickened bowed arc on immunoelectrophoresis, and by a localized band on immunofixation.

monocyte A type of leukocyte found in the peripheral blood.

monocytic Refers to the leukocyte type, monocytes.

monokine A soluble protein mediator.

mononuclear cell Cell types including the monocytes, promyelocytes, myelocytes, and blasts.

mononuclear-phagocyte system Formerly called the reticuloendothelial system (RES). This system is the body defense system and is composed of macrophages and a network of specialized cells of the spleen, thymus, and other lymphoid tissues.

monovalent An antigen with only one antigenic determinant.

morbidity A condition of being diseased; the ratio of sick to healthy persons or the number of cases of a specific illness in a designated population.

mortality The rate of death or ratio of the number of deaths to living individuals in a designated population.

M protein (*see* Monoclonal protein)

multiple myeloma A malignant disorder of plasma cells also known as plasma cell myeloma or Kahler's disease.

multipotential stem cell (MSC) Precursor cells in the bone marrow capable of differentiating into various blood cell (hematopoietic) types.

murine hybridoma The fusion product of a malignant and normal cell that produces large quantities of monoclonal antibodies.

myalgia Pain or tenderness in the muscles.

myelitis An inflammation of the spinal cord or bone marrow.

myeloma cell Plasma cells derived from malignant tumor strains.

myeloma clone A group of neoplastic cells that are descendants of a single, neoplastic cell.

myeloma kidney Abnormalities of the kidney associated with the neoplastic disorder multiple myeloma.

myelomatosis A term for multiple myeloma.

myeloperoxidase An important enzyme in the process of phagocytosis.

myocarditis An inflammation of the cardiac muscle tissue.

myosin One of the two main contractile proteins found in muscles.

nasopharyngeal carcinoma A malignancy involving the nose and throat.

natural killer cell (NK cells, previously called *null cells).* A population of effector lymphocytes that produces such mediators as interferon and interleukin 2.

natural resistance Innate or inborn.

necrosis The death of cells or a localized group of cells.

necrotizing vasculitis An inflammation of a vessel, such as a blood vessel, that results in tissue destruction.

neonatal septicemia A systemic disease caused by pathogenic microorganisms or their toxins in the blood of an infant up to 4 weeks old.

neonate An infant up to 4 weeks old.

neoplasm Any new and abnormal tissue such as a tumor.

neoplastic Refers to new, abnormal tissue growth.

nephelometry A laboratory assay method based on the measurement of the turbidity of particles in suspension. A nephelometer can be used for assays such as quantitating immunoglobulin concentrations in serum.

nephritis An inflammation of the kidney.

nephritogenic An agent or microorganism capable of causing an inflammation of the kidney.

nephropathy Any inflammatory, degenerative, or sclerotic disease of the kidneys.

nephrosis A condition of the kidney, particularly tubular degeneration, without the signs and symptoms of inflammation.

nephrotic syndrome A disorder of the kidneys characterized by a decreased concentration of albumin in the circulating blood, marked edema (swelling), increased protein in the urine (proteinuria), and increased susceptibility to infection.

nephrotoxic An agent such as a specific toxin that is destructive to kidney cells.

neurologic sequelae Morbid nervous system signs and symptoms that follow or are caused by a disease.

neurotoxic cytokine A substance that has the ability to destroy nervous tissue.

neutropenia A marked decreased in the neutrophil-type of leukocyte.

neutrophil A granulocyte-containing type of leukocyte.

NK cell (*see* Natural killer cell)

non-Hodgkin's lymphoma A condition of solid, malignant tumors of the lymph nodes and associated tissues or bone marrow that is not of the Hodgkin's type.

non-self A term covering micro-organisms as well as cells, organs, and other materials from a different animal or individual. The term is not generally applied to food or drugs, although they are sometimes involved in immunity.

nonsymptomatic An abnormal condition such as an infectious disease that does not manifest the signs and symptoms of the disorder.

normal flora Micro-organisms that normally inhabit areas of the body such as the skin, mucous membranes, and the intestinal tract.

normocytic, normochromic anemia A deficiency of erythrocytes; however, the erythrocytes present in the circulation are of normal size and have a normal color.

nosocomial Pertaining to a hospital. For example, a nosocomial infection is a hospital-acquired infection.

null cell (*see* Natural killer cells)

oncogene A transforming gene of cellular origin that is contained in retroviruses and associated with acute leukemias.

oncogenic Associated with tumor formation.

oocyst The encysted form of a fertilized gamete occurring in certain sporozoa; an immature ovum.

opportunistic infection A microbial disease that infects a debilitated host.

opsonization When the complement component C3b is attached to a particle, it promotes the adherence of phagocytic cells because of the C3 receptors. Antibody, if present, augments this by binding to Fc receptors.

oropharynx The part of the throat between the soft palate and the upper edge of the epiglottis.

osteoclast A giant, multinucleated cell formed in the bone marrow of growing bones. This cell is associated with reabsorption and removal of unwanted tissue.

osteomyelitis An inflammation of bone/bone marrow.

osteonecrosis The accelerated destruction of bone tissue.

osteoporosis Increased porosity of bone that causes softening and thinning of the bone.

otitis media Inflammation of the middle ear.

pancreatitis An inflammation of the structure with endocrine and exocrine functions located behind the stomach, between the spleen and duodenum.

papule A small, solid, elevated lesion of the skin.

paraprotein (*see* M protein or Monoclonal protein)

parenchymal Refers to the functional constituents of an organ as opposed to the framework (stroma).

parenteral Situation outside of the alimentary (oral) canal. Parenteral medications, for example, can be administered subcutaneously (beneath the skin), intramuscularly or intravenously.

parotid gland The largest of the three salivary glands located near the ear.

paroxysmal cold hemoglobinuria (PCH) A form of destruction of erythrocytes (red blood cells) caused by an IgG protein that reacts with the erythrocytes in colder parts of the body and subsequently causes complement components to irreversibly bind to erythrocytes. It is commonly seen as an acute transient condition secondary to viral infection.

paroxysmal nocturnal hemoglobinuria (PNH) A disorder in which the patient's erythrocytes act as a complement activator. The activation of complement results in excessive lysis of the patient's erythrocytes.

partial thromboplastin time (APTT) A coagulation procedure to detect factors that are active in the external mechanism (stage I) of blood coagulation.

passive hemagglutination technique (*see* Indirect hemagglutination technique)

pathogen A disease-causing microorganism or agent.

pathogenesis The origin of disease.

pathogenic (pathogenicity) The disease-producing potential of a microorganism.

perforation A hole or break in the wall or membrane of an organ or body structure.

periarteritis nodosa An inflammation of the layers of small and medium-sized arteries. This condition is manifested by a variety of systemic signs and symptoms, including febrile manifestations.

pericarditis An inflammation of the serous membrane lining of the sac surrounding the heart and the origins of the great blood vessels.

perinatal Preceding, during, or after birth.

perineal region The external region between the vulva and anus in the female or between the scrotum and anus in the male.

peritonitis An inflammation of the serous membrane covering the intestines and abdominal organs (viscera) and the abdominal cavity.

pernicious anemia An erythrocytic disorder associated with defective vitamin B_{12} uptake.

petechiae Small purple hemorrhagic spots on the skin or mucous membranes.

PG (*see* Prostaglandins)

phagocyte Any cell capable of engulfing and destroying foreign particles such as bacteria.

phagocytosis A form of endocytosis. This important body defense mechanism is the process in which specialized cells engulf and destroy foreign particles, such as microorganisms or damaged cells. Macrophages and segmented neutrophils (PMNs) are the most important phagocytic cells.

phagolysosome A vacuole (secondary lysosome) formed by the fusion of a phagosome and a primary lysome(s) in which microorganisms are killed and digested.

phagosome A membrane-bound vesicle in a phagocyte containing the phagocytized material.

pharyngitis An inflammation of the throat.

pharynx The throat.

phototherapy The use of ultraviolet light to accelerate the breakdown of bilirubin that has abnormally accumulated in the skin.

phytohemagglutinin A specific substance, a lectin, that is derived from plants and has the ability to agglutinate erythrocytes.

plasma The straw colored fluid component of blood in circulating or anticoagulated blood.

plasma cell A mature plasma cell found in small numbers in the bone marrow but not normally seen in the circulating blood.

plasma cell myeloma (*see* Multiple myeloma)

plasmacytoid Plasma cell-like.

plasmacytoid lymphocyte A cell that resembles a plasma cell.

plasmin A proteolytic enzyme with the ability to dissolve formed fibrin clots.

plasminogen The inactive precursor to plasmin, which is converted to plasmin by the action of substances such as urokinase.

platelet factor 3 An important factor associated with blood thrombocytes (platelets).

pleura The membrane covering the lungs, the walls of the thoracic cavity (chest), and diaphragm.

pleuritis An inflammation of the serous membrane lining, the pleura.

pluripotent (*see* Multipotential stem cells)

PMN (*see* Polymorphonuclear leukocyte)

pneumocystis carinii A protozoa that causes interstitial plasma cell pneumonia. This microorganism is frequently observed as an opportunistic pathogen in patients with acquired immunodeficiency syndrome (AIDS).

pol gene A gene of a retrovirus, such as HIV, that encodes for reverse transcriptase, endonuclease, and proteases activities.

polyarthritis Inflammation of several joints.

polyclonal gammopathy A dysproteinemia in which the products of a number of different cell types is demonstrated.

polyendocrinopathies A disease condition that involves several endocrine glands.

polymorphonuclear leukocyte A short-lived scavenger blood cell whose granules contain powerful bactericidal enzymes.

polymyositis Inflammation of several muscles at the same time. This condition is manifested by a number of signs and symptoms including pain, edema, deformity, and sleep disturbance.

polyneuropathy A disease involving several nerves.

polyserositis A condition of general inflammation of serous membrane with effusion (the escape of fluid). The inflammation is progressive and especially prevalent in the upper abdominal cavity.

posterior cervical In the back (dorsal surface) and associated with the vertebral bone of the neck.

postnatal After birth.

postoccipital lobe The back portion (lobe) of the cerebral hemisphere that is shaped like a three-sided pyramid.

postpartum A term referring to after birth.

pre-B cell An early, rapidly dividing mature B cell precursor.

precipitate The formation of a solid mass from previously soluble components. An alternate definition is to occur suddenly or unexpectedly.

prenatal A term that refers to prior to birth.

presentation of antigens The activity associated with the conveying of an altered antigenic molecule to T and B cells by macrophages. This process is necessary for most adaptive responses.

prime To give an initial sensitization to antigen.

primary antibody response An immunologic (IgM antibody) response following a foreign antigen challenge.

primary biliary cirrhosis Cirrhosis (interstitial inflammation of an organ) of the liver caused by chronic retention of bile. The causative agent (etiology) is unknown in the primary form of the disorder.

primary immunodeficiency Dysfunction in an immune organ such as the thymus.

primary immunoglobulin deficiency A genetically determined disorder associated with certain diseases.

primary lymphoid tissue or organ The bone marrow and thymus gland are classified as primary or central lymphoid tissues.

primitive stem cell The early form of uncommitted, multipotential blood cells that replicate themselves and generate more differentiated daughter cells.

procainamide A drug that functions as a cardiac depressant used in the treatment of cardiac arrhythmias.

prodromal period (prodrome, prodromal) The earliest or initial sign or symptom of a developing disease or disorder. For example, the prodromal period of an infectious disease manifested by rash would be the space of time between the earliest symptoms and the appearance of the rash or fever.

prognosis A forecast of the probable outcome of a condition, disorder, or disease.

progressive systemic sclerosis (PSS) A disorder of loss of tissue elasticity throughout the body that advances in severity over time.

prophylaxis A synonym for prevention.

prostaglandin A prostaglandin is a pharmacologically active derivative of arachidonic acid. Prostaglandins are naturally occurring unsaturated fatty acids that stimulate and suppress the effects of many inflammatory processes and stimulate the contraction of uterine and other smooth muscle tissues. Different prostaglandins are capable of modulating cell mobility and immune responses.

prostration A condition of extreme exhaustion (lack of strength or energy).

proteinuria Protein (albumin) in the urine.

proteolysis The breaking apart of a protein molecule.

proteolytic enzyme A substance able to break apart a protein molecule.

prothrombin time (PT) A blood coagulation test that assesses the process of clotting beginning with the formation of factor X.

protocol The steps that are usually followed in a situation such as laboratory testing or patient treatment.

proximal humeri The end portion of the upper bone of the arm that is nearest the center of the body (shoulder).

prozone phenomenon A possible cause of false negative antigen-antibody reactions caused by an excessive amount of antibody.

psychoneuroimmunology The relationship between the mind and the body that combines research in basic science with psychologic and psychosocial factors.

psychosocial factors Related to both psychologic and social factors.

PT *(see Prothrombin time)*

purpura An extensive area of red or dark purple discoloration of the skin.

pyelonephritis An inflammation of the kidney and pelvis region of the kidney (the funnel-shaped expansion of the upper end of the ureter into which the renal calices open).

pyoderma Any purulent (pus-producing) skin disease.

pyrogenic Microorganisms that cause the production of pus.

pyroglobulin An abnormal (IgM) globulin that precipitates on heating to 50° or 60° C but does not redissolve on cooling or intensified heating as typical Bence-Jones pyroglobulins do.

radioimmunoassay A laboratory technique involving the use of radioactive substances in the evaluation of immunoglobulins.

Raynaud's phenomenon (Raynaud's disease) A condition of episodic constriction of small arteries of the extremities (usually fingers or toes) induced by cold temperatures or emotional stress that would not affect an unafflicted person. The signs and symptoms of the condition include two forms: a pale appearance and numb feeling followed by redness and tingling or a swollen, red, and painful condition. Heat relieves the condition, if the stimulus was cold-induced.

reagin An antibody-like protein that binds to a test antigen such as cardiolipid-lecithin-coated cholesterol particles in the venereal disease research laboratory (VDRL) serologic method of testing for syphilis; or an old term for IgE with a specificity for allergens.

reagin antibodies Nontreponemal antibodies produced by a patient infected with *Treponemal pallidum* against components of their own or other mammalian cells.

recessive The term used to describe a gene which is not expressed unless it is in the homozygous form.

receptor A cell surface molecule that binds specifically to particular proteins or peptides in the fluid phase.

recirculation In reference to lymphocytes, mostly T cells, which pass from the circulating blood through the lymphatic system back to the circulating blood.

refractory anemia A form of anemia (decreased erythrocytes in the circulation) that is resistant to ordinary treatment.

regimen A schedule of treatment.

regional adenopathy Swelling or enlargement of the lymph nodes in a certain area or areas of the body.

relative lymphocytosis An increase of lymphocytes in the circulating blood in relationship to the total number of leukocytes in the circulation.

renal impairment Dysfunction of the kidneys.

renal insufficiency Inadequate functioning of the kidneys.

reticuloendothelial system (see Mononuclear phagocytic system)

retinal hemorrhage Extreme bleeding from the inner layer (the retina) into the fluid-filled interior of the eye.

retinitis An inflammation of the inner layer (the retina) of the eye.

retroauricular Behind the protruding portion of the external ear which surrounds the opening (auricle).

retrovirus A type of virus that carries a single, positive-stranded RNA and uses a special enzyme, reverse transcriptase, to convert viral RNA into DNA.

reverse passive hemagglutination A laboratory method that uses erythrocytes as an indicator cell to observe the absence of agglutination in the presence of antibodies.

reverse transcriptase An enzyme found in the single, positive-stranded RNA core of a retrovirus.

Reye's syndrome An acute and frequently fatal childhood disease that may follow a variety of common viral infections within several hours or days. The signs and symptoms of disease include persistent vomiting followed by delirium caused by edema of the brain, hypoglycemia, dysfunction of the liver, convulsions, and coma.

rheumatic fever A disease caused by the presence of the toxins produced by group A beta Streptococci.

Rh factor This blood group antigen, named for the rhesus monkey, was originally identified because an antibody agglutinated the erythrocytes of all rhesus monkeys and 85% of humans. The antibody was later discovered to be the Landsteiner-Wiener antibody, which is dissimilar from the Rh antibody.

rhinorrhea Watery discharge from the nose.

rouleaux (rouleaux formation) Pseudoagglutination or the false clumping of erythrocytes when the cells are suspended in their own serum. This phenomenon is caused by the presence of an abnormal protein in the serum, plasma expanders, e.g., dextran, or Wharton's jelly from cord blood samples. Rouleaux formation appears as rolls resembling stacks of coins upon microscopic examination.

rubella The viral cause of measles.

rubella syndrome A number of congenital anomalies such as mental retardation and cardiovascular defects caused by the rubella virus.

scarlet fever An acute infectious disease caused by group A Streptococcus. The rash and other signs and symptoms are caused by the erythema-producing toxin produced by the Streptococci.

sclerodactyly A chronic disorder characterized by progressive fibrosis of the fingers and toes.

scleroderma A progressive fibrosis beginning with the skin.

sebum The oily secretion of the sebaceous glands whose ducts open into the hair follicles.

secondary immunoglobulin deficiency An acquired disorder associated with certain diseases.

secondary lymphoid tissue or secondary lymphoid organs The secondary tissues include the lymph nodes, spleen, and Peyer's patches in the intestine.

self-limiting Confined, able to resolve in time.

senescence The process of growing old.

sensitivity The frequency of positive EIA results obtained in the testing of a population of individuals who are truly positive for antibody, e.g., anti-HIV.

sensitization Physical attachment of antibody molecules to antigens on the erythrocytic membrane.

sepsis Microbial infection throughout the systemic circulation.

septic arthritis An inflammation of the joints caused by the presence of pathogenic microorganisms.

septicemia The presence of pathogenic microorganisms in the blood.

sequelae A disease condition following or occurring as a consequence of another condition or event.

seroconversion The development of a demonstrable antibody response to a disease or vaccine.

seroepidemiologic The evidence of antibodies to a disease in a defined population.

seronegative The lack of evidence of an antibody to a disease.

serositis An inflammation of the membrane consisting of mesothelium, a thin layer of connective tissue, having lines enclosing the body cavities.

serum Straw-colored fluid present after blood clots.

serum electrophoresis The separation of proteins into five fractions on a medium such as paper or cellulose acetate. The separation is based on the rate of migration of these individual components in an electrical field.

serum sickness A hypersensitivity reaction following a single, large injection of serum from an animal of another species.

sex-linked A genetic trait associated with the X chromosome.

sialic acid Found on red blood cell membranes; produces a negative surrounding charge.

sickle cell anemia An inherited form of anemia caused by a genetically defective hemoglobin.

sIg (see Surface immunoglobulin)

silent carrier A carrier of a disease who manifests no clinically obvious symptoms or signs.

sinusitis An inflammation of the cavity in a bone, such as in the paranasal sinuses.

sinusoid A specialized capillary found in locations such as the bone marrow, spleen, and liver through which blood passes to reach the veins, allowing the lining macrophages to remove damaged or antibody-coated cells.

Sjögren's syndrome An autoimmune disorder manifested by enlargement of the parotid glands, chronic polyarthritis, and dryness of the conjunctiva, throat, and mouth.

SLE (see Systemic lupus erythematosus)

solid-phase assay A laboratory method in which one of the reactants is bound to surface.

soluble mediator (also called lymphokine). A substance secreted by monocytes, lymphocytes or neutrophils that provides the mechanism of cell-to-cell communication. Important lymphokines include: migration inhibitory factor (MIF), interleukin-2 (T cell growth factor), chemotactic factors, and interleukin-1.

somnolence A condition of prolonged drowsiness or a state resembling a trance.

sor gene A gene of a retrovirus, such as HIV. The product of the small open-reading frame is a protein that induces antibody production in the natural course of infection.

Southern blot analysis A laboratory technique used to detect the HIV-1 sequence in peripheral blood cells and tissues such as lymph nodes, liver, and kidney.

specificity
1. The ability of a particular antibody to combine with one antigen instead of another based on the fact that the binding sites of antibodies directed against determinants of one antigen are not complementary to determinants of another dissimilar antigen.
2. The proportion of negative EIA test results obtained in the population of individuals who actually lack the antibody in question, e.g., anti-HIV.

spirochete A type of bacteria with a twisted or spiral appearance when viewed microscopically.

spleen A large, glandlike organ located in the upper left quadrant of abdomen under the ribs. The spleen is the body's largest reservoir of mononuclear-phagocytic cells.

splenomegaly A markedly enlarged spleen.

stasis Stoppage of bleeding.

steric hindrance Mutual blocking of dissimilar antibodies with the same binding constant and directed against antigenic determinants located in close proximity on a cell's surface.

streptokinase An enzyme that dissolves clots by converting plasminogen to plasmin.

subclinical infection An early or mild form of a disease without visible signs.

substrate A substance upon which another substance such as an enzyme acts.

supernatant Fluid above the solid portion, e.g., cells in a centrifuged or sedimented specimen.

suppressor/cytotoxic (also referred to as T8 or Leu-2). A major phenotypic lymphocyte subset of T lymphocytes.

supraglottic larynx The area above the true vocal cords.

surface immunoglobulin (sIg) Immunoglobulin, at first cytoplasmic and later surface bound, is the key feature of B cells, through which they recognize specific antigens.

surrogate testing Procedures performed in place of specific tests for an infectious agent such as non-A, non-B hepatitis.

susceptibility Having little resistance, such as resistance to infectious disease.

symptom An indication of a disorder or disease, or a variation in normal body function.

symptomatic A deviation from usual function or appearance.

syncytia Giant, multinucleated groups or masses of cells.

syndrome A collection of symptoms that occur together.

synergistic The action of two or more agents that frequently produces a much greater effect than the expected sum of the individual agents.

systemic Throughout the body.

systemic circulation Blood circulation throughout the body.

systemic lupus erythematosus (SLE) An autoimmune disorder expressed as a group of multisymptom disorders that can affect practically every organ of the body.

systemic sclerosis Loss of tissue elasticity of vessels, such as blood vessels, throughout the whole body.

tabes dorsalis A slowly progressive degeneration of the nervous system caused by syphilis. In untreated patients this condition may appear from 5 to 20 years after the initial infection with *Treponema pallidum*.

tachycardia An abnormally fast heart rate.

tart cell When a blood preparation is microscopically examined for the presence of cells associated with systemic lupus erythematosus (SLE), tart cells may be seen. Tart cells usually represent monocytes that have phagocytized another whole cell or nucleus, often a lymphocyte. These cell formations can be mistaken for the classic LE cell connected with SLE.

T cell (*see* T lymphocyte)

TdT (*see* Terminal deoxynucleotidyl transferase)

telangiectasia A vascular lesion formed by the dilation of a group of capillaries and occasionally terminal arteries.

terminal deoxynucleotidyl transferase (TdT) An intracellular DNA polymerase found mainly in cortical, and therefore young, thymocytes. These cells are lost from the thymus following corticosteroid treatment.

thrombocytopenia A severe deficiency of circulating blood platelets (thrombocytes).

thrombophlebitis An inflammation of a vein that develops prior to the formation of a thrombus (clot).

thrombosis A condition of formation of a blood clot or thrombus.

thrombus A clot.

thymoma A tumor derived from the epithelial or lymphoid elements of the thymus.

thymosin (also called *thymic hormone*). A humoral factor secreted by the thymus which promotes the growth of peripheral lymphoid tissue.

thymus A primary or central lymphoid tissue that is responsible for processes of lymphocytes into the T type of cell. This ductless glandlike structure is located beneath the sternum (breastbone).

titer The concentration or strength of an antibody expressed as the highest dilution of the serum that produces agglutination, e.g., 1:4, 1:8, etc.

T lymphocyte or T cell The cells responsible for the cellular immune response and involved in the regulation of antibody reactions.

toxic shock syndrome A serious and potentially fatal disorder caused by toxins produced by *Staphylococcus aureus*.

toxoplasma gondii A protozoal micro-organism that can be transmitted from an infected mother to an unborn infant. The disease can result in encephalomyelitis.

trans A prefix meaning across, over, or through.

transaminase (ALT/SGPT) A surrogate test for non-A, non-B hepatitis.

transplacental hemorrhage The entrance of fetal blood cells into the maternal circulation.

treponemes (Treponema) A genus of spirochetes.

tubular cell injury Damage to cells of the renal tubules.

ubiquitous Existing everywhere.

ulcerative lesion An open sore.

unilateral blindness The lack of vision in one eye.

universal blood and body fluid precautions Specific regulations and practices, such as wearing gloves, that conform to current state and federal requirements. These precautions assume that *all* specimens, e.g., blood, have the potential for transmitting disease.

urticaria Hives.

vaccination A method of stimulating the adaptive immune response and generating memory and acquired resistance without suffering disease. A form of artificial active acquired immunity.

vaccine A suspension of killed or attenuated (inactivated) infectious agents administered for the purpose of establishing resistance to the disease.

variable region The antigen-binding portion of an immunoglobulin molecule.

variant lymphocyte A type of white blood cell that lacks the characteristics of a normal lymphocyte.

varicella A term for chickenpox.

varicosity A condition of having distended veins.

vasculitis An inflammation of a vessel such as a blood vessel.

vasoamine Vasoactive amines, e.g., histamine, 5-hydroxytryptamine, produced by mast cells, basophils, and platelets, and causing increased capillary permeability.

venereal route A sexually transmitted mode of infection.

viral capsid antigen (VCA) A "new" antigen expressed by B lymphocytes infected with Epstein-Barr virus in infectious mononucleosis.

viremia A systemic (blood) infection caused by a virus.

virion A complete virus particle.

virulence The degree of pathogenicity or ability to cause disease of a micro-organism.

Waldenstrom's primary macroglobulinemia (Waldenstrom's macroglobulinemia) A neoplastic proliferation of the lymphocyte-plasma cell system.

Wasserman test The first diagnostic serologic test for syphilis; no longer in use.

Index